BOARD REVIEW FROM MEDSCAPE

Case-Based Internal Medicine Self-Assessment Questions

www.acpmedicine.com

WebMD®

Director of Publishing	Cynthia M. Chevins
Director, Electronic Publishing	Liz Pope
Managing Editor	Erin Michael Kelly
Development Editors	Nancy Terry, John Heinegg
Senior Copy Editor	John J. Anello
Copy Editor	David Terry
Art and Design Editor	Elizabeth Klarfeld
Electronic Composition	Diane Joiner, Jennifer Smith
Manufacturing Producer	Derek Nash

Printed in the United States of America

ISBN: 0-9748327-8-2

Published by WebMD Inc.

Board Review from Medscape
WebMD Professional Publishing
111 Eighth Avenue
Suite 700
New York, NY 10011

1-800-545-0554

1-203-790-2087

1-203-790-2066

acpmedicine@webmd.net

The authors, editors, and publisher have conscientiously and carefully tried to ensure that recommended measures and drug dosages in these pages are accurate and conform to the standards that prevailed at the time of publication. The reader is advised, however, to check the product information sheet accompanying each drug to be familiar with any changes in the dosage schedule or in the contraindications. This advice should be taken with particular seriousness if the agent to be administered is a new one or one that is infrequently used. *Board Review from Medscape* describes basic principles of diagnosis and therapy. Because of the uniqueness of each patient and the need to take into account a number of concurrent considerations, however, this information should be used by physicians only as a general guide to clinical decision making.

Board Review from Medscape is derived from the *ACP Medicine* CME program, which is accredited by the University of Alabama School of Medicine and Medscape, both of whom are accredited by the ACCME to provide continuing medical education for physicians. *Board Review from Medscape* is intended for use in self-assessment, not as a way to earn CME credits.

EDITORIAL BOARD

CONTENTS

3 ENDOCRINOLOGY

4 GASTROENTEROLOGY

5 HEMATOLOGY

6 IMMUNOLOGY/ALLERGY

7 INFECTIOUS DISEASE

8 INTERDISCIPLINARY MEDICINE

9 METABOLISM

10 NEPHROLOGY

11 NEUROLOGY

12 ONCOLOGY

13 PSYCHIATRY

14 RESPIRATORY MEDICINE

15 RHEUMATOLOGY

PREFACE

The idea behind the creation of this book is to provide time-pressed physicians with a convenient way to measure and sharpen their medical knowledge across all of the topics in adult internal medicine, possibly with preparation for recertification as a final goal.

With this idea in mind, we have collected 981 case-based questions and created *Board Review from Medscape*. The list of topics is comprehensive, providing physicians an extensive review library covering all of adult internal medicine, as well as such subspecialties as psychiatry, neurology, dermatology, and others. The questions present cases of the kind commonly encountered in daily practice. The accompanying answers and explanations highlight key educational concepts and provide a full discussion of both the correct and incorrect answers. The cases have been reviewed by experts in clinical practice from the nation's leading medical institutions.

Board Review from Medscape is derived from the respected *ACP Medicine* CME program. A continually updated, evidence-based reference of adult internal medicine, *ACP Medicine* is also the first such comprehensive reference to carry the name of the American College of Physicians. At the end of each set of questions, we provide a cross-reference for further study in *ACP Medicine*. You can learn more about this publication on the Web at www.acpmedicine.com.

This review book has also been produced in a convenient PDF format, available on the Web at www.acpmedicine.com. This format allows you to purchase individual sections, if you so choose, and to leave the file(s) on your computer or handheld device for a quick look during free moments.

I hope you find this book helpful. Please feel free to send any questions or comments you might have to danfedermanmd@webmd.net. You will help us improve future editions.

Daniel D. Federman, M.D., M.A.C.P.
Founding Editor, *ACP Medicine*
The Carl W. Walter Distinguished Professor of Medicine
and Medical Education and Senior Dean for Alumni Relations and Clinical Teaching
Harvard Medical School

CLINICAL ESSENTIALS

Ethical and Social Issues

1. An 81-year-old woman recently became ill and is now dying of metastatic cancer. She wishes to have her life preserved at all costs. Her physician is concerned that such an effort would be medically futile and extremely costly. Until recently, the patient had an active social life, which included regular participation in many church activities. Her closest relatives are two nieces, whom she does not know well.

   At this time, it would be most appropriate for which of the following groups to become involved in decisions about this patient?

   - ❑ **A. Social workers**
   - ❑ **B. The patient's family**
   - ❑ **C. Clergy**
   - ❑ **D. Ethics committee**
   - ❑ **E. Risk management personnel**

   Key Concept/Objective: To understand that the patient's beliefs and support systems can often guide health care providers in engaging others in support of the patient

   The patient's active involvement in church activities may mean that she will be receptive to the involvement of clergy. Communication regarding prolongation of suffering by aggressive measures to preserve life at all costs and discussion of spiritual dimensions may help this patient resolve the issue. Although courts have generally upheld the wishes of individuals regardless of issues involving the utilization of resources, the appropriate use of resources continues to be a legitimate and difficult problem. *(Answer: C—Clergy)*

2. An 80-year-old woman presents with severe acute abdominal pain. She is found to have bowel ischemia, severe metabolic acidosis, and renal failure. She has Alzheimer disease and lives in a nursing home. Surgical consultation is obtained, and the surgeon feels strongly that she would not survive surgery.

   When you approach the patient's family at this time, what would be the best way to begin the discussion?

   - ❑ **A. Explain that DNR status is indicated because of medical futility**
   - ❑ **B. Find out exactly what the family members know about the patient's wishes**
   - ❑ **C. Explain that the patient could have surgery if the family wishes but that the patient would probably not survive**
   - ❑ **D. Discuss the patient's religious beliefs**
   - ❑ **E. Explain to the family that the patient is dying and tell them that you will make sure she is not in pain**

   Key Concept/Objective: To understand the duties of the physician regarding the offering of choices to patients and families in urgent situations when the patient is dying

   Although the issues underlying each of these choices might be fruitfully discussed with the family, ethicists have affirmed the duty of physicians to lead and guide such discussions

on the basis of their knowledge and experience. Health care providers should not inflict unrealistic choices on grieving families; rather, they should reassure them and describe the efficacy of aggressive palliative care in relieving the suffering of patients who are dying. In this case, a direct approach involving empathy and reassurance would spare the family of having to make difficult decisions when there is no realistic chance of changing the outcome. *(Answer: E—Explain to the family that the patient is dying and tell them that you will make sure she is not in pain)*

3. An 86-year-old man with Alzheimer disease is admitted to the hospital for treatment of pneumonia. The patient has chronic obstructive pulmonary disease; coronary artery disease, which developed after he underwent four-vessel coronary artery bypass grafting (CABG) 10 years ago; and New York Heart Association class 3 congestive heart failure. His living will, created at the time of his CABG, calls for full efforts to resuscitate him if necessary. A family meeting is scheduled for the next morning. At 2 A.M., a nurse discovers that the patient is blue in color and has no pulse; the nurse initiates CPR and alerts you regarding the need for emergent resuscitation. An electrocardiogram shows no electrical activity.

What should you do at this time?

- ❑ **A. Proceed with resuscitation because of the patient's living will**
- ❑ **B. Proceed with resuscitation until permission to stop resuscitation is obtained from the family**
- ❑ **C. Decline to proceed with resuscitation on the basis of medical futility**
- ❑ **D. Continue resuscitation for 30 minutes because the nurse initiated CPR**
- ❑ **E. Decline to proceed with resuscitation because the patient's previous living will is void, owing to the fact that it was not updated at the time of admission**

Key Concept/Objective: To understand the concept of medical futility as the rationale for not performing CPR

It would be medically futile to continue CPR and attempts at resuscitation, given the absence of ECG activity. In this case, the patient's likelihood of being successfully resuscitated is less than 1%, owing to his multiple medical conditions. *(Answer: C—Decline to proceed with resuscitation on the basis of medical futility)*

For more information, see Cassel CK, Purtilo RB, McParland ET: Clinical Essentials: II Contemporary Ethical and Social Issues in Medicine. ACP Medicine Online (www.acpmedicine.com). Dale DC, Federman DD, Eds. WebMD Inc., New York, July 2001

Reducing Risk of Injury and Disease

4. A 26-year-old woman presents to clinic for routine examination. The patient has no significant medical history and takes oral contraceptives. She smokes half a pack of cigarettes a day and reports having had three male sexual partners over her lifetime. As part of the clinic visit, you wish to counsel the patient on reducing the risk of injury and disease.

Of the following, which is the leading cause of loss of potential years of life before age 65?

- ❑ **A. HIV/AIDS**
- ❑ **B. Motor vehicle accidents**
- ❑ **C. Tobacco use**
- ❑ **D. Domestic violence**

Key Concept/Objective: To understand that motor vehicle accidents are the leading cause of loss of potential years of life before age 65

Motor vehicle accidents are the leading cause of loss of potential years of life before age 65. Alcohol-related accidents account for 44% of all motor vehicle deaths. One can experience

a motor vehicle accident as an occupant, as a pedestrian, or as a bicycle or motorcycle rider. In 1994, 33,861 people died of injuries sustained in motor vehicle accidents in the United States. The two greatest risk factors for death while one is driving a motor vehicle are driving while intoxicated and failing to use a seat belt. The physician's role is to identify patients with alcoholism, to inquire about seat-belt use, and to counsel people to use seat belts and child car seats routinely. In one study, 53.5% of patients in a university internal medicine practice did not use seat belts. Problem drinking, physical inactivity, obesity, and low income were indicators of nonuse. The prevalence of nonuse was 91% in people with all four indicators and only 25% in those with no indicators. Seat belts confer considerable protection, yet in one survey, only 3.9% of university clinic patients reported that a physician had counseled them about using seat belts. Three-point restraints reduce the risk of death or serious injury by 45%. Air bags reduce the risk of death by an additional 9% in drivers using seat belts. Because air bags reduce the risk of death by only 20% in unbelted drivers, physicians must tell their patients not to rely on air bags. *(Answer: B—Motor vehicle accidents)*

For more information, see Sox HC Jr.: Clinical Essentials: III Reducing Risk of Injury and Disease. ACP Medicine Online (www.acpmedicine.com). Dale DC, Federman DD, Eds. WebMD Inc., New York, July 2003

Diet and Exercise

5. A 78-year-old woman with hypertension presents for a 3-month follow-up visit for her hypertension. A year ago, she moved to a retirement community, where she began to eat meals more regularly; during the past year, she has gained 15 lb. She is sedentary. She weighs 174 lb, and her height is 5 ft 1 in. She is a lifelong smoker; she smokes one pack of cigarettes a day and has repeatedly refused to receive counseling regarding smoking cessation. She has occasional stiffness on waking in the morning. Her blood pressure is 120/80 mm Hg. She reports taking the prescribed antihypertensive therapy almost every day. She is concerned about her weight gain because this is the most she has ever weighed. She has reported that she has stopped eating desserts at most meals and is aware that she needs to reduce the amount of fat she eats. She has never exercised regularly, but her daughter has told her to ask about an aerobic exercise program. She has asked for exercise recommendations, although she does not know whether it will make much difference.

Which of the following would you recommend for this patient?

- ❑ A. **Attendance at a structured aerobic exercise program at least three times a week**
- ❑ B. **Membership in the neighborhood YMCA for swimming**
- ❑ C. **Walking three times a week, preferably with a partner**
- ❑ D. **Contacting a personal trainer to develop an individualized exercise program**
- ❑ E. **No additional exercise because she has symptoms of osteoarthritis**

Key Concept/Objective: To recognize that even modest levels of physical activity such as walking and gardening are protective even if they are not started until midlife to late in life

Changes attributed to aging closely resemble those that result from inactivity. In sedentary patients, cardiac output, red cell mass, glucose tolerance, and muscle mass decrease. Systolic blood pressure, serum cholesterol levels, and body fat increase. Regular exercise appears to retard these age-related changes. In elderly individuals, physical activity is also associated with increased functional status and decreased mortality. Although more studies are needed to clarify the effects of exercise in the elderly, enough evidence exists to warrant a recommendation of mild exercise for this patient, along with counseling concerning the benefits of exercise at her age. Walking programs increase aerobic capacity in individuals in their 70s with few injuries. Although structured exercise is most often recommended by physicians, recent studies demonstrate that even modest levels of physical activity such as walking and gardening are beneficial. Such exercise is protective even if it is not started until midlife or late in life. Because this patient is used to a sedentary lifestyle

and is not strongly motivated to begin exercising, compliance with exercise recommendations may be an issue. Lifestyle interventions appear to be as effective as formal exercise programs of similar intensity in improving cardiopulmonary fitness, blood pressure, and body composition. Exercise does not appear to cause or accelerate osteoarthritis. However, counseling concerning warm-ups, stretches, and a graded increase in exercise intensity can help prevent musculoskeletal problems as a side effect of exercise. *(Answer: C—Walking three times a week, preferably with a partner)*

6. A 50-year-old woman presents for a follow-up visit to discuss the laboratory results from her annual physical examination and a treatment plan. Her total serum cholesterol level is 260 mg/dl, which is up from 200 mg/dl the previous year. Her blood pressure is 140/100 mm Hg, which is up from 135/90 mm Hg; she weighs 165 lb, a gain of 12 lb from the previous year. Results from other tests and her physical examination are normal. Her height is 5 ft 3 in. She is postmenopausal and has been receiving hormonal replacement therapy for 2 years. You discuss her increased lipid levels and increased blood pressure in the context of her weight gain and dietary habits. When asked about her dietary habits, she says that she has heard that putting salt on food causes high blood pressure. She asks if she should stop putting salt on her food because her blood pressure is high.

How would you describe for this patient the relationship between sodium and hypertension?

- ❑ **A. Tell her that reducing sodium intake usually leads to significant reductions in blood pressure**
- ❑ **B. Tell her that reducing intake of sodium and fats while increasing intake of fruits, vegetables, and whole grains usually leads to significant reductions in hypertension**
- ❑ **C. Explain to her that decreasing sodium is only important in elderly patients**
- ❑ **D. Tell her that research studies are unclear about the role of sodium in hypertension**
- ❑ **E. Explain to her that antihypertensive medication is effective in reducing hypertension, making sodium reduction unnecessary**

Key Concept/Objective: To understand current evidence that supports the relationship between sodium and hypertension

The Dietary Approaches to Stop Hypertension (DASH) trial[1] demonstrated that the combination of eating fruits, vegetables, and whole grains along with reducing fat and sodium levels can lower systolic blood pressure an average of 11.5 mm Hg in patients with hypertension. Reductions in dietary sodium can contribute to substantial reductions in the risk of stroke and coronary artery disease. In addition, for this patient, a reduction in sodium intake will decrease urinary calcium excretion and thus reduce her risk of osteoporosis. Because the patient has asked about putting salt on food, she should also be counseled that 80% of dietary sodium comes from processed food. It is important to review these hidden sources of salt with patients who would benefit from sodium restriction. The average American diet contains more than 4,000 mg of sodium a day. There is no recommended daily allowance for sodium, but the American Heart Association (AHA) recommends that daily consumption of sodium not exceed 2,400 mg, with substantially lower sodium intake for patients with hypertension. *(Answer: B—Tell her that reducing intake of sodium and fats while increasing intake of fruits, vegetables, and whole grains usually leads to significant reductions in hypertension)*

1. Sacks FM, Svetkey LP, Vollmer WM, et al: Effects on blood pressure of reduced dietary sodium and the Dietary Approaches to Stop Hypertension (DASH) diet. DASH-Sodium Collaborative Research Group. N Engl J Med 344:3, 2001

7. A 64-year-old man comes to your clinic for a routine visit. He has a history of myocardial infarction, which was diagnosed 1 year ago. Since that time, he has been asymptomatic, and he has been taking all his medications and following an exercise program. His physical examination is unremarkable. He has been getting some information on the Internet about the use of omega-3 polyunsaturated fatty acids as part of a cardioprotective diet.

Which of the following statements is most accurate concerning the use of omega-3 fatty acids?

- ❑ A. **Consumption of omega-3 polyunsaturated fatty acids has been shown to decrease the incidence of recurrent myocardial infarctions**
- ❑ B. **Omega-3 polyunsaturated fatty acids have been shown to decrease low-density lipoprotein (LDL) cholesterol levels**
- ❑ C. **Consumption of omega-3 polyunsaturated fatty acids is inversely related to the incidence of atherosclerosis and the risk of sudden death and stroke**
- ❑ D. **Omega-3 polyunsaturated fatty acids have been shown to elevate triglyceride levels**

Key Concept/Objective: To understand the benefits of omega-3 polyunsaturated fatty acids

Omega-3 polyunsaturated fatty acids have been shown to have a cardioprotective effect. Consumption of omega-3 fatty acids is inversely related to the incidence of atherosclerosis and the risk of sudden death and stroke. In high doses, omega-3 fatty acids may reduce blood triglyceride levels, but in dietary amounts, they have little effect on blood lipids. Even in modest amounts, however, omega-3 fatty acids reduce platelet aggregation, thereby impairing thrombogenesis. They may also have antiarrhythmic and plaque-stabilizing properties. *(Answer: C—Consumption of omega-3 polyunsaturated fatty acids is inversely related to the incidence of atherosclerosis and the risk of sudden death and stroke)*

8. A 52-year-old woman is diagnosed with diabetes on a blood sugar screening test. She is started on a diet and undergoes education about diabetes. After a month, she comes back for a follow-up visit and asks you why she should eat complex carbohydrates instead of simple carbohydrates if they are all the same.

Which of the following statements about simple and complex carbohydrates is true?

- ❑ A. **Simple and complex carbohydrates are indeed of the same caloric value, and there is no advantage in using one over the other**
- ❑ B. **Simple carbohydrates have a higher glycemic index than complex carbohydrates, and they may decrease high-density lipoprotein (HDL) cholesterol levels**
- ❑ C. **Simple carbohydrates have a higher glycemic index than complex carbohydrates, and they may increase HDL cholesterol levels**
- ❑ D. **Simple carbohydrates have a lower glycemic index than complex carbohydrates, and they may decrease HDL cholesterol levels**

Key Concept/Objective: To understand the difference between simple and complex carbohydrates

Plants are the principal sources of carbohydrates. Simple carbohydrates include monosaccharides such as glucose, fructose, and galactose and disaccharides such as sucrose, maltose, and lactose. Sugars, starches, and glycogen provide 4 cal/g; because fiber is indigestible, it has no caloric value. Complex carbohydrates include polysaccharides and fiber. Carbohydrates contribute about 50% of the calories in the average American diet; half of those calories come from sugar and half from complex carbohydrates. Because sugars are more rapidly absorbed, they have a higher glycemic index than starches. In addition to provoking higher insulin levels, carbohydrates with a high glycemic index appear to reduce HDL cholesterol levels and may increase the risk of coronary artery disease. Food rich in complex carbohydrates also provides vitamins, trace minerals, and other valuable nutrients. *(Answer: B—Simple carbohydrates have a higher glycemic index than complex carbohydrates, and they may decrease high-density lipoprotein [HDL] cholesterol levels)*

9. A 52-year-old woman comes to your clinic to establish primary care. She has not seen a doctor in years. She describes herself as being very healthy. She has no significant medical history, nor has she ever used tobacco or ethanol. She underwent menopause 3 years ago. Her physical examination is unremarkable. You ask about her dietary habits and find that the amount of fat that she is eating is in accordance with the AHA recommendations for healthy adults. She does not drink milk. Results of routine laboratory testing are within normal limits.

Which of the following additional dietary recommendations would be appropriate for this patient?

- ❑ A. Take supplements of calcium, vitamin D, and vitamin A
- ❑ B. Take supplements of calcium and vitamin D, and restrict the amount of sodium to less than 2,400 mg a day
- ❑ C. Take supplements of iron, vitamin D, and vitamin A
- ❑ D. Continue with the present diet

Key Concept/Objective: To know the general recommendations for vitamin and mineral consumption

It is becoming clear that many Americans, particularly the elderly and the poor, do not consume adequate amounts of vitamin-rich foods. There is conflicting information regarding the effects that the use of vitamins and minerals has on health; some recommendations, however, have been accepted. Women of childbearing age, the elderly, and people with suboptimal nutrition should take a single multivitamin daily. Strict vegetarians should take vitamin B_{12}. Use of so-called megadose vitamins should be discouraged. Multivitamin supplements may also be necessary to avert vitamin D deficiencies, particularly in the elderly. Population studies demonstrate conclusively that a high sodium intake increases blood pressure, especially in older people. There is no conclusive evidence that sodium restriction is beneficial to normotensive persons. Pending such information, the AHA recommends that daily consumption of sodium not exceed 2,400 mg, and the National Academy of Sciences proposes a 2,000 mg maximum. Calcium intake is related to bone density; at present, fewer than 50% of Americans consume the recommended daily allowance of calcium. Routine administration of iron is indicated in infants and pregnant women. A high intake of iron may be harmful for patients with hemochromatosis and for others at risk of iron overload. *(Answer: B—Take supplements of calcium and vitamin D, and restrict the amount of sodium to less than 2,400 mg a day)*

10. A 34-year-old man comes to your clinic to establish primary care. He has no significant medical history. He takes no medications and does not smoke. His family history is significant only with regard to his father, who contracted lung cancer at 70 years of age. You discuss the benefits of exercise with the patient and encourage him to start a regular exercise program.

Which of the following assessment measures would be appropriate in the evaluation of this patient before he starts an exercise program?

- ❑ A. History, physical examination, complete blood count, and urinalysis
- ❑ B. History, physical examination, chest x-ray, and electrocardiogram
- ❑ C. History, physical examination, and echocardiography
- ❑ D. History, physical examination, exercise, and electrocardiography

Key Concept/Objective: To understand the evaluation of patients starting an exercise program

Physicians can provide important incentives for their patients by educating them about the risks and benefits of habitual exercise. A careful history and physical examination are central to the medical evaluation of all potential exercisers. Particular attention should be given to a family history of coronary artery disease, hypertension, stroke, or sudden death and to symptoms suggestive of cardiovascular disease. Cigarette smoking, sedentary living, hypertension, diabetes, and obesity all increase the risks of exercise and may indicate the need for further testing. Physical findings suggestive of pulmonary, cardiac, or peripheral vascular disease are obvious causes of concern. A musculoskeletal evaluation is also important. The choice of screening tests for apparently healthy individuals in controversial. A complete blood count and urinalysis are reasonable for all patients. Young adults who are free of risk factors, symptoms, and abnormal physical findings do not require further evaluation. Although electrocardiography and echocardiography might reveal asymptomatic hypertrophic cardiomyopathy in some patients, the infrequency of this problem makes routine screening impractical. The AHA no longer recommends routine exercise electrocardiography for asymptomatic individuals. *(Answer: A—History, physical examination, complete blood count, and urinalysis)*

For more information, see Simon HB: Clinical Essentials: IV Diet and Exercise. ACP Medicine Online (www.acpmedicine.com). Dale DC, Federman DD, Eds. WebMD Inc., New York, September 2003

Adult Preventive Health Care

11. A healthy 50-year-old mother of three moves to your town from an inner-city area where she received no regular health care. She has never had any immunizations, will be working as a librarian, and plans no international travel. History and physical examination do not suggest any underlying chronic illnesses.

Which of the following immunizations would you recommend for this patient?

- ❏ A. **Measles, mumps, rubella**
- ❏ B. **Hepatitis B**
- ❏ C. **Tetanus-diphtheria**
- ❏ D. **Pneumococcal**
- ❏ D. **All of the above**

Key Concept/Objective: To know the recommendations for routine adult immunization

Only 65 cases of tetanus occur in the United States each year, and most occur in individuals who have never received the primary immunization series, whose immunity has waned, or who have received improper wound prophylaxis. The case-fatality rate is 42% in individuals older than 50 years. This patient should therefore receive the primary series of three immunizations with tetanus-diphtheria toxoids. Because she was born before 1957, she is likely to be immune to measles, mumps, and rubella. She does not appear to fall into one of the high-risk groups for whom hepatitis A, hepatitis B, and pneumococcal vaccinations are recommended. *(Answer: C—Tetanus-diphtheria)*

For more information, see Snow CF: Clinical Essentials: V Adult Preventive Health Care. ACP Medicine Online (www.acpmedicine.com). Dale DC, Federman DD, Eds. WebMD Inc., New York, March 2002

Health Advice for International Travelers

12. A 43-year-old man with asymptomatic HIV infection (stage A1; CD4+ T cell count, 610; viral load, < 50 copies/ml) seeks your advice regarding immunizations for a planned adventure bicycle tour in Africa. He is otherwise healthy, takes no medications, and has no known allergies. He is known to be immune to hepatitis B but is seronegative for hepatitis A. His trip will last approximately 3 weeks and will include travel to rural areas and to areas beyond usual tourist routes. You counsel him about safe food practices, safe sex, and mosquito-avoidance measures.

What should you recommend for malaria prophylaxis?

- ❏ A. **No prophylaxis**
- ❏ B. **Chloroquine**
- ❏ C. **Pyrimethamine-sulfadoxine**
- ❏ D. **Mefloquine**
- ❏ E. **Amoxicillin**

Key Concept/Objective: To know the specific indications and options for malaria prophylaxis for the international traveler

Appropriate malaria chemoprophylaxis is the most important preventive measure for travelers to malarial areas. In addition to advice about the avoidance of mosquitos and the use of repellants, most visitors to areas endemic for malaria should receive chemoprophylax-

is, regardless of the duration of exposure. In most parts of the world where malaria is found, including Africa, chloroquine resistance is common, so chloroquine would not be recommended as prophylaxis for this patient. Pyrimethamine-sulfadoxine is no longer recommended for prophylaxis because of the associated risk of serious mucocutaneous reactions. Amoxicillin does not have known efficacy against *Plasmodium*. Mefloquine is the preferred agent for malaria chemoprophylaxis in areas of the world where chloroquine-resistant malaria is present. *(Answer: D—Mefloquine)*

13. A 56-year-old man seeks your advice regarding malaria prophylaxis before a planned 10-day business trip to New Delhi, India. His medical problems include atrial fibrillation and medication-controlled bipolar disorder. He has no known allergies; his regular medications include diltiazem and lithium.

What should you recommend to this patient regarding malaria prophylaxis?

❑ **A. No prophylaxis is required because his trip will be less than 14 days long**

❑ **B. Chloroquine**

❑ **C. Mefloquine**

❑ **D. Pyrimethamine-sulfadoxine**

❑ **E. Doxycycline**

Key Concept/Objective: To understand the options for prophylaxis of chloroquine-resistant malaria

Chloroquine-resistant malaria is widespread and occurs in India. Thus, chloroquine would not be appropriate. Pyrimethamine-sulfadoxine is generally not used for prophylaxis because of the risk of severe mucocutaneous reactions. Mefloquine and doxycycline are the most commonly used chemoprophylactic agents for travelers to chloroquine-resistant malarial areas. Although mefloquine is generally well-tolerated in prophylactic doses, underlying cardiac conduction abnormalities and neuropsychiatric disorders or seizures are generally considered contraindications for mefloquine use. Thus, daily doxycycline taken from the start of the travel period until 4 weeks after departure from malarial areas would be the best choice for malaria chemoprophylaxis for this patient. *(Answer: E—Doxycycline)*

14. A 48-year-old woman seeks your advice about prevention of traveler's diarrhea. Her only medical problems include diet-controlled diabetes mellitus and occasional candidal vaginitis. She will be visiting Bombay and several rural villages for a total of 8 days as an inspector of sewage-treatment facilities. Given her tight schedule, it is imperative that she not lose any time as a result of diarrhea. You counsel her about safe food practices, prescribe mefloquine for malaria prophylaxis, and immunize her appropriately.

Which of the following would be the best choice for prevention of traveler's diarrhea in this patient?

❑ **A. Loperamide daily**

❑ **B. Ciprofloxacin daily**

❑ **C. Doxycycline daily**

❑ **D. Trimethoprim-sulfamethoxazole daily**

❑ **E. Erythromycin daily**

Key Concept/Objective: To know the prophylactic options for traveler's diarrhea

Traveler's diarrhea is most commonly caused by bacteria (particularly enterotoxigenic *Escherichia coli*). Travelers should follow safe food practices and may take either chemoprophylaxis or begin treatment after onset. For the patient in this question (whose visit will be relatively short and who cannot afford to have her schedule interrupted by an episode of diarrhea), chemoprophylaxis is a reasonable approach. A quinolone, trimethoprim-sulfamethoxazole, bismuth subsalicylate, and doxycycline are all options. Resistance to trimethoprim-sulfamethoxazole is widespread, so this drug would be less than optimal. Vaginal candidiasis is a common complication of doxycycline (particularly in a patient

with diabetes and a history of candidal vaginitis), and therefore doxycycline would not be suitable for this patient. Of the choices, ciprofloxacin would be the best option. Loperamide or erythromycin would not be an appropriate choice for the chemoprophylaxis of traveler's diarrhea. *(Answer: B—Ciprofloxacin daily)*

15. A 35-year-old woman in excellent health is planning a trip to remote areas of Asia. She has not traveled abroad before, and she wants some information on travel-related illnesses and risks. She has had her childhood immunizations, and her tetanus immunization was updated last year. She has an aversion to immunizations and medications but will accept them if needed.

What is the most common preventable acquired infection associated with travel for this person?

- ❑ A. Malaria
- ❑ B. Typhus
- ❑ C. Hepatitis A
- ❑ D. Cholera
- ❑ E. Yellow fever

Key Concept/Objective: To understand the risks of infection associated with travel to various parts of the world

Travel-related risks of infection are dependent on which part of the world an individual will be traveling to, the length of stay, and any underlying predisposing medical factors. Hepatitis A is prevalent in many underdeveloped countries and is the most common preventable infection acquired by travelers. Malaria is also a risk for this individual, but it is not acquired as commonly as hepatitis A. Sexually transmitted diseases are a frequent risk for travelers and should be discussed with patients. Typhus vaccine is no longer made in the United States and is not indicated for most travelers. Cholera vaccination is not very effective and is not recommended for travelers. Yellow fever is not a risk for this individual, who will be traveling in Asia; yellow fever would be a risk if she were traveling to parts of Africa or South America. *(Answer: C—Hepatitis A)*

16. A 42-year-old male executive who works for a multinational company will be flying to several countries in Asia over a 2-week period. He has not traveled overseas before. His past medical history is significant for mild hypertension, for which he takes medication, and for a splenectomy that he underwent for injuries from an automobile accident. He had routine childhood immunizations, but he has received none since. The itinerary for his business trip includes 4 days in India, 5 days in Singapore, and 3 days in Malaysia.

Which of the following would NOT be recommended for this patient?

- ❑ A. Hepatitis A vaccination
- ❑ B. Meningococcal vaccination
- ❑ C. Yellow fever vaccination
- ❑ D. Malaria prophylaxis
- ❑ E. Tetanus booster

Key Concept/Objective: To understand pretravel evaluation and immunizations

Yellow fever is endemic in Africa and South America but not in Asia, and therefore, yellow fever vaccination is not recommended for this person. Medical consultation for travel should be obtained at least 1 month before travel to allow for immunizations. A travel itinerary and a general medical history should be obtained to define pertinent underlying medical conditions. Hepatitis A is the most common preventable acquired infection among travelers, and therefore, hepatitis A vaccine should be offered. Because this patient has undergone a splenectomy, meningococcal vaccination should be recommended because he is predisposed to more severe infections with encapsulated bacteria, specifically, more severe babesiosis or malaria. Malaria is a risk for travelers in this area of the world,

and therefore, chemoprophylaxis is recommended. A tetanus-diphtheria booster should be administered every 10 years, and boosters should be administered before travel. *(Answer: C—Yellow fever vaccination)*

17. A 26-year-old asymptomatic man who was recently diagnosed as being HIV positive will be traveling in South America. He has no planned itinerary and has not started any medications. He has had routine childhood immunizations and has not previously traveled overseas. He has a severe allergy to egg proteins.

Which of the following should this patient receive before he travels?

- ❑ **A. Oral typhoid vaccine**
- ❑ **B. Oral polio vaccine**
- ❑ **C. Yellow fever vaccine**
- ❑ **D. Measles vaccine**
- ❑ **E. Meningococcal vaccine**

Key Concept/Objective: To know the contraindications for common travel immunizations

Vaccines that contain live, attenuated viruses should not be given to pregnant women or persons who are immunodeficient or who are potentially immunodeficient. Oral typhoid and oral polio vaccines are both live, attenuated vaccines and should not be given to an HIV-positive individual. An alternative to both vaccines is the killed parenteral vaccines. Yellow fever is also a live vaccine; the risks of the use of this vaccine in HIV-infected patients have not been established. However, severe allergic reaction to egg proteins is a contraindication for yellow fever vaccinations, and therefore, that vaccine should not be given to this person. Some countries in South America may require proof of yellow fever vaccination, and the patient should be advised of this before travel. The one exception to the use of live, attenuated vaccines in immunocompromised individuals is measles vaccinations. Measles can be severe in HIV-positive patients, and therefore, measles immunization should be provided if the patient is not severely immunocompromised and if he was immunized for measles before 1980. *(Answer: D—Measles vaccine)*

18. A middle-aged couple is planning a 1-week trip to Africa. They are both in excellent health and are not taking any medications. They have previously been to Africa and were given mefloquine prophylactically for malaria because of the presence of chloroquine-resistant strains of malaria in this area. However, both had to discontinue the medication before completing the regimen because of severe side effects, which included nausea and dizziness.

Which of the following is an acceptable recommendation for the prevention of malaria for this couple?

- ❑ **A. Recommend no prophylaxis because their risk is minimal, owing to the length of their stay, and the side effects from prophylaxis outweigh the benefits**
- ❑ **B. Recommend chloroquine because its side effects are milder than those of mefloquine**
- ❑ **C. Recommend doxycycline and emphasize the need to use sun protection**
- ❑ **D. Recommend that additional general preventive measures such as the use of strong insect repellent, staying indoors in the evenings and at nighttime, and covering exposed areas are unnecessary when taking medications for prophylaxis**
- ❑ **E. Recommend seeking immediate medical attention for any febrile illnesses that occur during travel or within the first week upon return**

Key Concept/Objective: To understand general and chemoprophylatic measures for preventing travel-associated malaria

Malaria is prevalent in various parts of the world. Chloroquine resistance is increasing worldwide and is very common in sub-Saharan Africa. Mefloquine and malarone are

treatments of choice for chemoprophylaxis. Mefloquine's side effects are usually minor, but mefloquine can cause severe nausea and dizziness, which can lead some patients to discontinue treatment. Because even brief exposure to infected mosquitoes can produce malaria, travel in endemic regions, no matter how brief the duration, mandates the use of chemoprophylaxis in addition to general precautions, such as covering exposed skin, staying indoors in the evenings and at night, and using insect repellent. Doxycycline is an acceptable alternative to mefloquine and should be recommended when persons are traveling to regions in which chloroquine-resistant malaria is known to occur. Doxycycline increases photosensitivity skin reactions, and avoidance of sun exposure should be emphasized. Despite chemoprophylaxis, travelers can still contract malaria; symptoms begin 8 days to 2 months after infection. *(Answer: C—Recommend doxycycline and emphasize the need to use sun protection)*

For more information, see Weller PF: Clinical Essentials: VII Health Advice for International Travelers. ACP Medicine Online (www.acpmedicine.com). Dale DC, Federman DD, Eds. WebMD Inc., New York, January 2005

Quantitative Aspects of Clinical Decision Making

19. A 56-year-old black man presents to your office for evaluation. For the past 6 months, the patient has been experiencing fatigue and mild dyspnea on exertion. He has no pertinent medical history. He denies having chest pain, orthopnea, edema, fever, or chills, but he does state that he has developed intermittent numbness and tingling of his distal extremities. Physical examination is significant only for conjunctival pallor and decreased vibratory sensation in both feet. CBC reveals normal WBC and platelet counts, a hematocrit of 28%, and a mean corpuscular volume of 115 fl. Blood smear is significant for multiple hypersegmented neutrophils. Alcohol screening by history is negative. The patient takes no medications, and he denies having any risk factor for HIV infection. Further laboratory testing reveals normal liver function, a low reticulocyte count, and normal serum vitamin B_{12} and RBC folate levels.

Which of the following statements regarding the necessity of further testing for vitamin B_{12} deficiency is true?

- ❑ A. **Assuming the serum vitamin B_{12} test has a low sensitivity and high specificity, no further testing is needed**
- ❑ B. **Assuming the serum vitamin B_{12} test has a low sensitivity and low specificity, no further testing is needed**
- ❑ C. **Assuming the serum vitamin B_{12} test is 100% specific, no further testing is needed**
- ❑ D. **Considering this patient's high pretest probability for vitamin B_{12} deficiency and knowing that the vitamin B_{12} assay is not perfect (i.e., that it has a sensitivity of less than 100%), further testing is required**

Key Concept/Objective: To understand the importance of sensitivity and specificity and pretest probability in the interpretation of test results

The vast majority of tests used in the daily practice of medicine are less than perfect. For any given test, four possible results are possible. Of these results, two are true and two are false. The two true results are (a) a positive result when disease is present (true positive), and (b) a negative result when disease is absent (true negative). Two false results are always possible for any given test: (a) the test can be negative when disease is present (false negative), and (b) the test can be positive when disease is absent (false positive). A test with high sensitivity has mostly true positive results and few false negative results; a test with high specificity has mostly true negative results and few false positive results. In addition, clinicians need to recognize the importance of the likelihood of disease before using a test (i.e., pretest probability). If in a given patient the likelihood of disease is high (as in this patient with vitamin B_{12} deficiency), then only a test with 100% sensitivity would exclude the diagnosis. Because the sensitivity of the B_{12} assay is less than 100%, the clinician should continue to pursue this diagnosis if the patient has a high pretest probability.

Proceeding with a measurement of methylmalonic acid is indicated for this patient. *(Answer: D—Considering this patient's high pretest probability for vitamin B_{12} deficiency and knowing that the vitamin B_{12} assay is not perfect [i.e., that it has a sensitivity of less than 100%], further testing is required)*

20. A childhood friend who has recently become a father contacts you for advice. The pediatrician has informed him and his wife that their child has tested positive on a screening for phenylketonuria (PKU). Your friend would like you to comment on the accuracy of this screening test. You realize that PKU is a very uncommon illness in newborns in North America, occurring in less than one in 10,000 newborns. You also know that the commonly used test for the detection of PKU is highly sensitive and, therefore, almost never results in a false negative test. You know of no good data regarding the specificity of the test.

Which of the following statements is most appropriate as a response to this concerned father?

- ❑ A. **The child has PKU with 100% certainty**
- ❑ B. **Considering the high sensitivity of the test, false positive test results are very unlikely**
- ❑ C. **On the basis of the very low prevalence of PKU, further testing must be undertaken to determine whether or not the infant has this illness**
- ❑ D. **Additional testing, employing a test with even greater sensitivity, is needed**

Key Concept/Objective: To understand the importance of sensitivity and prevalence on the interpretation of test results

In the absence of perfectly sensitive or specific tests, clinicians need to be prepared to order tests in a sequential manner. A perfect test for screening should have both high sensitivity (i.e., the test would miss few diseased patients) and high specificity (i.e., few of the patients being tested would be incorrectly identified as having a disease). If asked to choose between a screening test with high sensitivity and one with high specificity, a highly sensitive test would be preferred to minimize false negative results; this high sensitivity usually comes at the expense of lower specificity. This case concerns a highly sensitive test that is applied to a large population (all newborns in the United States). Because of the high sensitivity of the test, very few cases of disease will be missed. However, a few newborns will be misidentified as having PKU, because the specificity of the test is less than perfect. To confirm the diagnosis suggested by the screening test, a confirmatory test that has higher specificity is needed (such tests are usually more expensive or difficult to perform). *(Answer: C—On the basis of the very low prevalence of PKU, further testing must be undertaken to determine whether or not the infant has this illness)*

For more information, see Haynes B, Sox HC: Clinical Essentials: VIII Quantitative Aspects of Clinical Decision Making. ACP Medicine Online (www.acpmedicine.com). Dale DC, Federman DD, Eds. WebMD Inc., New York, April 2004

Palliative Medicine

21. A 55-year-old man is discharged from the hospital after presenting with a myocardial infarction. Before discharge, an echocardiogram shows an ejection fraction of 20%. The patient is free of chest pain; however, he experiences shortness of breath with minimal physical activity. The patient and his family tell you that they have a neighbor who is on a hospice program, and they ask you if the patient could be referred for hospice.

Which of the following would be the most appropriate course of action for this patient?

- ❑ A. **Palliative care together with medical treatment of his condition**
- ❑ B. **Referral to hospice**
- ❑ C. **The prognosis is unknown at this time, so palliative care and hospice are not indicated; the patient should continue receiving medical care for his heart failure**

❑ D. **Pain is not a component of his disease at this time, so neither hospice nor palliative care are indicated; medical therapy should be continued**

Key Concept/Objective: To understand the indications for palliative care and hospice

This patient's condition is not terminal at this time, and he may benefit from symptomatic management. The palliative medicine model applies not only to patients who are clearly at the end of life but also to those with chronic illnesses that, although not imminently fatal, cause significant impairment in function, quality of life, and independence. Palliative medicine for patients with serious illness thus should no longer be seen as the alternative to traditional life-prolonging care. Instead, it should be viewed as part of an integrated approach to medical care. Hospice is one way to deliver palliative care. Hospice provides home nursing, support for the family, spiritual counseling, pain treatment, medications for the illness that prompted the referral, medical care, and some inpatient care. Palliative care differs from hospice care in that palliative care can be provided at any time during an illness; it may be provided in a variety of settings, and may be combined with curative treatments. It is independent of the third-party payer. Medicare requires that recipients of hospice spend 80% of care days at home, which means that to qualify for hospice, the patient must have a home and have caregivers capable of providing care. In addition, Medicare requires that recipients have an estimated survival of 6 months or less and that their care be focused on comfort rather than cure. *(Answer: A—Palliative care together with medical treatment of his condition)*

22. A 77-year-old African-American woman is admitted to the hospital with severe shortness of breath. She lives in a nursing home. The patient has a history of dementia and left hemiplegia. A chest x-ray shows a large pneumonia and several masses that are consistent with metastatic disease. The patient is a widow and does not have a designated health care proxy. You discuss the situation with her granddaughter, who used to live with her before the patient was transferred to the nursing home. She asks you to do everything that is in your hands to save her life. The rest of the family lives 2 hours from the hospital.

Which of the following would be the most appropriate course of action in the care of this patient?

❑ A. **Ignore the granddaughter's requests because any further medical care would be futile**

❑ B. **Ask the granddaughter to bring the rest of the family, and then discuss the condition and prognosis with them**

❑ C. **Follow the granddaughter's requests and proceed with mechanical ventilation if needed**

❑ D. **Obtain an ethics consult**

Key Concept/Objective: To understand cultural differences in approaching end-of-life issues

The ability to communicate well with both patient and family is paramount in palliative care. Patients whose cultural background and language differ from those of the physician present special challenges and rewards and need to be approached in a culturally sensitive manner. People from other cultures may be less willing to discuss resuscitation status, less likely to forgo life-sustaining treatment, and more reluctant to complete advance directives. For example, because of their history of receiving inappropriate undertreatment, African-American patients and their families may continue to request aggressive care, even in terminal illness. Further interventions in this patient may not be indicated, and the physician may decide that doing more procedures on the patient would be unethical; however, it would be more appropriate to have a discussion with the family and to educate them about the condition and prognosis. Not uncommonly, the family will understand, and a consensus decision to avoid further interventions can be obtained. If the medical condition is irreversible and the family insists on continuing with aggressive therapies, the physician may decide that further treatments would be inhumane; in such a circumstance, the physician is not obligated to proceed with those interventions. An ethical consult may also be helpful under these circumstances. *(Answer: B—Ask the granddaughter to bring the rest of the family, and then discuss the condition and prognosis with them)*

23. A 66-year-old man with Parkinson disease comes to your clinic for a follow-up visit. He was diagnosed with Parkinson disease 3 years ago. His wife tells you that he is very independent and is able to perform his activities of daily living. While reviewing his chart, you find that there are no advance directives.

Which of the following would be the most appropriate step to take with regard to a discussion about advance directives for this patient?

- ❏ **A. Postpone the discussion until his disease progresses to the point where the patient is unable to perform his activities of daily living, making the discussion more relevant**
- ❏ **B. Ask the patient to come alone on the next visit so that you can discuss these difficult issues without making the patient feel uncomfortable in the presence of his wife**
- ❏ **C. Wait until the patient has a life-threatening illness so that the discussion would be more appropriate**
- ❏ **D. Start the discussion on this visit**

Key Concept/Objective: To know the appropriate timing for discussing advance directives

Public opinion polls in the United States have revealed that close to 90% of adults would not want to be maintained on life-support systems without prospect of recovery. A survey of emergency departments found that 77% did not have advance directives, and of those patients who had one, only 5% had discussed their advance directives with their primary care physician. Primary care physicians are in an excellent position to speak with patients about their care preferences because of the therapeutic relationship that already exists between patient and doctor. Conversations about preferences of care should be a routine aspect of care, even in healthy older patients. Determination of the patient's preferences can be made over two or three visits and then updated on a regular basis. Reevaluation is indicated if the patient's condition changes acutely. In general, it is preferable that a close family member or friend accompany the patient during these discussions, so that these care preferences can be witnessed and any potential surprises or conflicts can be explored with the family. *(Answer: D—Start the discussion on this visit)*

24. A 66-year-old man with a history of amyotrophic lateral sclerosis comes to the emergency department with a pulmonary thromboembolism. The patient is unable to talk but can communicate with gestures; his cognitive function is preserved. When asked about advance directives, the patient expresses his wishes not to be mechanically ventilated or resuscitated but to focus on comfort care only. The family is present and disagrees with his decision, saying that he is not competent to make such a decision because of his medical condition. The patient's respiratory status suddenly deteriorates, and he becomes cyanotic and unresponsive. The family demands that you proceed with all the measures needed to save his life.

Which of the following would be the most appropriate intervention for this patient?

- ❏ **A. Proceed with intubation and obtain an ethics consult**
- ❏ **B. Follow the patient's wishes and continue with comfort measures only**
- ❏ **C. Proceed with intubation and life support while obtaining a court opinion on the patient's competence because of the possibility of litigation**
- ❏ **D. Proceed with life support interventions and follow the family's wishes**

Key Concept/Objective: To know the criteria for decision-making capacity

Decision-making capacity refers to the capacity to provide informed consent to treatment. This is different from competence, which is a legal term; competence is determined by a court. Any physician who has adequate training can determine capacity. A patient must meet three key criteria to demonstrate decision-making capacity: (1) the ability to understand information about diagnosis and treatment; (2) the ability to evaluate, deliberate, weigh alternatives, and compare risks and benefits; and (3) the ability to communicate a choice, either verbally, in writing, or with a nod or gesture. In eliciting patient preferences, the clinician should explore the patient's values. This patient met these three criteria when he made his decision about advance directives, and his wishes should be respected. There

is no need for an ethics consult under these circumstances. Fear of litigation should not influence the decision to follow the patient's wishes. *(Answer: B—Follow the patient's wishes and continue with comfort measures only)*

For more information, see Pann C: Clinical Essentials: IX Palliative Medicine. ACP Medicine Online (www.acpmedicine.com). Dale DC, Federman DD, Eds. WebMD Inc., New York, September 2003

Symptom Management in Palliative Medicine

25. A patient with terminal lung cancer on home hospice is brought to the hospital by his family for admission. He is agitated and confused, and his family is unable to care for him at home. Upon examination, the patient is disoriented and appears to be having visual hallucinations.

Which of the following statements is true regarding delirium in terminal patients?

- ❑ A. **Benzodiazepines are first-line therapy for treatment of delirium**
- ❑ B. **If the patient's condition is deemed terminal, there is no point in addressing the specific underlying cause of the dementia**
- ❑ C. **Physical restraints should generally be used for patient safety in the setting of delirium**
- ❑ D. **The subcutaneous route is a viable option for the administration of benzodiazepines**
- ❑ E. **Delirium generally occurs only in patients with underlying dementia**

Key Concept/Objective: To understand the treatment of delirium in the terminally ill patient

Pharmacologic treatment for relief of symptoms of delirium is best achieved through the use of antipsychotic agents such as haloperidol or risperidone. Benzodiazepines and sedatives should be used only if antipsychotic agents fail. In as many as 25% of terminally ill patients who experience delirium characterized by escalating restlessness, agitation, or hallucinations, relief is achieved only with sedation. Even in a terminally ill patient, treatment of the underlying cause (e.g., infection, hypoxemia) can be the best way to improve the delirium. Physical restraints can actually be a precipitating factor for delirium and should be avoided in the delirious patient whenever possible. In patients who cannot take oral medications and in whom a functional intravenous line is not available, the subcutaneous route is a rapidly effective way to administer certain medications, including midazolam. Patients with underlying dementia are predisposed to delirium, but delirium can occur in patients with other comorbidities. *(Answer: D—The subcutaneous route is a viable option for the administration of benzodiazepines)*

26. An 80-year-old man with very poor functional status who has a history of cerebrovascular accident presents to the emergency department from the nursing home with severe shortness of breath. Chest x-ray shows that he has severe pneumonia. The patient is intubated immediately and transferred to the ICU. His condition worsens over the next several days, despite aggressive therapy. His family decides that because of the severity of the patient's illness and his poor functional status before this illness, they want him taken off the ventilator. They approach you with this request.

Which of the following statements accurately characterizes ventilator withdrawal in this situation?

- ❑ A. **You should refuse the family's request on ethical grounds**
- ❑ B. **To protect the family's emotions, you should not allow them to be with the patient until after the endotracheal tube has been removed**
- ❑ C. **Pulse oximetry should be followed to help guide the family through the dying process**
- ❑ D. **You should demonstrate that the patient is comfortable receiving a lower fraction of inspired oxygen (F_IO_2) before withdrawing the endotracheal tube**

❑ E. **Such patients generally die within 30 minutes to an hour after the endotracheal tube is removed**

Key Concept/Objective: To understand how to appropriately perform the process of terminal ventilation withdrawal

Every physician has his or her own level of comfort with regard to terminal ventilation withdrawal. However, in a situation in which the family makes a very reasonable request and the patient's wishes are not known, the family's wishes should generally be followed. The family should be given the opportunity to be with the patient when the endotracheal tube is removed. The decision should be theirs to make. All monitors should be turned off at the initiation of the process. The patient's comfort will guide therapy. F_IO_2 should be diminished to 20%, and the patient should be observed for respiratory distress before removing the endotracheal tube. Distress can be treated with opioids and benzodiazepines. It is important to inform the family that a patient may live for hours to days after the ventilator is removed and to reassure them that all measures necessary to ensure comfort during the dying process will be used. *(Answer: D—You should demonstrate that the patient is comfortable receiving a lower fraction of inspired oxygen [F_IO_2] before withdrawing the endotracheal tube)*

27. A patient with severe dementia has developed worsening anorexia and nausea over the past 6 weeks. You have turned your attention to symptom management.

Which of the following statements accurately characterizes treatment of these complications of severe dementia?

❑ A. **Haloperidol has minimal effects against nausea**

❑ B. **Even though this patient has severe dementia, it would be unethical to withhold nutrition and hydration**

❑ C. **A feeding tube will reduce the risk of aspiration pneumonia**

❑ D. **Prochlorperazine relieves nausea by blocking serotonin at its site of action in the vomiting center of the brain**

❑ E. **Impaction may explain all the symptoms**

Key Concept/Objective: To understand the management of nausea and anorexia near the end of life

Haloperidol is highly effective against nausea and may be less sedating than many commonly used agents, such as prochlorperazine. Because of the terminal and irreversible nature of end-stage dementia and the substantial burden that continued life-prolonging care may pose, palliative care focused predominantly on the comfort of the patient is often viewed as preferable to life-prolonging measures by a substantial proportion of nursing [illegible] but it is never unethical to withhold nutrition and hydration if these are not helping the patient. There is no evidence that tube feeding reduces the risk of pneumonia in such patients, and it may even increase it. Dopamine-mediated nausea is probably the most common form of nausea, and it is the form of nausea most frequently targeted for initial symptom management. Prochlorperazine relieves dopamine-mediated nausea. Bowel impaction could easily explain the gradually worsening anorexia and nausea in a bedridden patient. *(Answer: E—Impaction may explain all the symptoms)*

28. In a palliative care unit, a patient with terminal ovarian cancer became dramatically less responsive several hours ago. Her breathing pattern has changed, and it appears that she is actively dying.

Which of the following statements accurately characterizes appropriate physician management during the last hours of living?

❑ A. **Subcutaneous hydration prevents the discomfort that terminal dehydration causes**

❑ B. **The body should be removed very soon after death for the emotional well-being of the family**

❑ C. **Scopolamine can be useful for diminishing pharyngeal secretions**

❑ D. **At this point, the unconscious patient is unaware of the surroundings**

❑ E. **Physician contact of the family after the death implies concern about improper management on the part of the physician**

Key Concept/Objective: To understand basic management principles that should be employed during the final hours of life

Dehydration in the final hours of living does not cause distress and may stimulate endorphin release that adds to the patient's sense of well-being. The removal of the body too soon after death can be even more upsetting to the family than the moment of death, so the family should be given the time they need with the body. Scopolamine, an anticholinergic, can diminish pharyngeal secretions and relieve the so-called death rattle: noisy respirations caused by secretions as they move up and down with expiration and inspiration. Always presume that the unconscious patient hears everything. This very well may be true and will be comforting to the family. The physician should consider contacting the family during the bereavement period by letter or visit. Physician contact during this period can help the family deal with grief and does not imply that a medical error was made. *(Answer: C—Scopolamine can be useful for diminishing pharyngeal secretions)*

For more information, see Carney MT, Rhodes-Kropf J: Clinical Essentials: X Symptom Management in Palliative Medicine. ACP Medicine Online (www.acpmedicine.com). Dale DC, Federman DD, Eds. WebMD Inc., New York, July 2002

Psychosocial Issues in Terminal Illness

29. A 64-year-old man presented to the emergency department complaining of substernal chest pressure that radiated to his left arm. Subsequent evaluation revealed that the patient had suffered myocardial infarction. He received appropriate treatment, and his condition improved. Over the first 2 days of his hospitalization, the patient expressed fears of death and was anxious. However, on hospital day 3, his fears and anxiety seem to subside.

Which of the following emotions does such a patient usually experience?

❑ A. Jubilance

❑ B. Acceptance

❑ C. Depression

❑ D. Denial

Key Concept/Objective: To know the sequence of emotions experienced by those coping with acute illness

Studies have been conducted in patients with myocardial infarction regarding the patients' emotional reactions to their illness. The general sequence of these emotions is fear and anxiety, stabilization, denial, confirmation of illness, and then despondency. It is important to be familiar with these concepts; patients in the denial stage have been known to sign themselves out of the hospital against medical advice. The physician should gently reassure the patient and remind the patient of the plan of treatment, the benefits of continued care, and the risks of deviating from the management plan. Family and friends should also be involved if possible. *(Answer: D—Denial)*

30. A 67-year-old woman is diagnosed as having adenocarcinoma of the breast, which has metastasized to bone. She has been admitted to the hospital for pain control. During hospitalization, the patient develops sadness and anhedonia accompanied by continued problems with her pain and frequent crying spells. You worry that she has developed depression and would like to provide symptomatic relief in the next few days.

Which of the following is NOT a use for methylphenidate (Ritalin) and pemolin (Cylert) in the palliative care setting?

- ❑ A. **Short-term treatment of depression**
- ❑ B. **To stimulate appetite**
- ❑ C. **To counteract opiate sedation**
- ❑ D. **To potentiate opiate analgesia**

Key Concept/Objective: To understand alternative medications that can hasten relief of symptoms of depression in the palliative care setting

Because standard therapies for depression typically require several weeks to take full effect, other treatment modalities have been sought for use as palliative care for those with depression and for short-term treatment. Methylphenidate and pemolin are psychostimulants that are useful for the short-term treatment of depression. They are also useful in counteracting opiate sedation, and they potentiate opiate analgesia. These medications may suppress appetite. *(Answer: B—To stimulate appetite)*

31. A 70-year-old woman has just lost her husband to prostate cancer. She comes to your office for a routine health maintenance visit. You note that she seems more reserved and less interactive than normal. You ask her how she is handling the loss of her husband.

What is the best predictor of later problems associated with abnormal grieving?

- ❑ A. **Inability to grieve immediately after loss (e.g., an absence of weeping)**
- ❑ B. **A close relationship with the deceased**
- ❑ C. **Unresolved issues with the deceased**
- ❑ D. **Somatic symptoms**

Key Concept/Objective: To know the best predictor of problems associated with abnormal grieving in a patient who has lost a loved one

Grief is the psychological process by which an individual copes with loss. One of the greatest losses—and stressors—that one may suffer is the loss of a spouse. There are many recognized features of normal grieving that can be mistaken for pathologic conditions. Normal grieving can include somatic symptoms, feelings of guilt, preoccupation with the deceased person, hostile reactions, irritability, and some disruption of normal patterns of behavior. The best predictor of later problems associated with abnormal grieving is an inability to grieve immediately after the loss, as evidenced by the absence of weeping. Other important predictors of abnormal grieving include prolonged hysteria that is excessive in terms of the patient's own cultural norms; overactivity in the absence of a sense of loss; and furious hostility against specific persons, such as caregivers, to the exclusion of the other concerns associated with normal grief. *(Answer: A—Inability to grieve immediately after loss [e.g., an absence of weeping])*

32. A 78-year-old man is brought to you by his family because he has not been acting himself since his wife passed away 2 months ago. The family is worried about him and states that he has become more reclusive and less active over the past few weeks. They even worry that he is hearing his dead wife's voice and seeing visions of her.

Which of the following features is NOT an aspect of normal grieving?

- ❑ A. **Somatic symptoms**
- ❑ B. **Guilt**
- ❑ C. **A feeling that one is hearing, is seeing, or is touched by the dead person**
- ❑ D. **Giving away personal belongings**

Key Concept/Objective: To be able to distinguish normal from abnormal grieving

Features of normal grieving are easily mistaken as pathologic. However, these features have been well established in those suffering serious loss, such as the loss of a spouse.

Somatic symptoms such as fatigue, gastrointestinal symptoms, and choking are prominent, as are feelings of guilt. Preoccupation with the image of the deceased can manifest as continual mental conversations with them as well as the feeling that one is hearing, seeing, or being touched by the dead person. Hostile reactions, irritability, and disruption of normal patterns of conduct are also common. Self-destructive behavior such as giving away belongings, ill-advised business deals, and other self-punitive actions are early indicators of abnormal grieving. Patients showing evidence of abnormal grieving should receive counseling to help bring their feelings into the open and facilitate recovery. *(Answer: D—Giving away personal belongings)*

33. A 34-year-old woman has lost her husband in a traffic accident. She comes to see you for a health maintenance visit but seems despondent. You speak with her at length, and it seems that she is suffering a normal grief reaction to the loss of her husband.

Which of the following will NOT facilitate this patient's grieving?

- ❑ **A. The opportunity for the patient to see her husband's remains**
- ❑ **B. The patient's returning to her job**
- ❑ **C. The patient's joining a self-help group**
- ❑ **D. The health care provider's pointing out that life must go on and that the patient should do her best to be cheerful**

Key Concept/Objective: To know measures that will facilitate normal grieving

The bereaved tend to be isolated from society. Many persons in our society are uncomfortable around people who are in grieving, and the bereaved are often encouraged—and subsequently force themselves—to suppress the manifestations of their grief. Survivors are at high risk for abnormal or complicated bereavement if their loved one died unexpectedly or suddenly, if the death was violent, and if no bodily remains were found. Seeing the body of the deceased facilitates grieving, and returning to one's job helps with recovery and return to normalcy. Self-help groups allow the bereaved to express feelings, relate to others with similar experiences, and rebuild self-esteem. Statements that negate or argue against grieving should be avoided. *(Answer: D—The health care provider's pointing out that life must go on and that the patient should do her best to be cheerful)*

34. A 78-year-old woman with widely metastatic ovarian cancer is admitted to the hospital for intractable pain. High doses of opiates are required to control her pain, but she is intermittently alert and interactive. Several family members visit her. During rounds, one of her sons asks you whether the patient's 8-year-old great-granddaughter should be brought to see her.

Which of the following is the most appropriate answer to this relative's question?

- ❑ **A. Children should not see loved ones in such a condition**
- ❑ **B. He should ask the patient**
- ❑ **C. The child's parents should decide**
- ❑ **D. The child should be asked if she would like to see her great-grandmother**

Key Concept/Objective: To understand that the visits of children can be of great comfort to terminally ill patients and that the best way to determine if a particular child should visit a patient is to ask the child if he or she would like to do so

Visits of children are among the most effective ways to bring comfort to the terminally ill patient. In addition, allowing children to be present during the dying process provides an opportunity for them to learn that death is not necessarily a terrifying or violent process. Although it is preferable that the entire family agree that it is appropriate for a child to see their dying relative, the best criterion for determining whether such a visit should occur is to ask the child if he or she would like to see the loved one. *(Answer: D—The child should be asked if she would like to see her great-grandmother)*

For more information, see Rhodes-Kropf J, Cassern NH: Clinical Essentials: XI Management of Psychosocial Issues in Terminal Illness. ACP Medicine Online (www.acpmedicine.com). Dale DC, Federman DD, Eds. WebMD Inc., New York, May 2002

Complementary and Alternative Medicine

35. A patient comes to your office and states that she is absolutely convinced that acupuncture will help her fibromyalgia. You would like to present data to her that either refute or support this practice.

Which of the following statements regarding complementary and alternative medicine (CAM) is false?

- ❑ A. **Critical reviews of published studies on CAM therapies from a number of countries have shown that they are almost universally positive**
- ❑ B. **Establishment of adequate control groups is frequently difficult**
- ❑ C. **The therapies themselves are not standardized and are therefore difficult to compare**
- ❑ D. **Studies are funded by special interest groups and therefore have potential to be biased**
- ❑ E. **Many patients do not feel a need to communicate their use of alternative medicine modalities to their physician**

Key Concept/Objective: To understand the inherent difficulties in obtaining and interpreting research information on CAM

One of the defining characteristics of alternative medicine is the paucity of definitive evidence supporting mechanism of action, efficacy, and safety. Although a number of clinical trials on CAM have been published, the overall quality of these trials is quite poor, primarily because of insufficient sample size and a lack of randomization and blinding. One concern is that only studies that report positive results make it to press. Another concern is that establishing adequate control groups is very difficult because, by their very nature, the therapies cannot preserve subject blinding. Another issue is that the therapies themselves lack standardization. For example, different forms of acupuncture may utilize completely unique sets of points for treatment of the same condition. If the physician is not aware that the patient is using some form of CAM, it can be very difficult to advise the patient properly. Many patients do not feel a need to communicate their use of CAM because of a perception that their physician would be unable to understand and incorporate that information into the treatment plan. Thus, it is very important that the physician inquire about the use of alternative medicine modalities. Physician funding for large-scale studies in CAM emanate almost exclusively from governmental resources. There is little private funding for large, well-controlled trials of most CAM treatment modalities. *(Answer: D—Studies are funded by special interest groups and therefore have potential to be biased)*

36. A patient in your clinic states that her entire family is using acupuncture for everything that ails them.

Which of the following statements regarding the practice of acupuncture is true?

- ❑ A. **Clear evidence supports the use of acupuncture for chemotherapy-induced vomiting**
- ❑ B. **There are essentially no adverse events associated with acupuncture**
- ❑ C. **Acupuncture was proven ineffective for postoperative vomiting**
- ❑ D. **Acupuncture likely has a role in smoking cessation**
- ❑ E. **Acupuncture works by stimulating nerves at the needle site**

Key Concept/Objective: To understand basic concepts of acupuncture and in which settings it has been proven to be useful

To date, no clear mechanism of action has emerged to explain the potential therapeutic response to acupuncture. In 1997, the National Institutes of Health held a Consensus

Development Conference on Acupuncture, which concluded that there is clear evidence to support the use of acupuncture for postoperative, chemotherapy-induced, and probably pregnancy-associated nausea and vomiting.[1] Current evidence does not support its use for smoking cessation. Performed correctly, acupuncture is quite safe. Rare case reports of serious adverse events, including skin infections, hepatitis, pneumothorax, and cardiac tamponade, seem to stem from inadequate sterilization of needles and practitioner negligence. *(Answer: A—Clear evidence supports the use of acupuncture for chemotherapy-induced vomiting)*

1. Acupuncture. NIH Consensus Statement 15(5):1, 1997

37. A 65-year-old woman with a medical history of paroxysmal atrial fibrillation with episodes of rapid response, congestive heart failure, and osteoarthritis comes to your office for a routine follow-up visit. She states that she has been taking herbs and nonherbal supplements to help alleviate the symptoms of menopause, combat depression and anxiety, and improve her arthritis.

Which of the following statements regarding CAM treatments is false?

- ❑ A. **St. John's wort (used to treat depression and anxiety) can decrease serum levels of digoxin**
- ❑ B. **Dong quai (used to treat the symptoms of menopause) can prolong the international normalized ratio (INR) in patients taking warfarin**
- ❑ C. **The cardioprotective effects of garlic are as yet unproven**
- ❑ D. **Kava kava (used to treat anxiety) may potentiate the effect of benzodiazepines and other sedatives**
- ❑ E. **Glucosamine and chondroitin have been proven to be ineffective in treating osteoarthritis**

Key Concept/Objective: To become aware of drug interactions of some very commonly used herbal and nonherbal supplements, as well as the effectiveness of these supplements

Several drug interactions are associated with herbal and nonherbal supplements: St. John's wort can decrease serum digoxin levels; dong quai can prolong INR; and kava kava is known to potentiate sedatives. The definitive beneficial effects of garlic in cardioprotection are unproven. Glucosamine and chondroitin are some of the few supplements for which there are data showing efficacy. Current data suggest symptomatic improvement for osteoarthritis of the hips and knees. There are data supporting the use of St. John's wort in the treatment of mild to moderate depression. *(Answer: E—Glucosamine and chondroitin have been proven to be ineffective in treating osteoarthritis)*

38. A patient with chronic back and neck pain reports that he has finally gotten some relief through a local chiropractor. He wants your opinion about the safety and efficacy of chiropractic therapy for such conditions.

Which of the following statements is false regarding chiropractic therapy?

- ❑ A. **Very little data support the use of chiropractic manipulation to treat hypertension, menstrual pain, or fibromyalgia**
- ❑ B. **Research may be insufficient to prove a benefit for patients with acute or chronic lower back pain**
- ❑ C. **Patients with coagulopathy should be advised against chiropractic therapy**
- ❑ D. **Patients who try chiropractic therapy become dissatisfied after the first several treatments**
- ❑ E. **Serious complications can occur with cervical manipulation**

Key Concept/Objective: To understand the efficacy and contraindications of chiropractic therapy

Chiropractic manipulation has been touted as a treatment for a number of conditions, including hypertension, asthma, menstrual pain, and fibromyalgia. However, very little

data support its use for these conditions. Much of the current use of chiropractic care stems from its utility in cases of low back pain. A number of controlled trials on chiropractic treatment for low back pain have been done, with conflicting results. A meta-analysis suggested that research was insufficient to prove a benefit for acute or chronic low back pain. In general, however, patient satisfaction is high with chiropractic therapy. Patients with coagulopathy, osteoporosis, rheumatoid arthritis, spinal neoplasms, or spinal infections should be advised against such treatments. Serious complications have been reported as a result of cervical manipulation, including brain stem or cerebellar infarction, vertebral fracture, tracheal rupture, internal carotid artery dissection, and diaphragmatic paralysis. It is therefore difficult to advocate routine use of cervical manipulation for treatment of head and neck disorders. *(Answer: D—Patients who try chiropractic therapy become dissatisfied after the first several treatments)*

39. One of your patients tells you that she attended a seminar on the use of mind-body interventions to treat various conditions. She has been using various methods to overcome problems with asthma, anxiety, and substance abuse.

Which of the following statements is false regarding mind-body interventions?

- ❑ **A. The success of hypnotherapy depends on patient attitude toward hypnosis**
- ❑ **B. Biofeedback is a relaxation technique in which the patient continually subjectively assesses his or her level of relaxation and makes appropriate adjustments**
- ❑ **C. Aromatherapy involves the use of essential oils to induce a relaxation response**
- ❑ **D. Mind-body interventions likely affect hormonal balance in a positive manner**

Key Concept/Objective: To understand various forms of mind-body interventions

Hypnotherapy is the induction of a trancelike state to induce relaxation and susceptibility to positive suggestion. Success of therapy likely depends on patient susceptibility and attitude toward hypnosis. Biofeedback involves self-regulation of the physiologic response to stress through relaxation techniques. Instrumentation (electroencephalography, electromyography, skin temperature/sweat monitors) is used to assess and guide therapy. Thus, biofeedback is one of the least subjective of the mind-body interventions. Aromatherapy involves the use of essential oils (e.g., jasmine and lavender) to induce a relaxation response. The proposed mechanism of action of mind-body interventions involves hormonal changes (e.g., a decrease in epinephrine levels) and reversal of the physiologic consequences of stress. Counteracting the physiologic effects of stress can presumably help combat the manifestations of various disease states. *(Answer: B—Biofeedback is a relaxation technique in which the patient continually subjectively assesses his or her level of relaxation and makes appropriate adjustments)*

40. A 54-year-old woman whom you have followed for years in clinic for benign hypertension, osteoporosis, and chronic low back pain returns for her annual examination. She has no new complaints, but she is interested in alternative forms of treatment for her low back pain.

Which of the following statements concerning chiropractic treatment is true?

- ❑ **A. Spinal manipulation is considered a first-line treatment for low back pain because there are no known side effects**
- ❑ **B. Studies have suggested that spinal manipulation is an effective treatment option for patients with chronic back pain**
- ❑ **C. Health care insurance plans do not cover chiropractic treatments**
- ❑ **D. Osteoporosis does not preclude this patient's use of chiropractic treatment for low back pain**

Key Concept/Objective: To understand the uses and limitations of chiropractic treatments

Health care insurance plans, including Medicare, cover many of the services performed during chiropractic visits. Most chiropractic visits are for musculoskeletal problems, including low back pain, neck pain, and extremity pain. Much of the current use of chiropractic care stems from its utility in cases of low back pain. A number of controlled trials on chiropractic treatment for low back pain have been done, with conflicting results. A recent systematic review suggested that spinal manipulation is effective and is a viable treatment option for patients with acute or chronic low back pain. Patient satisfaction also seems to be high with such therapy. Serious complications from lumbar spinal manipulation seem to be uncommon, although there are reports of cauda equina syndrome. Many patients, however, experience mild to moderate side effects, including localized discomfort, headache, or tiredness. These reactions usually disappear within 24 hours. Brain stem or cerebellar infarction, vertebral fracture, tracheal rupture, internal carotid artery dissection, and diaphragmatic paralysis are rare but have all been reported with cervical manipulation. Given the lack of efficacy data and the risk (although small) of catastrophic adverse events, it is difficult to advocate routine use of this technique for treatment of neck or headache disorders. Physicians should also recognize potential contraindications to chiropractic therapy. Patients with coagulopathy, osteoporosis, rheumatoid arthritis, spinal neoplasms, or spinal infections should be advised against such treatments. *(Answer: B—Studies have suggested that spinal manipulation is an effective treatment option for patients with chronic back pain)*

41. A 63-year-old man presents to your clinic for an initial evaluation. He has a history of coronary artery disease, congestive heart failure, atrial fibrillation, benign prostatic hyperplasia, and erectile dysfunction. His current medical regimen includes hydrochlorothiazide, metoprolol, enalapril, digoxin, coumarin, and terazosin. During the visit, the patient pulls out a bag of vitamins and herbal supplements that he recently began taking. He hands you several Internet printouts regarding the supplements and asks your advice.

Which of the following statements about dietary supplements is true?

- ❑ A. **Under the Dietary Supplement Health and Education Act (DSHEA), all supplements are now required to undergo premarket testing for safety and efficacy**
- ❑ B. **Because they are natural products, dietary supplements are uniformly safe, with no significant drug-drug interactions**
- ❑ C. **The dietary-supplement industry has little incentive for research because natural substances cannot be patented**
- ❑ D. **The Food and Drug Administration regulates dietary supplements under the same guidelines as pharmaceuticals**

Key Concept/Objective: To understand the potential for toxicity and drug-drug interactions associated with dietary supplements

The supplement industry has become a billion-dollar business, largely as a result of loosening of federal regulations. In 1994, DSHEA expanded the definition of dietary supplements to include vitamins, amino acids, herbs, and other botanicals. Furthermore, under DSHEA, supplements no longer require premarket testing for safety and efficacy. Dietary supplements, such as herbs, may have a significant profit potential, but the incentive for research is weakened by the fact that herbs, like other natural substances, cannot be patented. In addition, foods and natural products are regulated under rules different from those for pharmaceuticals, which must meet stringent standards of efficacy and safety. Although most dietary supplements are well tolerated and are associated with few adverse effects, the potential for harm from the lack of regulation can be seen from examples of misidentification of plant species, contamination with heavy metals, and addition of pharmaceutical agents. Overall, there is only limited evidence supporting the use of most dietary supplements. Most clinical trials have been small, nonrandomized, or unblinded. The potential for significant toxicity and drug interactions does exist. *(Answer: C—The dietary-supplement industry has little incentive for research because natural substances cannot be patented)*

For more information, see Dobs AS, Ashar BH: Clinical Essentials: XII Complementary and Alternative Medicine. ACP Medicine Online (www.acpmedicine.com). Dale DC, Federman DD, Eds. WebMD Inc., New York, November 2004

SECTION 1

CARDIOVASCULAR MEDICINE

Heart Failure

1. A 56-year-old man with a history of coronary artery disease and a documented ejection fraction of 40% by echocardiography presents for further management. At this visit, the patient denies having shortness of breath, dyspnea on exertion, orthopnea, or lower extremity edema. He has never been admitted to the hospital for congestive heart failure (CHF).

    According to the new American College of Cardiology/American Heart Association (ACC/AHA) guidelines for the evaluation and management of heart failure, in what stage of heart failure does this patient belong?

    ❑ A. Stage A

    ❑ B. Stage B

    ❑ C. Stage C

    ❑ D. Stage D

    Key Concept/Objective: To understand the new classification of heart failure proposed by the ACC/AHA

    The ACC/AHA classification is a departure from the traditional New York Heart Association (NYHA) classification, which characterizes patients by symptom severity. The aim of the new ACC/AHA guidelines is to identify patients at risk for developing heart failure. Early recognition of contributing risk factors, as well as the identification and treatment of asymptomatic patients with ventricular dysfunction, can prevent pathologic progression to symptomatic heart failure. Stage A identifies patients who are at high risk for developing heart failure but who have no apparent structural abnormality of the heart. Stage B denotes patients with a structural abnormality of the heart but in whom symptoms of heart failure have not yet developed. Stage C refers to patients with a structural abnormality of the heart and symptoms of heart failure. Stage D includes the patient with end-stage heart failure that is refractory to standard treatment. This patient has stage B heart failure. The goal of therapy is aimed at preventing progression to stage C or D. *(Answer: B—Stage B)*

2. A 67-year-old man presents for evaluation of worsening dyspnea. The patient reports that his symptoms have been worsening over the past several months. He also mentions that he has developed some swelling in his legs and notes that he is easily fatigued. His medical history is remarkable for type 2 (non–insulin-dependent) diabetes mellitus, presumed cytogenic cirrhosis, and "arthritis" in his hands. The patient denies ever using alcohol. On physical examination, the patient's vital signs are normal; examination of the jugular venous pulse shows the height to be 10 cm; no thyromegaly is present; pulmonary examination reveals faint basilar crackles; cardiac examination shows nondisplaced point of maximal impulse and no audible murmur; no hepatosplenomegaly is noted; and 2+ bilateral lower extremity edema is noted. An ECG is unremarkable. An echocardiogram reveals normal ejection fraction and normal valvular function. You order lab work that includes iron studies and make the diagnosis of hemochromatosis.

    What is the pathogenesis of heart failure in this patient?

    ❑ A. Ischemic cardiomyopathy

❑ B. **Infiltrative cardiomyopathy**

❑ C. **Valvular cardiomyopathy**

❑ D. **Idiopathic cardiomyopathy**

Key Concept/Objective: To recognize infiltrative cardiomyopathy as a cause of dyspnea in a patient with normal ejection fraction but symptoms of both left- and right-side heart failure

Infiltrative causes of ventricular dysfunction, which are usually associated with restrictive cardiomyopathy, include amyloidosis, hemochromatosis, and sarcoidosis. This patient's symptoms are the result of impaired diastolic filling leading to increased pulmonary venous pressure and subsequent symptoms of right heart failure (elevated jugular venous pulse and edema). It should be noted that patients with hemochromatosis may develop dilated cardiomyopathy. The pathogenesis of this patient's heart failure is the result of iron deposition in the heart, leading to impaired myocardial relaxation. The normal ECG and the absence of wall motion abnormalities on the echocardiogram make ischemic cardiomyopathy an unlikely diagnosis. The normal ejection fraction and normal size of the ventricles exclude the diagnosis of idiopathic cardiomyopathy. Finally, there is no echocardiographic evidence of valvular heart disease. *(Answer: B—Infiltrative cardiomyopathy)*

3. A 56-year-old patient with stage D ischemic cardiomyopathy comes to you for a second opinion. He is already receiving furosemide, an angiotensin-converting enzyme (ACE) inhibitor, a beta blocker, and spironolactone. He has been told by a specialist that he needs a device to avoid dying from an irregular heart rhythm.

What nonpharmacologic treatments are available for the prevention of sudden cardiac death in patients with ischemic cardiomyopathy?

❑ A. **Ventricular assist device (VAD)**

❑ B. **Implantable cardioverter defibrillator (ICD)**

❑ C. **Biventricular pacemaker**

❑ D. **Intra-aortic balloon pump (IABP)**

Key Concept/Objective: To understand that sudden cardiac death contributes significantly to the mortality of patients with heart failure

The management of heart failure has evolved from primarily noninvasive medical therapies to include invasive medical devices. In addition to contributing to worsening heart failure, ventricular arrhythmias are a likely direct cause of death in many of these patients; the rate of sudden cardiac death in persons with heart failure is six to nine times that seen in the general population. The use of ICDs for the primary prevention of sudden death in patients with left ventricular dysfunction has grown enormously in recent years. There is increasing evidence that ICD placement [illegible] mortality in patients with [illegible] cardiomyopathy, regardless of whether they have nonsustained ventricular arrhythmias. The role of these devices in patients with heart failure of a nonischemic cause has yet to be elucidated and is the subject of several ongoing trials. Biventricular pacing improves prognosis in patients with severe CHF but has no role in the management of lethal arrhythmias. Both IABP and VAD are mechanical devices utilized as a bridge to cardiac transplantation for patients with very severe CHF. *(Answer: B—Implantable cardioverter defibrillator [ICD])*

4. A 38-year-old man with stage C CHF remains symptomatic in spite of diuretic therapy. You are considering adding a second and perhaps even a third agent to his regimen.

Which of the following pharmacologic agents used in the management of heart failure lacks trial data indicating a mortality benefit and does not prevent maladaptive ventricular remodeling?

❑ A. **ACE inhibitors or angiotensin receptor blockers (ARBs)**

❑ B. **Spironolactone**

❑ C. **Beta blockers**

❑ D. **Digoxin**

Key Concept/Objective: To be aware of proven pharmacologic therapy aimed at counterbalancing the activation of the renin-angiotensin and sympathetic systems

Left ventricular dysfunction begins with an injury to the myocardium. The unanswered question is why ventricular systolic dysfunction continues to worsen in the absence of recurrent insults. This pathologic process, which has been termed remodeling, is the structural response to the initial injury. Mechanical, neurohormonal, and possibly genetic factors alter ventricular size, shape, and function to decrease wall stress and compensate for the initial injury. Remodeling involves hypertrophy, loss of myocytes, and increased fibrosis, and it is secondary to both neurohormonal activation and other mechanical factors. In patients with heart failure, ACE inhibitors have been shown to improve survival and cardiac performance, to decrease symptoms and hospitalizations, and to decrease or slow the remodeling process. ARBs block the effects of angiotensin II at the angiotensin II type 1 receptor site. ACC/AHA guidelines recommend the use of ARBs only in patients who cannot tolerate ACE inhibitors because of cough or angioedema; the guidelines stress that ARBs are comparable to ACE inhibitors but are not superior. Since publication of the guidelines, however, several key trials have reported successful intervention with ARBs in patients in stage A and stage B. The primary action of beta blockers is to counteract the harmful effects of the increased sympathetic nervous system activity in heart failure. Beta blockers improve survival, ejection fraction, and quality of life; they also decrease morbidity, hospitalizations, sudden death, and the maladaptive effects of remodeling. Aldosterone also works locally within the myocardium, contributing to hypertrophy and fibrosis in the failing heart. A large randomized trial has shown that the addition of low-dose spironolactone (25 mg daily) to standard treatment reduces morbidity and mortality in patients with NYHA class III and IV heart failure (stage C and D patients). A large randomized study demonstrated that digoxin was successful in decreasing hospitalization for heart failure—an important clinical end point—but did not decrease mortality. It has no role in preventing maladaptive ventricular remodeling. *(Answer: D—Digoxin)*

5. A 60-year-old woman with a history of hypertension and mild chronic obstructive pulmonary disease (COPD) presents with a new complaint of progressive dyspnea.

Which of the following would best support a definite diagnosis of left-sided systolic heart failure as the cause of this patient's new symptoms?

- ❑ A. **Grade IV to VI murmur at the apex that radiates to the axilla**
- ❑ B. **Fixed splitting of S_2**
- ❑ C. **Recumbent dyspnea**
- ❑ D. **Pulsus alternans**
- ❑ E. **S_4 gallop**

Key Concept/Objective: To understand the physical examination findings of left-sided systolic heart failure

Mitral regurgitation resulting from annular dilatation is commonly audible in systolic heart failure. However, the regurgitant murmur is generally no louder than grade II to grade III in intensity and will wax and wane, depending on the extent of left ventricular dilatation. Murmurs of greater intensity should suggest intrinsic rather than functional valve disease. Paradoxical splitting of S_2 can occur in systolic chronic heart failure as a result of either left bundle branch block or reversal of A_2 and P_2 caused by prolonged ejection of blood by the impaired left ventricle. Fixed splitting of S_2 is associated with atrial septal defect or right ventricular failure. Orthopnea is not specific to CHF. Patients with COPD also find it easier to breathe with the head of the bed and thorax elevated. A presystolic, or S_4, gallop indicates reduced compliance of the left ventricle but not a failing left ventricle per se. Pulsus alternans, characterized by alternating weaker and stronger pulsations in the peripheral arteries, indicates a diseased left ventricle with poor systolic function. Pulsus alternans will usually be accompanied by an S_3 gallop. *(Answer: D—Pulsus alternans)*

6. A 60-year-old man presents with progressive symmetrical lower extremity edema.

Which of the following findings would be inconsistent with a diagnosis of right-sided heart failure?

- ❏ A. The Kussmaul sign
- ❏ B. Prolonged prothrombin time
- ❏ C. Diarrhea
- ❏ D. Elevated bilirubin level
- ❏ E. Pulsus paradoxus

Key Concept/Objective: To understand the clinical findings of right-sided heart failure

In right ventricular failure, constrictive pericarditis, or tricuspid stenosis, the compromised right ventricle cannot accommodate the normal increased venous return that occurs during inspiration. This causes a rise, rather than the normal fall, in jugular venous pressure during inspiration (a positive Kussmaul sign). This sign is a subtle indicator of right ventricular dysfunction and may be seen even in the presence of normal jugular venous pressure. In patients with severe and chronic systemic venous congestion, the prothrombin time can be prolonged. Thus, an abnormal international normalized ratio does not automatically indicate liver disease. Similarly, chronic congestion may produce mild elevations in bilirubin and alkaline phosphatase levels. An elevation of transaminase levels is more likely to be associated with acute liver congestion with hypoxia and hepatocellular damage. Splanchnic congestion in right heart failure can lead to nausea, diarrhea, and malabsorption. Pulsus paradoxus consists of a greater than normal (10 mm Hg) inspiratory decline in systolic arterial pressure. It can occur in cases of cardiac tamponade, constrictive pericarditis, hypovolemic shock, pulmonary embolus, and COPD. It would not be expected in isolated right-sided heart failure. *(Answer: E—Pulsus paradoxus)*

7. A 54-year-old man presents to your clinic to establish primary care. He has a history of diabetes, CHF, and hypertension. His blood pressure is 160/90 mm Hg, 2+ edema is present, and mild crackles are heard in the bases of his lungs. He takes no medications.

Which of the following statements incorrectly characterizes attributes of the medications to be considered for this patient?

- ❏ A. Hydrochlorothiazide may exacerbate hyperglycemia
- ❏ B. Without a loading dose, the blood level of digoxin will plateau in 7 days
- ❏ C. Oral bioavailability of loop diuretics varies little from drug to drug
- ❏ D. Spironolactone has been associated with gynecomastia
- ❏ E. Nonsteroidal anti-inflammatory drugs (NSAIDs) may cause diuretic unresponsiveness

Key Concept/Objective: To understand the fundamental pharmacology and side effects of medications commonly used in the treatment of heart failure

Thiazides may precipitate or exacerbate hyperglycemia, worsen hyperuricemia, and decrease sexual function. The blood level of digoxin will plateau 7 days (four to five half-lives) after initiation of regular maintenance doses without loading, making this approach satisfactory for gradually increasing the digoxin levels of outpatients. The oral bioavailability of furosemide varies widely (10% to 100%), but absorption of torsemide and bumetanide is nearly complete, ranging from 80% to 100%. Of the potassium-sparing diuretics, spironolactone has been associated with gynecomastia; amiloride has been associated with impotence; and triamterene has been associated with kidney stones. Diuretic unresponsiveness may be caused by excessive sodium intake, use of agents that antagonize their effects (NSAIDs), chronic renal dysfunction, or compromised renal blood flow. *(Answer: C—Oral bioavailability of loop diuretics varies little from drug to drug)*

8. A patient with CHF asks about his prognosis.

Which of the following statements regarding the clinical course of CHF and the prognosis of patients with this condition is true?

❑ A. **Arrhythmias cause the majority of deaths in patients with CHF**

❑ B. **Signs of chronic right-sided heart failure portend a poorer prognosis**

❑ C. **A persistent fourth heart sound portends a poorer prognosis**

❑ D. **Annual mortality increases by 5% to 7% for each NYHA class (i.e., from class I to IV)**

❑ E. **Once heart failure has developed, sex has no prognostic significance**

Key Concept/Objective: To understand factors affecting the prognosis of patients with CHF

For patients with CHF, progressive heart failure accounts for the majority of deaths. Sudden cardiac death caused by ventricular tachycardia, fibrillation, bradycardia, or electromechanical dissociation occurs in 20% to 40% of patients with CHF. Syncope, a persistent third heart sound, signs of chronic right-sided heart failure, extensive conduction system disease, and ventricular tachyarrhythmias portend a poor prognosis. Annual mortality for patients with CHF caused by impaired systolic function is less than 5% for patients with asymptomatic left ventricular dysfunction; annual mortality is 10% to 20% for patients with mild to moderate symptoms (NYHA class II or III symptoms); it often exceeds 40% for patients with advanced class IV symptoms. Overall, female sex is associated with a better prognosis than male sex in CHF. *(Answer: B—Signs of chronic right-sided heart failure portend a poorer prognosis)*

9. A 65-year-old woman with long-standing hypertension has dyspnea associated with the classic symptoms and physical findings of CHF. Her chest x-ray shows signs of pulmonary edema. Her echocardiogram, however, shows slightly thickened myocardium and a normal left ventricular ejection fraction. A diagnosis of diastolic dysfunction is made.

Which of the following would improve this patient's symptoms?

❑ A. **Digoxin**

❑ B. **Furosemide**

❑ C. **Enalapril**

❑ D. **Metoprolol**

❑ E. **None of the above**

Key Concept/Objective: To understand the treatment of CHF caused by diastolic dysfunction

One important goal in the management of CHF is to distinguish CHF caused by systolic dysfunction from CHF caused by diastolic dysfunction, because therapies for the two differ distinctly. The goal of treatment for CHF caused by diastolic dysfunction is to reduce symptoms by lowering filling pressures without significantly compromising forward cardiac output. Symptom control is best achieved with nitrates and mild diuresis. Other goals of therapy are control of hypertension and tachycardia and alleviation of myocardial ischemia. No pharmacologic agents have been shown to effectively improve diastolic distensibility or mortality. *(Answer: B—Furosemide)*

10. A 55-year-old patient of yours presents for routine follow-up of CHF. An echocardiogram done 6 months ago showed a left ventricular ejection fraction of 20%. He feels quite well, has unlimited exercise tolerance while exercising on flat ground, and has dyspnea only with climbing more than two flights of stairs. His current regimen is enalapril, 40 mg/day, and furosemide, 40 mg b.i.d. On physical examination, his blood pressure is 135/80 mm Hg, his pulse is 88 beats/min, and his respirations are normal. The rest of his examination is remarkable only for moderate obesity and 1+ pretibial edema. He has heard that medications called beta blockers could be helpful for people with heart trouble and wonders if he should be taking them.

Which of the following statements regarding beta-blocker use is true?

❑ A. **Beta blockers are contraindicated in patients with CHF**

❑ B. **Beta blockers are contraindicated in this patient because his ejection**

fraction is so severely diminished

- ❑ D. **Beta blockers are not indicated in this patient because his blood pressure is already well controlled**
- ❑ E. **Beta blockers are not indicated in this patient because his CHF is well controlled by his current therapy**
- ❑ F. **Beta blockers are indicated in this patient**

Key Concept/Objective: To know the indications for use of beta blockers in patients with CHF

The use of beta blockers in CHF represents a major change in pharmacotherapy for this disease. These agents were once thought to be contraindicated because of their negative effects on cardiac inotropy (and they still are contraindicated in patients with NYHA class IV symptoms). It is now recognized that beta blockers play an important role in interrupting the catecholamine cascade that is brought on by the low flow state. They have significant benefit with regard to mortality for CHF patients with NYHA class II and class III symptoms. No specific beta blocker has been shown to be preferable to the others. *(Answer: F—Beta blockers are indicated in this patient)*

11. An 80-year-old man presents with dyspnea and is found to have CHF caused by systolic dysfunction. He also has mild renal insufficiency, with a creatinine level of 1.4.

Which of the following statements is true regarding ACE inhibitor therapy in this patient?

- ❑ A. **It is contraindicated because of his age**
- ❑ B. **It is contraindicated because of his renal insufficiency**
- ❑ C. **Angiotensin II receptor blockers are preferred for CHF in elderly patients**
- ❑ D. **ACE inhibitor therapy can be started, provided it is accompanied by careful monitoring of his creatinine and potassium levels**
- ❑ E. **ACE inhibitor therapy can be started but must be discontinued if his creatinine level rises above its current level**

Key Concept/Objective: To be able to identify patients with CHF for whom ACE inhibitor therapy is indicated

All patients with CHF should be on an ACE inhibitor unless there is a very good reason not to use one. The only patients with CHF in whom an ACE inhibitor cannot be used are those in whom an ACE inhibitor causes hypersensitivity, hyperkalemia, or cough or those with bilateral renal artery stenosis. Neither this patient's age nor his creatinine level is a con-[illegible] improved forward flow may actually increase his glomerular filtration rate and improve his renal function). His creatinine and potassium levels should be checked 1 to 2 weeks after starting the medication to ensure that the creatinine level has not increased by more than 25% and that his potassium level is less than 5.0 mmol/L. Preliminary data suggested that angiotensin II receptor blockers were preferred over ACE inhibitors in older patients, but a larger trial failed to confirm these results. *(Answer: D—ACE inhibitor therapy can be started, provided it is accompanied by careful monitoring of his creatinine and potassium levels)*

12. A 70-year-old woman presents to the emergency department with acute pulmonary edema with evidence of myocardial ischemia on ECG. In spite of maximal medical management, she develops cardiogenic shock. A second ECG shows ST segment elevation of 3 mm in the precordial leads. She has no contraindications to thrombolytic therapy.

Which of the following statements regarding thrombolytic therapy is true?

- ❑ A. **Thrombolytic therapy is indicated, but direct revascularization is preferable if it can be obtained quickly**
- ❑ B. **Thrombolytic therapy is contraindicated because of her age**

❑ C. **Thrombolytic therapy is contraindicated because of the presence of cardiogenic shock**

❑ D. **Thrombolytic therapy will establish antegrade coronary artery perfusion in 75% of cases**

❑ E. **Thrombolytic therapy is contraindicated because of the risks of bleeding associated with it**

Key Concept/Objective: To understand the indications for thrombolytic therapy in patients with cardiogenic shock caused by myocardial infarction

Patients who develop cardiogenic shock because of a myocardial infarction have dismal mortality rates; however, mortality can be lowered from 85% to less than 60% if flow can be reestablished in the infarct-related artery. Thrombolytic therapy is able to achieve this in about 50% of cases, making percutaneous angioplasty preferable; however, if angioplasty cannot be administered quickly or is not available, thrombolytic therapy is indicated. This patient's age is not a contraindication to thrombolytic therapy, nor is the presence of cardiogenic shock (patients with cardiogenic shock benefit most from thrombolytic therapy). *(Answer: A—Thrombolytic therapy is indicated, but direct revascularization is preferable if it can be obtained quickly)*

For more information, see Winakur S, Jessup M: 1 Cardiovascular Medicine: II Heart Failure. ACP Medicine Online (www.acpmedicine.com). Dale DC, Federman DD, Eds. WebMD Inc., New York, November 2003

Hypertension

13. A 42-year-old white man presents to your office as a new patient. He has been in good health and has not seen a physician in many years. While attending a local health fair recently, the patient was told that he had high blood pressure, and he was advised to seek medical help. He seeks your advice about hypertension. His blood pressure is 145/95 mm Hg.

Which of the following general statements about hypertension is false?

❑ A. **Hypertension is the most common chronic disorder in the United States, affecting 24% of the adult population**

❑ B. **Hypertension is a major risk factor for stroke, myocardial infarction, heart failure, chronic kidney disease, progressive atherosclerosis, and dementia**

❑ C. **For a normotensive middle-aged person in the United States, the lifetime risk of developing hypertension approaches 90%**

❑ D. **Hypertension is the third most common reason adults visit the doctor's office; it is surpassed only by visits for upper respiratory complaints and low back pain**

Key Concept/Objective: To understand the dramatic impact of hypertension on health care in the United States

Hypertension is the most common chronic disorder in the United States, affecting 24% of the adult population. In the year 2000, hypertension accounted for more than 1 million office visits to health care providers. The prevalence increases with age: for a normotensive middle-aged person in the United States, the lifetime risk of developing hypertension approaches 90%. With the increasing age of the population in most developed and developing societies, it seems safe to assume that hypertension will become steadily more widespread in the coming years. Hypertension is a major risk factor for stroke, myocardial infarction, heart failure, chronic kidney disease, progressive atherosclerosis, and dementia. Hypertension is the most common reason adults visit the doctor's office. *(Answer: D—Hypertension is the third most common reason adults visit the doctor's office; it is surpassed only by visits for upper respiratory complaints and low back pain)*

14. A 64-year-old black man presents to your office for routine follow-up care. You have treated him for many years for hypertension with a calcium channel blocker and a thiazide diuretic. His hypertension has been moderately well controlled with this regimen. He asks you whether having a home blood pressure monitor would be useful for his care.

Which of the following statements regarding ambulatory blood pressure monitoring (ABPM) is true?

❑ **A. ABPM is not useful in patients whose office blood pressure is normal and who have hypertensive target organ injury**

❑ **B. ABPM is not a useful tool in the evaluation of suspected autonomic dysfunction in patients with orthostatic hypotension**

❑ **C. Cross-sectional studies show that blood pressure averages obtained during office visits correlate better with the presence of target-organ injury (especially LVH) than those obtained with ABPM**

❑ **D. ABPM is useful in establishing a diagnosis of white-coat hypertension**

Key Concept/Objective: To understand the usefulness of ABPM

Cross-sectional studies show that blood pressure averages from ABPM correlate better with the presence of target-organ injury (especially left ventricular hypertrophy [LVH]) than office blood pressure averages. Also, prospective studies and population-based observational studies have shown that average blood pressure derived from ABPM predicts additional risk of cardiovascular (CV) events after adjustment for clinic or office blood pressure. ABPM is the best method to establish the presence of isolated clinic hypertension (so-called white-coat hypertension), which is defined as an elevation in BP that occurs only in the clinic setting, with normal BP in all other settings, in the absence of evidence of target-organ injury. Screening for white-coat hypertension is currently a reimbursable indication for ABPM by Medicare. Other uses for ABPM include assessment of hypotensive symptoms, episodic hypertension, and suspected autonomic dysfunction in patients with postural hypotension. ABPM is also useful in the evaluation of the occasional patient with hypertensive target-organ injury (LVH, stroke) whose office blood pressure is normal. *(Answer: D—ABPM is useful in establishing a diagnosis of white-coat hypertension)*

15. A 25-year-old black man presents to your office seeking to establish primary care. The patient has no complaints and denies any known medical history. His blood pressure is noted to be 185/115; otherwise, his physical examination is normal. After measuring the patient's blood pressure a total of four times during two office visits, you diagnose hypertension.

Which of the following statements regarding the initial evaluation of hypertension in this patient is true?

❑ **A. A retinal examination should now be performed on this patient**

❑ **B. Because this patient has been diagnosed with hypertension, obtaining a family history of hypertension or early CV disease is no longer useful**

❑ **C. During the initial examination, only a single careful blood pressure measurement is needed**

❑ **D. This patient has no findings consistent with secondary hypertension**

Key Concept/Objective: To understand the importance of the initial evaluation of hypertension

Secondary hypertension may be suspected on finding features that are not consistent with essential hypertension. Such features include age at onset younger than 30 years or older than 50 years; blood pressure higher than 180/110 mm Hg at diagnosis; significant target-organ injury at diagnosis; hemorrhages and exudates on fundus examination; renal insufficiency; LVH; poor response to appropriate three-drug therapy; and accelerated or malignant hypertension. The clinician should inquire about a family history of hypertension, premature CV disease, and disorders that would increase the possibility of secondary hypertension. The examination should include at least two standardized measurements of blood pressure with the patient in the seated position. Initially, blood pressure should also be measured in the opposite arm (to identify arterial narrowing, which can cause an inac-

curately low reading in one arm) and in the standing position, especially in diabetic patients and older patients (to identify orthostatic declines). Retinal examination should be performed, primarily to identify retinal changes of diabetes or severe hypertension (i.e., hemorrhages, exudates, or papilledema). *(Answer: A—A retinal examination should now be performed on this patient)*

16. A 51-year-old white man recently relocated to the area and presents to your office as a new patient. He denies having any history of medical problems. He made very infrequent visits to a primary care provider where he previously lived. He is on no medicines and denies having any significant family medical history. He is a current smoker with a 40 pack-year smoking history. His blood pressure is 170/95 mm Hg, and a fourth heart sound is present. His physical examination is otherwise unremarkable.

Which of the following statements regarding treatment of this patient's hypertension is true?

- ❑ **A. The most appropriate initial medical therapy for this patient is an alpha blocker**
- ❑ **B. The most appropriate initial medical therapy for this patient is a thiazide diuretic**
- ❑ **C. The most appropriate initial medical therapy for this patient is a thiazide diuretic in combination with another antihypertensive agent that works via a different blood pressure regulatory pathway**
- ❑ **D. To have this patient stop smoking cigarettes would have little or no effect on the control of his hypertension**

Key Concept/Objective: To understand the importance of appropriate drug therapy and lifestyle modifications in the treatment of hypertension

The Seventh Report of the Joint National Committee on Prevention, Detection, Evaluation, and Treatment of High Blood Pressure (JNC VII) recommends thiazide diuretics as initial drugs of choice for most patients with hypertension; this recommendation is based on the totality of data from randomized trials, including the Antihypertensive and Lipid Lowering Treatment to Prevent Heart Attack Trial (ALLHAT). The JNC VII report suggests initiation of therapy with two drugs rather than a single agent if the systolic blood pressure is higher than 20 mm Hg above the treatment goal or if the diastolic blood pressure is higher than 10 mm Hg above the goal. Generally, a two-drug regimen should include a diuretic appropriate for the level of renal function. The alpha-blocker arm of the ALLHAT trial was terminated early because of an almost twofold increase in the risk of heart failure, compared with the diuretic group. On the basis of these results, alpha blockers are no longer considered an appropriate initial therapy for hypertension. Tobacco use should be discouraged because, in addition to being a powerful CV risk factor, each cigarette smoked elevates blood pressure for 15 to 30 minutes, and multiple cigarettes can raise blood pressure for most of the day. *(Answer: C—The most appropriate initial medical therapy for this patient is a thiazide diuretic in combination with another antihypertensive agent that works via a different blood pressure regulatory pathway)*

17. A 40-year-old white woman whom you have been treating for resistant hypertension presents for routine follow-up. Laboratory results of screening tests were normal. There is electrocardiographic evidence of LVH. The patient's lipid profile is normal. The patient has been receiving a thiazide diuretic, a calcium channel blocker, and an ACE inhibitor at near maximal doses for several weeks. Her blood pressure today remains very elevated, at 175/100 mm Hg. She experienced a minimal response to titration of her antihypertensive medicines. With the exception of elevated blood presure and a fourth heart sound, the patient's physical examinations have been consistently normal. Today, the physical examination is unchanged, except that you notice a soft bruit in the left upper quadrant.

Which of the following statements regarding renovascular hypertension is true?

- ❑ **A. Renovascular hypertension is an exceptionally rare cause of hypertension in patients with treatment-resistant hypertension**
- ❑ **B. Stenosing lesions of the renal circulation cause hypertension through ischemia-mediated activation of the renin-angiotensin-aldosterone system**

❑ C. Fibromuscular disease is an uncommon cause of renovascular hypertension in patients of this age

❑ D. Atheromatous disease and fibromuscular disease are equally frequent causes of renovascular hypertension

Key Concept/Objective: To know the characteristics of renovascular hypertension that is mediated by atheromatous lesions and fibromuscular disease

Renovascular hypertension is the most common form of potentially curable secondary hypertension. It probably occurs in 1% to 2% of the overall hypertensive population. The prevalence may be as high as 10% in patients with resistant hypertension, and it may be even higher in patients with accelerated or malignant hypertension. Stenosing lesions of the renal circulation cause hypertension through ischemia-mediated stimulation of the renin-angiotensin-aldosterone axis. Fibromuscular disease is the most common cause of renovascular hypertension in younger patients, especially women between 15 and 50 years of age; it accounts for approximately 10% of cases of renovascular hypertension. Atheromatous disease is the most common cause of renovascular hypertension in middle-aged and older patients and accounts for approximately 90% of cases of renovascular hypertension. The prevalence of atheromatous renal artery disease increases with age and is common in older hypertensive patients, especially in those with diabetes or with atherosclerosis in other vascular beds. Most patients with atheromatous renal vascular disease and hypertension have essential hypertension. *(Answer: B—Stenosing lesions of the renal circulation cause hypertension through ischemia-mediated activation of the renin-angiotensin-aldosterone system)*

18. A 55-year-old man presents to establish primary care. His medical history is significant only for 40 pack-years of smoking. He drinks four beers a night. He is minimally physically active. On physical examination, the patient's blood pressure is 158/98 mm Hg, and he is moderately obese (body mass index, 27); the rest of his examination is normal. His laboratory examination, including a chem 7, CBC, TSH, and urinalysis, is normal, as is his electrocardiogram. Repeated blood pressure measurements over the next month are similar to the values first obtained.

With respect to this patient's blood pressure, what therapeutic option should be offered to this patient now?

❑ A. No treatment

❑ B. Continued monitoring for 6 months

❑ C. Lifestyle modifications, including decreased alcohol consumption, weight loss, smoking cessation, and moderate exercise for 6 months

❑ D. Pharmacologic therapy

Key Concept/Objective: To know the appropriate intervention, based on the patient's hypertensive stage and risk group

This patient has stage 1 (systolic, 140 to 159 mm Hg; diastolic, 90 to 99 mm Hg), or mild, hypertension. Given his smoking history, he has greater than or equal to 1 risk factor for CV disease, which puts him in risk group 2. On the basis of the JNC VI (Joint National Committee on Prevention, Detection, and Treatment of High Blood Presssure) recommendations, it is appropriate to try lifestyle modifications (weight loss, dietary modification such as adherence to the DASH [Dietary Approaches to Stop Hypertension] diet, and moderate exercise) for 6 months before starting medications. *(Answer: C—Lifestyle modifications, including decreased alcohol consumption, weight loss, smoking cessation, and moderate exercise for 6 months)*

19. The patient in Question 18 adhered to your recommendations, but his blood pressure remains elevated to the same degree. He is interested in controlling his blood pressure but is worried about the cost of medications.

What should be the first-line pharmacologic therapy for this patient?

❑ A. Lisinopril, 5 mg/day

❑ B. Extended-release diltiazem, 120 mg/day

❑ C. Amlodipine, 5 mg/day

❑ D. Hydrochlorothiazide, 25 mg/day

Key Concept/Objective: To know the recommended first-line medications for treatment of hypertension

Thiazide diuretics for the treatment of high blood pressure have been shown most consistently to have the best outcomes with respect to stroke and CV disease, mortality, and patient compliance. Given that the benefits of treating high blood pressure accrue only over the long term, the last of these attributes is especially important. Also, hydrochlorothiazide is by far the least expensive of all of the medications listed. *(Answer: D—Hydrochlorothiazide, 25 mg/day)*

20. Three months after starting therapy, the patient in Question 18 returns for follow-up. His blood pressure is 145/92 mm Hg, and blood pressure values that he has obtained outside the clinic are similar. He says that he has been taking hydrochlorothiazide as directed and has noted no unpleasant side effects. He is doing his best to adhere to the lifestyle modifications that you recommended.

What is the best step to take next in the management of this patient?

❑ A. Continue present management

❑ B. Add atenolol, 25 mg/day

❑ C. Double the dose of hydrochlorothiazide to 50 mg/day

❑ D. Add amlodipine, 5 mg/day

Key Concept/Objective: To understand the goals of antihypertensive therapy and to be able to select an appropriate second medication to achieve those goals

The goal for the treatment of hypertension is a blood pressure lower than 140/90 for most people (although this number is arbitrary, and some experts recommend still lower targets). Given that your patient is compliant with his current therapy and has done as much as he can to achieve lifestyle modification, it is appropriate to add a second agent. Atenolol is the best choice because of its low cost and proven mortality benefit. Doses of hydrochlorothiazide higher than 25 mg/day will not improve blood pressure control, and higher doses of hydrochlorothiazide have been associated with increased mortality. Amlodipine is a reasonable choice, but it is expensive, and there are no data to suggest that the calcium channel blockers improve mortality. *(Answer: B—Add atenolol, 25 mg/day)*

21. A 72-year-old woman comes to see you to establish care, after her previous physician retired. Her medical history is significant for diet-controlled diabetes and a myocardial infarction. She is taking aspirin, simvastatin, and amlodipine. On examination, her blood pressure is 170/95 mm Hg. She has an S_4 gallop and 1+ pretibial edema.

What should be the target blood pressure in the long term for this patient?

❑ A. < 150/90 mm Hg

❑ B. < 140/90 mm Hg

❑ C. < 130/85 mm Hg

❑ D. < 120/70 mm Hg

Key Concept/Objective: To know the goal for blood pressure control for patients with evidence of target-organ disease and diabetes

This patient has stage 2 (moderate) hypertension and is in risk group C because of her history of myocardial infarction and diabetes (either one alone would suffice to put her in this risk group). As such, her target blood pressure is less than 130/85 mm Hg. Note that

there is some evidence that lowering patients' diastolic blood pressure to less than 70 mm Hg is associated with increased mortality. *(Answer: C— < 130/85 mm Hg)*

22. Your nurse alerts you that a patient in your clinic has severely elevated blood pressure. The patient is a 45-year-old man without other significant medical history. The patient's blood pressure is 220/125 mm Hg; blood pressure measurements are essentially the same in both arms. The patient says that he is feeling fine. He has had no symptoms of flushing, sweating, or headache, nor has he had visual changes, focal weakness, numbness, chest pain, dyspnea, or decreased urine output. On examination, neurologic status is normal. An S_4 gallop and trace pretibial edema are noted. The lungs are clear to auscultation. An ECG shows sinus rhythm with LVH. There is no evidence of ischemia or infarction.

    How should you manage this patient?

    - ❑ **A. Administer sublingual nifedipine, 10 mg**
    - ❑ **B. Administer atenolol, 50 mg, and follow up in 24 hours**
    - ❑ **C. Prescribe atenolol, 50 mg, and follow up in 1 week**
    - ❑ **D. Admit him to the intensive care unit for cardiac and blood pressure monitoring and intravenous nitroprusside therapy**

    Key Concept/Objective: To be able to recognize and treat severe high blood pressure

    This patient has severe hypertension but no evidence of acute target-organ (brain, heart, aorta, kidney) damage or secondary causes of hypertension. In all likelihood, his hypertension has been long-standing, as suggested by his S_4 gallop and LVH. Thus, he is best managed by a long-acting antihypertensive and very close follow-up to ensure that the hypertension has not worsened. He should also be educated about the symptoms of target-organ damage and told to seek emergency care should they occur. Sublingual short-acting nifedipine has been associated with stroke, myocardial infarction, and death, and its use is very strongly discouraged. Because the patient does not have evidence of acute target-organ damage, hospital admission is not necessary. *(Answer: B—Administer atenolol, 50 mg, and follow up in 24 hours)*

    For more information, see Schwartz GL, Sheps SG: 1 Cardiovascular Medicine: III Hyptertension. ACP Medicine Online (www.acpmedicine.com). Dale DC, Federman DD, Eds. WebMD Inc., New York, January 2004

Atrial Fibrillation

23. A previously healthy 47-year-old woman presents with a complaint of palpitations of sudden onset. Her [illegible] atrial fibrillation (AF) with a ventricular response of 135 beats/min. Her cardiac examination is unremarkable except for an irregularly irregular pulse. She has no other medical problems and takes no medications. A transthoracic echocardiogram (TTE) is normal.

    Which of the following is the most likely classification of this patient's AF according to guidelines from the American College of Cardiology (ACC), the American Heart Association (AHA), and the European Society of Cardiology (ESC)?

    - ❑ **A. Permanent**
    - ❑ **B. Persistent**
    - ❑ **C. Recurrent**
    - ❑ **D. Lone**

    Key Concept/Objective: To understand the appropriate classification of AF

    The ACC/AHA/ESC guidelines include the following categories: recurrent—more than one episode of AF has occurred; lone—AF occurring in a patient younger than 60 years who has no clinical or echocardiographic evidence of cardiopulmonary disease; valvular—AF

occurring in a patient with evidence or history of rheumatic mitral valve disease or prosthetic heart valves is defined as valvular; paroxysmal—AF that typically lasts 7 days or less, with spontaneous conversion to sinus rhythm; persistent—AF that typically lasts longer than 7 days or requires pharmacologic or direct current (DC) cardioversion; permanent—AF that is refractory to cardioversion or that has persisted for longer than 1 year. Paroxysmal, persistent, and permanent AF categories do not apply to episodes of AF lasting 30 seconds or less or to episodes precipitated by a reversible medical condition. Reversible conditions include acute myocardial infarction, cardiac surgery, pericarditis, myocarditis, hyperthyroidism, pulmonary embolism, and acute pulmonary disease. *(Answer: D—Lone)*

24. A 75-year-old woman with a history of symptomatic, recurrent, persistent nonvalvular AF comes to your office. She has been told that there are several options for the treatment of her AF.

Which of the following is true regarding establishment and maintenance of normal sinus rhythm, as compared with pharmacologic rate control?

- ❑ **A. Establishment and maintenance of sinus rhythm provides no survival advantage**
- ❑ **B. Establishment and maintenance of sinus rhythm reduces thromboembolic risk**
- ❑ **C. Establishment and maintenance of sinus rhythm improves the degree of symptomatic impairment**
- ❑ **D. Conversion to normal sinus rhythm is rarely needed for patients with unstable angina, acute myocardial infarction, heart failure, or pulmonary edema**

Key Concept/Objective: To understand that establishment and maintenance of sinus rhythm is not superior to ventricular rate control in patients with AF

Several trials compared restoration of sinus rhythm with control of ventricular rate in patients with AF. Evaluated outcomes included overall mortality, stroke, symptoms, and quality of life. Contrary to the expectations of many experts, maintenance of sinus rhythm provided no survival advantage and possibly a higher mortality when compared with ventricular rate control. Maintenance of sinus rhythm frequently requires the use of antiarrhythmic medications that may precipitate ventricular arrhythmias, bradycardia, and depression of left ventricular function. It was further theorized that maintenance of sinus rhythm would reduce rates of thromboembolism and the need for anticoagulation; however, trial results demonstrated no significant reduction in thromboembolic risk. Peak exercise capacity may improve with maintenance of sinus rhythm, but the two treatment strategies result in a similar degree of perceived symptomatic impairment. Nevertheless, ventricular rate control frequently is not feasible because of the complications that patients experience while in AF. AF often cannot be tolerated by patients with unstable angina, acute myocardial infarction, heart failure, or pulmonary edema. *(Answer: A—Establishment and maintenance of sinus rhythm provides no survival advantage)*

25. An 81-year-old man with a history of symptomatic permanent AF presents to your office to discuss options for reestablishing sinus rhythm. He hopes to decrease his symptoms of dyspnea. In addition to AF, the patient has congestive heart failure and echocardiographically documented significant mitral regurgitation.

Which of the following is NOT a risk factor for cardioversion failure in this patient?

- ❑ **A. Duration of AF of longer than 1 year**
- ❑ **B. Older age**
- ❑ **C. Left atrial enlargement**
- ❑ **D. Normal-sized heart**

Key Concept/Objective: To know the risk factors associated with failed synchronized DC cardioversion

Although success rates are high with DC cardioversion, a number of risk factors for cardioversion failure have been identified. These include longer duration of AF (notably, longer than 1 year), older age, left atrial enlargement, cardiomegaly, rheumatic heart disease, and transthoracic impedance. Pretreatment with amiodarone, ibutilide, sotalol, flecainide, propafenone, disopyramide, and quinidine have been shown to increase DC cardioversion success rates. *(Answer: D—Normal-sized heart)*

For more information, see Aizer A, Fuster F: 1 Cardiovascular Medicine: IV Atrial Fibrillation. ACP Medicine Online (www.acpmedicine.com). Dale DC, Federman DD, Eds. WebMD Inc., New York, December 2003

Supraventricular Tachycardia

26. A 29-year-old white woman presents to the emergency department with the complaint that her heart is "racing away." The patient reports that this symptom began 1 hour ago and that it is associated with mild shortness of breath. She also reports having had similar episodes in her life, but she says they never lasted this long and that they usually abated with a simple cough. On examination, the patient's pulse is regular at 175 beats/min. Her lungs are clear, and she is in mild distress. Electrocardiography reveals atrioventricular nodal reentry tachycardia (AVNRT).

Which of the following statements regarding AVNRT is false?

- ❑ A. **Most cases of AVNRT begin with a premature ventricular contraction (PVC)**
- ❑ B. **Acute therapy includes carotid sinus massage and I.V. adenosine**
- ❑ C. **Long-term therapy includes beta blockers, calcium channel blockers, and digoxin**
- ❑ D. **Catheter ablation for AVNRT is clearly the procedure of choice for patients in whom drug therapy fails**

Key Concept/Objective: To understand the pathogenesis of and therapy for AVNRT

The normal AV node has a single transmission pathway. In two to three persons per 1,000 population, however, the AV node has both a normal (fast) pathway and a second (slow) pathway. In such persons, the sinus impulse is ordinarily transmitted over the fast pathway to the ventricle, and slow-pathway conduction is preempted. However, if an atrial premature complex (APC) occurs at a critical point in the conduction cycle, the impulse can become blocked in the fast pathway, thus allowing for anterograde (forward) conduction over the slow pathway and retrograde (backward) conduction over the fast pathway. This may produce a single echo beat (a beat that returns to the chamber of origin), or it may [illegible] of AVNRT [illegible] by careful analysis of the 12-lead ECG. Because retrograde conduction over the AV node is occurring more or less simultaneously with anterograde conduction to the ventricles, the P wave is either buried within the QRS complex or inscribed just after the QRS. AVNRT may respond to carotid sinus massage but is highly responsive to intravenous adenosine, beta blockers, or calcium channel blockers. If carotid massage fails to convert supraventricular tachycardia, the drug of choice is intravenous adenosine, which is effective in 95% of cases. A wide variety of drugs have proved effective for controlling episodes of AVNRT, including beta blockers, calcium channel blockers, and digoxin. Long-term drug therapy is associated with frequent recurrences and adverse effects, however. Catheter ablation for AVNRT has proved so safe and effective that it is clearly the procedure of choice for patients in whom drug therapy fails. Moreover, it can be offered to those patients with milder symptoms who prefer to avoid long-term drug therapy. *(Answer: A—Most cases of AVNRT begin with a premature ventricular contraction [PVC])*

27. A 19-year-old man presents to the emergency department complaining of dyspnea and palpitations of acute onset. He has been short of breath for 2 hours now but denies having any chest pain. He has never had these symptoms before, and he denies having any cardiac disorders in the past. He is taking no med-

icines and has no significant family history of sudden cardiac death or arrhythmias. On examination, the patient is tachycardic but the heartbeat is regular. The patient's lungs are clear. His blood pressure is 110/72 mm Hg, and he is afebrile. ECG reveals a narrow complex tachycardia with a retrograde P wave noted in the ST segment. You diagnose the patient as having atrioventricular reentry tachycardia (AVRT).

Which of the following statements regarding AVRT is true?

- ❑ A. **AVRT usually improves during pregnancy**
- ❑ B. **Because of the location of the reentrant pathway, catheter ablation is contraindicated**
- ❑ C. **During an episode of atrial fibrillation in a patient with Wolff-Parkinson-White (WPW) syndrome, the drug of choice for initial management is a calcium channel blocker**
- ❑ D. **Patients with WPW syndrome are at risk for sudden cardiac death from ventricular fibrillation**

Key Concept/Objective: To understand the pathogenesis and treatment of WPW syndrome

The most prominent manifestation of accessory atrioventricular pathways is the WPW syndrome. In this syndrome, the accessory pathway can be located at various regions around the tricuspid and the mitral atrioventricular rings, but it is most commonly sited at the left free wall of the mitral annulus. The basic mechanism of tachycardia in AVRT is similar to that of AVNRT. Electrical impulses can travel down both the AV node and the accessory pathway to activate the ventricles, with ventricular activation occurring earlier at sites near the accessory pathway than at sites activated normally (i.e., ventricular preexcitation). The most feared arrhythmia in the WPW syndrome involves atrial fibrillation with dominant conduction over an accessory pathway that has rapid conduction properties. These patients may experience extraordinarily rapid ventricular rates and are at risk for sudden cardiac death from ventricular fibrillation. Symptomatic tachyarrhythmias associated with the WPW syndrome generally begin in the teenage years or during early adulthood. Pregnancy may produce an initial attack in some women. Pregnancy can also be associated with an increasing frequency of attacks and more symptomatic episodes. Ventricular preexcitation may be evident on a baseline ECG as fusion complexes (WPW pattern). The WPW pattern comprises a short PR interval and an earlier-than-normal deflection on the QRS complex (delta wave). The ECG during AVRT will usually show a narrow complex with the retrograde P wave falling in the ST segment, because atrial activation occurs well after ventricular depolarization. The acute management of AVRT is similar to that for AVNRT: adenosine is the drug of choice, but calcium channel blockers or beta blockers are also effective. Long-term therapy for AVRT may be directed at interfering with conduction either through the AV node (i.e., with beta blockers or calcium channel blockers) or through the accessory pathway (i.e., with class IC or class III antiarrhythmic agents). The remarkable efficacy and safety of ablation make this mode of therapy more attractive than long-term drug therapy for symptomatic patients. Drug therapy carries the possibility of recurrent arrhythmias, including atrial fibrillation. Hence, ablation is currently recommended for all patients with symptomatic WPW. *(Answer: D—Patients with WPW syndrome are at risk for sudden cardiac death from ventricular fibrillation)*

For more information, see Tchou PJ, Trohman RG: 1 Cardiovascular Medicine: V Supraventricular Tachycardia. ACP Medicine Online (www.acpmedicine.com). Dale DC, Federman DD, Eds. WebMD Inc., New York, August 2004

Pacemaker Therapy

28. A 60-year-old man presents to his primary care physician for evaluation of dizziness and increased fatigue. An electrocardiogram is performed as part of his evaluation. The ECG demonstrates complete heart block, with a ventricular rate of 44 beats/min. The patient is referred for implantation of a pacemaker.

Which of the following is NOT an indication for implantation of a cardiac pacemaker?

- ❑ A. Temporary pacing in the setting of acute myocardial infarction complicated by conduction abnormalities and hemodynamic instability
- ❑ B. Resynchronization in the treatment of heart failure
- ❑ C. Type I second-degree atrioventricular (AV) block in an asymptomatic athlete
- ❑ D. Complete AV block
- ❑ E. Neurocardiogenic syncope with significant bradycardia

Key Concept/Objective: To know the various indications for cardiac pacing

Conduction abnormalities are common in the setting of acute myocardial infarction. Patients with acute inferior infarction can manifest a variety of abnormalities, including sinoatrial (SA) node dysfunction, first-degree AV block, type I second-degree block, and third-degree block at the level of the AV node. It is uncommon for any of these conduction disturbances to persist after the acute phase of the infarction. These patients often require temporary pacing if they manifest hemodynamic instability. Cardiac resynchronization therapy is an exciting new development in the treatment of heart failure. Complete AV block with bradycardia and the presence of symptoms is an indication for permanent cardiac pacing. Classic neurocardiogenic syncope involves sinus tachycardia followed by bradycardia, vasodilatation, and syncope. Some patients have primarily a vasodepressive (vasodilatation) syndrome, whereas others have a syndrome with a significant cardioinhibitory component (bradycardia). In the setting of bradycardia, cardiac pacemaker implantation is necessary. It is not uncommon for trained athletes to have type I second-degree AV block and be asymptomatic. Pacemaker therapy is not indicated. *(Answer: C—Type I second-degree atrioventricular (AV) block in an asymptomatic athlete)*

29. A 67-year-old female patient of yours is admitted to the hospital. She has a permanent pacemaker and sees a cardiologist. In reviewing her chart, you note that her pacemaker program code is VVI, with a lower rate of 60 beats/min.

Which of the following statements regarding this patient's pacemaker program code is false?

- ❑ A. Both the atria and ventricles are programmed to be paced
- ❑ B. The sensing lead is in the ventricle
- ❑ C. When the intrinsic heart rate falls below 60 beats/min, pacing will occur
- ❑ D. After a paced beat, the pacemaker clock resets and senses the next ventricular contraction
- ❑ E. VVI is also referred to as ventricular demand pacing or ventricular inhibited pacing

Key Concept/Objective: To understand the three-letter code for describing the basic functions of cardiac pacemakers

The three basic functions of a pacemaker—pacing, sensing, and action—are determined by basic pacemaker programming. In 1974, the American Heart Association and the American College of Cardiology proposed a three-letter code for describing the basic functions of pacemakers. Under the guidance of the North American Society of Pacing and Electrophysiology (NASPE) and the British Pacing and Electrophysiology Group (BPEG), this code evolved into the five-position code currently in use. The first position denotes the chamber or chambers paced; the second denotes the chamber or chambers sensed; the third denotes the action or actions performed; the fourth denotes rate response; and the fifth denotes multiple site pacing. The simplest mode of pacing is VVI, otherwise known as ventricular demand pacing or ventricular inhibited pacing. The most commonly used mode in dual-chamber pacing is DDD. The most basic timing cycle is the lower rate, which reflects how long the pacemaker will wait after a paced or sensed beat before initiating

pacing. If the pacemaker is set to VVI mode at a lower rate of 60 beats/min, then as long the interval between intrinsic beats is less then 1,000 msec, the pacemaker will reset the lower rate clock with each sensed QRS complex, and pacing will not occur. If, however, the intrinsic heart rate falls below 60 beats/min, the pacemaker's lower rate clock will time out before an intrinsic beat is sensed, and pacing will occur. After a paced beat, the lower-rate clock is reset and the cycle repeats. *(Answer: A—Both the atria and ventricles are programmed to be paced)*

30. A 56-year-old woman is admitted for implantation of a permanent pacemaker for management of sick sinus syndrome. The procedure is successful.

Which of the following statements regarding further care of this patient is true?

- ❑ A. **It is standard practice to discharge the patient the day of the procedure if no obvious complications occurred**
- ❑ B. **There is no need for telemetric monitoring if admitted**
- ❑ C. **A chest radiograph is routinely performed to verify lead position and to evaluate for pneumothorax**
- ❑ D. **The rate of adverse events associated with pacemaker implantation is 1%**
- ❑ E. **Once the pacemaker has been installed, there is no need for interrogating the device**

Key Concept/Objective: To understand the immediate complications associated with pacemaker implantation and appropriate postimplantation care

Overall, transvenous pacemaker implantation is both safe and well tolerated. The risk of major adverse events (e.g., death, myocardial infarction, stroke, and the need for emergency thoracotomy) is approximately 0.1%. Other complications sometimes encountered include pneuomothorax, vascular injury, cardiac perforation, tamponade, local bleeding, pocket hematoma, infection, and venous thrombosis. At most institutions, it is standard practice to admit patients for overnight observation after routine pacemaker implantation. Patients are monitored via continuous telemetry. We routinely obtain a portable chest x-ray and a 12-lead ECG immediately after implantation. The day after the procedure, the pacemaker is interrogated and the final settings confirmed. Posteroanterior and lateral chest x-rays are obtained both to verify the positioning of the leads and to rule out the possibility of a slowly accumulating pneumothorax. *(Answer: C—A chest radiograph is routinely performed to verify lead position and to evaluate for pneumothorax)*

31. A 76-year-old man with a permanent pacemaker is admitted to the hospital with a diagnosis of pneumonia. The patient unfortunately develops respiratory failure and is intubated. A central venous line is placed for administration of antibiotics and pressors. He improves clinically but develops fever. Blood cultures are positive for *Staphylococcus aureus*. Appropriate antimicrobial therapy is instituted, and the central line is removed. The patient remains febrile with persistently positive cultures.

Which of the following statements regarding pacemaker infection is true?

- ❑ A. **The most common organism causing pacemaker infection is *S. aureus***
- ❑ B. **Pacemaker infection is easily treated with appropriate antimicrobial therapy**
- ❑ C. **Patients with *S. aureus* bacteremia are not at significant risk for secondary pacemaker infection**
- ❑ D. **Infected pacemaker leads can simply be exchanged, as opposed to removing the entire unit**
- ❑ E. **Patients with infected pacemaker hardware need to be sent to a referral center with experience in removing these devices**

Key Concept/Objective: To understand that pacemaker infection requires special expertise and that patients should be referred to special centers with experience in device removal and pacemaker infection therapy

Bacterial infections can affect any part of the pacemaker system, and the consequences can be devastating. The most common pathogens are staphylococci, especially *S. epidermidis*. Once a pacemaker infection is established, it is difficult to eradicate with antibiotics; thus, infected pacemaker systems usually must be removed in their entirety. Patients with pacemakers in place who acquire *S. aureus* bacteremia are at significant risk for a secondary device infection. If an infection of an implanted cardiac device is suspected, prompt referral to an experienced center is critical. *(Answer: E—Patients with infected pacemaker hardware need to be sent to a referral center with experience in removing these devices)*

For more information, see Lowy J, Freedman RA: 1 Cardiovasculaar Medicine: VII Pacemaker Therapy. ACP Medicine Online (www.acpmedicine.com). Dale DC, Federman DD, Eds. WebMD Inc., New York, May 2004

Acute Myocardial Infarction

32. A 53-year-old black man presents to the emergency department with a complaint of chest pain of 2 hours' duration. The pain woke him from sleep. It is substernal and radiates to his left shoulder. The patient has vomited twice and is diaphoretic. He has no history of coronary artery disease but has hypertension and hypercholesterolemia.

Which of the following statements regarding acute myocardial infarction (MI) is false?

- ❑ **A. The presence of a severe stenosis (i.e., a stenosis ≥ 70% of the diameter of the artery), as seen on coronary angiography, correlates well with the most vulnerable sites for plaque rupture and occlusion of the coronary artery**
- ❑ **B. Within 10 minutes of arrival at the emergency department, a patient with symptoms suggestive of an MI should be evaluated; subsequently, the patient should be evaluated with a 12-lead electrocardiogram, and oxygen and aspirin should be administered**
- ❑ **C. Morphine sulfate is acceptable for pain control in a patient with an acute MI**
- ❑ **D. In the second International Study of Infarct Survival (ISIS-2) trial, aspirin was found to be nearly as effective as streptokinase in reducing 30-day mortality**

Key Concept/Objective: To understand the basic pathophysiology and the initial treatment of acute MI

Although to produce anginal symptoms, a stenosis of a coronary artery must be severe (i.e., ≥ 70% of the diameter of the artery), such stenoses tend to have dense fibrotic caps and are less prone to rupture than mild to moderate stenoses, which are generally more lipid laden. Studies of patients in whom angiography was performed before and after an MI revealed that in most cases, acute coronary occlusion occurred at sites in the coronary circulation with stenoses of less than 70%, as demonstrated on the preinfarction angiogram. A patient with symptoms suggestive of MI should be evaluated within 10 minutes after arrival in the emergency department. Early steps should include the assessment of hemodynamic stability by measurement of the patient's heart rate and blood pressure; the performance of a 12-lead ECG; and the administration of oxygen by nasal prongs, of I.V. analgesia (most commonly morphine sulfate), of oral aspirin, and of sublingual nitroglycerin if the blood pressure is greater than 90 mm Hg. *(Answer: A—The presence of a severe stenosis [i.e., a stenosis ≥ 70% of the diameter of the artery], as seen on coronary angiography, correlates well with the most vulnerable sites for plaque rupture and occlusion of the coronary artery)*

33. A 62-year-old white woman with a history of coronary artery disease presents to the emergency department with substernal, squeezing chest tightness of 2 hours' duration. The pain is identical to the pain she experienced with her first MI. On physical examination, the patient's heart rate is found to be 105 beats/min; a tachycardic regular rhythm without gallop is noted. The patient's lung fields are clear. A chest radiograph is normal, but ECG reveals ST segment elevation in leads I, aVL, V5, and V6.

Which of the following statements regarding the management of this patient is true?

- ❑ A. **Thrombolytic therapy has been studied in patients with ECG findings other than ST segment elevation or bundle branch block and has been found to be superior to conventional therapy**
- ❑ B. **Current recommendations are that the time between a patient's presentation to the emergency department and the administration of thrombolytic therapy not exceed 2 hours**
- ❑ C. **Coronary angiography is recommended in all patients after thrombolytic therapy has been administered, once they become hemodynamically stable**
- ❑ D. **Streptokinase therapy is contraindicated in patients who have recently received a dose of streptokinase because of antibodies that form against the drug**

Key Concept/Objective: To understand the basic principles of thrombolytic therapy

The time between a patient's presentation to the emergency department and the administration of thrombolytic therapy should not exceed 60 minutes. Front-loaded tissue plasminogen activator (t-PA) has been found to be superior to the other thrombolytic regimens. However, some physicians prefer the less expensive streptokinase therapy, particularly for patients at low risk of dying (e.g., those with uncomplicated inferior infarctions) and the elderly, who are more likely to have hemorrhagic complications with t-PA than with streptokinase. Streptokinase is contraindicated in patients who have recently received a dose of streptokinase because of antibodies that form against the drug; these antibodies limit the efficacy of repeat doses and increase the risk of allergic reactions. Thrombolytic therapy has been studied in patients with ECG findings other than ST segment elevation or bundle branch block and has been found to be either of no use or deleterious. Patients treated with thrombolytic therapy in whom complications do not occur are at low risk for reinfarction and death after discharge, and routine performance of coronary angiography and coronary angioplasty does not reduce the occurrence of these adverse events. Coronary angiography is recommended only for patients with hemodynamic instability or for patients in whom spontaneous or exercise-induced ischemia occurs. *(Answer: D—Streptokinase therapy is contraindicated in patients who have recently received a dose of streptokinase because of antibodies that form against the drug)*

34. A 49-year-old white man who presented to the emergency department with an ST segment elevation MI was given thrombolytics, oxygen, and aspirin. He is now free of chest pain and will be admitted to the coronary care unit for further monitoring.

Which of the following statements regarding adjuvant medical therapy for acute MI is false?

- ❑ A. **Early administration of beta blockers reduces the mortality and the reinfarction rate**
- ❑ B. **Unless contraindicated, angiotensin-converting enzyme (ACE) inhibitors are indicated in patients with significant ventricular dysfunction after acute MI**
- ❑ C. **When given within 6 hours after presentation to the hospital, I.V. nitroglycerin reduces mortality in patients with MI**
- ❑ D. **Prophylactic therapy with lidocaine does not reduce and may actually increase mortality because of an increase in the occurrence of fatal bradyarrhythmia and asystole**

Key Concept/Objective: To understand the adjuvant medical therapies available for patients with acute MI after reperfusion therapy has been administered

Early administration of beta blockers may reduce infarct size by reducing heart rate, blood pressure, and myocardial contractility. It is recommended that all patients with acute MI without contraindications receive I.V. beta blockers as early as possible, whether or not they receive reperfusion therapy. Several large, randomized, controlled clinical trials evaluated the use of ACE inhibitors early after acute MI; all but one trial revealed a significant reduction in mortality. To determine whether nitroglycerin therapy is beneficial in patients treated with reperfusion, 58,050 patients with acute MI in the ISIS-4 trial were randomized to receive either oral controlled-release mononitrate therapy or placebo; thrombolytic therapy was administered to patients in both groups. The results of this study revealed no benefit from the routine administration of oral nitrate therapy in this setting. Previously, routine prophylactic antiarrhythmic therapy with I.V. lidocaine was recommended for all patients in the early stages of acute MI. However, studies have revealed that prophylactic therapy with lidocaine does not reduce and may actually increase mortality because of an increase in the occurrence of fatal bradyarrhythmia and asystole. *(Answer: C—When given within 6 hours after presentation to the hospital, I.V. nitroglycerin reduces mortality in patients with MI)*

35. A 49-year-old white woman was admitted last night with an acute ST segment elevation MI. She underwent left heart catheterization with restoration of blood flow to her left circumflex artery and is currently in the CCU. She has received anticoagulation therapy and has been started on an ACE inhibitor, aspirin, and a beta blocker.

Which of the following statements regarding possible complications of acute MI is true?

- ❏ A. **The Atrial Fibrillation Follow-up Investigation of Rhythm Management (AFFIRM) trial showed that rhythm-control strategies provided a significant survival advantage when compared with rate-control strategies**
- ❏ B. **Beta blockers may reduce the early occurrence of ventricular fibrillation**
- ❏ C. **Severe mitral regurgitation is 10 times more likely to occur with anterior MI than with inferior MI**
- ❏ D. **When patients have right ventricular infarction, the left ventricle is almost always spared of any damage**

Key Concept/Objective: To know the complications associated with acute MI

Although lidocaine has been shown to reduce the occurrence of primary ventricular fibrillation, mortality in patients receiving lidocaine was increased because of an increase in fatal bradycardia and asystole, and prophylactic lidocaine is no longer recommended if defibrillation can rapidly be performed. Beta blockers may reduce the early occurrence of ventricular fibrillation and should be administered to patients who have no contraindications. The treatment of atrial fibrillation in acute MI should be similar to the treatment of atrial fibrillation in other settings. If atrial fibrillation recurs, antiarrhythmic agents may be used, although their impact on clinical outcomes is unproven. Mild mitral regurgitation is common in acute MI and is present in nearly 50% of patients. The posterior papillary muscle receives blood only from the dominant coronary artery (the right coronary artery in nearly 90% of patients); thrombotic occlusion of this artery may cause rupture of the posterior papillary muscle, resulting in severe mitral regurgitation. Although nearly all patients with right ventricular infarction suffer both right and left ventricular infarction, the characteristic hemodynamic findings of right ventricular infarction generally dominate the clinical course and must be the main focus of therapy. *(Answer: B—Beta blockers may reduce the early occurrence of ventricular fibrillation)*

36. A 55-year-old white man presented to the emergency department with crushing substernal chest pain of 1 hour's duration that radiated to his left arm; associated with this pain were dyspnea, diaphoresis, nausea, and vomiting. The patient's cardiac risk factors include hypertension of 10 years' duration, current tobacco use, and a strong family history of CAD. Examination findings were as follows: BP, 158/87 mm Hg; pulse, 105 beats/min; and lung crackles at bases. ECG showed an ST segment elevation of 3 mm in leads V2 through V5 with reciprocal ST segment depression in leads II, III, and aVF. Laboratory results

showed normal CK and troponin I levels and an LDL level of 120. After administration of O_2, aspirin, nitrates, and morphine, the chest pain subsided, but the ECG still shows an ST segment elevation in leads V2 through V5.

Which of the following would you consider for initial treatment of this patient?

❑ **A. Reperfusion therapy**

❑ **B. Statin therapy**

❑ **C. ACE inhibitor**

❑ **D. Glycoprotein IIb-IIIa inhibitor**

Key Concept/Objective: To understand the indications and contraindications for reperfusion therapy

This patient was initially treated for acute MI, and he now needs to receive reperfusion therapy as rapidly as possible to restore normal antegrade blood flow in the occluded artery. Reperfusion may be accomplished by thrombolytic therapy or by percutaneous transluminal coronary angioplasty (PTCA). In prospective trials, thrombolytic therapy has been shown to reduce mortality by 29% in patients with ST segment elevation who have been treated within 6 hours of the onset of chest pain. In prospective, randomized clinical trials comparing thrombolytic therapy with direct coronary angioplasty, direct coronary angioplasty was associated with lower morbidity and mortality than thrombolytic therapy. PTCA, therefore, is the preferred choice in facilities that have surgical backup where it can be performed quickly and that have a high angiographic success rate. Reperfusion therapy is contraindicated in patients who present with conditions that predispose them to significant bleeding. Thrombolytic therapy is contraindicated in patients who have ECG abnormalities other than ST segment elevation or bundle branch block. A complete and rapid assessment needs to be conducted to ensure that the right course of action is taken. The potential benefits of thrombolytic therapy may outweigh the risks of reperfusion therapy. *(Answer: A— Reperfusion therapy)*

37. The patient described in Question 36 has now been treated with thrombolytic therapy with t-PA.

Adding which of the following at or before the time of administration of thrombolytic therapy would likely improve this patient's outcome?

❑ **A. Statin therapy**

❑ **B. I.V. nitroglycerin**

❑ **C. Glycoprotein IIb-IIIa inhibitor**

❑ **D. I.V. beta-blocker therapy**

Key Concept/Objective: To understand the value of beta blockers early in the treatment of MI

A number of studies of beta-blocker therapy in patients with acute MI have documented improved patient outcomes, including reductions in hospital stay and improved long-term mortality. Early administration of beta blockers may reduce infarct size by reducing heart rate, blood pressure, and myocardial contractility, all of which diminish myocardial oxygen demand. Use of I.V. beta-blocker therapy as soon as possible is recommended for all patients with acute MI in whom beta-blocker therapy is not contraindicated, whether or not patients receive reperfusion therapy. Those with the largest infarcts benefit the most from the use of beta blockers. In the absence of side effects and contraindications, beta-blocker therapy should be continued indefinitely. *(Answer: D—I.V. beta-blocker therapy)*

38. A 56-year-old man presents to the emergency department with complaint of chest pain of 20 minutes' duration. The pain is severe, crushing, substernal, and without radiation. He has associated nausea and diaphoresis without vomiting. He has had no previous episodes of chest discomfort. He has not seen a doctor for over 20 years and takes no medications. He has smoked two packs of cigarettes a day for the past 35 years and has lived a sedentary lifestyle. His family history is remarkable for an MI in his father at 49 years of age. Physical examination reveals a thin man, sitting upright, breathing rapidly on 2 L of oxygen. His vital signs include the following: temperature, 98.8° F (37.1° C); pulse, 98 beats/min; respiratory rate, 22 breaths/min; blood pressure, 150/95 mm Hg. Cardiac examination reveals normal rate and rhythm without murmur, and neck veins are not elevated. Lungs are clear to auscultation. ECG shows normal sinus rhythm with occasional premature ventricular contractions and ST segment elevations of 0.2 mV in leads II, III, and aVF.

Which of the following interventions is NOT indicated for this patient at this time?

❑ A. **Morphine sulfate I.V.**

❑ B. **Lidocaine**

❑ C. **Aspirin**

❑ D. **Metoprolol**

❑ E. **Streptokinase**

Key Concept/Objective: To understand the initial management of acute MI

This patient meets criteria for acute MI with a characteristic history and ECG changes. Emergent therapy should include oxygen, aspirin, analgesia, nitrates, beta blockers, and early reperfusion. The prophylactic administration of antiarrhythmic agents in the absence of significant arrhythmias does not reduce mortality and may actually increase mortality through increased incidence of bradyarrhythmias and asystole. *(Answer: B—Lidocaine)*

39. The patient in Question 38 receives thrombolytic therapy with streptokinase within 30 minutes of the onset of his chest pain. Soon after administration of streptokinase, the ECG changes revert to baseline. He is monitored on telemetry for 48 hours without any arrhythmias. He is able to walk around the ward without difficulty.

Further diagnostic tests during the immediate discharge period should include which of the following?

❑ A. **Cardiac catheterization**

❑ B. **Nuclear imaging with pharmacologic stress**

❑ C. **Stress echocardiogram**

❑ D. **Low-level exercise treadmill test at 1 week post-MI**

❑ E. **Symptom-limited exercise treadmill test at 1 week post-MI**

Key Concept/Objective: To understand the post-MI risk-stratification strategies

The utility of cardiac catheterization post-MI has not been extensively studied, and patterns of practice vary widely. In the setting of a patient with acute MI who has successfully been treated with thrombolytic agents, the utility of post-MI catheterization has been studied in two clinical trials and has been found not to reduce the risk of reinfarction or death. The recommendation of the American College of Cardiology/American Heart Association is to use a submaximal exercise test at 5 to 7 days or a symptom-limited exercise test at 14 to 21 days. The stress echocardiogram and nuclear imaging are to be used in patients who are unable to exercise or in those whose baseline ECG has abnormalities, such as left bundle branch block or left ventricular hypertrophy with strain, that preclude interpretation of a stress test. The symptom-limited exercise treadmill test is recommended not in the immediate postdischarge period but at 3 to 6 weeks. Coronary angioplasty following positive exercise treadmill tests has been shown to improve the rates of nonfatal MI and unstable angina in the Danish Acute Myocardial Infarction (DANAMI) study. *(Answer: D—Low-level exercise treadmill test at 1 week post-MI)*

40. A 72-year-old woman is seen by her primary care physician. She reports 5 days of shortness of breath on exertion. Five days ago, she reported having several hours of chest discomfort, which she ascribed to indigestion, and did not seek medical attention. She currently denies any chest discomfort. Her medical history is remarkable for hypertension, type 2 diabetes mellitus, and obesity. Medications include glyburide and hydrochlorothiazide. She is a nonsmoker. Physical examination reveals a moderately obese

woman, seated in a chair, breathing comfortably. Vital signs are as follows: pulse, 90 beats/min; blood pressure, 145/90 mm Hg; respiratory rate, 20 breaths/min. Examination of the heart shows a regular rate and rhythm and the presence of an S_3 gallop. Neck veins cannot be assessed because of obesity. Lungs are clear to auscultation. Laboratory data are remarkable for a low-density-lipoprotein (LDL) cholesterol level of 135 mg/dl, a high-density-lipoprotein (HDL) cholesterol level of 41 mg/dl, and a triglyceride level of 220 mg/dl. ECG shows normal sinus rhythm; Q waves in V1, V2, and V3; and poor R-wave progression, which are new changes compared with an ECG of 2 years ago. Echocardiography reveals a depressed ejection fraction of 35% and no valvular pathology.

Which of the following medications is not likely to prolong survival in this patient?

- ❑ **A. Carvedilol**
- ❑ **B. Simvastatin**
- ❑ **C. Aspirin**
- ❑ **D. Enalapril**
- ❑ **E. Estrogen/progesterone**

Key Concept/Objective: To understand the pharmacotherapy of secondary prevention after acute MI

Beta blockers have been shown to increase survival and are recommended in all post-MI patients without contraindications. Carvedilol has been studied specifically in the setting of nondecompensated congestive heart failure and has been shown to prolong survival. Lipid-lowering therapy with HMG-CoA reductase inhibitors (statins) has been shown to reduce both cardiac and all-cause mortality. Treatment guidelines in patients with known coronary heart disease establish a treatment-goal LDL cholesterol level of less than 100 mg/dl. Aspirin therapy has been shown to have significant reductions in the rate of nonfatal MI, nonfatal stroke, and vascular death. ACE inhibitors have been shown to reduce mortality post-MI and are recommended in all patients with anterior MI or with clinical heart failure in the absence of hypotension. The recently published Heart and Estrogen/Progestin Replacement Study (HERS) showed no overall cardiovascular benefit at 5 years from estrogen/progestin replacement and an increase in early cardiovascular events compared with placebo. On the basis of this study, estrogen/progestin is not recommended as secondary prevention after acute MI. Women who are already taking hormone replacement therapy at the time of acute MI may continue to do so. *(Answer: E—Estrogen/progesterone)*

41. An 80-year-old man presents to the emergency department with chest pain of 30 minutes' duration. He has a history of an inferior MI that was treated with streptokinase 6 months ago. He has hypertension, with a controlled blood pressure of 130/80 mm Hg, and has not taken his medications for several days. He says his current symptoms are similar to those he experienced previously. His medical history is remarkable for gout, hypertension, and an ischemic stroke 8 years ago. Current medications include atenolol, aspirin, and allopurinol. The patient is afebrile, his blood pressure is 170/100 mm Hg, his pulse is 90 beats/min, and his respiratory rate is 20 breaths/min. He is diaphoretic and in apparent pain. Cardiovascular examination shows a regular rate and rhythm without murmur. Lungs are clear to auscultation. ECG shows ST segment elevation greater than 0.2 mV in V2 to V6.

Which of the following features in this case would be an absolute contraindication to thrombolytic therapy?

- ❑ **A. Failure to meet ECG criteria**
- ❑ **B. Age greater than 75 years**
- ❑ **C. History of stroke**
- ❑ **D. Elevated blood pressure**
- ❑ **E. There are no absolute contraindications**

Key Concept/Objective: To understand the indications and contraindications for thrombolytic therapy

The patient clearly meets ECG criteria for the administration of thrombolytic therapy: ST segment elevation greater than 0.1 mV in two contiguous leads. Age greater than 75 years

is not a contraindication to thrombolysis. There is increased mortality in this group with and without thrombolytic therapy. In patients older than 75 years, there is an increased risk of hemorrhagic stroke, but overall mortality is reduced in such patients without contraindications. A prior history of hemorrhagic stroke is an absolute contraindication to thrombolytics, but a history of an ischemic stroke more than 1 year before presentation is a relative contraindication. Severe uncontrolled hypertension (blood pressure > 180/110 mm Hg) is a relative contraindication to thrombolytic therapy, but this patient does not have that degree of hypertension. Because this patient has had exposure to streptokinase within the past 2 years, this agent should be avoided, as antibodies against the drug will reduce its efficacy and create potential for allergic reactions. *(Answer: E—There are no absolute contraindications)*

42. A 77-year-old woman presents with 2 hours of chest pain, which varies in intensity from mild to severe. Her pain is described as "pressure" felt over the left chest, with radiation to the left arm. It occurred at rest and is worsened by any activity. She has nausea without vomiting. Her medical history is remarkable for an inferior MI 5 years ago, diabetes, and hypertension. Her medications include lisinopril and metformin. Physical examination reveals a moderately obese woman in apparent discomfort. Vital signs include pulse, 84 beats/min; BP, 130/80 mm Hg; respiratory rate, 16; oxygen saturation, 96% on room air. Cardiac and lung examinations are normal. Her ECG shows Q waves in III and aVF; 2 mV ST segment depression in leads V3 to V6; and 1 mV ST segment elevation in V1. She is treated initially with oxygen, sublingual nitroglycerin, aspirin, metoprolol, and morphine, and her symptoms improve. She still rates her pain as moderate, and repeat ECG is unchanged.

Which of the following would NOT be an appropriate intervention for this patient?

- ❑ A. Low-molecular-weight heparin
- ❑ B. Cardiac catheterization
- ❑ C. Abciximab
- ❑ D. Thrombolytics
- ❑ E. Eptifibatide

Key Concept/Objective: To understand the management of acute coronary syndromes with a nondiagnostic ECG

This case represents an acute coronary syndrome that is not diagnostic for acute MI and does not represent chronic stable angina. Patients with nondiagnostic ECGs on presentation may have noncardiac chest pain, unstable angina, or MI. The use of low-molecular-weight heparin in this setting has been studied in several trials and has been shown to have a clear benefit. Glycoprotein IIb/IIIa inhibitors (abciximab, eptifibatide, and tirofiban) block the final common pathway of platelet aggregation and have been shown to reduce the risk of death, MI, and revascularization procedures. The use of cardiac catheterization in the setting of non–ST segment acute coronary syndromes has been shown to reduce the length of stay with initial hospitalization and the need for rehospitalization. In a recent trial, an invasive strategy combined with antiplatelet therapy was shown to reduce the rate of death or MI when compared with a noninvasive strategy. Current recommendations of the American College of Cardiology/American Heart Association include catheterization and revascularization of high-risk patients (defined by prior MI, left ventricular dysfunction, widespread ECG changes, or recurrent ischemia). Thrombolytics have been studied in the setting of acute coronary syndromes without ST segment elevation or bundle branch block and have been found to be deleterious, so they are contraindicated in this setting. *(Answer: D—Thrombolytics)*

For more information, see Berger PB, Orford JL: 1 Cardiovascular Medicine: VIII Acute Myocardial Infarction. ACP Medicine Online (www.acpmedicine.com). Dale DC, Federman DD, Eds. WebMD Inc., New York, September 2004

Chronic Stable Angina

43. A previously healthy 52-year-old man presents with complaints of intermittent substernal chest discomfort. The pain does not radiate. The symptoms occur with exercise, and they are not relieved by rest. The patient does not have shortness of breath. The resting ECG is normal. You determine that the patient has an intermediate pretest probability of having significant coronary artery disease, and you elect to have him undergo exercise ECG testing to further evaluate his symptoms.

Which of the following findings would be most highly suggestive of significant ischemic heart disease (IHD) on exercise ECG testing?

- ❑ **A. Chest discomfort before completion of the test**
- ❑ **B. Hypertension during the test**
- ❑ **C. An S_3 heart sound during the test**
- ❑ **D. A 0.5 mm ST segment depression during the test**

Key Concept/Objective: To understand the significant positive findings during exercise ECG testing

Recently published guidelines from the American College of Cardiology/American Heart Association/American College of Physicians (ACC/AHA/ACP) recommend exercise ECG as the diagnostic test of choice for the average patient with an intermediate pretest probability of IHD and a normal resting ECG. Exercise-induced falls in blood pressure or the development of an exercise-induced S_3 heart sound are strongly suggestive of ischemic left ventricular dysfunction. Specific exercise-induced ECG changes include changes ≥ 1 mm horizontal or downward-sloping ST segment depression or elevation during or after exercise. Exercise-induced changes in lead V5 are most reliable for the diagnosis of IHD. *(Answer: C—An S_3 heart sound during the test)*

44. A 56-year-old man with hypertension presents to your clinic for a routine health maintenance visit. He is asymptomatic and takes only hydrochlorothiazide. His blood pressure is 138/78 mm Hg. His total cholesterol level is 190 mg/dl, and his high-density liproprotein (HDL) cholesterol level is 36 mg/dl. He is a nonsmoker. He tells you he is concerned about IHD and that he has read about new methods to detect early disease, including CT imaging. He is interested in this screening test in hope of detecting any disease he may have before it becomes a problem.

How should you advise this patient with regard to electron-beam computed tomography (EBCT)?

- ❑ **A. You should tell him that EBCT is a safe and effective method of detecting early coronary artery disease**
- ❑ **B. You should recommend this test because it will hopefully alleviate his concerns about IHD**
- ❑ **C. You should recommend against this form of testing because his risk of heart disease can be equally well determined by the information already known about him**
- ❑ **D. You should recommend against this test because even if the test is negative, he would still have a high likelihood of having significant lesions**

Key Concept/Objective: To understand the limitations of new technology in the diagnosis of IHD

Although the sensitivity of EBCT for the diagnosis of significant coronary artery stenosis is high, the specificity of EBCT for significant coronary artery stenosis ranges from only 41% to 76%, yielding many false positive results. To date, no prospective, population-based studies have been performed to investigate a potential association between the calcium score derived from EBCT and the risk of future coronary events, and no studies have shown that screening for IHD with EBCT reduces mortality. Asymptomatic patients for whom EBCT results indicate a potentially high risk of cardiac events may suffer anxiety and unnecessary procedures as a result of the study. The ACC/AHA do not currently recommend EBCT and other imaging procedures, such as magnetic resonance imaging

angiography, in asymptomatic patients. *(Answer: C—You should recommend against this form of testing because his risk of heart disease can be equally well determined by the information already known about him)*

45. A 61-year-old woman was recently admitted to the hospital with acute coronary syndrome. She was found to have coronary artery disease that is not amenable to revascularization procedures. She is hypertensive and has hyperlipidemia. She smokes approximately 1 pack of cigarettes a day. She currently has stable angina. Medical therapy and lifestyle changes are recommended for this patient.

Which of the following statements is true regarding the management of this patient?

- ❑ A. **Clopidogrel and ticlopidine are equally effective in reducing future cardiovascular events**
- ❑ B. **Smoking cessation is as effective as or more effective than any current medical therapy in reducing the risk of future cardiovascular events**
- ❑ C. **Patients with chronic stable angina should be placed on statin therapy only if their low-density lipoprotein (LDL) cholesterol level is greater than 100 mg/dl**
- ❑ D. **It is clear that patients who walk for at least 1 hour five to seven times a week derive more benefit than patients who walk only for 30 minutes five to seven times a week**

Key Concept/Objective: To understand the management of patients with IHD and chronic stable angina

A systematic review of prospective cohort studies of smokers with IHD found a striking 29% to 36% relative risk reduction in all-cause mortality for patients who were able to quit smoking. The magnitude of the risk reduction for smoking cessation was as great as or greater than that expected to result from use of aspirin, statins, beta blockers, or angiotensin-converting enzyme (ACE) inhibitors. Patients with chronic stable angina should be encouraged to include moderate aerobic activity in their daily lives. Moderate physical activity consists of walking briskly for 30 minutes or more five to seven times a week or the equivalent. There are no studies demonstrating that ticlopidine reduces cardiovascular events in outpatients with chronic stable angina. Results of the Heart Protection Study indicate that all patients with chronic stable angina should be treated with a statin, barring specific allergy. *(Answer: B—Smoking cessation is as effective as or more effective than any current medical therapy in reducing the risk of future cardiovascular events)*

46. A 72-year-old male patient has long-standing IHD. He has significant angina that is stable but causes him considerable distress and limits his activities of daily living. You hope to improve his anginal symptoms.

For this patient, which of the following statements regarding the management of the symptoms of chronic stable angina is true?

- ❑ A. **Because of bronchospasm, beta blockers are usually not well tolerated in patients with chronic obstructive pulmonary disease**
- ❑ B. **Although both beta blockers and calcium channel blockers are effective in the treatment of angina, the combination of these two medicines offers little additional benefit**
- ❑ C. **Patients with left ventricular systolic dysfunction should never be started on calcium channel blockers because of their negative inotropic effects**
- ❑ D. **Nitrates should not be used as treatment for anginal symptoms within 24 hours of taking sildenafil for erectile dysfunction**

Key Concept/Objective: Understand the appropriate management of the symptoms of chronic stable angina

Beta blockers are generally well tolerated in patients with chronic obstructive pulmonary disease, although they may exacerbate bronchospasm in patients with severe asthma. Calcium channel blockers can be used as monotherapy in the treatment of chronic stable angina, although combinations of beta blockers and calcium channel blockers relieve angina more effectively than either agent alone. Calcium channel blockers are contraindicated in the presence of decompensated congestive heart failure, although the vasoselective dihydropyridine agents amlodipine and felodipine are tolerated in patients with clinically stable left ventricular dysfunction. Nitroglycerin and nitrates should not be used within 24 hours of taking sildenafil or other phosphodiesterase inhibitors used in the treatment of erectile dysfunction, because of the potential for life-threatening hypotension. *(Answer: D—Nitrates should not be used as treatment for anginal symptoms within 24 hours of taking sildenafil for erectile dysfunction)*

47. A 70-year-old man presents to establish care. His medical history is remarkable for hypertension and a myocardial infarction 3 years ago. His medications include aspirin, 325 mg daily; metoprolol, 100 mg twice daily; and isosorbide mononitrate, 120 mg daily. He reports that when walking more than one block he has substernal chest pressure, which is relieved by rest. He had a cardiac catheterization 2 months ago that showed a left main coronary artery stenosis of 80%, a proximal left anterior descending artery stenosis of 60%, and a 70% stenosis of the first obtuse marginal branch. The left ventricular ejection fraction (LVEF) was estimated at 45%.

Which of the following therapies would be most beneficial for this patient?

- ❑ A. **Continuing the patient's current medication regimen without modification**
- ❑ B. **Percutaneous transluminal angioplasty (PCTA)**
- ❑ C. **Coronary artery bypass graft (CABG)**
- ❑ D. **Enhanced external counterpulsation therapy (EECP)**
- ❑ E. **Transmyocardial revascularization procedure (TMR)**

Key Concept/Objective: To know the indications for coronary artery bypass surgery

CABG is recommended in patients with any of the following criteria: significant left main coronary artery disease, three-vessel disease (in patients with three-vessel disease, those with LVEF < 50% have the greatest survival benefit), and two-vessel disease with significant left anterior descending coronary artery involvement or abnormal LV function (LVEF < 50%). In patients with three-vessel disease and abnormal LVEF, the survival benefit and symptom relief of CABG are superior to those of PCTA or medical therapy. EECP involves leg cuffs that inflate and deflate to augment venous return. This therapy may be helpful in decreasing angina in patients who have refractory angina and are not candidates for revascularization. In TMR, a laser is used to create channels in the myocardium to relieve angina. This procedure has been shown to improve severe refractory angina in patients who could not be treated with conventional revascularization techniques (PCTA or CABG). For the patient described here, CABG is the preferred procedure. *(Answer: C—Coronary artery bypass graft [CABG])*

48. A 65-year-old woman presents to the emergency department with anterior chest pain that has been radiating to her left arm for the past 10 minutes. She had just run one block to catch a bus before she called the paramedics. Her pain was quickly relieved by two sublingual nitroglycerin tablets given by the paramedics. She said she has had similar pain with exertion over the past 3 years and has been using her husband's nitroglycerin occasionally. Her medical history is remarkable for diabetes. Her only medication is glyburide, 5 mg daily. Her blood pressure is 110/60 mm Hg; pulse, 80 beats/min; and respirations, 20 breaths/min. Examination reveals a moderately obese woman in no apparent distress. Heart rate and rhythm are regular, without murmur, and the lungs are clear to auscultation.

Which of the following medications should not be used to treat this patient's angina?

- ❑ A. **Metoprolol extended release, 100 mg p.o., q.d.**
- ❑ B. **Aspirin, 325 mg p.o., q.d.**

❑ C. **Nifedipine, 20 mg p.o., t.i.d.**

❑ D. **Isosorbide dinitrate, 10 mg p.o., t.i.d.**

❑ E. **Nitroglycerin sublingual, 0.4 mg, q. 5 min, p.r.n. chest discomfort**

Key Concept/Objective: To understand the agents used in the pharmacologic treatment of angina

Although not an antianginal, aspirin, 75 to 325 mg daily, should be used in all patients who have angina without specific contraindications, because it has been shown to reduce the risk of adverse cardiovascular events by 33%. Beta blockers, such as metoprolol, are the cornerstone of angina treatment because they are the only antianginals shown to reduce the risk of death and myocardial infarction. Diabetes and use of hypoglycemic medications are not contraindications to beta-blocker therapy, because there is no increase in hypoglycemic events or hypoglycemic unawareness with the use of beta blockers. Nitrates, such as isosorbide dinitrate and nitroglycerin, are effective antianginals, but they do not reduce the risk of cardiac events or death. Calcium channel blockers are effective antianginals. Short-acting agents such as immediate-release nifedipine may increase the risk of vascular events and are associated with hypotension, and therefore, they should be avoided. If calcium channel blockers are used, those agents with a long half-life or slow-release formulations should be used. *(Answer: C—Nifedipine, 20 mg p.o., t.i.d.)*

49. A 72-year-old man with a history of myocardial infarction 10 years ago and angina presents with complaints of recurrent chest pain, which he has been experiencing over the past 4 months. This pain is retrosternal, is brought on by exertion, and is relieved by rest. The patient has been taking aspirin, long-acting diltiazem, simvastatin, atenolol, and isosorbide dinitrate at maximal doses. His blood pressure is 130/80 mm Hg; pulse, 62 beats/min; and respirations, 16 breaths/min. Physical examination is normal. ECG shows normal sinus rhythm, with left bundle branch block.

Which of the following tests would be most useful in the evaluation of this patient's angina?

❑ A. **Exercise treadmill ECG**

❑ B. **Exercise treadmill cardiac nuclear imaging**

❑ C. **Exercise treadmill echocardiography**

❑ D. **Dobutamine echocardiography**

❑ E. **Cardiac catheterization**

Key Concept/Objective: To understand the modalities available for diagnostic testing and the utility of these tests in various patients

This patient has known coronary artery disease and angina that is refractory to maximal medical management. The diagnosis of angina is firmly established with high probability because this patient has known coronary artery disease and typical symptoms. The patient's baseline ECG has left bundle branch block, and therefore, exercise stress testing is not interpretable. Exercise treadmill cardiac nuclear imaging, exercise treadmill echocardiography, and pharmacologic stress echocardiography all have higher specificity and sensitivity than conventional exercise tolerance testing and give information about functional anatomy. However, the most useful test for this patient would be cardiac catheterization, because he has symptoms despite maximal medical management, is therefore highly likely to need revascularization, and needs to have his cardiac vascular anatomy defined with cardiac catheterization. *(Answer: E—Cardiac catheterization)*

50. A 60-year-old man with complaints of substernal chest pressure, brought on only by vigorous activity and relieved by rest, returns for a follow-up appointment. He takes no medications and has smoked one pack of cigarettes a day for 40 years. His blood pressure is 120/70 mm Hg; pulse, 75 beats/min; and respirations, 16. Examination reveals a thin man in no distress. Heart examination reveals a regular rhythm, with no murmurs. Jugular venous pressure is estimated at 5 cm, lungs are clear to auscultation, and extremities are without edema. The patient had an exercise treadmill thallium study that showed a small reversible defect, which prompted cardiac catheterization. This revealed a 70% stenosis of the circumflex artery. His ejection fraction was estimated at 60%. His serum LDL cholesterol is 120 mg/dl, and HDL cholesterol is 35 mg/dl.

Which of the following measures would not be appropriate in this setting?

❑ A. Atorvastatin, 80 mg p.o., q.d.

❑ B. Nitroglycerin, 0.4 mg sublingual, p.r.n. chest pain

❑ C. Coronary artery bypass graft (CABG)

❑ D. Ramipril, 10 mg p.o., q.d.

❑ E. Atenolol, 50 mg p.o., q.d.

Key Concept/Objective: To understand the management of single-vessel and two-vessel coronary artery disease (CAD)

Patients who have one- or two-vessel CAD without significant proximal left anterior descending artery stenosis, who have mild symptoms or have not received adequate antianginal therapy, and who have a small area of reversible ischemia do not benefit from revascularization with CABG or PCTA. Patients with known CAD should be treated to achieve a target LDL < 100 mg/dl. Beta blockers are effective antianginals and reduce mortality. Nitrates are useful as antianginals but do not alter mortality. Ramipril, 10 mg daily, was studied in the HOPE trial[1] and was found to significantly reduce the risks of death, myocardial infarction, and stroke. The patients in that study were older than 55 years, had known cerebrovasular disease or diabetes, had one cardiovascular risk factor (e.g., smoking, hypertension, hyperlipidemia), and did not have heart failure or known low ejection fraction. *(Answer: C—Coronary artery bypass graft [CABG])*

1. Yusuf S, Sleight P, Pogue J, et al: Effects of an angiotensin-converting- enzyme inhibitor, ramipril, on cardiovascular events in high-risk patients: The Heart Outcomes Prevention Evaluation Study Investigators. N Engl J Med 342:145, 2000

51. A 70-year-old man presents to his physician with complaints of chest tightness. The sensation is substernal, is brought on by exertion, and is relieved by rest. He is able to walk several blocks before he notes chest pressure. His medical history is remarkable only for hypertension and hyperlipidemia. His medications are hydrochlorothiazide, 25 mg daily, and aspirin, 325 mg daily.

Which of the following statements is true for this patient regarding exercise treadmill testing?

❑ A. It is helpful to rule out angina

❑ B. It is helpful to establish the diagnosis of angina

❑ C. It is helpful to either establish or exclude the diagnosis of angina

❑ D. It is helpful to neither establish nor exclude the diagnosis of angina

❑ E. It will not give any prognostic information about morbidity

Key Concept/Objective: To understand the pretest probability of angina and the effect of diagnostic testing on the posttest probability of angina

In this male patient, who is older than 65 years and has typical angina, the pretest probability of significant coronary atherosclerosis is 93% to 97%. Exercise treadmill ECG has limited sensitivity and specificity. Therefore, the posttest probability after a positive or a negative test is only a few percentage points different from the pretest probability in a patient such as this one, who has a high pretest probability of coronary artery disease. In this patient, then, exercise treadmill testing (ETT) is not helpful for diagnosing angina (suspicion was sufficiently high before a test was conducted), nor is it helpful in excluding the diagnosis (because a negative test would most likely be a false negative). Exercise testing is most useful for diagnosing coronary artery disease in patients with an intermediate pretest probability (e.g., 20% to 80%). The ETT does provide useful information about the severity of disease and prognosis. *(Answer: D—It is helpful to neither establish nor exclude the diagnosis of angina)*

For more information, see Sutton PR, Fihn SD: 1 Cardiovascular Medicine: IX Chronic Stable Angina. ACP Medicine Online (www.acpmedicine.com). Dale DC, Federman DD, Eds. WebMD Inc., New York, December 2004

Unstable Angina/Non–ST Segment Elevation MI

52. A 76-year-old woman presents to the emergency department for evaluation of nausea and mild epigastric pain that started suddenly 45 minutes ago. She denies having chest pain. Her medical history includes diabetes mellitus, hypertension, and hyperlipidemia. An electrocardiogram is interpreted as being normal.

    For this patient, which of the following statements regarding the diagnosis of unstable angina is false?

    - ❑ A. **Chest pain must be present to make a diagnosis of unstable angina**
    - ❑ B. **The physical examination is normal in many patients presenting with unstable angina**
    - ❑ C. **The initial serum troponin level is likely to be normal**
    - ❑ D. **Up to 60% of patients with unstable angina have normal ECGs**
    - ❑ E. **Serum myoglobin levels might be the first marker to be elevated in patients presenting with unstable angina**

    Key Concept/Objectives: To know that a significant portion of patients with unstable angina present in atypical fashion

    Approximately 35% to 50% of patients with unstable angina will not have chest pain as their presenting symptom. In the National Registry of Myocardial Infarction, which included 440,000 patients, one third had atypical symptoms. In the Alabama Unstable Angina Study of Medicare beneficiaries, which included over 4,000 patients, 51.7% of patients with unstable angina had the following atypical symptoms: dyspnea (69.4%), nausea (37.7%), diaphoresis (25.2%), syncope (10.6%), arm pain (11.5%), epigastric pain (8.1%), shoulder pain (7.4%), and neck pain (5.9%). Atypical symptoms were more common in young patients (i.e., those 25 to 40 years of age), the elderly (i.e., those older than 75 years), diabetic patients, and women. In many cases, the physical examination will be normal. Troponin I and T (TnI and TnT) are cardiac-specific subunits of the thin filament–associated troponin-tropomyosin complex, which regulates striated muscle contraction. Troponins have become the primary biomarkers in the evaluation of patients with acute coronary syndrome. These markers are detected in about one third of patients without elevation in the level of creatine kinase–myocardial band. Troponins may be detectable 3 to 4 hours after the onset of ischemic symptoms; they peak at 12 to 48 hours and persist for 4 to 10 days. Myoglobin is a nonspecific biomarker found in both cardiac and skeletal muscle. It is released rapidly in response to muscle injury and is detectable 2 hours after the onset of ischemia. Interestingly, a quarter of patients diagnosed with unstable angina/non–ST segment elevation myocardial infarction (NSTEMI) will go on to develop Q waves, and up to 60% may have a normal 12-lead ECG. *(Answer: A—Chest pain must be [illegible])*

53. A 69-year-old woman presents to the emergency department for evaluation of dyspnea and nausea. An ECG reveals ST segment depression of 1 mm in leads II, III, and aVF. The patient is given an aspirin, a beta blocker, and nitroglycerin sublingually, and the ST segment depression resolves. A diagnosis of unstable angina is made.

    For this patient, which of the following statements regarding antiplatelet therapy with a thienopyridine is false?

    - ❑ A. **Thienopyridines irreversibly bind the adenosine diphosphate (ADP) receptor on platelets, preventing fibrinogen binding and platelet aggregation**
    - ❑ B. **The use of ticlodipine has been limited by severe neutropenia and, rarely, thrombotic thrombocytopenic purpura**
    - ❑ C. **Clopidogrel should be stopped 5 to 7 days before the patient undergoes elective surgical revascularization**
    - ❑ D. **In patients undergoing percutaneous coronary intervention (PCI),**

guidelines recommend indefinite use of clopidogrel

❑ **E. Pretreatment with clopidogrel before PCI should be initiated more than 6 hours before the procedure**

Key Concept/Objectives: To understand the use of thienopyridines in unstable angina and as an adjunct in PCI

Thienopyridines irreversibly bind the ADP receptor on platelets, preventing fibrinogen binding and platelet aggregation. In the Clopidogrel for the Reduction of Events During Observation (CREDO) study, benefit was observed for patients who received combination therapy with aspirin and clopidogrel in a bolus load administered 6 to 24 hours before PCI. The principal adverse reaction that has limited the clinical use of ticlopidine is severe neutropenia and, rarely, thrombotic thrombocytopenic purpura, which may occur within the first 3 months of therapy. An important issue with clopidogrel is bleeding during surgery; for this reason, surgery should be avoided for 5 and preferably 7 days after the last dose, because of the prolonged duration of action. Patients with unstable angina/NSTEMI for whom a percutaneous coronary intervention is planned and who are not at high risk for bleeding should receive clopidogrel for at least 1 month and for up to 9 months. *(Answer: D—In patients undergoing percutaneous coronary intervention [PCI], guidelines recommend indefinite use of clopidogrel)*

For more information, see Kupersmith J, Raval A: 1 Cardiovascular Medicine: X Unstable Angina and Non–ST Segment Elevation Myocardial Infarction. ACP Medicine Online (www.acpmedicine.com). Dale DC, Federman DD, Eds. WebMD Inc., New York, February 2004

Diseases of the Aorta

54. A 68-year-old woman presents to your office for a routine follow-up visit. She has no complaints. Her medical history is notable for type 2 (non–insulin-dependent) diabetes mellitus and hypertension. She has a 60-pack-year history of cigarette smoking. The physical examination is notable for a 4 to 6 cm pulsatile, nontender abdominal mass. The patient denies having abdominal pain, and she has no family history of abdominal aortic aneurysm.

Which of the following is the best step to take next in the workup of this patient?

❑ **A. The patient should return every 3 months for serial physical examinations to follow the suspected aneurysm**

❑ **B. The patient should be immediately referred for surgical evaluation**

❑ **C. An abdominal ultrasound should be ordered to evaluate the possible aneurysm**

❑ **D. No further intervention is necessary**

Key Concept/Objective: To understand the importance of early detection of abdominal aortic aneurysms

Early recognition of abdominal aortic aneurysms can be lifesaving. Most abdominal aortic aneurysms produce no symptoms and are discovered during a routine physical examination or as a result of noninvasive screening. Periods of rapid expansion or impending rupture are often marked by severe discomfort in the lower abdomen or back; the pain may radiate to the buttocks, groin, or legs. Patients with impending or actual rupture must be managed as a surgical emergency in a manner similar to that of patients with major trauma. The fact that this patient is completely asymptomatic makes simple aortic imaging a more reasonable first step than urgent surgical referral. Current recommendations are for noninvasive screening of patients of appropriate age, which is typically defined as older than 65 years but younger if there is a significant family history of or risk factors for aneurysms. Abdominal ultrasonography is the most frequently used and most practical method. Ultrasonography has a sensitivity of nearly 100% for diagnosing aneurysms of

significant size and can discriminate size to within ± 3 mm. Assessment by physical examination alone is unreliable; therefore, an imaging study is needed to confirm the diagnosis of aortic aneurysm and, if present, to determine the size. Aneurysms larger than 6 cm in diameter are generally referred for surgery; those less than 4 cm in diameter are generally watched. *(Answer: C—An abdominal ultrasound should be ordered to evaluate the possible aneurysm)*

55. A 62-year-old man with long-standing hypertension presents to your office for evaluation of a nonproductive cough. He has had the cough for 2 or 3 months, and it is getting progressively worse. He is without other complaint. The patient's blood pressure is 168/94 mm Hg; other vital signs are unremarkable. A chest x-ray reveals a widening of the mediastinum. Spiral CT reveals a thoracic aortic aneurysm with impingement upon the trachea.

Which of the following statements regarding thoracic aortic aneurysms is true?

- ❑ **A. Aneurysms that are invading local structures should usually be resected**
- ❑ **B. In contrast to abdominal aortic aneurysms, the size of a thoracic aortic aneurysm is not a critical issue in terms of risk of rupture**
- ❑ **C. In contrast to abdominal aortic aneurysms, careful control of blood pressure is not a crucial issue for patients with thoracic aortic aneurysms**
- ❑ **D. Most thoracic centers recommend surgery for thoracic aortic aneurysms that exceed 7 cm in otherwise suitable surgical candidates**

Key Concept/Objective: To understand the importance of surgical referral for symptomatic thoracic aortic aneurysms

This patient has a cough secondary to impingement by a thoracic aortic aneurysm on his trachea. The fact that his cough is a new problem likely reflects expansion of his aneurysm. Aneurysms that are invading local structures or creating a marked vascular effect should usually be resected. Because size is a critical issue in terms of the risk of rupture, the initial size and potential growth of an aneurysm are important factors in the decision whether to operate on asymptomatic aneurysms. Careful control of blood pressure is crucial for all patients and may require medical therapy, particularly with beta blockers, which may also slow the rate of aneurysm growth. Currently, most thoracic centers recommend surgery for aneurysms that exceed 5.5 to 6 cm in an otherwise suitable surgical candidate. *(Answer: A—Aneurysms that are invading local structures should usually be resected)*

56. A 75-year-old male patient is seen in the emergency department with a severe midscapular pain. He has been experiencing this pain for 3 hours. His pain does not radiate, and he states that it has a "tearing quality." He has no shortness of breath, anterior chest pain, or change in pain with change in position. He denies having a personal or family history of heart disease, and he denies any history of chest pain. Current vital signs are unremarkable, with the exception of his blood pressure, which is 190/105 mm Hg. His pain does not respond to sublingual nitroglycerin and intravenous beta blockade. There is no difference in pulse or blood pressure between the upper extremities. Cardiac examination is normal, with the exception of a loud fourth heart sound. Electrocardiography reveals nonspecific ST-T wave changes, along with findings consistent with left ventricular hypertrophy. A chest x-ray reveals a widening of the mediastinum and a large cardiac silhouette without pleural effusions.

Which of the following is the most appropriate step to take next in the workup of this patient?

- ❑ **A. Initiate anticoagulation therapy immediately and activate the heart catheterization laboratory**
- ❑ **B. Order a stat spiral CT to rule out thoracic aortic dissection**
- ❑ **C. Order stat aortography to rule out thoracic aortic dissection**
- ❑ **D. Admit the patient for serial cardiac enzyme assays and ECGs to rule out myocardial infarction**

Key Concept/Objective: To understand the importance of rapid diagnosis of thoracic aortic dissection

The most typical presentation of type B dissection is onset of severe interscapular pain, which may radiate down the back toward the legs. Type B dissection is frequently accompanied by hypertension, whereas type A dissection more often occurs in the presence of normal or low blood pressure. Although myocardial infarction remains a possibility, this patient's history and examination are consistent with aortic dissection. In lieu of the considerable pretest likelihood of aortic dissection, anticoagulation should be withheld until dissection is ruled out by spiral CT or another acceptable imaging modality. Although aortography is still used in some hospitals, it is seldom the initial test for aortic dissection. The reported false negative rate for aortography is in the range of 5% to 15%. Spiral or ultrafast CT scanning gives even greater resolution than the older scanners and has a reported sensitivity and specificity for aortic dissection that exceed 95%. Blood pressure control is also an urgent consideration. *(Answer: B—Order a stat spiral CT to rule out thoracic aortic dissection)*

57. An 84-year-old man comes to your office complaining of a severe left temporal headache, which he has had for the past 2 days. In addition, the patient states that over the past 2 days, he has had a low-grade fever, fatigue, and loss of appetite. Upon questioning, the patient admits to muscle weakness and jaw pain with mastication but has no visual complaint. The physical examination is within normal limits, with the exception of a tender, palpable left temporal artery. Laboratory evaluation reveals a slight elevation in the white blood cell count and a marked elevation in the erythrocyte sedimentation rate.

Which of the following statements regarding giant cell arteritis is true?

❑ A. **Giant cell arteritis often affects the branches of the proximal aorta**

❑ B. **Giant cell arteritis commonly occurs in patients 50 years of age or younger**

❑ C. **Giant cell arteritis never results in complete blindness despite the high frequency of visual complaints**

❑ D. **Standard therapy for this arteritis is prednisone, 5 to 15 mg/day**

Key Concept/Objective: To recognize that giant cell arteritis affects the branches of the proximal aorta

Giant cell arteritis often affects the branches of the proximal aorta, particularly the branches supplying the head and neck, the extracranial structures (including the temporal arteries), and the upper extremities. Aortic involvement often coexists with temporal arteritis and polymyalgia rheumatica. This illness is more commonly seen in patients older than 50 years (the mean age at onset of disease is 67 years). A serious complication of this syndrome is blindness, which results when arteritis affects the ophthalmic artery. Progression to total blindness may be rapid. Visual symptoms of some type occur in as many as 50% of patients. Standard therapy for giant cell arteritis is high-dose glucocorticoid therapy (e.g., prednisone, 40 to 60 mg/day). *(Answer: A—Giant cell arteritis often affects the branches of the proximal aorta)*

58. A 68-year-old man with a long history of cigarette smoking presents for routine evaluation. On physical examination, he has a pulsatile abdominal mass. An ultrasound shows a 4.5 cm infrarenal aortic aneurysm. He reports no symptoms of abdominal pain or back pain.

What would you recommend for this patient?

❑ A. **Referral for surgical repair**

❑ B. **Aortogram for further evaluation of aneurysm**

❑ C. **Repeat ultrasound in 6 to 12 months**

❑ D. **Treatment with a beta blocker**

Key Concept/Objective: To understand the approach to the treatment of abdominal aortic aneurysms

Studies have shown that the likelihood of rupture is highest in patients with symptomatic or large aneurysms. Aneurysms smaller than 4 cm in diameter have a low risk (< 2%) of rupture. Aneurysms exceeding 10 cm have a 25% risk of rupture over 2 years. Current management strategies call for identification and observation of aneurysms that are asymptomatic and sufficiently small so as not to have a high risk of rupture. The median rate of expansion is slightly less than 0.5 cm a year. Aneurysms that are expanding more rapidly are more likely to rupture than stable aneurysms. Patients with aneurysms larger than 6 cm are generally referred for surgery, whereas patients with aneurysms smaller than 4 cm generally undergo observation. Evidence of expansion, particularly if the aneurysm is larger than 5 or 5.5 cm, is often taken as an indication to operate. This patient has an asymptomatic aneurysm 4.5 cm in diameter. It would be appropriate to assess its growth with ultrasonography over the next few years to see whether it is expanding more rapidly than expected. The rate of expansion is an important variable in assessing the risk of aneurysmal rupture. If the patient becomes symptomatic at any time, urgent imaging is appropriate. Aortography carries risk of contrast exposure and of atheromatous emboli, and it offers no advantages over ultrasonography for assessing the size of aneurysms. Beta blockers are not known to reduce the risk of rupture of abdominal aortic aneurysms. *(Answer: C—Repeat ultrasound in 6 to 12 months)*

59. A 53-year-old man presents for evaluation of severe chest pain. The pain has been present for 2 hours and is radiating down both arms. He reports no previous similar episodes of chest pain. On examination, he is diaphoretic. His blood pressure is 160/100 mm Hg bilaterally, and his pulse is 100 beats/min. Chest and cardiac examinations are normal. An electrocardiogram shows sinus tachycardia but no ST segment changes. A chest x-ray is unremarkable.

What would you recommend as the next step in the workup of this patient?

❑ A. **Aortogram**

❑ B. **Abdominal ultrasound**

❑ C. **Admission to cardiac care unit to rule out myocardial infarction**

❑ D. **Transesophageal echocardiography (TEE)**

❑ E. **Repeat chest x-ray**

Key Concept/Objective: To be able to recognize aortic dissection and to know the appropriate workup

This patient with hypertension has had a severe episode of chest pain, with the pain radiating to the arm. Aortic dissection should be strongly considered, and the patient should undergo urgent evaluation. The fact that there is no discrepancy in the blood pressure measurements in the patient's arms or that the patient's chest x-ray is unremarkable does not rule out the diagnosis of aortic dissection. Pulse deficits are seen in approximately 25% of patients with type A dissection and in perhaps 5% to 10% of patients with type B dissection. The chest x-ray of patients with aortic dissection typically shows widening of the mediastinal silhouette, and it may also demonstrate evidence of a pleural effusion, cardiomegaly, or congestive heart failure if severe aortic regurgitation is present. The chest x-ray is normal in more than 15% of cases. TEE has a high sensitivity and specificity in diagnosing aortic dissections. If it is not available on an urgent basis, a chest CT or MRI is useful in establishing a diagnosis. Aortography is seldom used as an initial test for aortic dissection. The reported false negative rate for aortography ranges from 2% to 5%. More important, aortography frequently fails to detect lesions such as intramural hematomas. In addition, it takes less time to obtain a TEE using a portable device than to move a patient to an angiography suite. *(Answer: D—Transesophageal echocardiography [TEE])*

60. Further testing of the patient in Question 59 reveals that he has a type B aortic dissection. He has no neurologic symptoms and his renal function is normal.

What would you recommend for this patient at this time?

❑ A. **Heparin drip**

❑ B. **Aggressive treatment of hypertension with beta blockers**

❑ C. **Aggressive treatment of hypertension with vasodilators**

❑ D. **Surgical repair of aneurysm with Dacron prosthesis**

❑ E. **Surgical repair with endoprosthesis**

Key Concept/Objective: To understand the treatment of type B aortic aneurysms

Emergency surgery is crucial for patients with type A aortic dissections. This patient has a type B dissection. Most such cases are managed medically by means of aggressive blood pressure control with beta blockers. If blood pressure is not adequately controlled after beta-blocker treatment, then vasodilators can be added to the beta blockers. Vasodilators should not be used in place of beta blockers. Surgery for type B dissection is indicated predominantly for patients with life-threatening complications requiring a surgical approach. Such conditions include ischemia of both kidneys, leading to reversible renal failure; the development of ischemic bowel; or ischemia involving an extremity. *(Answer: B—Aggressive treatment of hypertension with beta blockers)*

61. A 67-year-old man with type 2 diabetes and a long history of cigarette smoking develops severe exertional chest pain. Cardiac catheterization reveals three-vessel disease. Twenty-four hours later, he develops abdominal pain, painful toes, and a rash. On examination, he has purple discoloration of the second and fourth toes on his right foot and a lacy rash on both legs. Laboratory results are as follows: Hb, 13; HCT, 39; WBC, 9.0; BUN, 26; and Cr, 1.8.

What is the most likely diagnosis for this patient?

❑ A. **Contrast nephropathy**

❑ B. **Aortic dissection**

❑ C. **Atheromatous emboli syndrome**

❑ D. **Abdominal aortic aneurysmal rupture**

Key Concept/Objective: To be able to recognize atheromatous emboli syndrome

This patient experienced the onset of abdominal pain, purple toes, and livedo reticularis shortly after undergoing cardiac catheterization. These symptoms are consistent with atheromatous emboli syndrome. The patient also has renal insufficiency, a common feature of the syndrome. Contrast nephropathy is common in patients with diabetes, but that condition would not account for the cutaneous findings. Aortic dissection and rupture could cause abdominal pain and renal insufficiency, but that should not cause livedo reticularis or purple toes. The abdominal pain this patient experienced was most likely the result of pancreatitis caused by atheromatous emboli. *(Answer: C—Atheromatous emboli syndrome)*

For more information, see Eagle KA, Armstrong WF: 1 Cardiovascular Medicine: XII Diseases of the Aorta. ACP Medicine Online (www.acpmedicine.com). Dale DC, Federman DD, Eds. WebMD Inc., New York, November 2003

Pericardium, Cardiac Tumors, and Cardiac Trauma

62. A 24-year-old man presents to the emergency department complaining of chest pain. He reports having substernal chest pain of 2 days' duration. The pain is worse with inspiration and is alleviated by maintaining an upright position. He also reports having had a fever recently. His medical history and physical examination are unremarkable. An ECG shows 2 mm elevation of the ST segment in precordial leads, without reciprocal changes and with concomitant PR segment depression. An echocardiogram is normal.

What is the most likely diagnosis and the most appropriate treatment approach for this patient?

❑ A. **Acute pericarditis; start a nonsteroidal anti-inflammatory drug (NSAID)**

❑ B. **Acute pericarditis; start prednisone**

❑ C. Acute pericarditis; repeat echocardiogram in 1 week to confirm diagnosis

❑ D. ST elevation myocardial infarction; start thrombolytics

Key Concept/Objective: To understand the diagnosis and treatment of acute pericarditis

The clinical diagnosis of acute pericarditis rests primarily on the findings of chest pain, pericardial friction rub, and electrocardiographic changes. The chest pain of acute pericarditis typically develops suddenly and is severe and constant over the anterior chest. In acute pericarditis, the pain worsens with inspiration—a response that helps distinguish acute pericarditis from myocardial infarction. Low-grade fever and sinus tachycardia also are usually present. A pericardial friction rub can be detected in most patients when symptoms are acute. Electrocardiographic changes are common in most forms of acute pericarditis, particularly those of an infectious etiology in which the associated inflammation in the superficial layer of myocardium is prominent. The characteristic change is an elevation in the ST segment in diffuse leads. The diffuse distribution and the absence of reciprocal ST segment depression distinguish the characteristic pattern of acute pericarditis from acute myocardial infarction. Depression of the PR segment, which reflects superficial injury of the atrial myocardium, is as frequent and specific as ST segment elevation and is often the earliest electrocardiographic manifestation. Analgesic agents, salicylates, or NSAIDs are often effective in reducing pericardial inflammation. Corticosteroids should be reserved for severe cases that are unresponsive to other therapy, because symptoms may recur after steroid withdrawal. The absence of a significant effusion on echocardiography is not evidence against acute pericarditis. *(Answer: A—Acute pericarditis; start a nonsteroidal anti-inflammatory drug [NSAID])*

63. A 40-year-old woman is being evaluated for fever. She started having fever 6 weeks ago. Other symptoms include an erythematous rash, fatigue, and weight loss. Her medical history is significant for hypertension. She takes hydrochlorothiazide. On physical examination, the patient's temperature is found to be 100.6° F (38.1° C), a 3/6 murmur is noted in the mitral area, and an erythematous rash is seen on both legs. A complete blood count shows anemia; the patient's erythrocyte sedimentation rate (ESR) is elevated at 80 mm/hr. A transthoracic echocardiogram shows a 2 cm pedunculated mass in the left atrium.

Which of the following is the most likely diagnosis for this patient?

❑ A. Metastatic colon adenocarcinoma

❑ B. Cardiac rhabdomyosarcoma

❑ C. Papillary fibroelastoma

❑ D. Cardiac myxoma

Key Concept/Objective: To be able to recognize cardiac myxomas

Cardiac tumors may be either primary or secondary and either benign or malignant. Metastatic cardiac involvement occurs 20 to 40 times more frequently than primary tumors. Eighty percent of all primary cardiac tumors are benign; myxomas account for more than half of these in adults. Myxomas consist of scattered stellate cells embedded in a mucinous matrix. They are found in the cavities of the heart, attached to the endocardial wall or heart valves by either a narrow stalk or a broader pedicle. About 70% of myxomas are in the left atrium. Myxomas are most often manifested clinically by mechanical hemodynamic effects, which often simulate mitral or tricuspid stenoses or regurgitation. Intermittent obstruction of the valve orifice can lead to syncope or to remarkable changes in physical signs that are sometimes related to changes in body position. Another manifestation is a constitutional disturbance consisting of fatigue, fever, erythematous rash, myalgias, and weight loss, accompanied by anemia and an increased ESR. The constitutional symptoms may be caused by production of interleukin-6 by the myxoma. Papillary fibroelastomas are small tumors, usually attached to cardiac valves; they can be a cause of cardioembolic stroke. Rhabdomyosarcoma is a malignant primary tumor of the heart. About 10% of patients who die of malignant disease have metastatic cardiac involvement, but the metastases produce symptoms in only 5% to 10% of the affected patients. The most frequent clinical manifestation is pericardial effusion with cardiac tamponade. Extensive

solid tumor in and around the heart is less common but may resemble constrictive pericarditis or effusive-constrictive pericarditis. Invasion of the myocardium most often manifests clinically as arrhythmias; atrial flutter and atrial fibrillation are particularly common. *(Answer: D—Cardiac myxoma)*

64. A 16-year-old male becomes unresponsive immediately after being hit in the chest by a baseball in a local game. A family member reports that the patient has a "heart murmur." He takes no medications. The emergency medical service is called and finds the patient to be pulseless. Resuscitation attempts are started and are unfortunately unsuccessful.

Which of the following is the most likely mechanism behind this patient's cardiac arrest?

- ❑ A. **Impaired wall motion secondary to myocardial necrosis**
- ❑ B. **Ruptured myocardium and pericardial tamponade secondary to cardiac trauma**
- ❑ C. **Ventricular tachycardia secondary to hypertrophic cardiomyopathy**
- ❑ D. **Ventricular fibrillation secondary to trauma during repolarization**

Key Concept/Objective: To understand the mechanisms of blunt cardiac trauma

Cardiovascular injury may be either blunt (i.e., nonpenetrating) or penetrating. Automobile accidents are the most common cause of blunt cardiovascular trauma; gunshots and stabbings are the most common causes of penetrating trauma. Both types of injury can damage the myocardium, the valves, the coronary arteries, the pericardium, and the great vessels, especially the aorta. Myocardial contusion is the most common blunt injury. The right ventricle, because of its location immediately beneath the sternum, is the chamber most often involved. The pathologic changes in myocardial contusion consist of myocardial necrosis with hemorrhage, which may range in severity from scattered petechiae to intramural extravasations with associated transmural necrosis. In some instances, coronary arterial occlusion with secondary myocardial infarction is present. Seemingly innocuous blows to the chest by missiles such as baseballs or hockey pucks may cause sudden arrhythmic death, probably when they strike directly over the heart during the vulnerable portion of the T wave and induce ventricular fibrillation. The most important complication of myocardial contusion is cardiac arrhythmia. Hypotension, intracardiac thrombus, congestive heart failure, and cardiac tamponade occur occasionally. Blunt trauma may injure any of the cardiac valves and lead to valvular regurgitation. Traumatic valvular regurgitation is more likely to be recognized after the patient has recovered from the acute injury; it is less likely to play a major role in the early postinjury course. *(Answer: D—Ventricular fibrillation secondary to trauma during repolarization)*

65. A 23-year-old man reports a 3-day history of a constant left-sided chest pain, which worsens with inspiration and activity. His symptoms were preceded by several days of fatigue, rhinorrhea, and cough. He is worried that he has broken a rib from coughing. He reports no other symptoms and has no risk factors for cardiovascular disease. On examination, he is comfortable. Other findings on physical examination are as follows: blood pressure, 120/70 mm Hg; pulse, 94 beats/min; respiratory rate, 12 breaths/min; temperature, 100.2° F (37.9° C). His lungs are clear. Cardiovascular examination shows tachycardia, but otherwise the results are normal.

Which of the following should be the appropriate step to take next in this patient's workup?

- ❑ A. **Chest x-ray**
- ❑ B. **Complete blood count**
- ❑ C. **Arterial blood gas test**
- ❑ D. **Electrocardiogram**
- ❑ E. **None of the above**

Key Concept/Objective: To be able to recognize the presentation of acute benign viral pericarditis

This patient's presentation is classic for acute viral pericarditis: constant anterior chest pain that is worse with inspiration, tachycardia, and a low-grade fever. A pericardial fric-

tion rub is often heard when patients are symptomatic but may be missed on examination. The differential diagnosis includes pneumonia, spontaneous pneumothorax, and musculoskeletal pain; an electrocardiogram would be the appropriate first step in the evaluation. A finding of diffuse ST segment elevations without reciprocal changes or PR depressions would confirm the diagnosis of viral pericarditis. *(Answer: D—Electrocardiogram)*

66. The patient in Question 65 is found to have PR depressions on electrocardiography.

What should be the next step in this patient's management?

- ❑ A. **Hospital admission**
- ❑ B. **Treatment with antibiotics**
- ❑ C. **Treatment with NSAIDs**
- ❑ D. **Treatment with prednisone**
- ❑ E. **Treatment with codeine**

Key Concept/Objective: To understand the management of acute pericarditis

This patient has acute benign pericarditis. Anti-inflammatory medications, including aspirin, are usually effective for reducing pericardial inflammation and decreasing pain. Codeine or another narcotic may be added for pain relief if needed. Although prednisone is effective as well, steroids are generally reserved for patients who are unresponsive to other treatments, because symptoms may recur after steroid withdrawal. Most acute pericarditis is viral in origin. Patients do not require hospitalization unless they have other complications such as arrhythmia or tamponade. *(Answer: C—Treatment with NSAIDs)*

67. A 44-year-old man on long-term dialysis for lupus nephritis presents with progressive dyspnea on exertion. He has no chest pain or lower extremity edema, nor does he have any other symptoms. His weight has remained stable. Other results of his physical examination are as follows: blood pressure, 130/70 mm Hg; pulse, 84 beats/min; respiratory rate, 14 breaths/min. His neck veins are elevated, and the elevation increases upon inspiration. His lungs are clear. His cardiovascular examination is remarkable for an extra sound in early diastole, and he has no paradoxical pulse. His hematocrit is normal, and the results of pulmonary function studies and electrocardiography are unremarkable.

What would be the definitive diagnostic workup for this patient?

- ❑ A. **High-resolution chest CT**
- ❑ B. **Transthoracic echocardiogram**
- ❑ C. **Right and left cardiac catheterization**
- ❑ D. **Bronchoscopy**
- ❑ E. **A and C**

Key Concept/Objective: To be able to recognize constrictive pericarditis

Given this patient's symptoms and his history of dialysis, he most likely has constrictive pericarditis. Definitive diagnosis requires demonstration of a thickened pericardium and equalization of right and left heart pressures. Findings of elevated central pressures in the absence of other signs of congestive heart failure are very helpful. In contrast to cardiac tamponade, paradoxical pulse is present, and the Kussmaul sign can occasionally be seen. *(Answer: E—A and C)*

For more information, see Eagle KA, Armstrong WF: 1 Cardiovascular Medicine: XII Diseases of the Aorta. ACP Medicine Online (www.acpmedicine.com). Dale DC, Federman DD, Eds. WebMD Inc., New York, November 2003

Congenital Heart Disease

68. A 26-year-old woman is being evaluated for dyspnea, which she experiences when she engages in physical activity. She has been having these symptoms for the past 4 months. She denies having chest pain, orthopnea, or paroxysmal nocturnal dyspnea. The patient's medical history is significant for her having one episode of atrial fibrillation 1 month ago. Her physical examination shows fixed splitting of S_2 and a 2/6 systolic murmur in the pulmonic area. An electrocardiogram shows mild right axis deviation and an rSR′ pattern in V1. A chest x-ray reveals an enlarged right atrium and main pulmonary artery.

Which of the following is the most likely diagnosis for this patient?

- ❑ **A. Atrioventricular septal defect (AVSD)**
- ❑ **B. Ostium secundum atrial septal defect (ASD)**
- ❑ **C. Ventricular septal defect (VSD)**
- ❑ **D. Dextrotransposition of the great arteries**

Key Concept/Objective: To be able to recognize an ASD

ASDs occur in three main locations: the region of the fossa ovalis (such defects are termed ostium secundum ASDs); the superior portion of the atrial septum (sinus venosus ASDs); and the inferior portion of the atrial septum near the tricuspid valve annulus (ostium primum ASDs). The last two are considered to be part of the spectrum of AVSDs. Ostium secundum ASDs are the most common variety, accounting for over half of ASDs. Most patients with ostium secundum ASDs are asymptomatic through young adulthood. As the patient reaches middle age, compliance of the left ventricle may decrease, increasing the magnitude of left-to-right shunting. Long-standing atrial dilatation may lead to a variety of atrial arrhythmias, including atrial fibrillation. A substantial number of middle-aged patients report dyspnea. The hallmark of the physical examination in ASD is the wide and fixed splitting of the second heart sound. A systolic murmur (from increased pulmonary flow) is common. On electrocardiography, the QRS axis is usually normal in patients with ostium secundum ASD but may be slightly rightward, and an rSR′ pattern is common in the right precordial leads. The chest x-ray reveals an enlarged right atrium, right ventricle, and main pulmonary artery. The diagnosis is confirmed by echocardiography. AVSDs include a complex spectrum of disorders involving abnormalities of the atrioventricular septum and, frequently, the atrioventricular valves. Patients with AVSDs can present with symptoms and physical findings similar to patients with ostium secundum ASD. An additional pansystolic murmur can be found in patients with a complete AVSD. Left axis deviation is present in the majority of patients with AVSD; in contrast, right axis deviation is found in patients with ostium secundum ASD. The classic physical finding of a VSD is a harsh pansystolic murmur, heard best at the left lower sternal border. Electrocardiography may be normal or show evidence of left ventricular hypertrophy and a pattern of diastolic overload. Dextrotransposition of the great arteries is a cyanotic congenital cardiopathy. Survival beyond the first year without surgical repair is uncommon. *(Answer: B—Ostium secundum atrial septal defect [ASD])*

69. A 35-year-old man presents to a hospital with fatigue and fever of 3 weeks' duration. He denies having chest pain, dyspnea, or orthopnea. When giving his medical history, he reports that he has had a "heart murmur" since birth. On physical examination, the patient is found to have a temperature of 101° F (38.3° C); a 3/6 harsh murmur is heard in the left lower sternal border; and the presence of small, tender nodules are noted on two fingers. These are the only abnormal findings on physical examination.

Which of the following cardiac anomalies is most consistent with this patient's clinical presentation?

- ❑ **A. Ostium primum ASD**
- ❑ **B. Patent ductus arteriosus (PDA)**
- ❑ **C. Eisenmenger syndrome**
- ❑ **D. VSD**

Key Concept/Objective: To be able to recognize VSD

This patient has had an asymptomatic heart murmur for a long time, and he now presents with symptoms and signs consistent with infectious endocarditis. VSDs are among the most common congenital cardiac disorders seen at birth but are less frequently seen as isolated lesions in adulthood. This is because most VSDs in infants either are large and lead to heart failure, necessitating early surgical closure, or are small and close spontaneously. With the exception of patients who contract infective endocarditis or those with Eisenmenger syndrome, adults with VSD are asymptomatic. The classic physical finding of VSD is a harsh, frequently palpable, pansystolic murmur heard best at the left lower sternal border. Echocardiography is the procedure of choice for determining the location, size, and hemodynamic significance of a VSD. ASDs are characterized by the presence of wide and fixed splitting of the second heart sound. The murmur seen in PDA is a continuous murmur. Eisenmenger syndrome is a serious complication of long-standing left-to-right shunts, in which severe, irreversible pulmonary hypertension develops. The presence of cyanosis is characteristic; symptoms such as dyspnea and chest discomfort can be seen. *(Answer: D—VSD)*

70. A 40-year-old man comes to your office as a new patient to establish primary care. He is asymptomatic. His physical examination reveals an early systolic click and a 2/6 murmur in the aortic area. An ECG is normal. An echocardiogram shows a bicuspid aortic valve without significant flow obstruction. His ventricle size and function are normal.

Which of the following is the most appropriate therapeutic intervention for this patient at this time?

- ❑ A. **Instructions about endocarditis prophylaxis**
- ❑ B. **Aortic valve replacement**
- ❑ C. **Balloon valvuloplasty**
- ❑ D. **No intervention is required**

Key Concept/Objective: To understand the treatment of a bicuspid aortic valve

As much as 2% of the population have congenitally bicuspid aortic valves. A bicuspid aortic valve may present as an incidental finding on physical examination or echocardiography done for other reasons; as significant aortic stenosis (AS); as regurgitation; or as infective endocarditis. On physical examination, the cardinal sign of a bicuspid aortic valve is an early systolic ejection click. If no significant hemodynamic abnormality is present, either no murmur or a soft ejection murmur may be heard; a very mild murmur of aortic regurgitation (AR) is not uncommon, even with hemodynamically insignificant bicuspid aortic valves. AS or AR from any other cause will produce similar findings. Both the presence of a bicuspid aortic valve and its hemodynamic significance can be determined by echocardiography. Serial studies are useful in following the progression of the lesion. All patients with bicuspid aortic valves—even those with no significant stenosis or regurgitation should be given instructions regarding endocarditis prophylaxis. Patients with AR from a bicuspid valve who are asymptomatic and have normal systolic function are followed with echocardiograms and physical examinations at regular intervals. If they begin to show decreasing systolic function, symptoms of heart failure, or progressive dilation of the left ventricle, surgical replacement of the aortic valve is indicated. *(Answer: A—Instructions about endocarditis prophylaxis)*

71. A 15-year-old girl is being evaluated for a heart murmur. She is asymptomatic. On physical examination, her blood pressure is 174/104 mm Hg on her right arm. Her pulses are 2+ on her upper extremities. The femoral pulses are slightly lower in amplitude than the radial pulses. Her cardiac examination reveals a short midsystolic murmur in the left infrascapular area.

For this patient, which of the following is most likely to be found on additional studies?

- ❑ A. **Downward displacement of the tricuspid valve annulus toward the right ventricle apex on echocardiogram**
- ❑ B. **Stenotic pulmonic valve on echocardiogram**
- ❑ C. **Rib notching and dilatation of the aorta on chest x-ray**

❑ **D. Cardiomegaly and pulmonary engorgement on chest x-ray**

Key Concept/Objective: To be able to recognize aortic coarctation

In this patient, the findings on physical examination are consistent with coarctation of the aorta. Coarctation is a common cause of secondary hypertension. Although lower-extremity claudication may occur, patients are commonly asymptomatic. The cardinal feature on physical examination is the differences in pulses and blood pressures above the coarctation as compared to below the coarctation. In coarctation of the aorta, the femoral pulse will occur later than the radial pulse, and it is often lower in amplitude. Because of variations in anatomy, blood pressure should be evaluated in both arms and in either leg when evaluating for coarctation of the aorta. When the coarctation is distal to the origin of the left subclavian artery, both arms will be in the high-pressure zone and both legs in the low-pressure zone. However, some coarctations are proximal to the left subclavian. Thus, the left arm and both legs will be in the low-pressure zone, and the diagnosis may be missed if only the left arm is used for measuring blood pressure. In addition to differential blood pressures, physical examination may also reveal a murmur across the coarctation that can be best heard in the left infrascapular area. Dilatation of the aorta proximal and distal to the coarctation site may lead to a so-called 3 sign on chest x-ray. Rib notching is often present; this term refers to apparent effacement or so-called scalloping of the lower edges of ribs because of large, high-flow intercostal collateral vessels that develop as a compensatory mechanism to bypass the narrowing at the coarctation site. In patients with Ebstein anomaly, downward displacement of the tricuspid valve annulus toward the right ventricle apex is seen on echocardiogram. *(Answer: C—Rib notching and dilatation of the aorta on chest x-ray)*

72. A 32-year-old man presents to establish care. His medical history is unremarkable. On physical examination, the patient's blood pressure is 132/84 mm Hg, and his pulse is 88 beats/min. Cardiac examination reveals a soft systolic murmur, heard best at the left upper sternal border. The second heart sound is split and has no variability with respirations. There is no evidence of cyanosis.

What is the most likely diagnosis for this patient?

❑ **A. Coronary arteriovenous fistula**

❑ **B. Bicuspid aortic valve**

❑ **C. Ostium secundum defect**

❑ **D. Tetralogy of Fallot**

❑ **E. Pulmonary insufficiency**

Key Concept/Objective: To be able to recognize the presentation of ASD

This patient presents with a soft systolic murmur. The remarkable finding is that of a fixed-split second heart sound. This is seen in a number of clinical situations, related to either delayed closure of the pulmonary valve or early closure of the aortic valve. Delayed pulmonary valve can occur in ASD, right bundle branch block, pulmonary stenosis, pulmonary hypertension, and right ventricular failure. The aortic valve may close early in VSD or severe mitral insufficiency. The most common variant of the ASD is the ostium secundum. *(Answer: C—Ostium secundum defect)*

73. What would be the most appropriate initial diagnostic study for the patient in Question 72?

❑ **A. Left heart catheterization**

❑ **B. Transthoracic echocardiography**

❑ **C. Transesophageal echocardiography**

❑ **D. Cardiac MRI**

❑ **E. Right heart catheterization**

Key Concept/Objective: To understand the appropriate evaluation of ASD

The patient presented most likely has an ASD. The most appropriate initial test would be a transthoracic echocardiogram. If this test is not helpful, one might proceed to transesophageal echocardiography. Cardiac catheterization is reserved for situations in which ventricular failure, pulmonary hypertension, or both are clinically likely. *(Answer: B—Transthoracic echocardiography)*

74. A 23-year-old woman with Down syndrome (trisomy 21) presents to establish care. In general, she appears comfortable. There is no evidence of cyanosis. Her cardiac examination reveals a soft systolic murmur with a midsystolic click. The clinical diagnosis of mitral valve prolapse is made. The patient's mother wonders if there are any other cardiac issues.

Which congenital heart anomaly is this patient most likely to have?

- ❑ A. **Ostium primum defect**
- ❑ B. **PDA**
- ❑ C. **Tetralogy of Fallot**
- ❑ D. **Pulmonary stenosis**
- ❑ E. **Transposition of great vessels**

Key Concept/Objective: To be able to recognize cardiac manifestations of Down syndrome

Patients with Down syndrome have roughly a 40% chance of congenital cardiac anomalies. The most common are the endocardial cushion defects (especially ostium primum defects). They are also at risk for AR, tetralogy of Fallot, and pulmonary hypertension. Tetralogy of Fallot is much less common than the endocardial cushion defects. Interestingly, these patients are also at increased risk for mitral valve prolapse. *(Answer: A—Ostium primum defect)*

75. A 54-year-old man has been referred to you by a local dentist. He states that he has been told that he has a heart murmur, and the dentist recommended evaluation before planned dental extractions. On examination, the patient is found to have a III/VI systolic murmur along the right upper sternal border. Carotid upstroke is brisk. Transthoracic echocardiography reveals a bicuspid aortic valve. No allergies are noted.

What is the most appropriate action to take next for this patient?

- ❑ A. **No prophylaxis is necessary**
- ❑ B. **Prophylaxis with ceftriaxone, 1 g I.M. 1 hour before procedure**
- ❑ C. **Prophylaxis with azithromycin, 1 g p.o. 1 hour before procedure**
- ❑ D. **Prophylaxis with vancomycin, 1 g I.V. 1 hour before procedure**
- ❑ E. **Prophylaxis with amoxicillin, 2 g p.o. 1 hour before procedure**

Key Concept/Objective: To understand the appropriate use of prophylactic antibiotics

According to the most recent American Heart Association (AHA) recommendations, this patient is a candidate for prophylactic antibiotics, preferably amoxicillin. Most congenital cardiac malformations are deemed to be in the moderate-risk category. Complex cyanotic congenital anomalies are considered high risk (along with prosthetic valves and previous history of endocarditis). The exceptions, in which prophylaxis is not recommended, include isolated secundum ASD, surgical repairs of septal defects (both atrial and ventricular), and PDA. Refer to the AHA guidelines for full details on antibiotic choices and indications. *(Answer: E—Prophylaxis with amoxicillin, 2 g p.o. 1 hour before procedure)*

76. A 19-year-old woman presents with complaint of dyspnea on exertion and mild fatigue. She has no significant medical history. She does not use tobacco. She is on no regular medications. On examination, her lungs are clear. Cardiac examination reveals a II/VI systolic murmur at the second left intercostal space, which varies with inspiration.

What is the most likely diagnosis for this patient?

- ❑ A. **Pulmonary stenosis**
- ❑ B. **ASD**
- ❑ C. **VSD**
- ❑ D. **Bicuspid aortic valve**
- ❑ E. **Idiopathic hypertrophic subaortic stenosis**

Key Concept/Objective: To be able to recognize the clinical presentation of pulmonary stenosis

This patient presents with a systolic murmur that varies with respiration. This makes it likely that the etiology is right sided. Given the location, pulmonary stenosis is more likely than tricuspid regurgitation. These murmurs vary with respiration because filling of the right heart is significantly affected by inspiration (as blood is returning from outside the chest and is therefore influenced by the negative thoracic pressure). Treatment for this disorder is most commonly done via transcatheter balloon dilatation. *(Answer: A—Pulmonary stenosis)*

For more information, see Mahoney LT, Skorton DJ: 1 Cardiovascular Medicine: XV Congenital Heart Disease. ACP Medicine Online (www.acpmedicine.com). Dale DC, Federman DD, Eds. WebMD Inc., New York, October 2003

Peripheral Arterial Disease

77. A 35-year-old man with a history of superficial thrombophlebitis and bronchitis reports with bilateral foot pain of two days' duration. Over the past year, he has had several episodes of severe burning pain involving the foot arches and several toes. On a scale of 1 to 10, the severity of the pain is 7 to 9, and the pain persists both at rest and with ambulation. The patient smokes one to two packs of cigarettes a day, drinks one or two beers daily, and uses no illicit drugs. On examination, he is slender; his feet are red and cold, and there are ulcerations around the margins of several toenails. The femoral pulses are intact, and the dorsalis pedis and posterior tibialis pulses are absent bilaterally. The pain is not worsened by deep palpation. Microscopic capillaroscopy is negative for dilated capillaries.

What is the most likely diagnosis for this patient?

- ❑ A. **Plantar fasciitis**
- ❑ B. **Spinal stenosis**
- ❑ C. **Raynaud phenomenon**
- ❑ D. **Atherosclerotic claudication**
- ❑ E. **Thromboangiitis obliterans**

Key Concept/Objective: To know the features of thromboangiitis obliterans and to be able to distinguish this disorder from other diseases in the differential diagnosis of foot pain

Thromboangiitis obliterans (also called Buerger disease) causes inflammatory blockage of arterioles in the distal extremities and is seen in male smokers who are less than 40 years of age. Other typical features include a history of recurrent thrombophlebitis, rest pain, and findings of dependent rubor and an absence of distal pulses. Plantar fasciitis is usually not painful when the patient is at rest; it is exacerbated by weight bearing and deep palpation on examination and is not accompanied by loss of distal pulses. Spinal stenosis usually occurs in older patients and presents as lower extremity pain that is exacerbated by standing or walking and is relieved by rest. Atherosclerotic claudication is also seen in older patients. It follows a steadily progressive course, beginning with exercise-induced pain and progressing slowly (over months to years) to pain at rest. In addition, larger, more proximal vessels are usually affected, with corresponding exercise-induced pain in the buttocks, thighs, or calves. Raynaud phenomenon is seen mostly in women; it is caused by vasospasm of small arterioles, more often in the hands than in the feet. The vasospasm is

precipitated by cold or stress and causes sequential color changes in the digits from white to blue to red. These changes in color may be accompanied by a sensation of cold, numbness, or paresthesias but usually not severe pain. Peripheral pulses usually remain intact even during episodes of vasospasm. *(Answer: E—Thromboangiitis obliterans)*

78. A 63-year-old woman with a history of obesity, diabetes, hypertension, hyperlipidemia, and severe hip arthritis is found to have a foot ulcer. She does not know how long it has been present but reports nocturnal foot pain of several months' duration that improves when she dangles her foot over the edge of the bed. She denies having fever or leg swelling. On examination, an ulcer 2 cm in diameter is seen under the first metatarsal head of her left foot; the base of the ulcer is necrotic, and there is no visible granulation tissue. As the patient sits in the clinic chair, her distal extremities are seen to be a deep red, and the skin of the distal extremities is smooth and thin, without hair. She is able to detect a monofilament on sensory examination of the feet. The dorsalis pedis and posterior tibialis pulses cannot be palpated. Her ankle brachial index is 0.35.

What is the most likely cause of this patient's foot ulcer?

- ❑ **A. Diabetic neuropathy**
- ❑ **B. Venous stasis**
- ❑ **C. Vasculitis**
- ❑ **D. Arterial insufficiency**
- ❑ **E. Pyoderma gangrenosum**

Key Concept/Objective: To be able to recognize ulceration associated with arterial insufficiency

The findings of rest pain that worsens when the patient is in the horizontal position and an ankle brachial index of less than 0.4 suggest severe arterial insufficiency. Loss of distal pulses and trophic skin changes, such as loss of subcutaneous tissue and hair, are also suggestive of arterial insufficiency. In patients with arterial insufficiency, ulcers commonly occur on the feet, particularly in weight-bearing areas or at sites of trauma. These areas include the area under the metatarsal heads, the ends of toes and the area between the toes, and the heel. Diabetic nephropathy also can lead to ulceration in these areas, although in patients with diabetic nephropathy, the foot is usually insensate, and therefore such patients are unable to detect a monofilament on examination. Ulcers that result from venous stasis are usually associated with edema, skin thickening, and hyperpigmentation or erythema. The base of these ulcers usually contains red, bumpy granulation tissue. Vasculitic ulcers are often associated with systemic signs of disease. With vasculitic ulcers, livedo reticularis may be present on the legs and trunk; there is no loss of distal pulses, nor would vasculitis lower the ankle brachial index. Pyoderma gangrenosum is usually seen on the anterior calf. Onset is abrupt. Pyoderma gangrenosum ulcers have a violet undermined edge, a ragged heaped-up border, and a surrounding red halo. Pyoderma gangrenosum is not associated with loss of distal pulses nor with an altered ankle brachial index. *(Answer: D—Arterial insufficiency)*

79. A 63-year-old woman with diet-controlled diabetes, hypertension, and a 45-pack-year history of cigarette smoking has intermittent left leg claudication and exercise-induced calf pain, which occurs when she walks three to four blocks. Her ankle brachial index is 0.7.

The patient is most likely to experience which of the following adverse health outcomes in the next 5 years?

- ❑ **A. Myocardial infarction**
- ❑ **B. Hypoglycemic event**
- ❑ **C. Limb amputation**
- ❑ **D. Ischemic limb**
- ❑ **E. Lung cancer**

Key Concept/Objective: To understand the high risk of coronary disease in patients with atherosclerotic claudication

This woman most likely has atherosclerotic peripheral arterial occlusive disease. She has multiple risk factors for this disorder (hypertension, a history of cigarette smoking, and diabetes), she experiences exercise-induced claudication, and her ankle-brachial index is low. Most patients with peripheral vascular atherosclerosis also have coronary atherosclerosis; mortality in patients with peripheral vascular disease is usually caused by myocardial infarction or stroke. This patient's risk of myocardial infarction far outweighs her risk of developing limb ischemia or of requiring limb amputation. Although the risk of lung cancer is 10-fold higher in cigarette smokers than in nonsmokers, this patient is less still likely to develop lung cancer than myocardial infarction: annual deaths from myocardial infarction attributable to smoking are estimated at 170,000, whereas deaths from lung cancer that are attributable to smoking number 100,000. Moreover, this patient's coronary risk factors would place her more at risk than would be indicated by these statistics. Because this patient does not use hypoglycemic agents, she is unlikely to experience hypoglycemia. Although 2% to 4% of patients with intermittent claudication develop critical limb ischemia annually, death and morbidity from myocardial infarction are much more likely. *(Answer: A—Myocardial infarction)*

80. A 45-year-old woman is receiving enoxaparin and warfarin for deep vein thrombosis (DVT) of the right thigh, which developed after she underwent an abdominal hysterectomy 3 weeks ago. On day 5 of treatment, she reports abrupt onset of pain in her left leg. On examination, her blood pressure is 150/90 mm Hg; she has a regular heart rate of 95 beats/min without murmur; and she has lower extremity petechiae. Her left foot is pale, pulseless, and cold, and there is an absence of sensation. Results of laboratory testing are as follows: prothrombin time, 45; INR for prothrombin time, 2.0; platelets, 15; and hematocrit, 36.

Which of the following changes in this patient's medication regimen should be made next?

- ❑ **A. Increase the heparin dose**
- ❑ **B. Increase the warfarin dose**
- ❑ **C. Administer tissue plasminogen activator**
- ❑ **D. Discontinue heparin therapy**
- ❑ **E. Discontinue warfarin therapy**

Key Concept/Objective: To be able to recognize heparin-induced thrombocytopenia and associated acute arterial thrombosis and to understand that heparin must be discontinued immediately in patients with this condition

This patient is experiencing an acute arterial occlusion. Given her heparin use and her low platelet count, heparin-induced thrombocytopenia is the likely diagnosis. Discontinuance of heparin therapy as soon as possible is key in reversing this antibody-mediated process. Increasing the heparin dose or even continued exposure to low doses of heparin (as through heparin I.V. catheter flushes) will worsen, not improve, the arterial clotting and thrombocytopenia. Although therapy with catheter-directed tissue plasminogen activator (t-PA) is used for acute arterial occlusion in many cases, this patient's recent abdominal surgery is an absolute contraindication to t-PA therapy. This patient's low platelet count and her use of oral warfarin are relative contraindications to the use of thrombolytic therapy. She needs continued anticoagulation for her DVT and new arterial thrombus; therefore, warfarin should be continued at its currently therapeutic dosage. *(Answer: D—Discontinue heparin therapy)*

For more information, see Creager MA: 1 Cardiovascular Medicine: XVI Peripheral Arterial Disease. ACP Medicine Online (www.acpmedicine.com). Dale DC, Federman DD, Eds. WebMD Inc., New York, July 2001

Venous Thromboembolism

81. A 44-year-old man presents to your office complaining of right leg pain and swelling of 3 days' duration. The patient was well until he had a wreck while riding his dirt bike 1 week ago. The patient states that he injured his right leg in this accident. Initially, his leg was moderately sore on weight bearing, but swelling and persistent pain have now developed. On physical examination, you note an extensive bruise on the patient's right calf and 2+ edema from the foot to the midthigh. You suspect trauma-associated deep vein thrombosis (DVT).

Which of the following statements regarding DVT is true?

❑ A. **Thrombi confined to the calf are large and typically result in pulmonary venous thromboembolism (VTE)**

❑ B. **The postthrombotic syndrome is a rare sequela of DVT and is associated with low morbidity**

❑ C. **Most patients presenting with a new DVT have an underlying inherited thrombophilia**

❑ D. **The most common cause of inherited thrombophilia associated with this illness is activated protein C resistance (factor V Leiden)**

Key Concept/Objective: To understand the general features of DVT

Seventy percent of patients with symptomatic pulmonary embolism have DVT, which is usually clinically silent. Thrombi confined to calf veins are usually small and are rarely associated with pulmonary embolism. An inherited thrombophilic defect known as activated protein C resistance, or factor V Leiden, has now been established as the most common cause of inherited thrombophilia, occurring in about 5% of whites who do not have a family history of venous thrombosis and in about 20% of patients with a first episode of venous thrombosis. The second most common thrombophilic defect is a mutation (G20210A) in the 3′ untranslated region of the prothrombin gene that results in about a 25% increase in prothrombin levels. This mutation is found in about 2% of whites who have no family history of venous thrombosis and in about 5% of patients with a first episode of venous thrombosis. Elevated levels of clotting factors VIII and XI and of homocysteine also predispose patients to thrombosis. Although inherited thrombophilia is a well-described and important cause of venous thrombosis, the large majority of patients with venous thrombosis do not have an inherited thrombophilia. The postthrombotic syndrome occurs as a long-term complication in about 25% (and is severe in about 10%) of patients with symptomatic proximal vein thrombosis in the 8 years after the acute event, with most cases developing within 2 years. Clinically, the postthrombotic syndrome may mimic acute venous thrombosis but typically presents as chronic leg pain that is associated with edema and that worsens at the end of the day. Some patients also have stasis pigmentation, induration, and skin ulceration; a smaller number of patients have venous claudication on walking, caused by persistent obstruction of the iliac veins. *(Answer: D—The most common cause of inherited thrombophilia associated with this illness is activated protein C resistance [factor V Leiden])*

82. A 43-year-old man presents to the emergency department complaining of chest pain of 2 hours' duration. The patient denies having any dyspnea. He has no significant medical history, nor does he have a family history of early coronary artery disease. He is a nonsmoker and an avid jogger. His chest pain is constant, is pleuritic, and does not radiate. His chest x-ray is clear, and his ECG reveals only sinus tachycardia. Blood gas measurements reveal a partial pressure of oxygen (Po_2) of 58 mm Hg with a widened alveolar-arterial difference in oxygen ($A\text{-}aDo_2$). Helical CT reveals segmental and subsegmental filling defects in the right lung.

Which of the following statements regarding anticoagulation and thrombolysis for thromboembolism is true?

❑ A. **When using unfractionated heparin, the therapeutic range for the activated partial thromboplastin time (aPTT) is 2.5 to 3.5 times the normal value**

❑ B. **Low-molecular-weight heparin (LMWH) is safe and effective for the treatment of pulmonary thromboembolism**

❑ C. **Because of a delay in achieving a therapeutic INR with lower doses, a starting dose of warfarin should be no less than 10 mg**

❑ D. In contrast to other thrombolytic agents, recombinant tissue plasminogen activator (rt-PA) stimulates antibody production and can induce allergic reactions

Key Concept/Objective: To understand individual therapies for pulmonary thromboembolism

When using unfractionated heparin, the dose should be adjusted as necessary to achieve a therapeutic range, which for many aPTT reagents corresponds to an aPTT ratio of 1.5 to 2.5. The published research on LMWHs, which includes over 3,000 patients treated with either once-daily or twice-daily subcutaneous doses, has established this class of anticoagulants as being safe, effective, and convenient for treating venous thrombosis and pulmonary embolism. Evidence indicates that it might be safer to use a starting dose of 5 mg of warfarin because, compared with 10 mg, the 5 mg starting dose does not result in a delay in achieving a therapeutic INR and is associated with a lower incidence of supratherapeutic INR values during the first 5 days of treatment. Because streptokinase is a bacterial product, it stimulates antibody production and can prompt allergic reactions. Antistreptococcal antibodies, which are present in variable titers in most patients before streptokinase treatment, induce an amnestic response that makes repeated treatment with streptokinase difficult or impossible for a period of months or years after an initial course of treatment. *(Answer: B—Low-molecular-weight heparin [LMWH] is safe and effective for the treatment of pulmonary thromboembolism)*

83. A 72-year-old man presents to the hospital with a hip fracture. An orthopedist is planning surgical repair and asks you to see the patient in consultation for preoperative assessment and advice. In particular, the orthopedist asks you to assess the patient's need for prophylaxis against venous thrombosis and to comment on the best prophylactic regimen for the patient.

Which of the following statements regarding primary prophylaxis against venous thrombosis and thromboembolism is true?

❑ A. Oral anticoagulation is the method of choice for moderate-risk general surgical and medical patients

❑ B. Prophylactic therapy should typically be discontinued at the time of discharge for patients who have undergone major orthopedic surgery

❑ C. LMWH is more effective than standard low-dose heparin in patients undergoing elective hip surgery

❑ D. For patients undergoing genitourinary, neurologic, or ocular surgery, the most appropriate method of prophylaxis is oral anticoagulation

Key Concept/Objective: To know the correct methods of prophylaxis for venous thrombosis and thromboembolism in medical and surgical patients

Low-dose-heparin prophylaxis is the method of choice for moderate-risk general surgical and medical patients. It reduces the risk of VTE by 50% to 70% and is simple, inexpensive, convenient, and safe. Extended prophylaxis with LWMH or warfarin for an additional 3 weeks after hospital discharge should be considered after major orthopedic surgery. Extended prophylaxis is strongly recommended for high-risk patients (e.g., those with previous VTE or active cancer). LMWH is more effective than standard low-dose heparin in general surgical patients, patients undergoing elective hip surgery, and patients with stroke or spinal injury. For those undergoing genitourinary, neurologic, or ocular surgery, intermittent pneumatic compression, with or without graduated compression stockings, is effective prophylaxis against venous thrombosis and does not increase the risk of bleeding. *(Answer: C—LMWH is more effective than standard low-dose heparin in patients undergoing elective hip surgery)*

84. An 80-year-old patient of yours is scheduled to undergo total knee replacement. He is in excellent health, and except for osteoarthritis, his medical history is not significant. The orthopedic surgeon asks you for advice regarding VTE prophylaxis.

What would you advise for this patient?

- ❑ **A. LMWH is contraindicated because of the risk of bleeding; intermittent pneumatic compression devices would be preferable**
- ❑ **B. Intermittent pneumatic compression devices are contraindicated because of the location of the surgery; LMWH is preferable**
- ❑ **C. Aspirin, 325 mg q.d., should be started immediately after surgery**
- ❑ **D. LMWH and intermittent pneumatic compression devices are equally effective in preventing VTE after knee surgery**
- ❑ **E. The risk of VTE after knee replacement is so low as to make prophylax-is unnecessary**

Key Concept/Objective: To know the prophylaxis for DVT after knee-replacement surgery

LMWH and intermittent pneumatic compression devices have been shown to be equally effective in preventing DVT after knee-replacement surgery. Aspirin has been shown to decrease the risk of DVT after hip fracture, but its efficacy relative to LMWH or intermittent pneumatic compression devices has never been studied, and the standard of care for postoperative DVT prophylaxis in North America does not call for its use. After knee-replacement surgery, the risk of postoperative DVT is 10% to 20%, and the rate of fatal pulmonary embolism is 1% to 5%, so prophylaxis is indicated. Prophylaxis is also cost-effective. *(Answer: D—LMWH and intermittent pneumatic compression devices are equally effective in preventing VTE after knee surgery)*

85. A 28-year-old woman who is 18 weeks pregnant and is G1P0 is referred to you by her obstetrician for advice regarding management of a possible VTE diathesis. Although she has no personal history of VTE, she reports that her mother and a cousin both had blood clots during pregnancy; she does not know whether they were tested for clotting disorders. She is feeling well, and her physical examination is remarkable only for her pregnancy.

Which of the following actions would you take for this patient?

- ❑ **A. Educate her about the symptoms of VTE and advise her to seek care immediately if she notes one of them; otherwise, no further testing or treatment is necessary**
- ❑ **B. Start warfarin therapy with a target INR of 2 to 3**
- ❑ **C. Start LMWH, 100 anti-10a U/kg subcutaneously q.d.**
- ❑ **D. Start aspirin therapy, 325 mg q.d.**
- ❑ **E. Test for antithrombin-III deficiency; if she has the deficiency, start LMWH therapy**

Key Concept/Objective: To understand the management of inherited thrombophilias in pregnancy

It is possible that this woman has an inherited thrombophilia. Pregnant women with antithrombin-III deficiency have an especially high rate of VTE. If this patient tests positive, she should receive prophylactic anticoagulation therapy throughout the rest of her pregnancy. The benefits of prophylactic anticoagulation in pregnant women with protein C or protein S deficiency outweigh the risks only if they have a history of VTE. Because this patient has never had VTE, the results of testing her for these disorders would not lead to a change in management. In pregnant women with factor V Leiden mutation or G20210A prothrombin mutation, no anticoagulation therapy is recommended unless they develop a clot during the current pregnancy. In any case, LMWH is preferable to warfarin therapy because of the teratogenic effects of warfarin. Aspirin does not provide effective anticoagulation therapy for VTE. Although this woman should be educated about the signs and symptoms of VTE, this alone is not sufficient. *(Answer: E—Test for antithrombin-III deficiency; if she has the deficiency, start LMWH therapy)*

For more information, see Kearon C, Hirsch J: 1 Cardiovascular Medicine: XVIII Venous Thromboembolism. ACP Medicine Online (www.acpmedicine.com). Dale DC, Federman DD, Eds. WebMD Inc., New York, December 2003

SECTION 2

DERMATOLOGY

Cutaneous Manifestations of Systemic Diseases

1. A 56-year-old white man presents to you in clinic complaining of increasing shortness of breath. His symptom began several months ago and has gotten progressively worse over time. It is primarily exertional. On further review of systems, he reports chronic sinusitis, some fatigue, and a new nonpainful, nonpruritic rash on his lower extremities. His medical history is significant only for hypertension. On physical examination, you note nasal ulcerations and a mildly erythematous, papular rash with occasional nodules on his lower extremities. His pulmonary examination is notable for fine, bilateral crackles. Urine dipstick testing reveals proteinuria and hematuria. Among other tests, you order a blood test for cytoplasmic antineutrophil cytoplasmic antibodies (c-ANCA) and a chest x-ray. The chest x-ray reveals interstitial abnormalities bilaterally. A subsequent biopsy reveals a necrotizing granulomatous vasculitis. The c-ANCA is positive.

This patient's findings are most consistent with which of the following diagnoses?

- ❑ **A. Lymphomatoid granulomatosis**
- ❑ **B. Systemic lupus erythematosus (SLE)**
- ❑ **C. Wegener granulomatosis**
- ❑ **D. Churg-Strauss syndrome**

Key Concept/Objective: To know the clinical presentation of Wegener granulomatosis

Wegener granulomatosis is associated with both distinctive and nonspecific mucocutaneous signs. Palpable purpura is one of the most common skin findings, but ulcers, papules, nodules, and bullae have also been described. In addition to upper and lower pulmonary symptoms, saddle-nose deformity, nasal ulcerations, and septal perforation should suggest the diagnosis of Wegener granulomatosis. Definitive diagnosis is made by the demonstration of a necrotizing granulomatous vasculitis in a patient with upper and lower respiratory tract disease and glomerulonephritis. ANCA autoantibodies are often present. The absence of asthma makes the diagnosis of Churg-Strauss syndrome unlikely. Although SLE would explain the skin rash, the abnormal urine dipstick result, and the progressive shortness of breath, the presence of nasal ulcerations, ANCA autoantibodies, and necrotizing granulomatous vasculitis would not be explained by SLE. Patients with lymphomatoid granulomatosis present with a predominance of pulmonary and nervous system manifestations; tests for ANCA autoantibodies are usually negative. *(Answer: C—Wegener granulomatosis)*

2. A 48-year-old African-American man with a history of diabetes and hypertension presents to your clinic complaining of a rash on his leg. It has been present for several months and is progressively getting worse. His diabetes is poorly controlled; diabetic complications include both chronic renal insufficiency and retinopathy. On physical examination, you note an 8 cm atrophic patch with a yellow central area and enlarging erythematous borders.

This patient's symptoms are most consistent with which of the following cutaneous manifestations of diabetes?

- ❑ **A. Acanthosis nigricans**
- ❑ **B. Necrobiosis lipoidica**

❑ C. Scleroderma

❑ D. Erythrasma

Key Concept/Objective: To recognize necrobiosis lipoidica as a potential skin manifestation of diabetes

Necrobiosis lipoidica is a specific cutaneous manifestation of diabetes. Lesions consist of chronic atrophic patches with enlarging erythematous borders. The legs are most commonly affected. The center of lesions appears yellow because of subcutaneous fat that is visible through the atrophic dermis and epidermis. Occasionally, the lesions ulcerate. Necrobiosis lipoidica is often associated with diabetic nephropathy or retinopathy. Acanthosis nigricans has been reported in patients with insulin resistance syndrome; however, the lesions are velvety to the touch, are black in color, and are located predominantly in contact areas such as the axilla. Scleroderma causes subcutaneous infiltration of the skin, mostly in the trunk of patients with long-standing diabetes. Erythrasma is a fungal infection affecting the fifth intertriginous space. *(Answer: B—Necrobiosis lipoidica)*

3. A 29-year-old Japanese-American man comes to the emergency department complaining of a rash on his lower extremity. The rash began in a small area on his calf 1 day ago and has progressed rapidly. The patient has recently noticed erythematous streaks toward the groin. There is a large blisterlike lesion at the initial site. The patient also complains of fever and dizziness, which began a few hours ago. The patient's medical history is significant only for hemachromatosis. He has lived in the United States since he was 10 years old. He lives alone and works as a sushi chef at a local restaurant. On physical examination, the patient is ill appearing. His temperature is 102.5° F (39.2° C), his heart rate is 120 beats/min, and his blood pressure is 90/40 mm Hg. His left lower extremity is notable for hemorrhagic bullous lesions and erythema tracking into the groin, with inguinal lymphadenopathy.

Which of the following organisms is most likely responsible for this patient's condition?

❑ A ***Neisseria meningitidis***

❑ B. ***Staphylococcus aureus***

❑ C. ***Borrelia burgdorferi***

❑ D. ***Vibrio vulnificus***

Key Concept/Objective: To know the clinical presentation and risk factors for V. vulnificus infection

V. vulnificus **infection can present as two distinct clinical syndromes: one arises from minor trauma sustained while swimming in lakes or the ocean or while cleaning seafood. Cellulitis occurs, with lymphangitis and bacteremia. In patients with hepatic cirrhosis, a systemic infection can occur after eating raw oysters. These patients develop hemorrhagic bullae with leukopenia and disseminated intravascular coagulation (DIC). Other groups at risk for the systemic form of the disease are those with hemosiderosis, chronic alcohol abuse, and chronic liver disease other than cirrhosis.** ***B. burgdorferi*** **is the causative agent of Lyme disease; the characteristic rash is erythema chronicum migrans. The characteristic rash of** ***N. meningitidis*** **infection is petechiae, which in some patients progresses to purpura. Staphylococcal infections can produce bullous lesions, but these lesions are usually associated with severe cellulitis and are not usually hemorrhagic.** *(Answer: D—Vibrio vulnificus)*

4. A 37-year-old white woman presents to you in clinic complaining of skin changes. She notes that the changes began on her face and hands but that they are becoming widespread. She complains that her skin feels tight and is beginning to change the appearance of her face. Physical examination confirms her report, and you note pursed lips and bound-down skin on her nose, creating a beaklike appearance. You suspect scleroderma and order several laboratory tests for further workup.

In patients with progressive systemic sclerosis, the presence of antibodies to which of the following portends a poor prognosis?

❑ A. Scleroderma-70 (Scl-70)

❑ B. Anticentromere antibody

❑ C. Anti-Ro and anti-La

❑ D. Antiphospholipids

Key Concept/Objective: To understand the significance of antibodies to Scl-70 in a patient with scleroderma

Progressive systemic sclerosis, also known as systemic scleroderma, is a frequently fatal disease in which patients present with Raynaud phenomenon and sclerodactyly (induration of the skin of the digits). Cutaneous induration can become widespread. Involvement of the face can lead to a characteristic appearance with pursed lips and bound-down skin of the nose that creates a beaklike appearance. Patients with antibodies to Scl-70 have a poor prognosis, often succumbing to renal disease and malignant hypertension. Patients with anticentromere antibodies have a more slowly progressive variant of scleroderma known as the CREST syndrome, which is characterized by cutaneous calcinosis, Raynaud phenomenon, esophageal dysmotility, sclerodactyly, and telangiectasia; with time, pulmonary fibrosis, pulmonary hypertension, and right-sided heart failure develop. Anti-Ro and anti-La antibodies are more commonly associated with Sjögren syndrome and SLE. The presence of antiphospholipid antibodies are characterized clinically by recurrent venous and arterial thrombosis, recurrent fetal loss, and prolongation of partial thromboplastin time; these findings are most likely to be seen in patients with SLE. *(Answer: A—Scleroderma-70 [Scl-70])*

For more information, see Lebwohl M: 2 Dermatology: I Cutaneous Manifestations of Systemic Diseases. ACP Medicine Online (www.acpmedicine.com). Dale DC, Federman DD, Eds. WebMD Inc., New York, July 2003

Papulosquamous Disorders

5. A 24-year-old man comes to your office with complaints of a diffuse, mildly pruritic rash that developed over the past 1 to 2 weeks. Examination reveals a papular eruption involving the trunk and extremities. You suspect pityriasis rosea.

Which of the following statements regarding the clinical features of pityriasis rosea is false?

❑ A. Lesions typically occur on the trunk in a symmetrical fashion and form cleavage planes on the skin

❑ B. The development of a herald-patch lesion 7 to 10 days before the onset of the diffuse eruption helps establish the diagnosis

❑ C. Pityriasis rosea typically involves the palms and soles

❑ D. The disorder is usually self-limited

Key Concept/Objective: To understand the distinguishing features of pityriasis rosea

Pityriasis rosea is a self-limited, exanthematous disease that manifests as oval papulosquamous lesions typically distributed in a symmetrical fashion over the trunk and extremities. The exact etiology is unclear, but viral triggers have been suggested. The eruption is usually preceded by a primary lesion consisting of a slightly raised, salmon-colored oval patch with fine scaling (the "herald patch"). Lesions tend to follow lines of cleavage on the skin and may appear on the back in a typical "fir tree" or "Christmas tree" distribution. The differential diagnosis of pityriasis rosea lesions includes secondary syphilis, tinea corporis, and tinea versicolor. The appearance of lesions on the palms and soles is more typical of secondary syphilis and may help distinguish this rash from pityriasis rosea. If there is high suspicion of syphilis or if the diagnosis is unclear, a serologic test for syphilis is warranted. The lesions of pityriasis rosea typically resolve spontaneously in 6 to 8 weeks. *(Answer: C—Pityriasis rosea typically involves the palms and soles)*

6. ***For an otherwise healthy individual with typical pityriasis rosea, which of the following would NOT be an appropriate option for treating symptoms?***

- ❑ A. **Low-potency topical steroids for lesions on the trunk**
- ❑ B. **Oral antihistamines**
- ❑ C. **Oral erythromycin**
- ❑ D. **Use of ultraviolet B (UVB) or exposure to sunlight early in the course of the eruption**
- ❑ E. **Retinoic acid**

Key Concept/Objective: To understand the treatment options for pityriasis rosea

Pityriasis rosea is typically self-limited, but several treatment options exist. Foremost, patients should be reassured and educated about the benign nature of the disease. If pruritis is a prominent symptom, oral antihistamines are usually effective. Low-potency topical steroids have been shown to be of benefit. Exposure to ultraviolet light has been shown to shorten the duration of the eruption, especially if treatment is started within the first week of onset. A single trial demonstrated that a 14-day course of oral erythromycin was safe and led to complete resolution of the eruption within 2 weeks in a third of patients. Retinoic acid has not commonly been employed to treat pityriasis rosea. *(Answer: E—Retinoic acid)*

7. A 40-year-old man comes to clinic complaining of an itchy rash on his wrist and hands, which he first noted 3 weeks ago. He has a history of hypertension but has otherwise been healthy. Skin examination reveals several small, polygonal papules on the dorsa of both hands and on the flexor surface of the left wrist. A few of the wrist lesions appear in a linear distribution. You also notice a papular lesion on the buccal mucosa; a white, lacy pattern appears on the surface of the lesion.

Which of the following is the most likely diagnosis?

- ❑ A. **Psoriasis**
- ❑ B. **Lichen planus**
- ❑ C. **Tinea versicolor**
- ❑ D. **Pityriasis rosea**
- ❑ E. **Candidiasis**

Key Concept/Objective: To know the typical appearance of lichen planus

Lichen planus is a localized or generalized inflammatory mucocutaneous eruption consisting of violaceous, flat-topped, polygonal papules; it occurs most commonly in patients 30 to 60 years of age. The etiology is unknown, but a variety of drugs (e.g., beta blockers, methyldopa, and nonsteroidal anti-inflammatory drugs) have been reported to cause lichenoid reactions in the skin. Common sites of involvement include the flexor surfaces of the wrists, the dorsal surfaces of the hands, the sacrum, oral mucous membranes, and the genitalia. Mucous membrane lesions typically have a white, reticulated appearance on the papule surface (Wickham striae), which helps establish the diagnosis. Linear lesions that appear in areas of local skin trauma (the Koebner phenomenon) are also typical. Patients usually complain of mild itching. Over 50% of patients with cutaneous lesions experience involvement of the oral mucosa. This finding, along with the typical appearance and distribution of the lesions, helps distinguish it from the other conditions listed. Patients with acute lichen planus have a good prognosis, but the chronic form may last for several years. Treatment generally consists of emollients and topical steroids, but systemic steroids may also be of use. A corticosteroid in a vehicle that adheres to the mucosal surface (e.g., Orabase) is useful for treating mouth lesions. *(Answer: B—Lichen planus)*

8. A 59-year-old man with long-standing psoriasis has had a recent worsening of his disease. About 2 weeks ago, several new psoriatic lesions developed; this was followed by diffuse skin involvement with erythema and subsequent scaling. The patient complains of skin tightness, pruritus, fever, and malaise of 2 days' duration. You suspect an exfoliative erythroderma reaction.

Which of the following statements regarding this patient's condition is true?

- ❑ A. **The majority of cases are spontaneous and are not associated with an underlying skin condition or systemic illness**
- ❑ B. **Dehydration and high-output cardiac failure secondary to transepidermal water loss can occur**
- ❑ C. **Bacterial infection is the likely cause**
- ❑ D. **The condition most commonly occurs in females younger than 20 years**

Key Concept/Objective: To understand that erythroderma is a potentially serious generalized skin reaction that can occur in patients with underlying dermatologic or systemic disease

This patient has exfoliative erythroderma, which is a generalized scaling erythematous dermatitis involving all or almost all of the cutaneous surface. The condition most commonly occurs in patients with underlying dermatoses such as psoriasis, atopic dermatitis, drug eruptions, or contact dermatitis. It may occur in patients with other systemic illnesses, including lymphoma and leukemia. It most commonly occurs in patients older than 40 years and is twice as common in men than in women. In severe cases, hospitalization may be necessary to treat significant fluid losses that occur as a result of disruption of the skin barrier. Treatment includes restoration of fluid and electrolytes and prevention of large, insensible fluid losses through the skin. Wet dressings applied over intermediate-strength topical steroid preparations are useful. Although infection is not the primary cause of the disorder, there is substantial risk of secondary skin infection, which may warrant the use of systemic antibiotics. *(Answer: B—Dehydration and high-output cardiac failure secondary to transepidermal water loss can occur)*

For more information, see Abel EA: 2 Dermatology: II Papulosquamous Disorders. ACP Medicine Online (www.acpmedicine.com). Dale DC, Federman DD, Eds. WebMD Inc., New York, June 2002

Psoriasis

9. A 26-year-old woman presents to your primary care clinic for the evaluation of a rash. The patient has no significant medical history and is not taking any medications. The family history is unrevealing. Physical examination reveals sharply demarcated, erythematous scaling plaques at both elbows and knees. Examination of the fingernails reveals groups of tiny pits. A presumptive diagnosis of psoriasis is made.

Which of the following statements regarding the epidemiology of psoriasis is accurate?

- ❑ A. **Psoriasis occurs more commonly in women than in men**
- ❑ B. **On average, onset of psoriasis occurs during the fifth decade**
- ❑ C. **In northern latitudes, exacerbations of psoriasis commonly occur during the spring and summer**
- ❑ D. **In persons with earlier age of onset, psoriasis is more likely to be severe**

Key Concept/Objective: To understand the epidemiology of psoriasis

The estimated prevalence of psoriasis ranges from 0.5% to 4.6% worldwide. The reasons for the geographic variation in prevalence are unknown, but climatic factors and genetics may play a role. On the basis of a survey mailed to 50,000 households, the prevalence in the United States is estimated to be 2.6%. Psoriasis can occur in patients of any age, with some cases being reported at birth and others being reported in patients older than 100 years. The average age of onset is 23 years in the United States. Psoriasis occurs with equal frequency in men and women. In populations in which there is a high prevalence of psoriasis, onset tends to occur at an earlier age. In persons with earlier age of onset, psoriasis is more likely to be severe, with involvement of a large area of skin surface. It has long been known that psoriasis improves when patients are exposed to sunny climates and to regions of lower latitude. In northern latitudes, exacerbation of psoriasis commonly occurs during

the fall and winter. *(Answer: D—In persons with earlier age of onset, psoriasis is more likely to be severe)*

10. An 18-year-old college student presents to the student health clinic for evaluation of a rash. The patient was recently evaluated for sore throat and diagnosed with streptococcal pharyngitis. Physical examination reveals small, scaling erythematous papules on the trunk and bilateral extremities.

This patient's clinical presentation is most consistent with which clinical variant of psoriasis?

❑ **A. Plaque-type**

❑ **B. Guttate**

❑ **C. Erythrodermic**

❑ **D. Pustular**

Key Concept/Objective: To be able to differentiate among the clinical variants of psoriasis

Nearly 90% of psoriasis patients have plaque-type psoriasis, a form that is characterized by sharply demarcated, erythematous scaling plaques. The elbows, knees, and scalp are the most commonly affected sites. The intergluteal cleft, palms, soles, and genitals are also commonly affected, but psoriasis can involve any part of the body. Lesions frequently occur in a symmetrical pattern of distribution. Many patients have only one or a few lesions that persist for years and that occasionally resolve after exposure to sunlight. Other patients can be covered with plaques that become confluent, affecting nearly 100% of the body surface area. Nail involvement is common, particularly in patients with severe disease. The second most common form of psoriasis, guttate psoriasis, affects fewer than 10% of patients and is characterized by the development of small, scaling erythematous papules on the trunk and extremities. This form of psoriasis often occurs after streptococcal infection. Patients with plaque-type psoriasis can develop guttate psoriasis. Conversely, patients with guttate psoriasis frequently develop plaque-type psoriasis.

Erythrodermic psoriasis is a severe form of psoriasis that often affects the entire cutaneous surface. Patients present with an exfoliative erythroderma in which the skin is very red and inflamed and is constantly scaling. Patients are acutely ill, their skin having lost all protective function. Loss of temperature control, loss of fluids and nutrients through the impaired skin, and susceptibility to infection make this a life-threatening condition. Some patients present with erythrodermic psoriasis de novo; others develop erythrodermic psoriasis after having typical plaque-type or guttate psoriasis. Erythrodermic psoriasis can occur after withdrawal of systemic corticosteroids, after phototherapy burns, as a result of antimalarial treatment, as a result of a drug-induced hypersensitivity reaction, or for no apparent reason. Erythrodermic psoriasis has been associated with cutaneous T cell lymphoma.

Pustular psoriasis, another severe form of the disease, can occur in patients with preexisting psoriasis or it can arise de novo. Pustular psoriasis can be generalized (von Zumbusch-type) or localized to the palms and soles. In either case, the condition is severe and debilitating. In generalized pustular psoriasis, the body is covered with sterile pustules. As with erythrodermic psoriasis, the protective functions of the skin are lost, and patients may succumb to infection or hypovolemia and electrolyte imbalance caused by loss of fluid through the skin. Although fever and leukocytosis are commonly found in patients with pustular psoriasis, the possibility of infection should not be overlooked; patients with pustular psoriasis have died of staphylococcal sepsis. As with erythrodermic psoriasis, pustular psoriasis is most commonly precipitated by withdrawal of systemic corticosteroids, but it can also result from therapy with antimalarial drugs or lithium, and it can develop spontaneously. *(Answer: B—Guttate)*

11. A 32-year-old woman presents to clinic to establish primary care. She has recently relocated from another city. The patient's medical history is significant for psoriasis, for which she has been treated with methotrexate, 20 mg a week for 6 years.

Which of the following should NOT be done to monitor for methotrexate toxicity?

❑ **A. Monitoring of liver function tests (LFTs)**

❑ **B. Liver biopsy**

❑ C. Monitoring of the complete blood cell count (CBC)

❑ D. Bone marrow biopsy

Key Concept/Objective: To understand monitoring for methotrexate toxicity in patients with psoriasis

The antimetabolite methotrexate was considered effective for the treatment of psoriasis because of its antimitotic effect on proliferating keratinocytes. However, tissue culture studies have suggested that activated lymphoid cells in the lymph nodes, blood, and skin are a likely target of methotrexate; proliferating macrophages and T cells are 100 times more sensitive to methotrexate than proliferating epithelial cells. These findings may be relevant to the mechanism of action of methotrexate in other immunologically based disorders, including psoriatic arthritis, rheumatoid arthritis, and Crohn disease. Methotrexate is best given in a single weekly oral dose of up to 30 mg or in three divided doses at 12-hour intervals during a 24-hour period (e.g., at 8:00 A.M., at 8:00 P.M., and again at 8:00 A.M.).

Side effects of methotrexate therapy include bone marrow suppression, nausea, diarrhea, stomatitis, and hepatotoxicity. Methotrexate is teratogenic and can cause reversible oligospermia. Evaluation by tests of liver function, renal function, and blood elements must be made before and throughout the course of methotrexate therapy. Cases of pancytopenia after low-dose methotrexate therapy underscore the hazards of use of the drug in patients with renal insufficiency or in patients who are concomitantly receiving drugs that increase methotrexate toxicity.

The use of liver biopsy to monitor patients on methotrexate has been a source of great controversy. Liver biopsies are not routinely performed in patients with rheumatoid arthritis who are undergoing treatment with methotrexate, but liver biopsy has been advocated in patients with psoriasis. Patients with psoriasis who are treated with methotrexate are more prone to hepatic fibrosis, possibly because of their underlying disease or because of the concomitant treatments they are given. Current guidelines call for the use of liver biopsy in patients with psoriasis who have received a cumulative dose of 1 to 1.5 g of methotrexate and who do not have a history of liver disease or alcoholism. Biopsy should be performed early in the course of treatment in patients with a history of hepatitis C, alcoholism, or other liver disease. Risk factors for hepatotoxicity include heavy alcohol intake, obesity, a history of diabetes or hepatitis, and abnormal results on liver function testing.

Although methotrexate causes bone marrow suppression, routine bone marrow biopsies are not indicated. Close monitoring with a monthly CBC is needed. *(Answer: D—Bone marrow biopsy)*

12. A 32-year-old high school teacher reports a mildly itchy new rash over the past week. He has been generally healthy, although he did take a course of penicillin for culture-positive streptococcal pharyngitis several weeks ago. He does not smoke, drinks alcohol only occasionally, and has been monogamous with his wife over the 5 years they have been married. He has had no fever, chills, eye symptoms, anorexia, nausea, diarrhea, bloody stool, abdominal pain, penile sores or discharge, dysuria, or joint pains. On examination, the patient is afebrile, with multiple sharply demarcated scaly papules 3 to 10 mm in diameter distributed symmetrically on his trunk, arms, palms, and penis. There are no target lesions or oral lesions, and no lymphadenopathy is found.

What is the most likely cause of this patient's rash?

❑ A. Primary HIV infection

❑ B. Secondary syphilis

❑ C. Reiter syndrome

❑ D. Guttate psoriasis

❑ E. Drug reaction

Key Concept/Objective: To be able to recognize guttate psoriasis

This is a classic presentation of guttate psoriasis, with onset after a recent streptococcal infection; a symmetrical distribution involving trunk, extremities, palms, and penis; and

well-demarcated, small, scaly, erythematous papules. In contrast, the rash of primary HIV infection is a maculopapular, diffuse eruption, with poorly defined borders and no scaling, usually accompanied by low-grade fever, malaise, lymphadenopathy, and other flu-like symptoms. Secondary syphilis can cause a scaly rash that may include the palms and soles, but the rash is not itchy and is usually accompanied by lymphadenopathy and/or oral lesions. Secondary syphilis is also accompanied by a positive rapid plasma reagin test. Reiter syndrome usually presents as a tetrad of arthritis, urethritis, conjunctivitis/uveitis, and mucocutaneous lesions. The skin and nail lesions of Reiter syndrome can be difficult to distinguish clinically from psoriasis. For example, the balanitis of Reiter syndrome can look scaly or pustular as in psoriasis; the keratoderma blennorrhagicum can cause a scaly or pustular rash on the palms or soles that can be indistinguishable from psoriasis; and Reiter syndrome nail changes (ridging, pitting, onycholysis) can mimic psoriasis. Though this patient does have penile lesions that could be confused with balanitis, he does not have the rest of the tetrad of symptoms. Most patients with Reiter syndrome also describe a preceding diarrheal illness or sexually transmitted infection, which this patient did not report. Drug reactions usually occur sooner after use of antibiotics than was seen in this patient, who took penicillin several weeks before his rash developed. Additionally, though drug reactions are often symmetrical, they are usually more diffuse, maculopapular eruptions and are worse on the trunk than on the extremities. If scaly at all, a drug reaction is then usually diffuse, involving the entire skin surface with an erythroderma or exfoliative dermatitis rather than with the small, discrete papules seen in this patient. *(Answer: D—Guttate psoriasis)*

13. A 62-year-old man wishes to continue oral therapy begun by another physician for onychomycosis. He reports disfigured nails over the past year, and he began daily oral ketoconazole 2 months ago without much change in the appearance of his nails. His past medical history includes hyperuricemia, chronic neck and back pain, sciatica, and excessive alcohol ingestion. On review of systems, he also reports finger stiffness and pain, especially in the distal interphalangeal (DIP) joints of multiple fingers. On examination, the patient's fingers are red, tender, and slightly swollen, appearing somewhat sausage-shaped, without obvious synovitis. Multiple fingernails show deep longitudinal ridging with some pitting, thickening, yellowish discoloration, and onycholysis. The distal ends of multiple fingers are encased in heaped-up scale, debridement of which reveals necrotic tissue underneath. No lymphadenopathy is found in the neck, axillae, or epitrochlear areas. Laboratory testing shows mild anemia with a normal white blood cell count; negative rheumatoid factor, rapid plasma reagin, and antinuclear antibody tests; and a mildly elevated uric acid and ESR. Hand x-rays show erosions in some DIP joints without hyperostosis or bone-cyst formation.

Which of the following is the most likely diagnosis for this patient?

❑ **A. Chronic gout**

❑ **B. Osteoarthritis**

❑ **C. [illegible]**

❑ **D. Rheumatoid arthritis**

❑ **E. Systemic lupus erythematosus (SLE)**

Key Concept/Objective: To be able to recognize psoriatic arthritis

Arthritis involving DIP joints and associated with characteristic psoriatic fingernail changes, including pitting, yellow discoloration, onycholysis, ridging, and subungual hyperkeratosis, is most likely to be psoriatic arthritis. Elevated uric acid and mild iron deficiency anemia can also accompany psoriasis because of high skin turnover. Careful examination of this patient's scalp, umbilicus, gluteal fold, and groin may reveal more characteristic scaly plaques. Chronic gouty arthritis can occur with chronic elevations of uric acid, but it is usually accompanied by tophi, seen on examination as gross deformities in or near the affected joints, and punched-out erosions with overhanging cortical bone (also called "rat-bite" lesions) adjacent to tophaceous deposits, seen on x-ray: findings that are not present in this patient. Additionally, gouty arthritis would not explain the skin findings. Osteoarthritis, like psoriatic arthritis, can affect DIP joints; but unlike psoriatic arthritis, osteoarthritis will cause Heberden nodes at the DIP joints and will dis-

play x-ray findings of hyperostosis and sometimes bone-cyst formation. Rheumatoid arthritis usually spares the DIP joints and causes a spongy swelling of synovial tissue at the metacarpophalangeal and/or wrist joints. SLE can present with rash and joint problems. Unlike the rash of psoriasis, that of SLE characteristically appears on the face or other sun-exposed areas and produces localized red plaques, follicular plugging, atrophy, and telangiectasias: quite unlike the isolated periungual scaling seen in this patient. The arthropathy of SLE does not cause bony erosions. *(Answer: C—Psoriatic arthritis)*

14. A 23-year-old man presents with worsening pain and swelling in his right ankle, which he has had for the past month. He is otherwise healthy, though he admits to an unhealthy lifestyle, including night-shift work, heavy alcohol use on the weekends, and occasional unprotected sex with men, though he has had none in the past 12 months. He denies any history of sexually transmitted disease or intravenous drug use, diarrheal illness, fever, chills, weight loss, dysuria, penile discharge, or other joint pains. On examination, he is in no apparent distress. Removal of his baseball cap reveals a 6 × 15 cm patch of a sharply demarcated, erythematous, scaly rash on his anterior scalp and forehead. Skin and nail examination reveals no further rashes in the groin, gluteal fold, or umbilicus and no nail pitting. A few 1 cm nodes are found in his neck and groin. His right ankle is normal in color but swollen and boggy, with decreased range of motion and mild tenderness to palpation. Biopsy of his scalp suggests psoriasis.

What other testing should be performed on this patient?

- ❑ **A. HIV test**
- ❑ **B. Uric acid level**
- ❑ **C. Urethral, anal, and pharyngeal swabs for gonorrhea**
- ❑ **D. HLA-B27 test**
- ❑ **E. Antinuclear antibody test**

Key Concept/Objective: To understand that new psoriasis can be associated with HIV infection, especially in patients who have risk factors for sexually transmitted disease or who have examination findings that suggest HIV infection

This patient is presenting with new-onset psoriasis and likely psoriatic arthritis. He also has a risk factor for HIV infection (unprotected sex with men), as well as unexplained lymphadenopathy. More careful examination may reveal other clues to HIV infection, including oral candidiasis, oral hairy leukoplakia, gingivitis, or seborrheic dermatitis. HIV testing is most wise in this case. Though gout can affect the ankle joint, there is usually much greater pain and inflammation associated with acute gouty arthritis. Furthermore, uric acid levels are not always helpful in making a diagnosis of gout, because they can be normal in up to 25% of patients with gout. Swabs for gonorrhea can be helpful in diagnosing septic arthritis, though as with gout, the involved joint is usually more obviously inflamed (warm, red, very tender to any movement). HLA-B27 testing has no role in the diagnosis or treatment of psoriatic arthritis. The HLA-B27 test is often positive in patients with Reiter syndrome, although this patient does not have the classic tetrad of symptoms (see Question 12). Antinuclear antibody test is not warranted, because this patient does not have any symptoms or findings that suggest SLE. *(Answer: A—HIV test)*

For more information, see Abel EA: 2 Dermatology: III Psoriasis. ACP Medicine Online (www.acpmedicine.com). Dale DC, Federman DD, Eds. WebMD Inc., New York, June 2002

Eczematous Disorders, Atopic Dermatitis, Ichthyoses

15. A 35-year-old woman presents to clinic complaining of a pruritic rash on her hands. She denies recently changing the detergents and soaps she uses, and she does not wear jewelry. She admits to being under a great deal of stress at work over the past few days. Examination is notable for small, clear vesicles on the sides of her fingers, and there is associated evidence of excoriation.

What is the most likely diagnosis for this patient?

❑ A. **Nummular eczema**

❑ B. **Contact dermatitis**

❑ C. **Dyshidrotic eczema (pompholyx)**

❑ D. **Seborrheic dermatitis**

Key Concept/Objective: To know the differential diagnosis of eczematous disorders and to recognize the presentation of dyshidrotic eczema

Eczema is a skin disease characterized by erythematous, vesicular, weeping, and crusting patches associated with pruritus. The term is also commonly used to describe atopic dermatitis. Examples of eczematous disorders include contact dermatitis, seborrheic dermatitis, nummular eczema, and dyshidrotic eczema (pompholyx). Contact dermatitis is very common and can be induced by allergic or irritant triggers. The distribution of the rash in contact dermatitis coincides with the specific areas of skin that were exposed to the irritant (e.g., in patients sensitive to nickel, rashes may appear on fingers on which rings containing nickel are worn; in patients sensitive to detergent, rashes may appear on areas covered by clothing containing detergent). This patient does not have a history of any particular exposure, and the rash occurs only on the sides of several fingers. Seborrheic dermatitis is also common and is characterized by involvement of the scalp, eyebrows, mustache area, nasolabial folds, and upper chest. Nummular eczema is characterized by coin-shaped patches occurring in well-demarcated areas of involvement. This patient most likely suffers from dyshidrotic eczema, which tends to occur on the side of the fingers, is intensely pruritic, and often flares during times of stress. The treatment includes compresses, soaks, antipruritics, and topical steroids. Severe cases may require systemic steroids. *(Answer: C—Dyshidrotic eczema [pompholyx])*

16. A 21-year-old man presents to the acute care clinic complaining of itching. He states that since childhood, he has had a recurrent rash characterized by "red, itchy, dry patches" of skin. Sometimes the rash is associated with "little bumps." Examination of his skin reveals erythematous, scaling plaques on the flexural surfaces of his arms with associated excoriations. You suspect the patient has atopic dermatitis.

Of the following findings, which is NOT among the major diagnostic criteria of atopic dermatitis?

❑ A. **Personal or family history of atopy**

❑ B. **Pruritus**

❑ C. **Chronic or chronically recurring dermatosis**

❑ D. **Elevated serum IgE level**

Key Concept/Objective: To recognize the clinical presentation of atopic dermatitis and to know the major diagnostic criteria

Atopic dermatitis is a clinical diagnosis. The major diagnostic criteria for atopic dermatitis include a personal or family history of atopy (including asthma, allergic rhinitis, allergic conjunctivitis, and allergic blepharitis); characteristic morphology and distribution of lesions (usually eczematous patches in flexural areas in adults and extensor surfaces in children who crawl; lichenification can occur with nodule formation in chronic cases); pruritus (virtually always present); and a chronic or chronically recurring course. An elevated serum IgE level is not a major diagnostic criterion. This patient is somewhat unusual in that his childhood atopic dermatitis has persisted past puberty (this occurs in only 10% to 15% of cases). *(Answer: D—Elevated serum IgE level)*

17. An 18-year-old woman presents for treatment of chronic dry skin and scaling. The rash typically involves the extensor surfaces of her extremities. She notes that she has had this condition since infancy and that her father has it as well. Her medical records indicate that she has been diagnosed with ichthyosis vulgaris by a dermatologist.

Which of the following statements is false?

❑ A. **The ichthyoses are a group of diseases characterized by abnormal cornification of the skin leading to excessive scaling**

- ❑ B. **Ichthyosis can be an acquired condition associated with endocrinopathies, autoimmune diseases, HIV infection, lymphomas, and carcinomas**
- ❑ C. **The most common form of ichthyosis is acquired ichthyosis**
- ❑ D. **Treatment of ichthyosis includes emollients and keratolytics**

Key Concept/Objective: To know the presentation of ichthyosis vulgaris and to be familiar with the ichthyoses

Etiologies of the ichthyoses are diverse, but the ichthyoses share common manifestations and treatments. The most common form is ichthyosis vulgaris, which is inherited in an autosomal dominant fashion (as seen in this patient); disease onset occurs in patients 3 to 12 months of age. Other forms of ichthyoses include recessive X-linked ichthyosis, lamellar ichthyosis, congenital ichthyosiform erythroderma, epidermolytic hyperkeratosis, and acquired ichthyosis. Acquired ichthyosis is associated with multiple disorders, including HIV infection and endocrinopathies; it can also occur as a paraneoplastic syndrome that is usually associated with lymphomas and carcinomas. Epidermolytic hyperkeratosis is the most difficult form to treat because therapeutic agents can induce blistering. Standard therapies are emollients (such as petrolatum) and keratolytics (such as lactic acid with or without propylene glycol). Antimicrobial agents are also frequently used to combat the odor and other complications of bacterial colonization of the affected skin. *(Answer: C—The most common form of ichthyosis is acquired ichthyosis)*

For more information, see Stevens SR, Cooper KD, Kang K: 2 Dermatology: IV Eczematous Disorders, Atopic Dermatitis, and Ichthyoses. ACP Medicine Online (www.acpmedicine.com). Dale DC, Federman DD, Eds. WebMD Inc., New York, March 2002

Contact Dermatitis and Related Disorders

18. A 45-year-old woman with a history of malaise, weight loss, and recurrent upper respiratory infections of several months' duration was picnicking with friends. Within a few minutes, most of the picnickers realized that they were developing a pruritic, erythematous skin reaction on skin exposed to the lush ground cover around them. One person belatedly recognized the plant as poison ivy. The patient, however, did not develop a reaction.

What is the most likely reason for this patient's failure to develop a reaction?

- ❑ A. **She had anergy related to weight loss**
- ❑ B. **She had impaired T cell immunity related to as yet undiagnosed AIDS**
- ❑ C. **She had not been previously exposed to the allergen found in poison ivy**
- ❑ D. **She was wearing sunscreen, which formed a barrier to the allergen**
- ❑ E. **Before the picnic, she had taken a dose of diphenhydramine for her persistent rhinorrhea**

Key Concept/Objective: To understand immediate-type sensitivity and the role that a history of previous exposure to an allergen plays in making a diagnosis

This woman did not experience an immediate reaction to poison ivy, which is a type I immediate hypersensitivity reaction mediated by circulating antibodies; in this case, the reaction would have been to toxicodendron antigens associated with poison ivy, poison oak, and sumac. Although it is possible that the patient had impaired immunity secondary to weight loss or possibly to HIV infection, even in these cases the immediate type I hypersensitivity reaction would likely occur. A barrier cream would not protect a patient from a contact dermatitis; the cream would only be an additional vector for the spread of the hapten or allergen. Although a dose of diphenhydramine before exposure to an allergen may diminish an allergic reaction, the primary reaction would still occur. *(Answer: C—She had not been previously exposed to the allergen found in poison ivy)*

19. A 30-year-old salesman in a party supply store that specializes in balloons develops a severe pruritic erythematous diffuse skin reaction after eating avocado.

What is the most likely explanation for this patient's reaction?

- ❑ **A. Delayed type IV reactivity to the avocado as the primary allergen**
- ❑ **B. Immediate type I reactivity to the avocado as the primary allergen**
- ❑ **C. Irritant contact dermatitis reaction to the avocado**
- ❑ **D. Immediate type I cross-reactivity reaction to the avocado with primary latex allergy as the underlying allergic cause**
- ❑ **E. IgM-mediated allergic reaction**

Key Concept/Objective: To understand natural rubber and latex allergy and cross-reactivity with certain fruits, including avocados, chestnuts, kiwi, and bananas

The patient has a history of exposure to latex through his work with balloons, and he develops a systemic pruritic reaction after eating avocado. The immediate reaction time rules out a type IV reaction, which usually takes 12 to 48 hours to occur. This patient would not be having an irritant reaction, because his exposure reaction is diffuse, not focal, as would be the case with irritant contact dermatitis. The latex allergic reaction is mediated through IgE, not IgM. *(Answer: D—Immediate type I cross-reactivity reaction to the avocado with primary latex allergy as the underlying allergic cause)*

20. ***What is the best method of distinguishing irritant contact dermatitis from allergic contact dermatitis?***

- ❑ **A. History of exposure frequency**
- ❑ **B. Examination of clinical features and distribution of rash**
- ❑ **C. Patch testing**
- ❑ **D. Histologic evaluation of skin biopsy of rash**
- ❑ **E. Family and travel history**

Key Concept/Objective: To understand the value of patch testing in distinguishing irritant contact dermatitis from allergic contact dermatitis

Determining the etiology of a contact dermatitis is difficult. The gold standard is patch testing, although its sensitivity and specificity vary with the tested allergen. Although history of exposure and examination of the distribution and quality of the reaction are valuable, the best method of distinguishing a contact irritant reaction from an allergic contact reaction is patch testing. The histologies of contact irritant dermatitis and allergic dermatitis are identical, and therefore, histologic evaluation would not be useful in determining whether a reaction is allergy-related. *(Answer: C—Patch testing)*

21. A 43-year-old woman with a long history of chronic actinic dermatitis was experiencing frequent upper respiratory infections, weight loss, and malaise. She was pleased that her chronic actinic dermatitis was improving to the point of being nearly resolved but was concerned about her recurrent infections and weight loss. She presented to a physician, who diagnosed HIV in her blood; the patient had a high viral load count and a very low helper T cell count. The physician started her on didanosine (DDI), zidovudine (AZT), and indinavir. A week later, the patient felt better, but there was evidence of her rash recurring in its previous pattern of distribution.

What is the probable reason for the recurrence of this patient's dermatitis?

- ❑ **A. Allergic reaction to DDI**
- ❑ **B. Allergic reaction to AZT, DDI, and the antiretroviral therapy**
- ❑ **C. Cytomegalovirus dermatitis**
- ❑ **D. T cell–mediated dermatitis**
- ❑ **E. Kaposi sarcoma manifesting in the same distribution pattern as the previous chronic actinic dermatitis**

Key Concept/Objective: To understand the important role of the T cell in the pathophysiology of chronic actinic dermatitis

In this case, a woman with a chronic actinic dermatitis mediated by type IV hypersensitivity via the T cells is compromised through development of AIDS. After therapy that restores her T cell function, she again develops dermatitis. A cytomegalovirus dermatitis would not have the same pattern, type, and distribution as chronic actinic dermatitis. Kaposi sarcoma would be more focal and distinctly pigmented, very unlike chronic contact dermatitis. Although allergic dermatitis can often be seen in the sites of previous skin trauma, such a reaction to the HIV drugs at a time of impaired T cell immunity would be hard to explain, especially in the absence of previous exposure to the medications. *(Answer: D—T cell–mediated dermatitis)*

22. A 24-year-old female emergency department nurse with a history of spina bifida with resultant neurogenic bladder and spastic paresis of the legs died of anaphylactic shock after intercourse during which her partner used a condom.

Which of the following is the most likely cause of this patient's shock?

- ❑ **A. Peritonitis after rupture of the bladder**
- ❑ **B. Allergic anaphylactic reaction to latex in her partner's condom**
- ❑ **C. Allergic anaphylactic reaction to a meal consumed less than an hour before death**
- ❑ **D. Blood loss associated with retroperitoneal hemorrhage for which she was predisposed because of the underlying spina bifida**
- ❑ **E. Sepsis from a urinary tract infection (UTI)**

Key Concept/Objective: To be able to recognize latex allergy

Risk factors for development of a natural rubber and latex (NRL) allergy include exposure through the workplace, which in this case involves use of latex gloves in the emergency department. Spina bifida patients have a 30% to 65% prevalence of NRL allergy. Cross-sensitization to NRL through exposure to chestnuts, kiwi, bananas, or avocado is also recognized. The reaction is mediated by IgE and the T cell. In this case, the latex in the partner's condom was the most likely allergen to cause anaphylaxis. *(Answer: B—Allergic anaphylactic reaction to latex in her partner's condom)*

For more information, see Taylor JS: 2 Dermatology: V Contact Dermatitis and Related Disorders. ACP Medicine Online (www.acpmedicine.com). Dale DC, Federman DD, Eds. WebMD Inc., New York, March 2001

Cutaneous Adverse Drug Reactions

23. A 23-year-old man presented with fever and sore throat; physical examination revealed an erythematous oropharynx and cervical lymphadenopathy. The patient had no known history of drug allergy. He was started on an empirical regimen of amoxicillin for streptococcal pharyngitis. Three days later, he returned to your office complaining that his symptoms had continued and that he had developed a rash. An erythematous maculopapular rash was noted on physical examination. A monospot test was performed. The results come back positive.

Which of the following statements regarding this patient's exanthematous drug eruption is true?

- ❑ **A. Persistence of fever is not helpful in determining whether the symptoms are the result of an allergic reaction, because fever is common in simple exanthematous eruptions**
- ❑ **B. Systemic corticosteroids are always required to treat this drug eruption**
- ❑ **C. After the patient's infectious process resolves, he will be able to tolerate all β-lactam antibiotics, including ampicillin**

❑ D. **In patients with viral infections, the mechanism of exanthematous eruption caused by ampicillin is IgE-mediated mast cell degranulation**

❑ E. **This patient's rash can be expected to progress to a vesicular stage before resolution**

Key Concept/Objective: To understand that ampicillin-amoxicillin–related exanthematous eruptions that occur in patients with viral infections do not appear to be IgE-mediated and that patients can tolerate penicillins and cephalosporins once the infection resolves

The etiology of the ampicillin rash that occurs in association with a viral infection is unknown, but the rash does not appear to be IgE-mediated. Patients can tolerate all β-lactam antibiotics, including ampicillin, once the infectious process has resolved. Fever is not associated with simple exanthematous eruptions. These eruptions usually occur within 1 week after the beginning of therapy and generally resolve within 7 to 14 days. The exanthem's turning from bright red to brownish red marks resolution. Resolution may be followed by scaling or desquamation. The treatment of simple exanthematous eruptions is generally supportive. For example, oral antihistamines used in conjunction with soothing baths may help relieve pruritus. Topical corticosteroids are indicated when antihistamines do not provide relief. Systemic corticosteroids are used only in severe cases. Discontinuance of the offending agent is recommended. *(Answer: C—After the patient's infectious process resolves, he will be able to tolerate all β-lactam antibiotics, including ampicillin)*

24. A 35-year-old woman with HIV was recently started on trimethoprim-sulfamethoxazole for *Pneumocystis carinii* prophylaxis. She now presents with fever, sore throat, malaise, and a desquamating rash on her trunk. Laboratory studies are notable for the following abnormalities: serum creatinine, 2.1 mg/dl; aspartate transaminase (AST), 215 mg/dl; and alanine transaminase (ALT), 222 mg/dl.

Which of the following statements regarding the care of this patient is true?

❑ A. **She may become hypothyroid as a result of the development of autoimmune thyroiditis within 2 months after the initiation of symptoms**

❑ B. **In the future, she should avoid sulfonylureas, thiazide diuretics, furosemide, and acetazolamide**

❑ C. **An elevated serum IgE level confirms the diagnosis of hypersensitivity syndrome reaction**

❑ D. **Her first-degree relatives have the same risk of experiencing a hypersensitivity syndrome reaction as the general population**

Key Concept/Objective: To understand the basic pathophysiology, epidemiology, and clinical [illegible]

Sulfonamide antibiotics can cause hypersensitivity syndrome reactions in susceptible persons. This kind of adverse drug reaction is caused by the accumulation of toxic metabolites; it is not the result of an IgE-mediated reaction. The primary metabolic pathway for sulfonamides involves acetylation of the drug to a nontoxic metabolite and renal excretion. An alternative metabolic pathway, quantitatively more important in patients who are slow acetylators, engages the cytochrome P-450 mixed-function oxidase system. These enzymes transform the parent compound to reactive metabolites—namely, hydroxylamines and nitroso compounds, which produce cytotoxicity independently of preformed drug-specific antibody. In most people, detoxification of the metabolite occurs. However, hypersensitivity syndrome reactions may occur in patients who are unable to detoxify this metabolite (e.g., those who are glutathione deficient). Other aromatic amines, such as procainamide, dapsone, and acebutolol, are also metabolized to chemically reactive compounds. The risk of first-degree relatives' developing hypersensitivity reactions to sulfonamides is higher than in the general population. Cross-reactivity should not occur between sulfonamides and drugs that are not aromatic amines (e.g., sulfonylureas, thiazide diuretics, furosemide, and acetazolamide); therefore, these drugs can be safely used in the future. Most systemic manifestations of the hypersensitivity reaction syndrome occur at the time

of skin manifestations. However, a subgroup of patients may become hypothyroid as part of an autoimmune thyroiditis up to 2 months after the initiation of symptoms. *(Answer: A—She may become hypothyroid as a result of the development of autoimmune thyroiditis within 2 months after the initiation of symptoms)*

25. A 19-year-old female college student is taking ampicillin and clavulanate for pharyngitis. After 5 days of treatment, she develops a generalized erythematous maculopapular rash. She is given a monospot test, and the result is positive.

For this patient, which of the following statements is true?

- ❑ A. **Exanthematous rashes may occur in up to 80% of patients with infectious mononucleosis that is treated with ampicillin**
- ❑ B. **The patient should undergo skin testing with penicilloyl polylysine and graded desensitization before any treatment with penicillins**
- ❑ C. **Treatment should include changing to a macrolide antibiotic**
- ❑ D. **The patient is experiencing a type II, or cytotoxic, hypersensitivity reaction**
- ❑ E. **The rash will worsen until ampicillin is stopped**

Key Concept/Objective: To be able to recognize typical ampicillin rash

The causal mechanism of an exanthematous ampicillin rash in the setting of a concurrent viral illness is unclear. It does not appear to be mediated by IgE, so β-lactams can be tolerated and sensitivity testing is not warranted. Although stopping ampicillin is suggested, the rash will generally resolve even if ampicillin is continued. *(Answer: A—Exanthematous rashes may occur in up to 80% of patients with infectious mononucleosis that is treated with ampicillin)*

26. ***In contrast to exanthematous rashes, which of the following is true of urticaria that develops after drug exposure?***

- ❑ A. **Type I immediate hyersensitivity reactions cause all urticarial rashes**
- ❑ B. **In severe reactions with angioedema and bronchospasm, plasmapheresis should be initiated early in treatment**
- ❑ C. **Urticarial rashes remain fixed for up to several days and may recur in the same location with repeated exposure to the causative drug**
- ❑ D. **Because of the risk of severe reactions, patients with drug-induced urticaria should not undergo skin testing or desensitization**
- ❑ E. **Biopsy should be considered for urticarial lesions that persist for longer than 24 hours**

Key Concept/Objective: To know the complications associated with urticarial rashes

For lesions that persist for longer than 24 hours, consideration should be given to the use of biopsy to exclude vasculitis. Biopsy may show deposits of IgM and C3 immune complexes within the lesions. Besides being associated with type I reactions, urticaria may occur with type III hypersensitivity reactions and as a result of nonimmunologic release of histamine caused by certain drugs, such as morphine. Treatment of severe allergic reactions includes epinephrine, antihistamines, bronchodilators, corticosteroids, and supportive treatment with fluids and pressors if needed. Patients can be desensitized if there is no therapeutic alternative to the causative drug. *(Answer: E—Biopsy should be considered for urticarial lesions that persist for longer than 24 hours)*

27. A 55-year-old woman has a well-demarcated reddish brown macular rash on her arm. The lesion recurs periodically and resolves slowly, with some persisting hyperpigmentation. She is otherwise healthy and takes no medications except an occasional laxative.

Which of the following is the most likely diagnosis for this patient?

- ❑ **A. Urticaria**
- ❑ **B. Lichen planus**
- ❑ **C. Pemphigus**
- ❑ **D. Fixed drug eruption**
- ❑ **E. Contact dermatitis**

Key Concept/Objective: To be able to diagnose fixed drug eruption in the appropriate setting

Fixed drug eruptions may occur after ingestion of several over-the-counter medications, including phenolphthalein laxatives and ibuprofen. After an exacerbation, a refractory period may occur during which reexposure does not produce a recurrence of the rash, so the diagnosis may be elusive. The most common site of involvement is the genitalia, so fixed drug eruptions must be distinguished from various sexually transmittable afflictions. *(Answer: D—Fixed drug eruption)*

28. ***Which of the following is true concerning the development of cutaneous necrosis in a patient taking warfarin?***

- ❑ **A. Skin lesions appear weeks to months after beginning treatment**
- ❑ **B. The pretibial area is the most common site**
- ❑ **C. Lesions generally occur only when the INR exceeds 3.5**
- ❑ **D. Treatment includes heparinization**
- ❑ **E. Patients with lupus anticoagulant or antithrombin III deficiency are predisposed**

Key Concept/Objective: To understand the pathogenesis and treatment of warfarin-induced skin necrosis

Patients with protein C or protein S deficiency may be predisposed to develop warfarin-induced skin necrosis. They develop a paradoxical hypercoagulable state at the onset of treatment because of suppression of protein C anticoagulant activity, resulting in venous thrombosis and necrosis 3 to 5 days later. Fatty areas are most frequently affected. Heparin, vitamin K, and fresh frozen plasma are the mainstays of treatment. *(Answer: D—Treatment includes heparinization)*

29. One month after starting phenytoin after a head injury, a 24-year-old man developed a low-grade fever, cervical lymphadenopathy, and a generalized erythematous maculopapular rash with subsequent exfoliation in some areas.

Which of the following statements is true of this condition?

- ❑ **A. It is commonly associated with penicillins and ACE inhibitors**
- ❑ **B. Limited laboratory investigation consisting of a complete blood count and a urinalysis is warranted**
- ❑ **C. Graves disease is a late complication**
- ❑ **D. First-degree relatives of the patient are at increased risk for similar reactions**
- ❑ **E. After the cutaneous reactions, rechallenge and desensitization are advised before reinstituting therapy**

Key Concept/Objective: To be able to recognize the signs and complications of hypersensitivity syndrome

Hypersensitivity syndrome is a potentially serious reaction occurring from 1 week to several weeks after exposure to aromatic anticonvulsants (e.g., phenytoin, carbamazepine),

sulfonamides, or other drugs with an aromatic amine chemical structure (procainamide). Inheritable defects in the metabolic pathways for these agents may place close relatives at increased risk as well. Eosinophilia, hepatitis, and interstitial nephritis may be detected initially, and autoimmune thyroiditis can cause late hypothyroidism. The rash may range from an exanthem to severe Stevens-Johnson syndrome or toxic epidermal necrolysis. Because these reactions are severe (and not IgE-mediated), patients and family members are advised to avoid the causative drug and drugs that are chemically similar to it. *(Answer: D—First-degree relatives of the patient are at increased risk for similar reactions)*

For more information, see Shear NH, Knowles S, Shapiro L: 2 Dermatology: VI Cutaneous Adverse Reactions. ACP Medicine Online (www.acpmedicine.com). Dale DC, Federman DD, Eds. WebMD Inc., New York, March 2004

Fungal, Bacterial, and Viral Infections of the Skin

30. A 6-year-old boy comes with his mother to your clinic with a scalp lesion. He developed this lesion a few weeks ago. On physical examination, the patient has an area of alopecia on his scalp; associated with the alopecia is a painful inflammatory mass with pus and sinus tracts. A skin specimen treated with potassium hydroxide (KOH) shows the presence of dermatophytes. A Gram stain shows no bacterial organisms.

What is the likely diagnosis for this patient, what is the causal organism, and how should his condition be treated?

- ❑ A. **Kerion; *Microsporum* or *Trycophyton*; oral griseofulvin**
- ❑ B. **Bacterial abscess; *Staphylococcus aureus*; oral dicloxacillin**
- ❑ C. **Fungal and bacterial coinfection; *Trychophyton* and *Staphylococcus aureus*; oral itraconazole and dicloxacillin**
- ❑ D. **Sebaceous tumor; surgical removal**

Key Concept/Objective: To understand the clinical picture and treatment of kerion

Tinea capitis occurs primarily in children. Only *Microsporum* and *Trychophyton* species can cause tinea capitis. Zoophilic species, such as *Microsporum* or *Trycophyton*, can provoke intense inflammation, which can result in a kerion—a painful, boggy mass in which follicles may discharge pus and in which sinus tracts form. Crusting and matting of adjacent hairs are common, and cervical lymph nodes may enlarge. The diagnosis is confirmed by obtaining a sample from the lesion, treating it with KOH (which digests the keratin of the skin and hair), and examining it under the microscope for the presence of organisms. Although a bacterial infection or coinfection needs to be considered in the differential diagnosis, the presence of pus in this case is related to the intense inflammatory reaction against the fungus and does not necessarily mean that the patient has a bacterial infection. Oral therapy is necessary when treating fungal infections involving the hair or hair follicles or in extensive lesions. The agents of choice for the treatment of tinea capitis are griseofulvin and terbinafine. *(Answer: A—Kerion;* Microsporum *or* Trycophyton; *oral griseofulvin)*

31. A 26-year-old white man presents to a walk-in clinic complaining of a rash on his back. He noticed the rash 4 or 5 weeks ago. He describes small, whitish lesions that are not painful and do not itch on his back. On physical examination, the patient is seen to have several small, dark macules that coalesce on his upper back. When the lesions are scratched, fine scales are produced.

How should you proceed in the management of this patient?

- ❑ A. **A fungal culture from the lesion should be obtained**
- ❑ B. **A skin biopsy should be performed**
- ❑ C. **The lesions should be scraped and a KOH stain should be performed**
- ❑ D. **The patient should be started on oral terbinafine**

Key Concept/Objective: To know the clinical picture of and diagnostic approach to tinea versicolor

This patient's presentation is consistent with tinea versicolor. Tinea (or pityriasis) versicolor is a yeast infection caused by *Malassezia furfur*. The lesions are small, discrete macules that tend to be darker than the surrounding skin in light-skinned patients and hypopigmented in patients with dark skin. They often coalesce to form large patches of various colors ranging from white to tan. Scratching the lesions produces a fine scale. This infection most commonly involves the upper trunk, but the arms, axillae, abdomen, and groin may also be affected. To confirm the diagnosis, a KOH preparation of scrapings from the lesions can be done, which can demonstrate pseudohyphae and yeasts resembling spaghetti and meatballs. Because these yeasts form part of the normal cutaneous flora, growth of the organism on cultures from the skin is not very helpful diagnostically. Treatment of tinea versicolor involves applying selenium sulfide shampoo topically. An alternative is the use of topical azoles such as ketoconazole, miconazole, and clotrimazole. For patients who have difficulty using topical agents, oral ketoconazole or fluconazole is an alternative. Terbinafine is not active against yeasts. *(Answer: C—The lesions should be scraped and a KOH stain should be performed)*

32. A 34-year-old man comes to your office complaining of a skin ulcer. He first noticed a skin lesion 6 or 7 days ago. It started as a small, painless papule on his right arm. Over the next few hours, the lesion enlarged, and the patient noticed significant swelling around the lesion. After a few days, he developed a black eschar, which sloughed the day before the visit, leaving a painless ulcer. On physical examination, the patient has a painless ulcer measuring 2 × 2 cm that is surrounded by significant edema and that has a tender, epitrochlear node. A Gram stain of the ulcer shows broad gram-positive rods. The patient is not allergic to penicillin. You have heard of similar cases in a local hospital.

What is the next step in the treatment of this patient?

- ❑ **A. Start penicillin V, 500 mg p.o., q.i.d., for 60 days and send cultures and serology to confirm your clinical diagnosis; change antibiotics according to the culture results**
- ❑ **B. Start ciprofloxacin, 500 mg p.o., q.d., for 10 days and send cultures and serology to confirm your clinical diagnosis; change antibiotics according to the culture results**
- ❑ **C. Start amoxicillin, 500 mg p.o., t.i.d., for 10 days and send cultures and serology to confirm your clinical diagnosis; change antibiotics according to the culture results**
- ❑ **D. Start ciprofloxacin, 500 mg p.o., q.i.d., for 60 days and send cultures and serology to confirm your clinical diagnosis; change antibiotics according to the culture results**

Key Concept/Objective: To know the appropriate treatment of cutaneous anthrax

Anthrax was very rare in the United States until 2002, when spores of *Bacillus anthracis* were sent through the mail as an act of terrorism. Except for cases associated with bioterrorism, humans usually develop anthrax from exposure to affected animals or their products. Occasionally, laboratory-acquired cases can occur. The cutaneous form develops when spores enter the skin through abrasions and then transform into bacilli, which produce edema and necrosis. After an incubation period of about 1 to 7 days, a painless, pruritic papule forms at the entry site. Over the next few hours, the lesion enlarges and a ring of erythema appears. Painless edema surrounds the lesion, often spreading to the adjacent skin and soft tissue. In the center of the lesion, a black eschar appears and sloughs within 1 to 2 weeks, leaving a shallow ulcer that heals with minimal scarring. Regional lymph nodes often enlarge, causing pain and tenderness. *B. anthracis* is a broad, encapsulated gram-positive rod, which can be seen on a Gram stain of material from the skin lesion. It grows readily on blood agar media. Skin biopsies reveal necrosis, hemorrhage, and edema. Organisms are demonstrable with tissue Gram stain or immunohistochemical staining. Because serologic testing requires acute and convalescent blood specimens, such testing is unhelpful for immediate diagnosis but may establish a retrospective diagnosis of a suspected but unconfirmed case. The treatment for cutaneous anthrax that is not associated

with bioterrorism is a regimen of penicillin V or amoxicillin for 7 to 10 days. In this patient, there is a chance that anthrax is related to a bioterrorist attack because similar cases have been seen in the past few days; therefore, ciprofloxacin should be started. The recommended regimen for cases associated with bioterrorism is 60 days because of the possibility of simultaneous aerosol exposure. *(Answer: D—Start ciprofloxacin, 500 mg p.o., q.i.d., for 60 days and send cultures and serology to confirm your clinical diagnosis; change antibiotics according to the culture results)*

For more information, see Hirschmann JV: 2 Dermatology: VII Fungal, Bacterial, and Viral Infections of the Skin. ACP Medicine Online (www.acpmedicine.com). Dale DC, Federman DD, Eds. WebMD Inc., New York, March 2003

Parasitic Infestations

33. A 22-year-old graduate student recently returned from a trip to central Mexico. She subsequently developed several nontender nodules on her lower back that intermittently drain brown fluid. She received treatment with dicloxacillin, without improvement. On examination, she has five purple, firm nodules that measure approximately 2 cm; the nodules have tiny central openings that intermittently drain serosanguineous fluid.

    What would you do next for this patient?

    - ❑ A. **Give her a 10-day course of oral cephalexin**
    - ❑ B. **Give her a 10-day course of oral levofloxacin**
    - ❑ C. **Excise a nodule for pathologic evaluation**
    - ❑ D. **Give her a 10-day course of I.V. gentamicin**
    - ❑ E. **Apply fatty bacon over the nodules**

    Key Concept/Objective: To be able to identify and manage patients with myiasis

    This patient has just returned from an area endemic for the botfly. The nodules with a central punctum that intermittently drain are a characteristic of infestation with larvae of that insect. Not infrequently, patients with myiasis are misdiagnosed as having bacterial furunculosis and are managed with a variety of antibiotics that have no effect. It is important to consider the diagnosis of myiasis because occluding the punctum with fatty bacon causes the larvae to protrude. The larvae can then be removed with forceps. Other occlusive substances, such as petroleum jelly and nail polish, have also been effective. Excising the nodule for pathologic evaluation is not needed. *(Answer: E—Apply fatty bacon over the nodules)*

34. A 37-year-old woman presents with intense perineal itching. On examination, she has both red papules and blue macules on the inner thighs. In addition, there are excoriated, crusted lesions in the same region. Tiny tan swellings are seen at the bases of some of the pubic hair shafts.

    What is your diagnosis?

    - ❑ A. **Dermatitis herpetiformis**
    - ❑ B. **Genital herpesvirus**
    - ❑ C. **Pediculosis**
    - ❑ D. **Scabies**
    - ❑ E. **Contact dermatitis**

    Key Concept/Objective: To know the distinguishing characteristics of diseases that cause pruritic skin lesions

    This patient has pediculosis pubis, caused by *Phthirus pubis*. Its characteristic blue-gray macules (maculae ceruleae) are caused by the pubic lice sucking blood from the dermis. The tan swellings are nits: lice eggs cemented to the hair shaft. None of the other diseases

listed have these findings. Scabies is caused by a burrowing mite that can at times be seen as a line in the stratum corneum. The mite's eggs are deposited in the burrows rather than as nits. Dermatitis herpetiformis is an autoimmune vesicular dermatitis characterized by grouped vesicles symmetrically distributed over the extensor skin surfaces. Genital herpes can be pruritic but is more often painful. Contact dermatitis can cause pruritic lesions but is not caused by a parasitic infestation. *(Answer: C—Pediculosis)*

35. A 32-year-old man returns from a vacation to the Caribbean. He spent time swimming and sunbathing at the local beaches. He now has intensely pruritic skin lesions on the abdomen. Examination reveals several serpiginous thin lines in the skin.

Which of the following organisms is most likely responsible for this disease?

- ❑ A. **Botfly larvae**
- ❑ B. **Avian schistosome free-swimming larvae (cercariae)**
- ❑ C. **Hookworm larvae**
- ❑ D. **Thimble jellyfish larvae**
- ❑ E. **Sandfleas**

Key Concept/Objective: To understand the causes and presentations of skin lesions that can occur during travel to tropical regions

Tungiasis (sandflea cutaneous infestation), seabather's eruption (infestation with larvae of the thimble jellyfish), swimmer's itch (infestation with cercarial larvae of an avian schistosome), and cutaneous larva migrans (infestation with hookworm larvae) can all cause intensely pruritic skin lesions. It is the migration of larval hookworms that causes the serpiginous or linear tracks in the skin. Tungiasis causes erythematous edematous papules in clusters. Seabather's eruption presents as a pruritic dermatitis in areas covered by swimwear. Swimmer's itch is a papulovesicular eruption on exposed skin sites. The larvae of the botfly cause myiasis, a nonpruritic nodular skin lesion mimicking an infected cyst or abscess. *(Answer: C—Hookworm larvae)*

36. Two months after returning from an expedition to the Amazon, a 42-year-old archeologist notices a red-brown papule on her nose. On skin examination, she is suntanned. She also has a verrucous nodule with early ulceration where she first noted the papule on the nose.

What would you do for this patient at this point?

- ❑ A. **Perform biopsy of the nodule for histopathology**
- ❑ B. **Treat with oral sodium stibogluconate (a pentavalent antimony compound)**
- ❑ C. **Ablate with cryosurgery**
- ❑ D. **Inject the nodule intralesionally with antimonials**
- ❑ E. **Treat with oral ivermectin**

Key Concept/Objective: To understand the presentation of cutaneous leishmaniasis and its management

This patient's clinical examination and course fit the diagnosis of New World cutaneous leishmaniasis. The differential diagnosis includes various inflammatory and neoplastic disorders, including squamous cell carcinoma. The safest course in this case would be to perform biopsy of the lesion to confirm the diagnosis. Once the diagnosis is confirmed, the patient could be treated with oral sodium stibogluconate. Old World leishmaniasis is usually limited to the skin and can be treated with cryosurgery, heat therapy, or intralesional injection of antimonials. Ivermectin is therapy for scabies, pediculosis, and cutaneous larva migrans. *(Answer: A—Perform biopsy of the nodule for histopathology)*

37. A 17-year-old boy living at home with his parents presents with an intensely pruritic papulovesicular eruption involving the hands and wrists. Skin scrapings identify eggs and waste products of *Sarcoptes scabiei.*

Which of the following management options is most appropriate?

- ❑ **A. Treat the patient and symptomatic household members with permethrin 5% cream, and tell them to wash all clothing and linens with which they have come in contact over the past 2 days**
- ❑ **B. Treat the patient and all household members with permethrin 5% cream, and tell them to wash all clothing and linens with which they have come in contact over the past 2 days**
- ❑ **C. Treat the patient and symptomatic household members with permethrin 5% cream, and tell them to wash all clothing and linens with which they have come in contact over the past 10 days**
- ❑ **D. Treat the patient and all household members with permethrin 5% cream, and tell them to wash all clothing and linens with which they have come in contact over the past 10 days**
- ❑ **E. Treat the patient and symptomatic household members with lindane lotion, and tell them to wash all clothing and linens with which they have come in contact over the past 10 days**

Key Concept/Objective: To understand the treatment of scabies

Both permethrin 5% cream and lindane are effective therapies for scabies. However, treatment involves more than just choosing a scabicidal agent. Because the skin flakes that are shed by patients contain large numbers of mites, fomites can spread. The recommendation is to treat all members of the household, not just those who are symptomatic. The organism's ability to survive for 48 hours away from a host dictates thorough laundering of materials that might have been contaminated within the previous 2 days. *(Answer: B—Treat the patient and all household members with permethrin 5% cream, and tell them to wash all clothing and linens with which they have come in contact over the past 2 days)*

For more information, see Abel EA: 2 Dermatology: VIII Parasitic Infestations. ACP Medicine Online (www.acpmedicine.com). Dale DC, Federman DD, Eds. WebMD Inc., New York, March 2001

Vesiculobullous Diseases

38. A 45-year-old man comes to your clinic complaining of skin and mouth lesions. Painful oral ulcers started to appear in his mouth 1 month ago. Over the past week, he has also noticed some skin lesions on his upper chest and back. He has no significant medical history and is not taking any medications. His physical examination is unremarkable except for the presence of several superficial tender ulcers on his oral mucosa and six superficial coin-sized lesions on his back and chest, which are surrounded by normal skin. The Nikolsky sign is positive.

On the basis of clinical presentation, which of the following is the most likely diagnosis for this patient?

- ❑ **A. Bullous pemphigoid**
- ❑ **B. Pemphigus vulgaris**
- ❑ **C. Pemphigus foliaceus**
- ❑ **D. Porphyria cutanea tarda**

Key Concept/Objective: To know the typical presentation of pemphigus vulgaris

Pemphigus is characterized by blisters that arise within the epidermis and by a loss of cohesion of the epidermal cells. Pemphigus vulgaris is the most common form of pemphigus. It can develop at any age but usually occurs in persons between 30 and 60 years

old. Pemphigus vulgaris usually begins with chronic, painful, nonhealing ulcerations in the oral cavity. Skin lesions can also be the initial manifestation, beginning as small fluid-filled bullae on otherwise normal-looking skin. The blisters are usually flaccid because the overlying epidermis cannot sustain much pressure. Bullae therefore rupture rapidly, usually in several days, and may be absent when the patient is examined. Sharply outlined, coin-sized, superficial erosions with a collarette of loose epidermis around the periphery of the erosions may appear instead. The upper chest, back, scalp, and face are common sites of involvement. A characteristic feature of all active forms of pemphigus is the Nikolsky sign, in which sliding firm pressure on normal-appearing skin causes the epidermis to separate from the dermis. Pemphigus foliaceus usually begins with crusted, pruritic lesions resembling corn flakes on the upper torso and face; oral involvement is very rare. Bullous pemphigus is characterized by recurrent crops of large, tense blisters arising from urticarial bases. Porphyria cutanea tarda appears as blistering lesions in sun-exposed areas, typically on the dorsa of hands. *(Answer: B—Pemphigus vulgaris)*

39. A 40-year-old man comes to clinic complaining of skin lesions. His symptoms started 6 weeks ago, with crusted lesions localized on his face, back, and chest; he denies having any oral lesions. He has no medical history and is not taking any medications. On physical examination, the patient has several crusted lesions on his face, upper chest, and back. Results of a skin biopsy are consistent with pemphigus foliaceus.

Of the following, which is the most appropriate treatment for this patient?

- ❑ **A. Plasmapheresis**
- ❑ **B. Intravenous immunoglobulin**
- ❑ **C. Cyclophosphamide**
- ❑ **D. Prednisone**

Key Concept/Objective: To understand the treatment of pemphigus foliaceus

Initial therapy for pemphigus is determined by the extent and rate of progression of lesions. Localized, slowly progressive disease can be treated with intralesional injections of corticosteroids or topical application of high-potency corticosteroids. New lesions that continue to appear in increasing numbers can be controlled in some cases with low-dose systemic corticosteroids (prednisone, 20 mg/day). Patients with extensive or rapidly progressive disease are treated with moderately high doses of corticosteroids. If disease activity persists despite high doses of corticosteroids, one of the following approaches should be considered for rapid control: plasmapheresis; intravenous immunoglobulin; or pulse therapy with high-dose intravenous methylprednisolone. Although pemphigus foliaceus is less severe than pemphigus vulgaris, the doses of medications required for treatment of both diseases are similar. *(Answer: D—Prednisone)*

40. A 30-year-old woman comes to clinic complaining of blisters on her body. She started developing these lesions a week ago. The lesions consist of very pruritic, small blisters on her arms, buttocks, and back. She says she had a similar lesion a few months ago that resolved on its own after a few weeks. Physical examination is significant for multiple small papules and vesicles on the elbows, buttocks, and lower back; there are signs of previous scratching. A skin biopsy specimen shows microabscesses at the tips of dermal papillae and granular deposits of IgA on the basement membrane zone.

On the basis of this patient's clinical presentation, what is the most likely diagnosis, and what treatment would you prescribe?

- ❑ **A. Erythema multiforme; prednisone**
- ❑ **B. Pemphigus vulgaris; prednisone**
- ❑ **C. Dermatitis herpetiformis; dapsone**
- ❑ **D. Pemphigus foliaceus; azathioprine**

Key Concept/Objective: To know the clinical presentation and management of dermatitis herpetiformis

Dermatitis herpetiformis is a vesiculobullous disease characterized by intensely pruritic, small vesicles that are grouped in small clusters and typically appear on the extensor aspects of extremities and on the buttocks, scalp, and back. The condition is believed to be an immune-mediated disorder and is associated with abnormal granular deposits of IgA at the basement membrane zone and with asymptomatic, gluten-sensitive, spruelike enteropathy. The disease is chronic, with periods of exacerbation and remission. Lesions may clear if patients follow a strict gluten-free diet. Dermatitis herpetiformis responds rapidly and dramatically to dapsone. Erythema multiforme is characterized by the presence of target lesions; it commonly affects mucosal surfaces. The histologic findings include subepidermal edema and a deep perivascular mononuclear infiltrate, sometimes with granular deposits of C3 or IgM. Pemphigus vulgaris and foliaceus show acantholysis; on immunofluorescence, intercellular autoantibodies, IgG, IgM, or IgA is seen. *(Answer: C—Dermatitis herpetiformis; dapsone)*

For more information, see Abel EA, Bystern JC: 2 Dermatology: IX Vesiculobullous Diseases. ACP Medicine Online (www.acpmedicine.com). Dale DC, Federman DD, Eds. WebMD Inc., New York, July 2003

Malignant Cutaneous Tumors

41. A 64-year-old retired Navy officer presents to clinic for a routine health maintenance visit. He has no complaints, but when asked about a pinkish papular lesion near the corner of his left eye, he states that it has been present "for years" and that it has become irritated on occasion with minor trauma or rubbing. The lesion is 4 to 5 mm in diameter and appears pearly. You recommend that the patient undergo biopsy because you are concerned about the possibility of basal cell carcinoma (BCC).

Which of the following epidemiologic and clinical statements is NOT true of BCC?

- ❑ A. **BCC is the most common skin cancer**
- ❑ B. **The vast majority of BCCs occur on the head and neck**
- ❑ C. **Based on appearance, this patient's lesion is likely a nodular BCC**
- ❑ D. **Metastatic disease and deaths associated with BCC have been reported**
- ❑ E. **BCC arises from cells in the dermis**

Key Concept/Objective: To understand fundamental aspects of basal cell carcinoma, a form of nonmelanoma skin cancer

Malignant tumors can arise from cells of any layer of the skin, and epidermal skin cancers are the most common cancers in humans. Basal cell carcinoma (BCC) and squamous cell carcinoma (SCC) arise from keratinocytes of the epidermis, whereas malignant melanoma arises from the melanocytes of the epidermis. Because BCC and SCC share many features, they are often lumped together under the term nonmelanoma skin cancer. BCC is the most common skin cancer and is more prevalent in people with lighter skin pigmentation. Over 90% of BCC lesions appear on the head and neck. Sun exposure is the most important risk factor. The two most common forms are nodular BCC (which is likely the type that this patient demonstrates) and superficial BCC, which appears as a pink patch of skin. Although rare, metastases and death from BCC have been known to occur, and any suspicious lesions (especially long-standing ones in a sun-exposed area that easily bleed with minor trauma) should be excised and submitted for pathologic examination. *(Answer: E—BCC arises from cells in the dermis)*

42. A 50-year-old construction worker with hypertension presents for a return office visit. His blood pressure appears well controlled, and you are discussing other health maintenance issues as you examine him. You notice several rough-surfaced, irregularly shaped lesions on his face, scalp, and dorsa of the hands. On closer inspection, they appear hyperkeratotic and have a small rim of surrounding erythema. He says they are not painful, do not itch, and have been appearing over the course of years.

Which of the following statements regarding this patient's risk of skin cancer is true?

- ❑ A. The lesions are precursors to melanoma and should be removed
- ❑ B. This patient's risk of developing a cutaneous malignancy in relation to the lesions is less than 2%, and he should be reassured that they are completely benign
- ❑ C. Treatment of the lesions by methods such as cryotherapy, curettage, or topical chemotherapy has been found to be effective in preventing the progression of such lesions to carcinoma
- ❑ D. Small squamous cell carcinomas arising in the areas described are more likely to metastasize than are more undifferentiated lesions developing in non–sun-exposed areas
- ❑ E. The most important risk factor in the development of these lesions is family history

Key Concept/Objective: To know that actinic keratosis is a potential precursor to squamous cell carcinoma of the skin

This patient has hyperkeratotic lesions typical of actinic keratosis in sun-exposed areas. Actinic keratosis is seen in areas of chronically sun-damaged skin and is considered a precursor lesion to the development of SCC. The majority of patients with actinic keratosis have multiple lesions, and the risk of SCC in these patients is estimated to be as high as 20%. Thus, it is important that the patient be followed regularly and evaluated by a dermatologist: the removal of these lesions through various techniques can prevent progression to cancer. Small SCCs that arise from actinic keratosis lesions are actually less likely to metastasize than more atypical SCCs, such as those that are poorly differentiated or appear in non–sun-exposed areas or oral or genital mucosa. Sunlight exposure is the most important risk factor for developing actinic keratosis and SCC, although radiation, chemical burns, and chronic nonhealing wounds may also predispose to squamous cell cancer. *(Answer: C—Treatment of the lesions by methods such as cryotherapy, curettage, or topical chemotherapy has been found to be effective in preventing the progression of such lesions to carcinoma)*

43. A 59-year-old white woman with rheumatoid arthritis who was treated in the past with methotrexate and courses of steroids presents for evaluation of a mole on her chest. She states that it has been present for years but that, in the past 6 to 8 months, she noticed more irregularity at the borders and an increase in the size of the lesion. Examination reveals an asymmetrical lesion approximately 8 mm in diameter that is variably pigmented from brown to black. You recommend biopsy of the lesion because you are concerned about malignant melanoma.

If a primary cutaneous melanoma is confirmed, which of the following factors would be the most important with regard to outcome in this patient?

- ❑ A. Evolution of the lesion from a dysplastic nevus
- ❑ B. History of immunosuppressive therapies
- ❑ C. Tumor diameter greater than 6 mm
- ❑ D. Tumor thickness
- ❑ E. Location of the melanoma

Key Concept/Objective: To understand the importance of tumor thickness as a prognostic factor in primary cutaneous melanoma

Malignant melanoma is the most aggressive of the primary cutaneous malignancies, and the clinician should have a high index of suspicion when evaluating moles with the characteristics of melanoma. The "ABCD" mnemonic is useful for remembering the features of melanoma: *a*symmetry, *b*order irregularity, *c*olor variation, and *d*iameter greater than 6 mm. Such features warrant biopsy of the lesion. In this patient, the change in the size of a mole over time also warrants prompt evaluation. The single strongest prognostic factor in melanoma is stage of disease at the time of diagnosis. Staging takes into account tumor size, nodal involvement, and distant metastases. For primary tumors, the most consistent factor predictive of outcome is tumor thickness, as described by the Breslow depth.

Patients with dysplastic nevi are at increased risk for the development of melanomas; the presence of dysplastic nevi does not consistently relate to the prognosis of patients with melanoma. *(Answer: D—Tumor thickness)*

44. A 35-year-old white man presents at a walk-in clinic with a complaint of lesions in his mouth and over his trunk. These lesions developed over the past several months. His medical history is unremarkable. He states that he is homosexual, that he has practiced unsafe sex in the past, and that he has had the same partner for the past 18 months. He denies having previously had any sexually transmitted diseases, but he says he has not had regular health care visits since high school. On examination, you note numerous purple-red, oval papules distributed on the trunk and two deep-purple plaques on the soft palate and buccal mucosa. The patient also has several small, firm, nontender, palpable lymph nodes in the posterior cervical, axillary, and inguinal chains. Results of routine blood work are unremarkable except for a white blood cell count of 3,000 cells/mm^3 and a differential with 5% lymphocytes.

Which of the following statements regarding our current knowledge of Kaposi sarcoma (KS) is false?

- ❑ **A. Human herpesvirus 8 (HHV-8) plays an etiologic role exclusively in HIV-associated KS**
- ❑ **B. Visceral organ (i.e., lung and GI tract) involvement is relatively common in HIV-associated KS**
- ❑ **C. If HIV infection is confirmed, initiation of highly active antiretroviral therapy (HAART) in this patient would likely lead to dramatic improvements in the lesions during the first few months of therapy**
- ❑ **D. Male sex is a significant risk factor for the condition, especially in the classic form of the disease**
- ❑ **E. Total CD4$^+$ T cell count is the most important factor predictive of survival in the form of this disease associated with HIV**

Key Concept/Objective: To be able to recognize KS and appreciate important aspects of its diagnosis and treatment

This patient is a homosexual man who presents with skin and oral lesions typical of KS. The additional findings of generalized lymphadenopathy and lymphopenia strongly suggest that the patient is infected with HIV. In its classic form, KS affects elderly men, primarily of Mediterranean descent, and manifests as violaceous plaques and nodules on the lower extremities. The disease was rare in the United States before the AIDS epidemic. Among HIV-infected patients, homosexual men have by far the highest incidence of KS. Recently, it has been shown that HHV-8 can be detected in all variants of KS, suggesting an etiologic role. HIV-associated KS presents as oral lesions or cutaneous lesions on the upper body. They often follow the skin lines in a pityriasis rosea-like distribution. KS can involve the pulmonary and gastrointestinal systems and can cause hemorrhage at these sites. As such, a chest x-ray and fecal occult blood test should be considered when evaluating patients newly diagnosed with HIV-associated KS. The single most important prognostic factor in HIV-associated KS is the CD4$^+$ T cell count. Large tumor burdens, lymphedema, and pulmonary involvement also portend a poorer outcome. HAART is often first-line therapy in treating KS, especially in a patient with newly diagnosed AIDS. The improvement in viral load and CD4$^+$ T cell counts is often accompanied by regression of KS lesions. Other therapeutic options include radiation, intralesional chemotherapy injections, and systemic chemotherapy, including liposomally encapsulated anthracyclines such as doxorubicin and daunorubicin. *(Answer: A—Human herpesvirus 8 [HHV-8] plays an etiologic role exclusively in HIV-associated KS)*

45. A middle-aged woman comes to clinic complaining of a long-standing rash involving her chest and left thigh, which she first noted over a year ago. She says the areas are chronically red and scaly and are occasionally mildly pruritic. She has not been able to identify any precipitating factors or irritants that have come into contact with those particular areas. She states that exposure to the sun has intermittently made the lesions improve to an extent. Approximately 6 months ago, she was prescribed a topical steroid cream, which did seem to cause improvement of the rash, but the rash soon returned after discontinuation. She thought that the rash likely represented psoriasis, and she had not been overly concerned about it until recently, when she has noticed that the lesions had become larger and more prominent. On examination, you note a large erythematous, scaly patch on the trunk. The lesion on the upper thigh is a thicker plaque that is deeper red in color. Skin biopsy reveals atypical lymphoid cells in the epidermis that have hyperconvoluted (cerebriform) nuclei. There is also a bandlike lymphocytic infiltrate in the upper dermis. A diagnosis of mycosis fungoides is made on the basis of the histologic report.

Which of the following clinical and therapeutic statements is NOT characteristic of this disorder?

- ❑ **A. The rash is caused by a cutaneous lymphoma that is most commonly of B cell origin**
- ❑ **B. The condition can be associated with generalized erythroderma and circulating atypical lymphocytes with cerebriform nuclei**
- ❑ **C. Early-stage disease that is confined to patches or plaques in the skin is primarily treated with topical therapy involving steroids or chemotherapeutic agents**
- ❑ **D. Ulcerations from the cutaneous lesions should be monitored closely and treated aggressively because sepsis originating from these lesions is a common cause of death in these patients**
- ❑ **E. Patients with visceral involvement have a poor prognosis; the median survival is 2.5 years**

Key Concept/Objective: To be able to recognize the clinical manifestations of cutaneous T cell lymphoma (CTCL)

Non-Hodgkin lymphomas may primarily involve the skin and present as chronic, erythematous patches or plaques. The vast majority of these are T cell in origin and are known as cutaneous T cell lymphomas (CTCLs). Mycosis fungoides is the name commonly applied to this condition, although there are other variants. Five percent of patients with CTCL present with Sézary syndrome and have generalized erythroderma and circulating atypical T cells (Sézary cells); this condition represents the leukemic variant of CTCL. CTCL can be difficult to diagnose, given its indolent course and the fact that its appearance is similar to those of other benign inflammatory conditions of the skin, including psoriasis, eczema, contact dermatitis, and drug reactions. The lesions typically appear in a bathing trunk distribution. Staging of the disease is based on the surface area of skin involved with patches or plaques and the involvement of lymph nodes, visceral organs, and blood. Early-stage disease is primarily treated with topical therapy (such as corticosteroids, nitrogen mustard, or carmustine) and radiation of the lesions. Advanced disease is associated with a poor prognosis. The most serious complications of CTCL are infections: sepsis from ulcerated cutaneous tumors is a common cause of death in these patients. *(Answer: A—The rash is caused by a cutaneous lymphoma that is most commonly of B cell origin)*

For more information, see Halpern AC: 2 Dermatology: X Malignant Cutaneous Tumors. ACP Medicine Online (www.acpmedicine.com). Dale DC, Federman DD, Eds. WebMD Inc., New York, October 2002

Benign Cutaneous Tumors

46. A 56-year-old white man presents to your office for evaluation of bumps on his upper back and chest. His wife reports that he has had them for years, but they seem to be increasing in number. He states that they do not itch or hurt. Examination reveals several sharply circumscribed papules measuring from 2 mm to 2 cm in diameter on the patient's upper back and chest. The lesions are light brown and have a stuck-on appearance. Closer examination reveals follicular plugging.

What is the most likely diagnosis for this patient?

- ❑ **A. Nevus cell nevus**
- ❑ **B. Pigmented basal cell carcinoma**
- ❑ **C. Seborrheic keratosis**
- ❑ **D. Dermatosis papulosa nigra**

Key Concept/Objective: To be able to recognize seborrheic keratosis and to be familiar with the differential diagnosis of lesions with a similar appearance

This patient's lesions are consistent with seborrheic keratosis (seborrheic wart). Seborrheic keratosis is a very common epithelial tumor that tends to occur on the upper trunks of light-skinned adults. They occur more frequently with increasing age. The color can range from dirty yellow to dark brown, and their size varies from 1 mm to several cm. They may be rough or smooth but often have a waxy surface. Dermatosis papulosa nigra is similar to seborrheic keratosis but tends to occur in dark-skinned individuals (this patient is white) and is usually localized on the face. In addition, dermatosis papulosa nigra tends to present at an earlier age than does seborrheic keratosis. The differential diagnosis of seborrheic keratosis also includes lentigo, warts, nevus cell nevus, and pigmented basal cell carcinoma. Inflamed seborrheic keratosis can be difficult to distinguish from malignant melanoma and squamous cell carcinoma. Transient development of seborrheic keratosis has been associated with inflammatory skin conditions such as drug-related erythroderma and psoriasis. The sign of Leser-Trelat is transient eruptive seborrheic keratosis that is associated with internal malignancy (especially adenocarcinoma); the validity of this sign is a subject of debate. *(Answer: C—Seborrheic keratosis)*

47. A 35-year-old woman presents with a lump on her back. She is worried about having cancer. The lump has been there for several months and has grown some over time. Otherwise, the patient is in good health and takes no medications. There is no family history of malignancy. Examination is notable for a firm, rubbery nodule measuring 1 cm on her upper back. The nodule seems to be just under the surface of the skin and is not fixed in place. The borders are smooth, there is no abnormal pigmentation, and there is a small pore in the center of the lesion. You tell the patient she most likely has an epidermoid cyst, and you attempt to reassure her.

Which of the following is NOT a treatment option for epidermoid cysts?

- ❑ **A. Systemic antibiotics and warm-water compresses if the cyst becomes infected or inflamed**
- ❑ **B. Incision of the cyst with a pointed scalpel, and expression of the cyst wall and its contents**
- ❑ **C. Excision of the entire cyst**
- ❑ **D. Cryotherapy**

Key Concept/Objective: To be able to recognize the presentation of an epidermoid cyst and to be familiar with treatment options for such a lesion

Epidermoid cysts, or wens, are common and appear to be derived from hair follicles. They are frequently found on the back as firm nodules measuring 0.2 to 5.0 cm in diameter. They are slow-growing and often have a central pore. They are asymptomatic unless they become inflamed or infected. In such cases, the patient should receive antibiotics and have warm-water compresses applied three or four times a day. After the inflammation or infection has resolved, the patient can have the cyst removed. Removal in other cases is usually for cosmetic reasons. The cyst may recur if the cyst wall is not removed. Therefore, treatment options include simple incision and expression of the cyst's contents and wall or, for more fibrotic cysts, surgical excision of the entire cyst. Cryotherapy is not useful for removal of the cyst. Pilar cysts are very similar in appearance to wens but have a semifluid, malodorous core. Milia are smaller and firmer than wens, and they tend to be located on the face and in scars. Treatment is similar for all these cysts. *(Answer: D—Cryotherapy)*

48. A 56-year-old farmer presents for a routine health examination. He states that he has been doing well. On examination, you note that the patient has some sun damage to his skin and that he has a dark complexion. There is a hyperpigmented, slightly raised lesion measuring 1 cm on his left forearm. There is no lymphadenopathy in his arm or axilla. The patient states that he does not really remember noticing this lesion before; he denies using any sunscreen. You are worried that the lesion on his forearm may be a dysplastic nevus or melanoma.

Which of the following features of this patient's hyperpigmented lesion would NOT make it more likely to be a dysplastic nevus or melanoma?

❑ A. Small size (< 5 mm)

❑ B. Flatness

❑ C. Irregular pigmentation

❑ D. Indistinct borders

Key Concept/Objective: To understand the features of hyperpigmented lesions that make them more likely to be a dysplastic nevus or melanoma than a nevus cell nevus (melanocytic nevus)

Nevus cell nevus (melanocytic nevus) is the most common skin tumor, and most young adults have 20 to 40 of these lesions. The incidence increases with age up to the second or third decade, then declines. These nevi are more common in sun-exposed areas. It is important to realize that the risk of melanoma increases with the number of melanocytic nevi. However, the presence of even one dysplastic nevus increases a person's risk of melanoma. Therefore, it is important to be familiar with the appearance of dysplastic nevi (the features of which are similar to those of melanoma). Features include large size (> 5 mm), flatness, irregular pigmentation, asymmetry, and indistinct borders. *(Answer: A—Small size [< 5 mm])*

49. A woman brings her 13-year-old son to your clinic for evaluation of multiple lumps and bumps. She states that her husband had similar problems and died of a nervous system disease. She does not remember the name of her husband's disease, but notes that his tumors were at times large and painful and that on numerous occasions he had to have some surgically removed. The patient has just experienced his "growth spurt" and is having some troubles with acne. He denies having any pain but admits that other children make fun of him at school. On examination, you note multiple large, skin-colored, pedunculated tumors. He also has evidence of acne, and there is a tan, oval macule measuring 3 cm on his chest. You believe he may have neurofibromatosis-1 (NF-1, also known as von Recklinghausen disease).

Which of the following statements about neurofibromatosis is false?

❑ A. There are two major forms, NF-1 and neurofibromatosis-2 (NF-2)

❑ B. Both NF-1 and NF-2 are inherited in an autosomal recessive pattern

❑ C. NF-1 is characterized by neurofibromas, café au lait spots, iris hamartomas (Lisch nodules), neurologic impairment, and bone abnormalities

❑ D. NF-2 is less common and is characterized by bilateral acoustic neuromas; skin findings are less common than in NF-1

Key Concept/Objective: To understand the key features of the two major forms of neurofibromatosis and their pattern of inheritance

It is most likely that this patient has NF-1 (von Recklinghausen disease) and that he inherited it from his father. Neurofibromas typically appear at puberty and are progressive, as are the other manifestations of neurofibromatosis. Such manifestations include café au lait spots; Lisch nodules; involvement of the spine and peripheral nerves with tumors; neurologic impairment; bony abnormalities; and a predisposition to malignancy. NF-2 is characterized by bilateral acoustic neuromas; NF-2 usually presents as hearing loss in the second or third decade of life. This form of neurofibromatosis is less common than NF-1 and is less likely to present with skin findings. Other features of NF-2 include meningiomas, gliomas, and cataracts. Both of these forms of neurofibromatosis are inherited in an autosomal dominant fashion, with near complete penetrance. *(Answer: B—Both NF-1 and NF-2 are inherited in an autosomal recessive pattern)*

50. A 17-year-old African-American adolescent presents with swelling of her earlobes; she had them pierced a few months ago. She can no longer put her earrings on and is distraught about her appearance. She notes that the involved areas itch and burn. Examination is remarkable for hyperpigmented, shiny, smooth tumors measuring 1 to 2 cm that are located around the areas of her ear piercing. There are small, crablike extensions from the lesions. There is no evidence of erythema or purulence. You believe the patient has developed keloids at the sites of her ear piercing.

Which of the following statements about keloids is false?

- ❑ A. **They are more common in African Americans, Hispanics, and those with a family history of keloids**
- ❑ B. **Cryotherapy is ineffective**
- ❑ C. **Intralesional steroids can flatten the keloids**
- ❑ D. **Risk factors for the development of keloids include wound tension, ear piercing, healing by second intention, young age, and deep laceration**

Key Concept/Objective: To understand the presentation of keloids, to know those who are at greatest risk for developing them, and to be aware of some of the common methods of treatment

Keloids represent an abnormal response to tissue injury, manifested as delayed, excessive proliferation of scar tissue. They do not regress and often cause pain, burning, and pruritus. They are more common in African Americans, Hispanics, and those with a family history of keloids. Risk factors for their development include wound tension, ear piercing, healing by second intention, young age, and deep laceration. Intralesional steroids administered at doses of 10 to 40 mg/ml every month for up to 6 months have been shown to effectively flatten keloids, although several side effects may occur. Cryotherapy given as a 30-second application once a month for 3 months has been found to be a safe and effective treatment. *(Answer: B—Cryotherapy is ineffective)*

For more information, see Abel EA: 2 Dermatology: XI Benign Cutaneous Tumors. ACP Medicine Online (www.acpmedicine.com). Dale DC, Federman DD, Eds. WebMD Inc., New York, July 2002

Acne Vulgaris and Related Disorders

51. A 16-year-old female patient comes to your office complaining of acne, which she has had for 3 years. The lesions have been small in size, not painful, and not swollen, and they have not progressed over this period. She says the acne is bothering her, and she would like to be treated. On physical examination, the patient is found to have multiple comedones measuring 0.5 to 1 mm that are open and closed on the face. Her arms, chest, and shoulders are not involved. There are no inflammatory lesions and no cysts. She is not sexually active.

Which of the following is the most appropriate treatment for this patient?

- ❑ A. **Educate the patient about diet and about trying to avoid chocolate and fatty meals**
- ❑ B. **Start oral doxycycline**
- ❑ C. **Start topical retinoids**
- ❑ D. **Start oral isotretinoin**
- ❑ E. **Start oral contraceptives**

Key Concept/Objective: To know the appropriate treatment of comedonal acne

Comedones consist of keratinized cells and sebum. Comedonal acne consists of a predominance of open and closed comedones, without inflammatory findings such as erythematous papules, pustules, nodules, or cysts. The treatment for this form of acne should be directed toward improving the abnormal follicular keratinization process. The best option is topical retinoids, such as tretinoin or adapalene. Also, comedolytic agents such as salicylic acid may be used. Oral agents are not indicated in this mild and noninflammatory form of the disease. There is no role for dietary change in the management of acne. Oral contraceptives can be beneficial for patients with acne; these agents are ideal in women who are seeking birth control methods and in women who are not candidates for or have not responded to other treatments. *(Answer: C—Start topical retinoids)*

52. A 23-year-old man has a 5-year history of severe acne with scarring. His acne involves the face, shoulders, and chest. He has been treated in the past with multiple courses of topical agents, including retinoids, benzoyl, topical antibiotics, and oral antibiotics for 1 year. His lesions have not improved significantly through these agents. On physical examination, the patient has multiple large cysts and abscesses that are confluent and form sinus tracts.

Which of the following options are indicated in the management of this patient?

- ❑ **A. Change the oral antibiotic being used, because the presence of a resistant organism is very likely**
- ❑ **B. Refer to a physician who is authorized to administer oral isotretinoin to consider starting this therapy**
- ❑ **C. Start antiandrogenic therapy (e.g., spironolactone)**
- ❑ **D. Perform a fungal culture of the lesions to exclude *Malassezia* folliculitis**
- ❑ **E. Reassure the patient that acne is a disease of adolescents and that his symptoms should improve in the next few months**

Key Concept/Objective: To know the indications for oral isotretinoin

Acne conglobata is a severe, scarring form of acne, with cysts, abscesses, and sinus tracts. This form of acne responds poorly to topical agents or oral antibiotics alone. Intralesional injections of corticosteroids and drainage of the abscesses are temporarily helpful, but these patients usually need oral isotretinoin for lasting improvement. Oral isotretinoin is the most effective agent available for the treatment of acne. It results in long-lasting remissions or cures in the majority of patients treated; however, it can produce severe side effects, so it should be used for severe forms of the disease only. To be able to prescribe and administer isotretinoin, physicians and pharmacists must be authorized and registered by the manufacturers of isotretinoin. *Malassezia* folliculitis does not respond to typical acne therapies with erythematous acneiform papules; however, it usually affects the extremities and is not characterized by the presence of abscess or sinus tracts. The resistance of *Propionibacterium acnes* to antibiotics has been well documented; however, antibiotic resistance is uncommon when benzoyl peroxide is used concomitantly with antibiotics. Furthermore, the severe form of acne seen in this patient usually does not respond to topical or antibiotic therapy. *(Answer: B—Refer to a physician who is authorized to administer oral isotretinoin to consider starting this therapy)*

53. A 21-year-old woman presents to the emergency department complaining of severe abdominal pain, which she has been experiencing for 2 days. The pain is epigastric and is accompanied by nausea and vomiting. Her medications include isotretinoin and oral contraceptives. She is sexually active and says she is using condoms in addition to oral contraceptives. On physical examination, the patient has moderately severe acne on her face and chest, and she has cheilitis. Her abdominal examination is remarkable for tenderness in the epigastrium with decreased bowel sounds.

Of the following, which one is the most likely diagnosis?

- ❑ **A. Ectopic pregnancy**
- ❑ **B. Peptic ulcer disease**
- ❑ **C. Ovarian cyst torsion**
- ❑ **D. Acute pancreatitis**
- ❑ **E. Appendicitis**

Key Concept/Objective: To know the side effects of isotretinoin

Isotretinoin use is associated with important side effects. Some of the reported side effects are cheilitis, dryness of mucous membranes and skin, myalgias, pseudotumor cerebri, and hypercholesterolemia. Triglyceride levels can rise significantly: enough to cause acute pancreatitis, which is the most likely diagnosis in this case. Because teratogenicity occurs with even a single dose of isotretinoin, patients should undergo pregnancy testing repeatedly and should use two different methods of contraception. There have been reports of depres-

sion and suicide in isotretinoin-treated patients. This association remains controversial, but this risk must be discussed with the patient before starting therapy. *(Answer: D—Acute pancreatitis)*

54. A 16-year-old female patient comes to your office complaining of pimples. She states that the pimples appeared on her face 2 to 3 months ago. She has also noticed some deepening of her voice and the appearance of an increasing amount of hair on her chin and breasts. Her menses were regular until 4 or 5 months ago, when she started noticing irregular and short-lasting periods. On physical examination, the patient has papules and pustules on her face. Hirsutism is noted on her face, arms, breasts, and infraumbilical area, and she has an enlarged clitoris.

Which of the following is the most appropriate step to take next in the treatment of this patient?

- ❑ **A. Evaluate the patient for the possibility of ovarian or adrenal tumors**
- ❑ **B. Start oral contraceptives for presumed polycystic ovarian syndrome (PCOS) and provide reassurance**
- ❑ **C. Start low-dose hydrocortisone for presumed late-onset congenital adrenal hyperplasia and follow up in 2 months**
- ❑ **D. Start benzoyl peroxide with topical metronidazole in the morning and topical retinoids at night**
- ❑ **E. Administer a pregnancy test and consider isotretinoin therapy**

Key Concept/Objective: To know the secondary causes of acne

Acne is very common in the adolescent population; however, it is important to recognize acne as a secondary manifestation of a primary process. Acne can be caused by medications such as isoniazid, corticosteroids, phenytoin, lithium, and progestins. Acne can also be a manifestation of androgen excess; this patient had acne of rapid onset, and there were other manifestations of androgen excess, such as changes in her voice, oligomenorrhea, clitoromegaly, and hirsutism. This rapid onset is characteristic of tumors producing androgens, which are frequently located in the ovarian or adrenal glands. Levels of testosterone, free testosterone, and dehydroepiandrosterone sulfate should be measured; if the results are high, imaging studies are indicated. PCOS can cause oligomenorrhea, hirsutism, and acne; however, it should not cause clitoromegaly or voice changes. Late-onset congenital adrenal hyperplasia (CAH)—21-hydroxylase deficiency in particular—is in the differential diagnosis. However, it would be atypical for it to present in such a rapid manner. If the workup for the presence of a tumor is negative, further workup for CAH would be indicated. *(Answer: A—Evaluate the patient for the possibility of ovarian or adrenal tumors)*

For more information, see Lebwohl M: 2 Dermatology: XII Acne Vulgaris and Related Disorders. ACP Medicine Online (www.acpmedicine.com). Dale DC, Federman DD, Eds. WebMD Inc., New York, November 2002

Disorders of Hair

55. A 38-year-old man presents to your clinic complaining of hair loss. He reports that the hair loss began several years ago but is more noticeable now. His hair has been thinning out on the sides as well as on the top of his head. He reports that several family members have the same problem.

Which of the following is the most appropriate therapy for this patient's condition?

- ❑ **A. Topical 2% minoxidil applied to the scalp twice daily**
- ❑ **B. Medium- to high-potency topical steroids applied daily**
- ❑ **C. Topical immunotherapy with the sensitizing chemical diphencyprone**
- ❑ **D. Short-contact topical therapy with 0.25% anthralin cream applied daily**

Key Concept/Objective: To be able to recognize and appropriately treat androgenetic alopecia

Androgenetic alopecia is the most common type of nonscarring hair loss affecting the crown. It results from a genetically determined end-organ sensitivity to androgens. It is often referred to as common baldness, male-pattern alopecia, and female-pattern alopecia. Androgenetic alopecia affects at least 50% of men by 50 years of age and 50% of women by 60 years of age. Men have more androgen than women and therefore are usually affected earlier and more severely. Male-pattern alopecia often starts in persons between 15 and 25 years of age. Male-pattern alopecia has two characteristic components, bitemporal recession and vertex balding, which in pronounced cases can progress to complete balding of the crown. Depending on the severity of the condition, management of androgenetic alopecia ranges from watchful inactivity to medical and surgical treatment; a hairpiece or wig may be used in the most refractory cases. Minoxidil is applied twice daily with a dropper, spread over the top of the scalp, and gently rubbed in. The drug should be tried for at least a year. Minoxidil acts by initiating and prolonging anagen. It produces visible hair growth in approximately one third of male and female patients, fine-hair growth in approximately one third, and no growth in approximately one third. It is more effective as a preventive agent, retarding hair loss in approximately 80% of patients. Topical steroid therapy, topical immunotherapy, and use of anthralin cream are therapeutic choices for the treatment of alopecia areata. *(Answer: A—Topical 2% minoxidil applied to the scalp twice daily)*

56. A 42-year-old woman presents to the walk-in clinic complaining of hair loss. She notes the hair loss mostly on the top of her head but also on the sides. She reports a history of hypertension and diabetes but is currently on no medications. On review of systems, she reports some menstrual irregularities but is otherwise without complaint. She has tried some over-the-counter products for facial hair growth, but they have not helped the hair loss on her scalp. She would like to try something "prescription strength."

Of the following, which is the most appropriate step to take next in the treatment of this patient?

- ❑ A. **Begin therapy with topical 2% minoxidil applied twice daily and see her again in 3 to 6 months**
- ❑ B. **Begin daily therapy with ethinyl estradiol-ethynodiol diacetate and see her again in 6 weeks**
- ❑ C. **Explain the risks and benefits of hormone replacement therapy for perimenopausal symptom relief and see her again in 1 to 2 months**
- ❑ D. **Screen the patient for hyperandrogenism and see her again in 1 to 2 weeks**

Key Concept/Objective: To be able to differentiate simple androgenetic alopecia from hyperandrogenism

The constellation of symptoms seen in this patient should raise concern about the possibility of excess circulating androgen. The diagnosis of androgenetic alopecia is usually obvious from the clinical pattern of hair loss from the top of the head. In some men, a female pattern of alopecia causes diagnostic confusion but has no other significance. In women, a male pattern of alopecia (i.e., bitemporal recession and vertex balding) in association with menstrual irregularities, acne, hirsutism, and a deep voice is significant. The virilism indicates significant hyperandrogenism, the cause of which must be identified and treated. Local therapy with either topical minoxidil or ethinyl estradiol-ethynodiol diacetate is reasonable for women with a diagnosis of androgenetic alopecia; however, in this case, the cause of virilism should be thoroughly investigated before initiating any therapy. *(Answer: D—Screen the patient for hyperandrogenism and see her again in 1 to 2 weeks)*

57. A 32-year-old woman presents to your office complaining of hair loss. The hair loss is occurring all over her head and seems to spare no area. She notes that it worsens when she showers, and she has begun showering every other day in an attempt to decrease the hair loss. She has been healthy all her life, and other than an uneventful pregnancy and vaginal delivery 3 months ago, she has no medical history.

This patient's clinical presentation and history are most consistent with which of the following hair disorders?

❑ A. Androgenetic alopecia

❑ B. Telogen effluvium

❑ C. Alopecia areata

❑ D. Cicatricial alopecia

Key Concept/Objective: To know the clinical presentation of telogen effluvium

Telogen effluvium is the most common form of diffuse alopecia. It presents as a generalized shedding of telogen hairs from normal resting follicles. The basic cause of telogen effluvium is a premature interruption of anagen, which leads to an increase in the number of hairs phased into telogen. When the 3-month telogen period ends, new anagen hairs grow in and numerous telogen hairs fall out. Patients may need reassurance that this apparent loss of hair is actually a sign of regrowth. Acute telogen effluvium can be caused by childbirth, febrile illnesses, surgery, chronic systemic diseases, crash diets, traction, severe emotional stress, and drug reactions. It can also be a physiologic reaction in neonates. During acute telogen effluvium, pull tests are positive all over the scalp, yielding two to 10 club hairs. Telogen effluvium is often accompanied by bitemporal recession; this is a useful diagnostic sign in women. The acute form usually ends within 3 to 6 months. The diagnosis is usually made on the basis of the history of an initiating event 3 months before the onset of shedding. No treatment is needed for acute telogen effluvium, because the hair invariably regrows within a short time. Alopecia areata is characterized by patchy areas of hair loss, not the diffuse hair loss seen in this patient. The pattern of hair loss in this female patient is not consistent with androgenetic alopecia (thinning of hair in the crown). The lack of skin changes makes the possibility of cicatricial alopecia remote. *(Answer: B—Telogen effluvium)*

For more information, see Whiting DA: 2 Dermatology: XIII Disorders of Hair. ACP Medicine Online (www.acpmedicine.com). Dale DC, Federman DD, Eds. WebMD Inc., New York, January 2003

Diseases of the Nail

58. A 36-year-old man comes to your clinic for the first time for a check-up. He has no active complaints. Review of systems is negative. His medical history is significant only for hypertension. He neither smokes nor drinks. His only medication is hydrochlorothiazide. Physical examination is unremarkable except for the presence of digital clubbing bilaterally. You asked the patient about this finding, and he says his nails have always looked like this and that his father had similar nails.

What would be an appropriate workup for this patient?

❑ A. Obtain a chest x-ray to rule out intrathoracic pathology

❑ B. Obtain an echocardiogram to rule out congenital heart disease

❑ C. Order hand x-rays to further document the presence of clubbing

❑ D. No further workup is necessary

Key Concept/Objective: To understand the differential diagnosis of clubbing

When the normal angle between the proximal nail fold and the nail plate exceeds 180°, digital clubbing is present. The morphologic changes of clubbing typically include hypertrophy of the surrounding soft tissue of the nail folds as a result of hyperplasia of dermal fibrovasculature and edematous infiltration of the pulp tip. Clubbing may be hereditary, or it may be seen in association with several underlying disease states, such as hypertrophic pulmonary osteoarthropathy, chronic congestive heart failure, congenital heart disease associated with cyanosis, polycythemias associated with hypoxia, Graves disease, chronic hepatic cirrhosis, lung cancer, and Crohn disease. This patient has no signs of diseases associated with clubbing, he has had clubbing for many years, and he has a family history of clubbing; therefore, further workup is not indicated. When clubbing is unilateral, consideration should be given to underlying causes of impaired circulation. *(Answer: D—No further workup is necessary)*

59. A 22-year-old woman presents to a walk-in clinic complaining of pain and swelling on one of her fingers. The swelling and pain are located on the second finger of her right hand, just proximal to her nail. She has also noticed some pus coming from this area. The symptoms started 3 days ago. She reports that she has been cutting her cuticle constantly for cosmetic reasons. Examination reveals erythema, swelling, and purulence of the nail fold of her second finger, and the area is very tender to palpation.

What is the appropriate treatment for this patient's condition?

- ❑ **A. Drainage of the focal abscess and administration of oral antibiotics active against *Staphylococcus aureus***
- ❑ **B. Oral fluconazole therapy for presumed *Candida paronychia***
- ❑ **C. Administration of steroid cream for presumed contact dermatitis affecting the nail fold**
- ❑ **D. Hand x-ray to rule out osteomyelitis**

Key Concept/Objective: To understand the differential diagnosis and management of paronychia

The nail folds are the cutaneous soft tissue that houses the nail unit, invaginating proximally and laterally to encompass the emerging nail plate. The term paronychia denotes inflammation of the nail folds. Paronychia may be acute or chronic and may occur secondary to a variety of conditions, including contact dermatitis, psoriasis, bacterial infections, and fungal infections. The cuticle is a thin, keratinized membrane that serves as a seal to protect the nail fold from exposure to external irritants, allergens, and pathogens. Bacterial paronychia is usually acute in nature. It is characterized by swelling, erythema, discomfort, and sometimes purulence. The most common etiologic pathogen is *Staphylococcus aureus*. Treatment requires drainage of a focal abscess, if present, and oral antibiotic therapy. Chronic paronychia results from chronic irritant dermatitis and loss of cuticle from trauma or nail-care practices; it also occurs secondary to candidal infection. *(Answer: A—Drainage of the focal abscess and administration of oral antibiotics active against* Staphylococcus aureus*)*

60. A 33-year-old man comes to your clinic complaining of weight loss. He has also been experiencing occasional diarrhea. He started to have these symptoms 4 months ago. He says he has been trying to eat more, but he is still losing weight. Physical examination shows bitemporal wasting, diffuse cervical lymphadenopathy, and proximal white subungual lesions. These lesions show dermatophytes on potassium hydroxide (KOH) staining.

What is the most likely diagnosis for this patient?

- ❑ **A. Graves disease**
- ❑ **B. HIV infection**
- ❑ **C. Lymphoma**
- ❑ **D. Inflammatory bowel disease**

Key Concept/Objective: To know the clinical presentation of white proximal onychomycosis

Onychomycosis, the most common infection of the nail, is a fungal infection characterized by nail-bed and nail-plate involvement. Dermatophyte onychomycosis is the most common type of fungal nail infection. The most characteristic clinical features of dermatophyte onychomycosis are distal onycholysis, subungual hyperkeratosis, and a dystrophic, discolored nail plate. Because this combination of features is also seen in persons with nail psoriasis, accurate diagnosis may require KOH preparation and fungal culture. The clinical presentation of proximal white subungual onychomycosis has been reported in association with systemic immunosuppression, including immunosuppression associated with HIV disease. The presence of this pattern of onychomycosis should prompt an evaluation for HIV disease. This patient has a very high probability of having HIV infection, given the clinical presentation. *Candida* onychomycosis is far less common than dermatophyte onychomycosis and is also often associated with immunosuppression. *(Answer: B—HIV infection)*

For more information, see Del Rosso JQ, Daniel CR III: 2 Dermatology: XIV Diseases of the Nails. ACP Medicine Online (www.acpmedicine.com). Dale DC, Federman DD, Eds. WebMD Inc., New York, February 2003

Disorders of Pigmentation

61. A 34-year-old African-American woman comes to your clinic for evaluation of dark spots on her face. These dark patches have been appearing over the past 2 or 3 months. She denies having any itching or other symptoms in this area. She has no history of similar skin lesions in the past. The patient has just delivered a healthy baby girl by cesarean section. She has no significant medical history; her only medication is a multivitamin. Physical examination shows hyperpigmented patches in the malar region bilaterally. The rest of her skin examination is normal.

What is the most likely diagnosis, and how would you treat this patient?

❑ A. **Lentigines; start hydroquinone**

❑ B. **Melasma; start a sunscreen and hydroquinone**

❑ C. **Postinflammatory hyperpigmentation; start azelaic acid**

❑ D. **Vitiligo; start topical corticosteroids**

Key Concept/Objective: To know the clinical picture and treatment of melasma

Melasma is a common acquired symmetrical hypermelanosis characterized by irregular light-brown to gray-brown macules involving the face. Melasma is commonly observed in females; men constitute only 10% of the cases. It occurs more commonly in geographic regions that receive intense ultraviolet radiation, such as tropical or subtropical regions. Clinically, the light-brown patches are commonly evident on the malar prominences, forehead, chin, nose, and upper lip. The patches may have a centrofacial or mandibular distribution. Current treatments for melasma include broad-spectrum sunscreens, hydroquinone formulations, azelaic acid, kojic acid, α-hydroxy acid products, retinoic acid, retinol, superficial chemical peels, and microdermabrasion. Although all these therapies improve melasma, none are curative. It is essential for patients to adhere to a regimen of daily sun protection. A lentigo is a well-circumscribed, brown-black macule that appears at birth or early childhood. Postinflammatory hyperpigmentation is characterized by an acquired increase in cutaneous pigmentation secondary to an inflammatory process; there is no such history in this patient. Vitiligo is a common skin disorder characterized by one or more patches of depigmented skin. *(Answer: B—Melasma; start a sunscreen and hydroquinone)*

62. A 16-year-old white male comes to your clinic for evaluation of skin pigmentation. For the past 6 weeks, he has been experiencing progressive dark pigmentation in both arms. He denies having had such an illness in the past. The patient has acne, which was first diagnosed 2 years ago. His acne affects his face and upper back. He says he is not taking any medications except for an "acne pill." Physical examination is remarkable for the presence of comedones and pustules on his face and upper back. The patient also has hyperpigmented skin in both arms. No other skin lesions are present; the rest of the examination is normal.

Which of the following is the most likely diagnosis for this patient?

❑ A. **Postinflammatory hyperpigmentation**

❑ B. **Addison disease**

❑ C. **Erythema dyschromicum perstans**

❑ D. **Drug-induced hyperpigmentation**

Key Concept/Objective: To recognize hyperpigmentation as a possible side effect of different medications

Medications are a common cause of cutaneous hyperpigmentation. Lesions may be localized or generalized. Medications can also cause hyperpigmentation of the oral mucosa and

nails. Medications causing drug-induced hyperpigmentation include oral contraceptives, hormone replacement therapies, antibiotics, antidepressants, antiviral agents, antimalarials, antihypertensives, and chemotherapeutic agents. This patient has acne, for which he is taking medication. This medication could be minocycline or tetracycline—antibiotics that are commonly used for treatment of acne and that can cause hyperpigmentation. This makes drug-induced hyperpigmentation the most likely etiology. Postinflammatory hyperpigmentation can be a sequela of several dermatologic conditions, including acne; however, the hyperpigmentation in this patient is not located where the acne lesions are. Addison disease can cause hyperpigmentation on the skin and mucosal surfaces; however, this patient has no other signs and symptoms of this disorder. Erythema dyschromicum perstans is an acquired benign condition characterized by the presence of slate-gray to violaceous macules. The lesions are usually symmetrically distributed and vary in size from small macules to very large patches. Common sites of involvement include the face, neck, trunk, and upper extremities. This patient's clinical picture is not consistent with this disorder. *(Answer: D—Drug-induced hyperpigmentation)*

63. A 40-year-old African-American woman with a history of hypertension comes to your clinic for a follow-up visit. She is in her usual state of health. Her only medication is hydrochlorothiazide. Physical examination reveals an area of hypopigmented skin measuring 5 × 7 cm on her right foot.

Which of the following is the most likely diagnosis for this patient, and what further workup is indicated?

- ❑ A. **Albinism; skin biopsy**
- ❑ B. **Vitiligo; no further workup is indicated**
- ❑ C. **Vitiligo; complete blood count, sedimentation rate, comprehensive metabolic panel, and autoantibody tests**
- ❑ D. **Idiopathic guttate hypomelanosis; skin biopsy**

Key Concept/Objective: To know the clinical picture and appropriate work-up of vitiligo

Vitiligo is a common acquired, idiopathic skin disorder characterized by one or more patches of depigmented skin caused by loss of cutaneous melanocytes. Onset may begin at any age, but peak incidences occur in the second or third decade of life. There is no racial predilection; females are affected more often than males. Vitiliginous lesions are typically asymptomatic depigmented macules without signs of inflammation. Occasionally, they may show signs of inflammation or pruritus. Areas of depigmentation vary in size from a few millimeters to many centimeters. In view of the association of vitiligo with myriad other autoimmune diseases, the routine evaluation of a patient should include a thorough history and physical examination. Recommended laboratory tests include a complete blood count, sedimentation rate, comprehensive metabolic panel, and autoantibody tests (antinuclear antibody, thyroid peroxidase, and parietal cell antibodies). Albinism is an uncommon congenital disorder characterized by hypopigmentation of the hair, eyes, and skin. Idiopathic guttate hypomelanosis is a common asymptomatic disorder characterized by hypopigmentation and depigmented polygonal macules ranging from approximately 2 to 8 mm in diameter. *(Answer: C—Vitiligo; complete blood count, sedimentation rate, comprehensive metabolic panel, and autoantibody tests)*

64. A 1-year-old boy is being evaluated for recurrent pneumonia. His history includes three episodes of pneumonia and one episode of skin infection. His family history is unremarkable. Physical examination shows ocular hypopigmentation; there are also two areas of skin hypopigmentation, one on his face and one on his left arm. His peripheral blood smear is remarkable for the presence of giant cytoplasmic granules in the neutrophils.

Which of the following is the most likely diagnosis for this patient?

- ❑ A. **Chédiak-Higashi syndrome**
- ❑ B. **Prader-Willi syndrome**
- ❑ C. **Hermansky-Pudlak syndrome**
- ❑ D. **Cross-McKusick-Breen syndrome**

Key Concept/Objective: To know the classic features of Chédiak-Higashi syndrome

Chédiak-Higashi syndrome is characterized by recurrent infections, peripheral neuropathy, and oculocutaneous hypopigmentation. This disorder leads to death at an early age as a result of lymphoreticular malignancies or infections. The presence of giant lysomal granules in the neutrophils is characteristic of Chédiak-Higashi syndrome. Prader-Willi syndrome is a developmental syndrome characterized initially by mental retardation, neonatal hypotonia, and poor feeding, followed by hyperphagia and obesity. Patients have ocular abnormalities and skin and hair hypopigmentation consistent with oculocutaneous albinism. Hermansky-Pudlak syndrome presents as a hemorrhagic diathesis. Skin and hair color varies from white to light brown. Freckles and lentigines develop with age. Cross-McKusick-Breen syndrome is characterized by hypopigmentation, microphthalmia, nystagmus, and severe mental and physical retardation. *(Answer: A—Chédiak-Higashi syndrome)*

65. A 22-year-old woman requests birth control pills. She has just moved to the United States from Poland with her new husband. She has no history of illness or current illness and has not seen a doctor in a long time. On examination, multiple flat, brown, uniformly pigmented 1 to 3 cm macules, as well as several fleshy, almost pedunculated, nodules are seen on her left leg, hip, and buttock. These lesions stop abruptly at midline on her back. None of these lesions are seen elsewhere on her body. She recalls having these all her life.

Which of the following steps will be useful in the management of this patient's skin lesions?

- ❑ **A. No further interventions are required**
- ❑ **B. Referral for genetic counseling**
- ❑ **C. Ophthalmologic screening**
- ❑ **D. Diagnostic skin biopsy**
- ❑ **E. Topical steroid therapy**

Key Concept/Objective: To recognize segmental neurofibromas and café au lait spots as the result of a focal mutation (type 5 neurofibromatosis) that is not associated with systemic or heritable disease

Type 5 neurofibromatosis manifests as skin lesions in a focal dermatomal segment caused by a localized mutation occurring during embryonic development. It does not carry the risk of the CNS tumors, cortical cataracts, or multiorgan system involvement seen with other types of neurofibromatosis. Additionally, focal dermatomal mutations do not affect the germline cells and are therefore not heritable, in contrast to the autosomal dominant pattern of inheritance of the other neurofibromatosis disorders. Therefore, there is no need for genetic counseling. Although ophthalmologic screening can confirm neurofibromatosis type 1 by finding Lisch nodules (iris hamartomas), this screening is not necessary in patients with type 5 neurofibromatosis because there is no associated eye disorder. Diagnosis of type 5 neurofibromatosis is made by inspection of the skin lesions, and no biopsy is required. Topical steroids have no effect on café au lait spots or neurofibromas. *(Answer: A—No further interventions are required)*

66. A 5-year-old girl is brought to the office by her mother after a fall that caused a forehead laceration. The fall was unwitnessed and occurred during the care of a babysitter. The child has been in good health, though she has been slower than other children her age in reaching the usual milestones in cognitive development. On examination, the patient is a fair-skinned, dark-haired child with a streak of gray hair on the left scalp. She has a 2 cm laceration on her forehead, with considerable associated swelling. Several papules are apparent on her face. A Wood lamp examination reveals four pale, elongated macules on her trunk.

Which disorder best accounts for the findings in this case?

- ❑ **A. Neurofibromatosis**
- ❑ **B. Pityriasis alba**
- ❑ **C. Vitiligo**

❑ D. Piebaldism

❑ E. Tuberous sclerosis

Key Concept/Objective: To be able to recognize tuberous sclerosis by a finding of hypopigmented macules in the setting of likely mental retardation, seizures, and facial angiofibromas

Tuberous sclerosis presents in infants and young children with a classic triad of hypopigmented, ash-leaf-shaped macules (including those in the scalp, which cause gray streaks of hair), mental retardation, and seizures, though the last two can be absent. This child's unwitnessed fall could have been a seizure, and her slowness to attain developmental milestones may be a sign of mental retardation. The finding of facial neurofibromas, skin-colored-to-red papules, is pathognomonic. In contrast, skin findings in neurofibromatosis include hyperpigmented, not hypopigmented, macules, as well as nodular neurofibromas in distributions other than the face. Pityriasis alba affects young children, usually those with dark skin. The lesions are usually on the face and may begin with subtle erythema and slightly raised borders. The lesions then become scaly, hypopigmented macules with indistinct borders and regress spontaneously after several months. Vitiligo causes depigmentation of skin and hair that develops in older children and young adults, usually those of darker skin color. Associated conditions include autoimmune endocrine disorders but not seizures or retardation. Piebaldism causes a white forelock in 90% of patients, as well as amelanotic macules on the trunk, extremities, and mucous membranes. These are present at birth and remain stable over time, unlike vitiligo, which develops later in life and is often progressive. *(Answer: E—Tuberous sclerosis)*

67. A 24-year-old Hispanic woman has been using oral contraceptives and was treated with ciprofloxacin for a bladder infection several months ago. She presents with concerns about some spots on her face that she would like to have removed. The spots appeared suddenly over the past few weeks. They are not itchy or painful. On examination, the patient has blotchy, hyperpigmented, brown macules over the central face, without scaling or induration, involving the nose, nasolabial folds, upper lip, cheeks, and forehead. There are no lesions on the oral mucosa and no rashes elsewhere on her body.

What is the most likely cause of this patient's hyperpigmented lesions?

❑ A. Melasma

❑ B. Tinea faciei

❑ C. Lichen planus

❑ D. Lupus erythematosus

❑ E. Drug-induced sun sensitivity

Key Concept/Objective: To recognize melasma in patients with risk factors and characteristic skin findings

Melasma causes hyperpigmented macules in the central areas of the face. Risk factors for melasma include dark skin, female gender, oral contraceptive use, pregnancy, and sun exposure. Tinea faciei can cause hyperpigmented lesions on the face, but these are usually scaly, with annular accentuation of hyperpigmentation and central clearing. Lichen planus is usually quite itchy and usually occurs in locations such as the wrists, back, shins, and buccal mucosa, but it can also involve the eyelids, tongue, lips, or scalp. Lichen planus is usually more violaceous in color and contains fine, parallel, lacy white lines called Wickham striae. Lupus can cause a malar rash, which is usually erythematous rather than brown and usually confluent rather than blotchy, with some associated fine scaling. Like melasma, this classic malar rash can worsen with sun exposure, but it spares the nasolabial folds. Drug-induced sun sensitivity should also spare the nasolabial folds and upper lip because these areas receive less sun exposure than do other areas of the face. *(Answer: A—Melasma)*

For more information, see Grimes PE: 2 Dermatology: XV Disorders of Pigmentation. ACP Medicine Online (www.acpmedicine.com). Dale DC, Federman DD, Eds. WebMD Inc., New York, February 2003

SECTION 3

ENDOCRINOLOGY

Testes and Testicular Disorders

1. A 76-year-old man is being evaluated for osteoporosis. He had a hip fracture 4 weeks ago. A dual-energy absorptiometry scan showed a decrease in bone mineral density consistent with osteoporosis. The serum concentration of total testosterone is in the low-normal range.

Which of the following is the most accurate description of the physiologic changes in testosterone seen with senescence?

❑ A. **With aging, there is a large decrease in serum total testosterone level; this decrease is related to a decrease in the concentration of sex hormone-binding globulin (SHBG)**

❑ B. **With aging, there is a relatively small decrease in serum total testosterone level; free testosterone decreases to a greater degree; SHBG increases**

❑ C. **With aging, serum estradiol concentration increases secondary to a decrease in the total testosterone concentration**

❑ D. **With aging, the total testosterone level remains unchanged**

Key Concept/Objective: To understand the physiologic changes in testosterone levels seen with aging

As men age, their serum total testosterone concentration decreases. The decrease in the serum concentration of total testosterone is very gradual and of relatively small magnitude. SHBG, however, increases with increasing age, so the free testosterone concentration decreases to a greater degree than the total. By 80 years of age, according to cross-sectional studies, the free testosterone concentration is one half to one third that at 20 years of age. The decrease in testosterone appears to result from both decreased luteinizing hormone (LH) secretion and decreased responsiveness of the Leydig cells. The serum estradiol concentration also decreases with increasing age. *(Answer: B—With aging, there is a relatively small decrease in serum total testosterone level; free testosterone decreases to a greater degree; SHBG increases)*

2. A 36-year-old man comes to your clinic complaining of lack of energy. He was diagnosed with diabetes 2 years ago. Review of systems is positive for decreased libido and energy for the past several months. He has been married for 3 years. He and his wife have been trying to conceive a child for the past year. Physical examination shows decreased pubic and axillary hair; his testicular volume is 15 ml. Total testosterone levels are low; LH and follicle-stimulating hormone (FSH) are in the low-normal range. The prolactin level is normal.

Which of the following would be the most appropriate test in the evaluation of this patient?

❑ A. **Testicular biopsy**

❑ B. **Head MRI**

❑ C. **Testicular ultrasound**

❑ D. **Karyotype**

Key Concept/Objective: To be able to recognize secondary hypogonadism

Male hypogonadism can occur as a consequence of a disease of the testes (primary hypogonadism) or as a consequence of a disease of the pituitary or hypothalamus (secondary hypogonadism). The clinical findings of hypogonadism result from either decreased spermatogenesis or decreased testosterone secretion. The sole clinical finding of decreased spermatogenesis is infertility. In contrast, decreased testosterone secretion causes a wide variety of clinical findings; specific findings depend on the stage of life in which the deficiency occurs. In adults, common manifestations are decreases in energy, libido, sexual hair, muscle mass, and bone mineral density, as well as the presence of anemia. Once the diagnosis of hypogonadism is suspected on the basis of symptoms and physical examination, the diagnosis must be confirmed by documenting decreased production of sperm or testosterone. If hypogonadism is confirmed, the next step is to measure LH and FSH levels. Elevated serum concentrations of LH and FSH indicate primary hypogonadism, whereas subnormal or normal values indicate secondary hypogonadism. In patients with secondary hypogonadism, MRI of the sellar region is indicated. This patient has secondary hypogonadism, so testicular biopsy and ultrasound are not indicated. Furthermore, testicular biopsy usually provides no more information about spermatogenesis than does sperm analysis. Karyotype should be considered in the evaluation of some congenital disorders, such as Klinefelter syndrome; however, this disorder causes primary hypogonadism. *(Answer: B—Head MRI)*

3. A 55-year-old man presents to your clinic complaining of swollen breasts. His symptoms started 3 or 4 months ago, when he noticed tenderness and swelling in both breasts. His medical history includes congestive heart failure and hypertension. His medications are benazepril, metoprolol, furosemide, and spironolactone. Review of systems is positive only for occasional dyspnea on exertion. Physical examination shows bilateral gynecomastia in the periareolar area, with some tenderness to palpation. Testicular examination is normal.

Which of the following would be the best step to take next in the evaluation and management of this patient?

❑ **A. Liver ultrasound**

❑ **B. Mammography**

❑ **C. Testicular ultrasound**

❑ **D. Cessation of spironolactone**

Key Concept/Objective: To know that spironolactone can cause gynecomastia

Gynecomastia is the development of glandular breast tissue in a man. In most cases of gynecomastia, the stimulation of glandular tissue appears to result from an increased ratio of estrogen to androgen. Mechanisms behind this change in the estrogen-to-androgen ratio include exposure to exogenous estrogen, increased estrogen secretion, increased peripheral conversion of androgens to estrogens, and inhibition of androgen binding. The diagnosis of gynecomastia is confirmed by physical examination. Mammography is usually unnecessary. Gynecomastia is generally bilateral, although it is occasionally unilateral. If the tissue is tender, the gynecomastia is more likely to be of recent origin. Gynecomastia must be distinguished from carcinoma of the breast. Breast cancer should be suspected when the breast enlargement is unilateral, nontender, not centered directly under the nipple, and hard. Many drugs that cause gynecomastia appear to do so by binding to the androgen receptor and thereby blocking endogenous testosterone. Spironolactone is one of these drugs. Although gynecomastia can be a sign of testicular cancer or cirrhosis, there is no other evidence of these disorders in this patient, and further imaging studies would not be indicated at this time. The most likely etiology is gynecomastia secondary to spironolactone, and the best intervention would be to stop this medication and then reevaluate the patient. *(Answer: D—Cessation of spironolactone)*

For more information, see Snyder PJ: 3 Endocrinology: II Testes and Testicular Disorders. ACP Medicine Online (www.acpmedicine.com). Dale DC, Federman DD, Eds. WebMD Inc., New York, September 2003

The Adrenal

4. A 44-year-old African-American woman presents to your clinic with a complaint of weight gain. She reports increasing weight gain over the past year despite any noticeable change in her dietary intake. She notes that most of the added weight is around her abdomen. During the review of symptoms, she notes recent onset of amenorrhea without associated hot flushes. All women in her family experienced menopause after 50 years of age. On physical examination, the patient is hypertensive, with a blood pressure of 152/94 mm Hg. You notice that she has classic moon facies with purple abdominal striae.

Which of the following statements regarding the testing for Cushing syndrome is true?

❑ **A. The single best biochemical marker of Cushing syndrome is an elevation in the 8:00 A.M. cortisol count of greater than 20 µg/dl**

❑ **B. Patients with a random plasma adrenocorticotropic hormone (ACTH) level of greater than 10 pg/ml should undergo a corticotropin-releasing hormone (CRH) challenge**

❑ **C. A random plasma ACTH level greater than 10 µg/ml is indicative of ACTH-dependent Cushing syndrome**

❑ **D. Patients with ACTH-independent Cushing syndrome should undergo inferior petrosal sinus sampling**

Key Concept/Objective: To understand the diagnosis of Cushing syndrome

The classic clinical presentation of Cushing syndrome includes central obesity, striae, moon facies, supraclavicular fat pads, diabetes mellitus, hypertension, hirsutism and oligomenorrhea in women, and erectile dysfunction in men. The diagnosis of Cushing syndrome is principally clinical. Typically, patients will have some, but not all, of the clinical manifestations of Cushing syndrome. The diagnosis is confirmed by an elevation in urinary free cortisol excretion on 24-hour urine testing; this is the single best biochemical marker of Cushing syndrome. Once the diagnosis is secure, the first step in the differential diagnosis is to determine whether the condition is ACTH-dependent or ACTH-independent. This is most easily done by measuring the level of circulating plasma ACTH. Although an ACTH level greater than 10 pg/ml indicates ACTH dependence, this threshold will fail to identify 5% of ACTH-dependent cases. Consequently, patients with a random plasma ACTH level of less than 10 pg/ml should undergo a corticotropin-releasing hormone challenge. Patients with ACTH-dependent Cushing syndrome should undergo an inferior petrosal sampling procedure to search for a gradient in ACTH levels between blood draining the pituitary gland (inferior petrosal sinus blood) and peripheral antecubital blood. An ACTH gradient of greater than 3 between simultaneously sampled central and peripheral blood confirms a pituitary etiology for Cushing syndrome. If the gradient is less than 3, the search for an ectopic source of ACTH should be undertaken. *(Answer: C—A random plasma ACTH level greater than 10 µg/ml is indicative of ACTH-dependent Cushing syndrome)*

5. A woman was admitted this morning in the medical intensive care unit for elective cholecystectomy. Before surgery, her physical examination, including vital signs, was normal. The procedure went well, and there were no noticeable complications. However, 3 hours after returning to her room, she was noted to be unresponsive and her blood pressure was barely palpable. She was intubated for respiratory failure. Her blood pressure has been refractory to intravenous fluids and pressors. You are consulted to help in the workup of suspected adrenal insufficiency.

Which of the following statements regarding adrenal insufficiency is true?

- ❑ **A. The most common cause of adrenal insufficiency in the United States is tuberculosis**
- ❑ **B. The critical test for the diagnosis of chronic adrenal insufficiency is the cosyntropin test**
- ❑ **C. Chronic secondary adrenal insufficiency is treated with hydrocortisone and fludrocortisone, whereas chronic primary adrenal insufficiency is treated with hydrocortisone alone**
- ❑ **D. In idiopathic or autoimmune adrenal insufficiency, CT of the abdomen shows enlarged adrenal glands**

Key Concept/Objective: To understand the diagnosis and treatment of adrenal insufficiency

Primary adrenal insufficiency results from destruction of the adrenal cortex. The list of causes of primary adrenal insufficiency is long. In the industrialized nations, idiopathic or autoimmune adrenal destruction is the most common cause. Secondary adrenal insufficiency results from disruption of pituitary secretion of ACTH. By far the most common cause of secondary adrenal insufficiency is prolonged treatment with exogenous glucocorticoids. The acute syndrome is closely analogous to cardiogenic or septic shock and involves reduced cardiac output and a dilated and unresponsive vascular system. Symptoms include prostration, as well as all of the signs and symptoms of the shock syndrome. With both chronic and acute syndromes, the diagnosis should be suspected on clinical grounds but requires laboratory confirmation. The critical test for the diagnosis of chronic adrenal insufficiency is the cosyntropin stimulation test. Synthetic ACTH (cosyntropin) is administered in a 250 μg intravenous bolus, and plasma cortisol levels are measured 45 and 60 minutes afterward. Values greater than 20 μg/dl exclude adrenal insufficiency as a cause of the clinical findings. Values less than 20 μg/dl suggest that adrenal compromise could be a contributing factor. In this situation, treatment with a glucocorticoid is mandatory until the clinical situation is clarified with more precision. The differential diagnosis of adrenal insufficiency requires the discrimination of primary and secondary causes. The most useful test for this is measurement of the circulating plasma ACTH level. ACTH levels greater than normal define primary disease; values in the normal range or below define secondary disease. Primary chronic adrenal insufficiency is treated with 12 to 15 mg/m^2 of oral hydrocortisone a day. Hydrocortisone is best given as a single daily dose with breakfast. Fludrocortisone is given at a dose of 0.1 mg a day. Chronic secondary adrenal insufficiency is treated in the same way as chronic primary disease but with replacement of hydrocortisone only, not aldosterone. *(Answer: B—The critical test for the diagnosis of chronic adrenal insufficiency is the cosyntropin test)*

6. A 32-year-old man presents to your clinic for evaluation of headaches. He has had episodic pounding headaches for 6 months. He never had headaches like this before in his life. He denies using illicit drugs. He has no family history of hypertension. On physical examination, the patient is hypertensive, with a blood pressure of 180/105 mm Hg. No further abnormalities are noted. You begin a workup for secondary causes of hypertension.

Which of the following statements regarding pheochromocytomas is true?

- ❑ **A. 90% of pheochromocytomas are malignant**
- ❑ **B. Almost all patients with pheochromocytomas have episodic hypertension, making diagnosis difficult in a single clinic visit**
- ❑ **C. The incidence of pheochromocytoma is increased in patients with multiple endocrine neoplasia type 1**
- ❑ **D. Treatment of pheochromocytoma is surgical; alpha blockade should be induced with phenoxybenzamine, beginning 7 days before surgery**

Key Concept/Objective: To understand the clinical presentation and treatment of pheochromocytoma

The primary disease of the adrenal medulla is pheochromocytoma; 90% of pheochromocytomas occur in the adrenal medulla. The main clinical manifestation of pheochromocytomas is hypertension. The hypertension can be sustained or episodic; the two forms occur with equal frequency. The incidence of pheochromocytoma is markedly increased in several genetic syndromes: multiple endocrine neoplasia type 2a and type 2b; and the phakomatoses, including neurofibromatosis, cerebelloretinal hemangioblastosis, tuberous sclerosis, and Sturge-Weber syndrome. The treatment of pheochromocytoma is surgical. Before the surgical procedure, complete alpha blockade should be induced to avoid intraoperative hypertensive crisis. Preparation should begin 7 days before the planned procedure, using phenoxybenzamine at an initial dosage of 10 mg by mouth twice daily. The dose should be increased daily so that by the seventh day, the patient is taking at least 1 mg/kg/day in three divided doses. *(Answer: D—Treatment of pheochromocytoma is surgical; alpha blockade should be induced with phenoxybenzamine, beginning 7 days before surgery)*

7. A 32-year-old man presents to your clinic as a new patient to establish primary care. He has a 2-year history of hypertension, which is managed with a calcium channel blocker. He has no knowledge of the cause of his hypertension. He is currently without complaints and only wants a refill on his medication. His physical examination is unremarkable, but laboratory results show hypokalemia.

Which of the following statements regarding hyperaldosteronism is true?

- ❑ A. **The most common causes of secondary hyperaldosteronism are congestive heart failure and cirrhosis with ascites**
- ❑ B. **Treatment of primary adrenal hyperaldosteronism is spironolactone**
- ❑ C. **Patients with primary adrenal hyperaldosteronism usually present with hypertension, hypokalemia, and metabolic acidosis**
- ❑ D. **Diagnosis of primary adrenal hyperaldosteronism is confirmed by elevations in the levels of both renin and aldosterone**

Key Concept/Objective: To understand the clinical presentation, diagnosis, and treatment of hyperaldosteronism

Hyperaldosteronism can be primary or secondary. In primary hyperaldosteronism, there is disordered function of the renin-aldosterone feedback axis; in secondary hyperaldosteronism, the renin-aldosterone axis responds normally to chronic intravascular volume deficiency. Primary hyperaldosteronism is caused by benign adrenal adenomas, which are typically unilateral and are usually less than 2.5 cm in diameter. They secrete aldosterone independently of renin-angiotensin stimulation. Patients present with hypertension. Primary adrenal hypersecretion of aldosterone is thought to account for about 2% of cases of hypertension. Laboratory testing shows hypokalemia and metabolic alkalosis, with a serum sodium level that is usually in the high normal range. Diagnosis is confirmed by demonstrating normal or elevated plasma aldosterone levels (> 14 ng/dl) in the presence of suppressed stimulated plasma renin activity (< 2 ng/ml/hr). The treatment of primary adrenal hyperaldosteronism is unilateral adrenalectomy, preferably by a laparoscopic procedure. Secondary hyperaldosteronism may or may not be associated with hypertension. Probably the most common causes are chronic heart failure and cirrhosis of the liver with ascites. *(Answer: A—The most common causes of secondary hyperaldosteronism are congestive heart failure and cirrhosis with ascites)*

For more information, see Loriaux DL: 3 Endocrinology: IV The Adrenal. ACP Medicine Online (www.acpmedicine.com). Dale DC, Federman DD, Eds. WebMD Inc., New York, October 2004

Calcium Metabolism and Metabolic Bone Disease

8. A 54-year-old woman comes to your clinic for a routine visit. She has no active complaints. Her medical history is positive only for mild asthma and arterial hypertension. Her only medications are albuterol,

which she administers with a measured-dose inhaler as needed, and an angiotensin-converting enzyme inhibitor. She smokes one pack of cigarettes a day. She has a strong family history of osteoporosis. Her physical examination is unremarkable. You have a discussion with her regarding her risk of osteoporosis, and you decide to obtain a dual-energy x-ray absorptiometry (DEXA) scan for screening. The results show a T score of –2.6. Her creatinine and albumin levels are normal, her liver function tests are normal except for a slightly elevated alkaline phosphatase level, and her calcium level is 11 mg/dl.

What is the most appropriate step to take next in the treatment of this patient?

- ❑ **A. Start bisphosphonate, calcium, and vitamin D, and reassess in 6 months**
- ❑ **B. Measure the parathyroid hormone (PTH) level with a two-site immunoradiometric assay (IRMA, or so-called intact PTH) and assess 24-hour urinary calcium output**
- ❑ **C. Order CT scans of the chest and abdomen to look for an occult malignancy**
- ❑ **D. Start hormone replacement therapy with estrogens and progestins**

Key Concept/Objective: To understand the appropriate initial evaluation of a patient with hypercalcemia

This patient presents with mild, asymptomatic hypercalcemia. The most common cause of hypercalcemia in outpatients is hyperparathyroidism. The differential diagnosis of hypercalcemia is extensive. Once hypercalcemia is confirmed, the next step is to measure the serum PTH concentration. Several PTH assays are commercially available. The most commonly utilized test is the intact PTH. Other helpful tests include blood urea nitrogen (BUN), serum creatinine, alkaline phosphatase, and serum inorganic phosphorus assays; an electrolyte panel; and an assessment of 24-hour urinary calcium output. If the levels of PTH are elevated or inappropriately normal, the hypercalcemia is said to be PTH mediated. When PTH levels are suppressed, the hypercalcemia is said to be non–PTH mediated. Patients with hyperparathyroidism typically have a serum calcium concentration of less than 12 mg/dl; mild to moderate hypophosphatemia; and non–anion gap acidosis (from renal tubular acidosis). Urinary calcium excretion is usually increased; in these patients, the reduction of fractional calcium excretion by PTH is overcome by the high filtered calcium load, which may result in nephrolithiasis. The levels of alkaline phosphatase can be elevated as well. Before starting a more extensive evaluation in this patient, it is necessary to exclude the possibility of primary hyperparathyroidism. *(Answer: B—Measure the parathyroid hormone [PTH] level with a two-site immunoradiometric assay [IRMA, or so-called intact PTH] and assess 24-hour urinary calcium output)*

8. A 45-year-old man with a history of primary hyperparathyroidism comes to your clinic for a follow-up visit. He was diagnosed 3 years ago after routine blood tests revealed an elevation in calcium level. He has no complaints. Review of systems is negative, and his physical examination is unremarkable. His family history is negative for similar problems. His calcium level is 11.5 mg/dl. A DEXA scan shows a T score of –2 at the hip.

What is the most appropriate treatment regimen for this patient?

- ❑ **A. Observation, with routine follow-up visits that include assessment of calcium levels and DEXA scans**
- ❑ **B. Start a bisphosphonate**
- ❑ **C. Refer to an experienced surgeon for parathyroid surgery**
- ❑ **D. Administer calcium, 1,000 to 1,500 mg/day, and vitamin D, 400 to 800 IU/day**

Key Concept/Objective: To understand the surgical indications for hyperparathyroidism

Treatment of the patient with hyperparathyroidism must take into account the degree of the hypercalcemia, the presence of symptoms, and the severity of any end-organ damage.

Because many patients with hyperparathyroidism are either asymptomatic or minimally symptomatic, there is controversy over which patients require definitive therapy with surgery. The 2002 National Institutes of Health Workshop on Asymptomatic Primary Hyperparathyroidism defined the following indications for surgical intervention: (1) significant bone, renal, gastrointestinal, or neuromuscular symptoms typical of primary hyperparathyroidism; (2) elevation of serum calcium by 1 mg/dl or more above the normal range; (3) marked elevation of 24-hour urine calcium excretion (> 400 mg); (4) decreased creatinine clearance (reduced by 30%); (5) significant reduction in bone density (T score < –2.5); (6) consistent follow-up is not possible or is undesirable because of coexisting medical conditions; and (7) age less than 50 years. Because of this patient's age, surgery is indicated. *(Answer: C—Refer to an experienced surgeon for parathyroid surgery)*

10. A 66-year-old woman presents to a walk-in clinic with muscle spasms. She complains that for the past 2 days she has had muscle spasms in her hands, arms, and legs. She has a medical history of cervical Hodgkin lymphoma, which was treated with radiation. She does not take any medications or vitamins. On physical examination, the Trousseau sign is positive. Her calcium level is 6.8 mg/dl; the albumin level is normal.

On the basis of this patient's history, what is the most likely diagnosis, and what should be the treatment?

- ❑ A. **Hypoparathyroidism secondary to radiation therapy; start PTH injections**
- ❑ B. **Vitamin D deficiency secondary to poor intake and lack of sunlight; start calcitriol**
- ❑ C. **Vitamin D deficiency secondary to poor intake and lack of sunlight; start cholecalciferol**
- ❑ D. **Hypoparathyroidism secondary to radiation therapy; start calcium and calcitriol**

Key Concept/Objective: To understand the most common causes of hypocalcemia and its treatment

Hypocalcemia is defined as a serum calcium level of less than 9 mg/dl. Hypocalcemia is most often related to disorders of the parathyroid glands. Removal of or vascular injury to the parathyroids during neck surgery can result in hypoparathyroidism, which is manifested by hypocalcemia, hyperphosphatemia, and inappropriately low concentrations of PTH. Autoimmune destruction of the parathyroid glands may be seen in other autoimmune conditions, such as polyglandular syndrome type 1. Certain infiltrative diseases, such as hemochromatosis, may also adversely affect parathyroid function, as may external beam radiation to the neck. In this patient, the history of radiation to the neck suggests the possibility of hypoparathyroidism secondary to radiation injury. Despite the fact that vitamin D deficiency is common in elderly patients, serum calcium concentrations are usually not severely affected thanks to compensatory increases in PTH levels. In patients with symptoms associated with hypocalcemia (e.g., neuromuscular irritability), calcium volume should be repleted with a slow intravenous infusion of calcium salts. In most patients, vitamin D should also be provided. If dietary deficiency is suspected, plain cholecalciferol is adequate. In cases of hypoparathyroidism, however, calcitriol will be required. *(Answer: D—Hypoparathyroidism secondary to radiation therapy; start calcium and calcitriol)*

11. A 55-year-old woman comes to your office with the results of a screening DEXA scan. Her T score is –2.7. She has not had any symptoms and denies having any previous fractures. She underwent menopause 3 years ago. Six months ago, she underwent mammography and had a Pap smear, both of which were negative. She has no family history of breast cancer. Her physical examination, including examination of the breasts, is normal. Her laboratory workup shows no evidence of conditions that are secondary causes of osteoporosis.

What is the most appropriate recommendation regarding the management of this patient's osteoporosis?

❑ A. **Start bisphosphonate therapy, start calcium and vitamin D therapy, and recommend exercise**

❑ B. **Start hormone replacement therapy, start calcium and vitamin D therapy, and recommend exercise**

❑ C. **Start calcitonin, calcium, and vitamin D therapy, and recommend exercise**

❑ D. **Do not start therapy until the osteoporosis becomes symptomatic**

Key Concept/Objective: To understand the appropriate management of osteoporosis

Osteoporosis is defined as decreased bone mass (or density) with abnormal skeletal microarchitecture that increases the risk of fracture. The diagnostic criteria of the World Health Organization are based on the results of standardized bone mass measurements: osteoporosis is present when the bone mineral density (BMD) is decreased to more than 2.5 standard deviations below that of a normal, young control population (T score). Osteopenia is present when the BMD falls between –1.0 and –2.5 from peak bone mass. In patients with osteoporosis, an adequate amount of calcium should be provided. This patient should take 1,000 to 1,500 mg of calcium a day. Also, the patient should receive 400 to 800 IU of vitamin D. Osteoporosis is most often treated with antiresorptive agents; these drugs include bisphosphonates, estrogen, selective estrogen receptor modulators (e.g., raloxifene), and calcitonin. All of these agents reduce fracture rates substantially, but estrogen and bisphosphonates appear to produce the greatest improvement in bone density. Until recently, estrogen replacement therapy was widely recommended as first-line therapy for both prevention and treatment of osteoporosis. Advocates argued that estrogen directly corrected the chief pathophysiologic defect of the menopause-estrogen deficiency. They also cited other benefits, such as relief from vasomotor disturbances, mood swings, sleep disturbance, and urogenital atrophy. Estrogen therapy was also thought to offer cardiovascular benefits, possibly related to its positive effects on plasma lipid levels. Recently, the multicentric Women's Health Initiative study was stopped prematurely because of a significant increase in the risk of breast cancer, myocardial infarction, strokes, and thromboembolic events. As a result of these findings, estrogen should no longer be considered the optimal first-line preventive or therapeutic agent for osteoporosis. Bisphosphonates should be considered the optimal choice for the initial therapy for osteoporosis. Calcitonin's effects on bone density appear to be weaker than those of estrogen or the bisphosphonates. Raloxifene can be used for osteoporosis prevention and treatment; it appears to have a less potent effect on bone density than either estrogens or bisphosphonates. *(Answer: A—Start bisphosphonate therapy, start calcium and vitamin D therapy, and recommend exercise)*

For more information, see Inzucchi SE: 3 Endocrinology: VI Diseases of Calcium Metabolism and Metabolic Bone Disease. ACP Medicine Online (www.acpmedicine.com). Dale DC, Federman DD, Eds. WebMD Inc., New York, March 2003

Genetic Diagnosis and Counseling

12. A 37-year-old man presents to the local emergency department with a swollen and tender right calf. The patient has had these symptoms for 4 days. He denies having undergone any trauma. He has no history of cancer, and he has had no similar episodes in the past. He denies having a family history of venous thrombosis. Ultrasound confirms deep vein thrombosis, and the patient is provided with appropriate anticoagulation. Several days later, the patient sees you for a follow-up visit. The laboratory studies made in the emergency department included a factor V Leiden mutation analysis.

Which of the following statements is true regarding this patient's test for factor V Leiden mutation?

❑ A. **The clinical setting and the patient's risk factors for deep vein thrombosis have no bearing on the decision to conduct factor V Leiden mutation testing**

❑ B. **It is estimated that 25% of whites and 50% of those with venous thromboembolism are heterozygous for factor V Leiden mutation**

❑ C. **Factor V Leiden mutation analysis is a DNA test with low sensitivity, low specificity, and high positive predictive value for this mutation**

❑ D. **Factor V Leiden mutation analysis is a DNA test with high sensitivity, low specificity, and low positive predictive value for this mutation**

Key Concept/Objective: To understand the limitations and characteristics of DNA-based testing

The clinical setting and risk factors given for a particular patient have great implications on the use of genetic testing. Although factor V Leiden is the most common known thrombophilic risk factor, only a small proportion of patients with this genetic disorder ever experience an episode of thrombosis (the risk of thrombosis is 2.4-fold greater in those with the mutation than in those without the mutation). It is estimated that 5% of whites are heterozygous for factor V Leiden and that approximately 20% of all persons with venous thromboembolism are heterozygous for factor V Leiden. Factor V Leiden mutation analysis, the most commonly ordered genetic test, is an example of a direct DNA-based test with 100% sensitivity but low specificity and low positive predictive value. *(Answer: D—Factor V Leiden mutation analysis is a DNA test with high sensitivity, low specificity, and low positive predictive value for this mutation)*

13. A 21-year-old man comes to your office to establish primary care. He states that he has been generally healthy but that he has multiple colon polyps. He states that he tested positive for familial adenomatous polyposis (FAP). He says that his former physician told him that this illness can run in families, and he asks your opinion on whether or not his family needs further testing.

Which of the following statements regarding FAP and the* APC *gene mutation is true?

❑ A. **Persons with the *APC* gene mutation develop colorectal adenomas starting at around age 30**

❑ B. **FAP is an autosomal dominant disorder with 50% to 70% penetrance of the disease-causing gene mutation**

❑ C. **Presymptomatic testing has never been shown to reduce morbidity or increase life expectancy**

❑ D. **Testing of the *APC* gene has been shown to be cost-effective when used to identify carriers of the *APC* gene mutation among at-risk relatives of individuals with FAP**

Key Concept/Objective: To understand the value and utility of presymptomatic genetic testing

FAP is a devastating, life-shortening condition when it is not recognized. FAP is an autosomal dominant disorder with 100% penetrance of the disease-causing gene. Persons with an *APC* gene mutation develop adenomas in the colorectum starting at around 16 years of age; in these individuals, the number of adenomas increases to hundreds or thousands, and colorectal cancer develops at a mean age of 39 years. The mean age at death is 42 years in those who go untreated. Testing of the *APC* gene has been shown to be cost-effective when used to identify carriers of the disease-causing *APC* gene mutation among at-risk relatives of individuals with FAP. Early diagnosis via presymptomatic testing reduces morbidity and increases life expectancy through improved surveillance and timely prophylactic colectomy. FAP is an example of a condition in which presymptomatic testing may be lifesaving. *(Answer: D—Testing of the* APC *gene has been shown to be cost-effective when used to identify carriers of the* APC *gene mutation among at-risk relatives of individuals with FAP)*

14. A 23-year-old female patient presents to your office for a routine annual visit. She mentions that her mother tested positive for the "breast cancer genes." She asks you for general information regarding these tests and about the need for her and her family to be tested for these mutations.

Which of the following statements is correct regarding* BRCA1 *and* BRCA2 *testing?

❑ A. **It is clear that all women should have genetic testing for the *BRCA1* and *BRCA2* mutations, because the efficacy of measures to reduce cancer risk for individuals with these mutations is well described**

❑ B. **In general, breast cancer is a simple disorder caused by heritable gene mutations only**

❑ C. **Only 5% to 10% of cases of breast cancer are attributed to mutations in single genes, including *BRCA1* and *BRCA2***

❑ D. **If this patient tests negative for the *BRCA1* and *BRCA2* mutations, she will have no future need for routine breast cancer screening**

Key Concept/Objective: To understand the importance and limitations of testing for BRCA *mutations*

The efficacy of measures to reduce cancer risk for individuals with *BRCA1* and *BRCA2* cancer-predisposing mutations is unknown. Breast cancer, like such other common disorders as coronary artery disease, diabetes mellitus, and Alzheimer disease, is regarded as a complex disorder. Complex disorders have multiple etiologies, including heritable single genes, multiple genes with an additive effect that interact with often undefined environmental influences, and acquired environmental or genetic changes. Single heritable genes may represent a relatively small contribution to the overall incidence and morbidity from common diseases, including breast cancer, which affects one in nine women. Only 5% to 10% of cases of breast cancer are attributed to mutations in single genes, including *BRCA1* and *BRCA2*. For a woman whose relatives have a known *BRCA1* mutation but who has tested negative for the mutation known to be in the family, the chance of the development of breast cancer is still one in nine. This patient therefore has the same need for close surveillance as women in the general population. *(Answer: C—Only 5% to 10% of cases of breast cancer are attributed to mutations in single genes, including* BRCA1 *and* BRCA2*)*

15. A 24-year-old man with a history of increasing muscle cramps, myalgias, and calf muscle hypertrophy was recently diagnosed with Becker muscular dystrophy (BMD) through muscle biopsy. The lab report of the patient's leukocyte DNA analysis, however, states, "no mutation known to be associated with BMD found." On further questioning, you discover that the patient has a reportedly healthy 2-year-old daughter; a 16-year-old maternal cousin who recently began suffering from muscle cramps similar to those of the patient; a sister in her teens who is reportedly healthy; a mother with a "big heart"; and a maternal grandfather who died of an unspecified heart problem 20 years ago. You suggest further genetic linkage analysis and counseling for this patient and his extended family.

Which of the following facts would serve as the basis of your recommendation?

❑ A. **Even though the patient cannot pass on the gene for BMD, his apparently healthy sister might be a carrier**

❑ B. **This patient's offspring and other relatives are at risk for BMD, and a genetic linkage analysis would help define their genotypic risk status**

❑ C. **Analysis of family members might help define the mutation in this patient and therefore help guide his therapies**

❑ D. **You should not suggest further counseling or testing because the lack of a specific gene mutation in the proband means you will not be able to determine the degree to which the patient's asymptomatic relatives are at risk**

❑ E. **The mother's mutation probably represents germline mosaicism; linkage analysis would help determine both her risk and her other children's risk**

Key Concept/Objective: To understand the pattern of inheritance of X-linked diseases and to know their implications

Because dystrophinopathies are inherited in an X-linked recessive manner, the risk to the siblings of a proband depends upon the carrier status of the mother. In this case, the moth-

er is an obligate heterozygote (because both her son and nephew have a disease-causing gene). As such, she is a carrier with a 50% chance of transmitting the *BMD* mutation to each of her children. Her sons who inherit the mutation will develop clinical symptoms of BMD; her daughters who inherit the mutation will be carriers. Were men with BMD to have daughters, those daughters would be carriers; were men with BMD to have sons, those sons would inherit their father's *BMD* mutation. When it is likely that a family member of a pregnant woman has the *BMD* gene, prenatal testing of the fetus for the presence of the gene is possible; such testing involves a search for linked markers. It is important that all female carriers be identified so that they can be advised of their risk for dilated cardiomyopathy and that the appropriate surveillance can be provided. Unfortunately, there is no therapy for BMD. *(Answer: B—This patient's offspring and other relatives are at risk for BMD, and a genetic linkage analysis would help define their genotypic risk status)*

16. A 34-year-old banker has just finished 6 months of warfarin therapy after a pulmonary embolus resulting from deep vein thrombosis. During her hospital stay, she was told she has a factor V Leiden mutation, which makes her prone to clotting. Her husband and two children have now all been tested as well; those test results are as follows:

Patient: Arg 506 Gln; increased activated protein C (APC) resistance
Husband: Normal
Daughter 1: Arg 506 Gln; increased APC resistance
Son 1: Normal

On the basis of these test results, what steps should be taken now?

- ❑ **A. The proband and the daughter carrying her mutant allele will require anticoagulation for a minimum of 6 months to 2 years**
- ❑ **B. The patient and her family should be advised that heterozygosity for factor V Leiden is associated with neither an increase in mortality nor a reduction in normal life expectancy**
- ❑ **C. The daughter with a factor V Leiden mutation should be counseled not to take oral contraceptives**
- ❑ **D. The family should be tested for other thrombophilic disorders as well, such as lupus anticoagulant**
- ❑ **E. The proband should be counseled about her need for anticoagulant therapy if she should choose to become pregnant again**

Key Concept/Objective: To understand that in cases involving factor V Leiden mutation, treatment decisions should be guided by the clinical situation of each patient and family member, not the presence or absence of a mutation

Heterozygosity for the factor V Leiden allele confers only a mildly increased risk of thrombosis. Routine testing of family members at risk is not recommended. In the absence of evidence that early diagnosis of the heterozygous state reduces morbidity or mortality, the decision to test family members who are at risk should be made on a case-by-case basis. Individuals requesting screening for factor V Leiden should be counseled regarding the implications of the diagnosis. Specifically, they should be informed that although the factor V Leiden mutation is an established risk factor, it does not predict the occurrence of pathologic thrombosis with certainty, even among heterozygotes of the same family. With this in mind, symptomatic individuals with a known factor V Leiden mutation should be screened for other potentially comorbid thrombophilias. Finally, the minimum period that symptomatic patients with factor V Leiden mutations should remain on anticoagulant therapy is unclear; current recommendations are that they receive therapy for a minimum of 6 months. *(Answer: B—The patient and her family should be advised that heterozygosity for factor V Leiden is associated with neither an increase in mortality nor a reduction in normal life expectancy)*

17. A 12-month-old baby is brought in for a well-baby visit, during which the baby is noted to have leukokoria (a white pupillary reflex). On further evaluation, it is determined that the child has an ablatable, unifocal retinoblastoma, with an *RB1* cancer-predisposing mutation in a tumor and no evidence of a germline *RB1* in white cell DNA. The parents are concerned about the risk of retinoblastoma if they have other children.

Regarding these parents' concern, which of the following statements is true?

- ❑ A. **Absence of a germline *RB1* mutation on the patient's DNA screening reduces the risk in the rest of the family to chance; there is no need for further family testing**
- ❑ B. **Both parents should be screened; if a germline mutation is not identified, the risk to future siblings is not increased**
- ❑ C. **The patient's future siblings may be at increased risk and should have aggressive surveillance and genetic screening**
- ❑ D. **The patient's future siblings would not be at increased risk, but the patient's offspring would be and should be screened for *RB1* mutations prenatally**
- ❑ E. **Testing for *RB1* is presymptomatic, and the patient—but not future siblings—will need continued aggressive surveillance to ensure that another retinoblastoma does not arise de novo**

Key Concept/Objective: To understand genetic mosaicism

The gold standard for detecting *RB1* gene defects is gene sequencing, which detects mutations in 80% of patients. Because the proband does not have a germline mutation for *RB1*, there is most likely a genetic mosaicism for the mutation, which must have arisen as a postzygotic event. This means that the parents and future siblings are not at increased risk for retinoblastoma, but the patient's children would be (they would have a 3% to 5% risk). DNA-based testing of the proband's children, however, could reduce the need for screening for retinoblastoma. Without DNA screening, offspring would need to be reevaluated regularly by an ophthalmologist. Children who test negative for an *RB1* mutation could be spared unnecessary screening protocols. It is important to note that DNA screening for *RB1* is predispositional, and even patients who have unilateral retinoblastoma with *RB1* cancer-predisposing mutations in a tumor and no evidence of a germline *RB1* cancer-predisposing mutation are at increased risk for developing additional tumors. *(Answer: D—The patient's future siblings would not be at increased risk, but the patient's offspring would be and should be screened for* RB1 *mutations prenatally)*

18. A 25-year-old Ashkenazi Jewish woman is concerned about her risk of breast cancer. Her 60-year-old mother was recently diagnosed with stage II breast cancer and underwent bilateral mastectomy. Her grandmother was killed in World War II, so she does not know whether her grandmother had breast cancer. She read in a newspaper article that the prevalence of *BRCA1* and *BRCA2* genes is increased in Ashkenazi Jewish women and that, as a result, this population is at increased risk for breast cancer. Now she would like to be tested for these genes because she is concerned about her risk status and [illegible] whether she needs a prophylactic mastectomy.

Of the following statements, which would be appropriate to tell this patient?

- ❑ A. **Testing for the *BRCA1* and *BRCA2* genes is not indicated, because the efficacy of measures to reduce risk in asymptomatic patients, even those with a mutation, is not known**
- ❑ B. **You would be happy to arrange for *BRCA* mutation screening, but she should undergo testing in conjunction with appropriate genetic counseling**
- ❑ C. **It would be more appropriate for the patient's mother to be tested first; if a cancer-predisposing mutation were found, then—and only then—would genetic testing for the patient be appropriate**
- ❑ D. **Testing in this patient is not indicated; even if she tests negative for an inherited cancer-predisposing mutation in the *BRCA1* or *BRCA2* gene, she may still have a mutation in another gene that predisposes to breast cancer**

❑ E. **It is very important that the patient and her family undergo genetic analysis of both the *BRCA* loci and other cancer-predisposing loci as soon as possible, because her mother's breast cancer demonstrates that her family is at increased risk**

Key Concept/Objective: To understand the role of testing in determining whether a disease-modifying gene is contributing to a complex disorder

BRCA1 **or** ***BRCA2*** **mutations are more likely to be found in families of Ashkenazi Jewish ancestry; in families in which a family member was diagnosed with breast cancer before 50 years of age; and in families in which a family member was diagnosed with bilateral breast cancer, ovarian cancer, or both breast cancer and ovarian cancer. It is important to note, however, that** ***BRCA1*** **and** ***BRCA2*** **mutations cause only a small increase in the overall incidence of breast cancer. In patients undergoing genetic testing because of a suggestive family history, it is highly recommended that there be pretest and posttest counseling. If a cancer-predisposing mutation is identified,** ***BRCA1*** **or** ***BRCA2*** **mutation analysis is more informative for unaffected relatives. However, depending on the type of analysis done, mutations of uncertain clinical significance may be identified; such findings are difficult (at best) to interpret. If a cancer-predisposing mutation is found in the mother, the patient should be counseled not to desist from rigorous screening for breast cancer.**

Given the high prevalence of breast cancer in the general population and in the Ashkenazi Jewish population in particular, regardless of this patient's ***BRCA*** **status, a negative result would not indicate that she is at reduced risk relative to that of the general population. Furthermore, in individuals from high-risk ethnic groups, such as Ashkenazi Jews, it might be reasonable to test for all the cancer-predisposing mutations known to be common in that population, even if a single cancer-predisposing mutation had already been identified in an affected family member. Unfortunately, there are no unique interventions of proven benefit for those individuals in whom a genetic susceptibility to breast cancer is found, beyond the routine mammography screening recommended for women of average risk beginning at 40 or 50 years of age. Additional recommendations for women in higher risk categories are made on the basis of presumptive benefit and have not yet been supported in clinical studies.** *(Answer: C—It would be more appropriate for the patient's mother to be tested first; if a cancer-predisposing mutation were found, then—and only then—would genetic testing for the patient be appropriate)*

For more information, see Pagon RA: 3 Endocrinology: VIII Genetic Diagnosis and Counseling. ACP Medicine Online (www.acpmedicine.com). Dale DC, Federman DD, Eds. WebMD Inc., New York, May 2002

Hypoglycemia

19. A 32-year-old man presents to your clinic for a routine follow-up visit. He complains of intermittent episodes of shaking, palpitations, sweating, and anxiety. The episodes generally occur between meals. He has a friend who is a hypoglycemic and is on a special diet, and he wonders if he too may have low blood sugar. While in the waiting room, he develops symptoms, and your nurse obtains a blood glucose level. The result is 74 mg/dl.

What is the most appropriate step to take next in the workup of this patient?

❑ A. **Admit the patient to the hospital for a prolonged fast**

❑ B. **Send the patient for an endoscopic ultrasound, looking for insulinoma**

❑ C. **Measure the insulin and C-peptide levels, assess for insulin antibodies, and have the patient follow up in 1 month**

❑ D. **Refer the patient directly to surgery for resection of presumed insulinoma**

❑ E. **No further workup for hypoglycemic disorder is necessary at this time**

Key Concept/Objective: To understand that a normal serum glucose concentration in a symptomatic patient rules out hypoglycemic disorders

A normal serum glucose concentration, reliably obtained during the occurrence of spontaneous symptoms, eliminates the possibility of a hypoglycemic disorder; no further evaluation for hypoglycemia is required. Glucometer measurements made by the patient during the occurrence of symptoms often are unreliable, because nondiabetic patients usually are not experienced in this technique and the measurements are obtained under adverse circumstances. However, a reliably measured capillary glucose level that is in the normal range eliminates the possibility of hypoglycemia as the cause of symptoms. Normoglycemia during symptoms cannot be ascribed to spontaneous recovery from previous hypoglycemia. In fact, the reverse is true; symptoms ease before the serum glucose achieves a normal level. Workup for insulinoma is not warranted. *(Answer: E—No further workup for hypoglycemic disorder is necessary at this time)*

20. A 53-year-old woman presents to your clinic complaining of transient episodes of diaphoresis, asthenia, near syncope, and clouding of thought process; she has had these symptoms for several months. These episodes most commonly occur several hours after she eats. She has no other significant medical history and takes no medications. A prolonged fast is begun, during which the patient becomes symptomatic. Her serum glucose concentration at the time is 43 mg/dl. The insulin level is elevated, and no insulin antibodies are present. The C-peptide level is high, and tests for the use of sulfonylureas and meglitinides are negative.

What is the most effective therapy for this patient's condition?

- ❑ A. **Observe the patient and schedule a follow-up fast 2 to 3 months from now**
- ❑ B. **Adjust the patient's diet to include smaller, more frequent meals**
- ❑ C. **Obtain a transabdominal ultrasound and refer the patient to surgery for resection**
- ❑ D. **Begin diazoxide, 400 mg t.i.d., and verapamil, 180 mg q.d., and have the patient appear for a follow-up visit in 3 months**
- ❑ E. **Begin phenytoin and octreotide and have the patient appear for a follow-up visit in 3 months**

Key Concept/Objective: To understand the diagnosis and treatment of insulinoma

Insulinoma is characterized by hypoglycemia caused by elevated levels of endogenous insulin. Confirmation of the diagnosis requires exclusion of hypoglycemia from exogenous sources. Once a biochemical diagnosis of insulinoma is made, the next step is localization. The effective modalities are center dependent and include abdominal ultrasound, [illegible] scan. After localization, the treatment of choice for insulinomas is surgical removal. Depending on the lesion, surgery may range from enucleation of the insulinoma to total pancreatectomy. Medical therapy is less effective than tumor resection but can be used in patients who are not candidates for surgery. The most effective medication for controlling symptomatic hypoglycemia is diazoxide, which lowers insulin production. Other medications for insulinomas include verapamil, phenytoin, and octreotide. *(Answer: C—Obtain a transabdominal ultrasound and refer the patient to surgery for resection)*

21. A 31-year-old woman presents to the emergency department complaining of episodes of dizziness, lightheadedness, palpitations, sweats, anxiety, and confusion. On the morning of admission, she reports that she almost passed out. Her husband, who is a diabetic patient who requires insulin, checked her blood sugar level and noted it to be low. Her symptoms resolved after drinking some orange juice. She is admitted to the hospital for a prolonged fast. After 18 hours, she becomes symptomatic, and her blood is drawn. The serum glucose concentration is 48 mg/dl, the serum insulin level is high, and test results are negative for insulin antibodies. The C-peptide level is low, and tests for sulfonylurea and meglitinides are negative.

Which of the following is the most likely diagnosis for this patient?

❑ A. **Insulinoma**

❑ B. **Factitial hypoglycemia**

❑ C. **Noninsulinoma pancreatogenous hypoglycemia syndrome (NIPHS)**

❑ D. **Insulin autoimmune hypoglycemia**

Key Concept/Objective: To be able to recognize the patient with factitial hypoglycemia

Factitial hypoglycemia is more common in women and occurs most often in the third or fourth decade of life. Many of these patients work in health-related occupations. Factitial hypoglycemia results from the use of insulin or drugs that stimulate insulin secretion, such as sulfonylureas or meglitinides. The possibility of factitial hypoglycemia should be considered in every patient undergoing evaluation for a hypoglycemic disorder, especially when the hypoglycemia has a chaotic occurrence—that is, when it has no relation to meals or fasting. The diagnosis of factitial hypoglycemia can usually be established by measuring serum insulin, sulfonylurea, and C-peptide levels when the patient is hypoglycemic. In a patient whose hypoglycemia results from covert use of a hypoglycemic agent, the agent will be present in the blood. In insulin-mediated factitial hypoglycemia, the serum insulin level is high and the C-peptide level is suppressed, usually close to the lower limit of detection, as seen in this patient. *(Answer: B—Factitial hypoglycemia)*

22. A 38-year-old man is brought to the emergency department after a generalized seizure. Blood glucose in the field is noted to be 45 mg/dl. The complete blood count and results of a blood chemistry 7 panel are normal, with the exception of a low glucose level. A head CT is negative, and a lumbar puncture reveals no evidence of infection. After the patient is stabilized and able to give a history, he tells you that he has been experiencing episodes of dizziness, confusion, headache, blurred vision, and weakness for the past month. The episodes always occur about 2 hours after he eats. He has no other significant medical history and takes no medications. He is admitted. Results of a supervised 72-hour fast are normal.

Which of the following is the probable diagnosis for this patient?

❑ A. **NIPHS**

❑ B. **Insulinoma**

❑ C. **Factitial hypoglycemia**

❑ D. **Insulin autoimmune hypoglycemia**

Key Concept/Objective: To be able to distinguish NIPHS from insulinoma

NIPHS is a recently described entity. Like insulinoma, it affects patients across a broad age range (16 to 78 years) and causes severe neurohypoglycemia, with loss of consciousness and, in some cases, generalized seizures. Unlike insulinoma, it occurs predominantly in males (70%). Histologic analysis of pancreatic tissue from patients with NIPHS shows cells budding off ducts, seen best by chromogranin A immunohistochemical staining. Islet cell hypertrophy is also evident. No gross or microscopic tumor has been identified in any patient with NIPHS. Symptoms of NIPHS occur primarily in a postprandial state, usually 2 to 4 hours after eating. Although patients with insulinoma may experience symptoms postprandially, they also have symptoms during food deprivation. It is extremely rare for insulinoma patients to have symptoms solely in the postprandial state. Results of supervised 72-hour fasts have always been negative in NIPHS patients. A negative 72-hour fast in a patient with insulinoma is a rare occurrence. Gradient-guided partial pancreatectomy has been effective in relieving symptoms in patients with NIPHS, though recurrence of hypoglycemia after a few symptom-free years has been reported in a few patients. *(Answer: A—NIPHS)*

For more information, see Service FJ: 3 Endocrinology: IX Hypoglycemia. ACP Medicine Online (www.acpmedicine.com). Dale DC, Federman DD, Eds. WebMD Inc., New York, May 2002

Obesity

23. A 42-year-old white woman comes to your office to establish primary care. She reports no previous medical history except "fibroids," for which she underwent a vaginal hysterectomy. She currently takes no medications. The results of physical examination are as follows: blood pressure, 136/81 mm Hg; heart rate, 87 beats/min; weight, 180 lb (82 kg); height, 5'7" (1.71 m). Other than the fact that she appears obese, there are no pertinent findings on physical examination. You are concerned with the long-term implications related to her being overweight.

On the basis of the available data, what is the calculated body mass index (BMI) for this patient?

❑ A. 28

❑ B. 24

❑ C. 32

❑ D. 34

Key Concept/Objective: To understand how to calculate BMI

Measures that were once used to determine excess mortality risk of obesity included the percentage of what was termed desirable weight or ideal body weight, which was based on data from the life-insurance industry. This form of measurement has been replaced by a classification system that attempts to allow comparison of weights independent of stature across populations. It is based on the BMI, which is calculated by dividing the body weight (in kilograms) divided by height (in meters) squared. In nonselected populations, BMI does correlate with percentage of body fat, but this relationship is independently influenced by sex, age, and race. In this patient, BMI is calculated as follows: 82 kg ÷ (1.71 m × 1.71 m) = 28 kg/m^2. *(Answer: A—28)*

24. A 38-year-old woman who is a longtime patient of yours comes to the clinic for her annual appointment. Despite multiple attempts at dietary and behavior modification, she has been gaining weight regularly since she was 23 years of age. In addition to obesity, she has moderately controlled hypertension and glucose intolerance and worsening osteoarthritis in her knees bilaterally. She requests to be placed on a more intensive weight-loss therapy.

On the basis of this patient's current BMI of 36 kg/m^2, which of the following would likely be the most appropriate therapy?

❑ **A. 3 to 6 months of intensive dietary restriction**

❑ **B. 3 to 6 months of intensive dietary restriction and exercise**

❑ **C. Initiation of pharmacologic therapy**

❑ **D. Referral for bariatric surgery**

Key Concept/Objective: To understand how BMI determines treatment of obese patients

The approach to the treatment of obesity is similar to that of other chronic conditions, such as hypertension, hypercholesterolemia, and diabetes. Patients are first managed with lifestyle measures for 3 to 6 months. For obesity, these lifestyle interventions include improved diet and increased activity. For patients whose weight does not change with lifestyle intervention alone or whose weight loss is insufficient to lower their long-term health risk, consideration is then given to pharmacologic or surgical management. A National Institutes of Health expert panel has suggested that patients whose BMI is 30 kg/m^2 or more or who have a BMI of 27 kg/m^2 or more plus obesity-related risk factors (i.e., diabetes, hypertension, or hyperlipidemia) could be considered for pharmacologic therapy. Patients with a BMI of 40 kg/m^2 or more or a BMI of 35 kg/m^2 or more plus obesity-related risk factors could be considered for surgical therapy. In this patient, the combination of hypertension, glucose intolerance, osteoarthritis, and a BMI greater than 35 kg/m^2 warrants referral for bariatric surgery. *(Answer: D—Referral for bariatric surgery)*

25. A 46-year-old African-American man presents to your office for a routine visit. On his last visit, which was 18 months ago, he was noted to be mildly hypertensive and obese. He underwent blood test screening for high lipid levels, thyroid disease, and glucose intolerance; all results were normal. His chief complaint today is excess fatigue. He reports that he frequently falls asleep during the day, occasionally when driving a car. He also reports occasional morning headaches.

Which of the following approaches are more likely to disclose the cause of this patient's fatigue?

- ❑ **A. Repeat thyroid function tests**
- ❑ **B. Transthoracic echocardiogram**
- ❑ **C. Pulmonary function tests**
- ❑ **D. The patient should be asked about his sleeping habits and referred for a sleep study**

Key Concept/Objective: To understand that sleep apnea is a common complication of obesity

In epidemiologic studies, persons who are overweight or obese and have central adiposity are at increased risk for hyperlipidemia, hypertension, and cardiovascular disease mortality. Sleep apnea is likely underdiagnosed in overweight and obese patients and should be strongly considered in patients with complaints of fatigue, daytime somnolence, snoring, restless sleep, and morning headaches. In this patient, the results of repeat thyroid function tests are likely to be normal, given this patient's constellation of symptoms and the fact that the results of recent testing were normal. Although fatigue can be attributed to primary cardiac or pulmonary disease, neither would explain the daytime somnolence and the morning headaches. *(Answer: D—The patient should be asked about his sleeping habits and referred for a sleep study)*

26. A 35-year-old white woman comes to your office requesting your opinion on how to lose weight. She has no known complications or associated comorbidities secondary to obesity. She read on the Internet that approaches to weight loss are based on the calculation of BMI. She tells you that because her BMI is 33 kg/m^2, medical therapy is indicated. Her sister has had great success taking orlistat, having lost 20 lb without having any significant side effects.

Which of the following statements regarding the use of orlistat therapy in this patient is true?

- ❑ **A. Orlistat is generally safe and well tolerated by most patients; the patient should be started on orlistat therapy in conjunction with a diet-and-exercise program**
- ❑ **B. The patient should be started on orlistat therapy; there is no need to prescribe**
- ❑ **C. Orlistat is generally safe, but a significant number of patients experience side effects; the patient should be started on orlistat therapy in conjunction with a diet-and-exercise program**
- ❑ **D. Orlistat is poorly tolerated by most patients and has life-threatening side effects**

Key Concept/Objective: To know the side effects of orlistat

Diet and exercise are the cornerstones of any weight loss program. Medication, including orlistat, should be considered as an adjunct to diet and exercise. Orlistat inhibits lipases in the gastrointestinal lumen, thereby antagonizing triglyceride hydrolysis and reducing fat absorption by roughly 30%. Gastrointestinal side effects may occur in up to 80% of patients when they begin therapy with orlistat (such side effects are also seen in 50% to 60% of patients given placebo), but this incidence diminishes with time. Symptoms include abdominal discomfort, flatus, fecal urgency, oily spotting, and fecal incontinence. When administered to patients who adhere to a low-fat diet, orlistat is generally well tolerated. Other than the gastrointestinal symptoms, orlistat is well tolerated without any other significant side effects. In one study, only 2.4%, 3.1%, and 1.6% of orlistat-treated patients had documented below-normal levels of β-carotene, vitamin D, and vitamin E, respectively. Nevertheless, orlistat should not be given to patients with existing malabsorptive states, and it is recommended that a daily multivitamin supplement be taken by patients during therapy. *(Answer: C—Orlistat is generally safe, but a significant number of patients* *experience side effects; the patient should be started on orlistat therapy in conjunction with a diet-and-exercise program)*

For more information, see Purnell JQ: 3 Endocrinology: X Obesity. ACP Medicine Online (www.acpmedicine.com). Dale DC, Federman DD, Eds. WebMD Inc., New York, June 2003

SECTION 4

GASTROENTEROLOGY

Esophageal Disorders

1. A 55-year-old man with long-standing gastroesophageal reflux disease (GERD) is found to have Barrett esophagus on a routine upper GI endoscopy. Four-quadrant biopsies show no dysplasia. He takes proton pump inhibitor (PPI) therapy every day, and he reports that his heartburn is under reasonable control. His physical examination is unremarkable.

What would you recommend regarding the treatment of this patient's Barrett esophagus?

- ❑ **A. Start an endoscopic surveillance program to look for dysplastic lesions**
- ❑ **B. Increase the PPI dose to maximally suppress acid secretion**
- ❑ **C. Refer for antireflux surgery to decrease the chances of progression to esophageal adenocarcinoma**
- ❑ **D. Refer for esophagectomy**

Key Concept/Objective: To understand the treatment of Barrett esophagus

Barrett esophagus is a sequela of chronic GERD in which the stratified squamous epithelium that normally lines the distal esophagus is replaced by abnormal columnar epithelium. The diagnosis of Barrett esophagus is established when the endoscopist sees columnar epithelium lining the distal esophagus. Regular endoscopic surveillance for esophageal cancer has been recommended in patients with Barrett esophagus. Esophageal biopsy specimens are taken during surveillance endoscopy primarily to identify dysplasia, a histologic diagnosis suggesting a premalignant lesion. For fit patients with identified high-grade dysplasia, three management options are available: esophagectomy, endoscopic ablative therapy, or intensive surveillance (withholding invasive therapy until the biopsies show adenocarcinoma). This patient has no active dysplasia, so invasive therapy is not indicated; he needs active surveillance. There is no evidence that increasing the doses of PPI helps with the dysplastic changes. Several studies have shown that antireflux surgery does not effect a permanent cure for GERD in the majority of patients (they still need to take PPI after the surgery), and surgery is no better than medication for preventing the peptic and neoplastic complications of GERD. *(Answer: A—Start an endoscopic surveillance program to look for dysplastic lesions)*

2. A 36-year-old woman comes to a walk-in clinic complaining of dysphagia. She has not seen a doctor in many years. She says her swallowing difficulty started 10 days ago. She has lost 30 lb in the past 6 months. She also complains of diarrhea with bloody stools and decreased visual acuity. She has had occasional fevers for the past 4 or 5 months. An enzyme-linked immunosorbent assay (ELISA) is positive for HIV; the patient's $CD4^+$ T cell count is 25 cells/mm^3. Her physical examination reveals fever and cachexia. Her funduscopic examination shows evidence of retinitis. There is no thrush in the mouth cavity. The patient's chest and abdominal examinations are unremarkable; her cardiovascular examination shows tachycardia; and her stools are heme positive. Endoscopy reveals one large (12 cm), shallow ulceration in the esophagus, surrounded by normal-appearing mucosa.

What is the most likely organism causing this patient's esophagitis?

- ❑ **A. Epstein-Barr virus**
- ❑ **B. Herpes simplex virus (HSV)**

❑ C. *Candida* esophagitis

❑ D. Cytomegalovirus (CMV)

Key Concept/Objective: To identify the most common etiologic agents for infectious esophagitis

Most esophageal infections are caused by *Candida*, HSV, or CMV, either alone or in combination. These organisms rarely infect the esophagus of normal persons but often cause esophagitis in patients whose immune system has been compromised by AIDS, by advanced malignancy, or by organ transplantation and the subsequent administration of immunosuppressive drugs. Other conditions that can be associated with esophagitis are diabetes, alcoholism, corticosteroid therapy, scleroderma, achalasia, and esophageal strictures. Dysphagia and odynophagia are the presenting symptoms in the majority of patients. CMV esophagitis often is only one component of a generalized CMV infection, and some 20% to 40% of patients with CMV esophagitis have systemic symptoms. In contrast, candidal and HSV esophagitis usually are not associated with infection in other organs, and systemic symptoms caused by these pathogens are uncommon. Oral lesions, thrush, or ulcers are commonly found in patients with candidal or HSV esophagitis, but not in those with CMV esophagitis. Epstein-Barr virus has not been associated with esophagitis. CMV tends to cause discrete, shallow esophageal ulcerations that are very elongated (up to 15 cm in length) and surrounded by normal-appearing mucosa. Some patients with AIDS can develop large esophageal ulcers in which no pathogenic organism can be identified by culture or biopsy. These ulcers resemble CMV ulcers. They do not respond to antibiotics; steroids and thalidomide have been used with success. Tissue sampling is necessary to differentiate these giant CMV ulcerations from the giant idiopathic esophageal ulcerations that can be associated with HIV infection. In this patient, the presence of a large solitary esophageal ulcer, signs of colitis and retinitis (suggesting a disseminated CMV infection), and the absence of mouth lesions make CMV the most likely diagnosis. *(Answer: D—Cytomegalovirus [CMV])*

For more information, see Spechler SJ: 4 Gastroenterology: I Esophageal Disorders. ACP Medicine Online (www.acpmedicine.com). Dale DC, Federman DD, Eds. WebMD Inc., New York, March 2003

Peptic Ulcer Diseases

3. A 57-year-old white man presents with a 2-week history of gnawing epigastric pain that seems to be relieved with food and antacid. His medical history is significant for hypertension. His medications include hydrochlorothiazide and 81 mg enteric-coated aspirin. He does not smoke.

Which of the following statements regarding ulcerogenesis is true?

❑ A. **The prevalence of *Helicobacter pylori* infection is much higher in patients with peptic ulcer disease than in age-matched control subjects, and it is clear that the presence of *H. pylori* is sufficient to cause peptic ulcers**

❑ B. **Epidemiologic studies suggest that nonsteroidal anti-inflammatory drugs (NSAIDs) vary in their propensity to cause ulcers; the risk of ulcer is dependent on dosage, but that risk is moderated by buffering and enteric coating**

❑ C. **Gastrinoma causes 10% of all peptic ulcers**

❑ D. **Idiopathic peptic ulcers account for up to 20% of gastric and duodenal ulcers in the United States**

Key Concept/Objective: To understand the pathogenesis of peptic ulcer diseases

Up to 20% of gastric and duodenal ulcers in the United States occur in patients who have no evidence of *H. pylori* infection, who deny taking NSAIDs, and who have normal serum gastrin concentrations. These ulcers are referred to as idiopathic peptic ulcers. The prevalence of *H. pylori* infection of the stomach is much higher in patients with duodenal ulcers

and, to a somewhat lesser extent, in patients with gastric ulcers than in age-matched control subjects. In addition, cure of *H. pylori* infection with antimicrobial therapy markedly reduces recurrences of duodenal and gastric ulcers. The etiologic mechanism linking *H. pylori* infection and ulcerogenesis is not yet absolutely established, for the following reasons: (1) voluntary ingestion of *H. pylori* led to gastric *H. pylori* infection and to gastritis but not to ulcers; (2) duodenal or gastric ulcers develop in only 10% to 20% of individuals with *H. pylori* gastritis, implying that only certain people with additional genetic, anatomic, physiologic, or environmental risk factors are predisposed to ulcers or that only certain *H. pylori* strains are ulcerogenic; (3) *H. pylori* induces diffuse inflammation in the stomach, yet the strongest link between *H. pylori* and peptic ulcer is with focal duodenal bulbar ulcer; and (4) gastric *H. pylori* infection is as common in women as in men, yet duodenal ulcer is two to three times less common in women. Currently, *H. pylori* can be considered the most important risk factor for duodenal and gastric ulcers, but it is clear that the mere presence of *H. pylori* in the stomach is not sufficient to cause peptic ulcers. Epidemiologic studies suggest that NSAIDs vary in their ability to cause ulcers, but this issue is complicated by the difficulty of comparing equipotent doses of NSAIDs. All prescription or over-the-counter NSAIDs should be considered ulcerogenic, with the risk of ulcer dependent on dosages and other patient-related factors, particularly advanced age and previous ulcer history. Even low doses of aspirin used for prophylaxis of cardiovascular disease (75 to 325 mg/day) are ulcerogenic in humans. Neither buffering of aspirin nor enteric coating appears to reduce the incidence of clinically detected ulcer formation. Gastrinoma causes less than 1% of all peptic ulcers. Peptic ulcers develop in 95% of patients with gastrinoma (Zollinger-Ellison syndrome); ulcers occur most commonly in the duodenal bulb but are also seen in the postbulbar duodenum, jejunum, lower esophagus, and stomach. Multiple ulcers are present in up to 25% of cases of Zollinger-Ellison syndrome. *(Answer: D—Idiopathic peptic ulcers account for up to 20% of gastric and duodenal ulcers in the United States)*

4. Two months ago, a 53-year-old white man was diagnosed by esophagogastroduodenoscopy (EGD) as having an uncomplicated duodenal ulcer. At that time, the patient tested positive on rapid urease testing and was appropriately treated with a clarithromycin-based regimen for *H. pylori*. He now returns with recurrent epigastric pain. He has no other medical conditions. He has been maintained on a proton pump inhibitor. He denies using NSAIDs. His vital signs and physical examination are unremarkable. His complete blood count, serum electrolyte levels, and serum calcium level are all within normal limits. He is referred for an upper GI series and is found to have a recurrent duodenal ulcer. The patient's fasting gastrin level is 500 pg/ml (normal value, < 100 pg/ml).

For this patient, which of the following statements is true?

- ❑ A. An upper GI series that is diagnostic of a bulbar duodenal ulcer will preclude endoscopy
- ❑ B. Treatment failure with clarithromycin-based regimens occurs in approximately 30% of cases of *H. pylori* infection
- ❑ C. A positive serum antibody test (sensitivity and specificity > 90%) would indicate persistent infection and require retreatment with metronidazole, tetracycline, and bismuth, as well as continuation of a proton pump inhibitor
- ❑ D. Ulcers refractory to pharmacotherapy are seen in acid hypersecretory states; this patient's fasting gastrin level is diagnostic of the Zollinger-Ellison syndrome

Key Concept/Objective: To understand the diagnostic modalities used in peptic ulcer disease

Despite having a lower sensitivity and specificity than endoscopy, an upper GI series using barium and air (double contrast) may be favored by primary care physicians and patients over referral for endoscopy for suspected uncomplicated ulcer. An upper GI series offers lower cost, wider availability, and fewer complications. However, for troublesome and undiagnosed dyspepsia, an upper GI series may be superfluous, because a normal result will often necessitate endoscopy (endoscopy is more sensitive than radiography) and because an upper GI series showing a gastric ulcer will also necessitate endoscopy and biopsy to exclude gastric malignancy. In many patients, only a finding of a duodenal bul-

bar ulcer on an upper GI series will preclude endoscopy.

Antimicrobial agents with activity against *H. pylori* include metronidazole, tetracycline, amoxicillin, and clarithromycin. A 2-week course of a three-drug regimen that includes a proton pump inhibitor, clarithromycin, and amoxicillin has a success rate approaching 90%. The major causes of treatment failure are poor compliance with the regimen and clarithromycin resistance; the latter occurs in around 10% of current strains and is increasing with increased macrolide use in the population. Breath testing is more useful than serology in diagnosing failure of eradication of *H. pylori* or reinfection in patients who were previously treated for *H. pylori* infection, because the serology will usually remain positive for several months even after successful treatment. A fasting serum gastrin concentration can be used to screen for an acid hypersecretory state resulting from Zollinger-Ellison syndrome. Antisecretory drugs (especially proton pump inhibitors) can also raise serum gastrin levels modestly (to 150 to 600 pg/ml). Definitive documentation of an acid hypersecretory state requires quantitative gastric acid measurement (gastric analysis). *(Answer: A—An upper GI series that is diagnostic of a bulbar duodenal ulcer will preclude endoscopy)*

5. A 54-year-old man with a history of COPD and tobacco abuse presents for evaluation of burning epigastric pain and melena. The epigastric pain has persisted for several weeks; the melena began several hours ago. His current medical regimen includes albuterol and ipratropium bromide nebulizers, long-term oral steroids, and theophylline. He also reports that he recently used an NSAID for joint pain. On physical examination, the patient's heart rate is 115 beats/min and his blood pressure is 98/45 mm Hg. There is evidence of orthostasis. Abdominal examination does not demonstrate tenderness, rebound, or rigidity. A complete blood count is significant for a hematocrit of 39%; serum electrolytes are within normal limits. The patient is admitted for volume resuscitation. EGD is performed, and the patient is found to have a gastric ulcer with a visible vessel. The lesion is treated by injection of epinephrine.

For this patient, which of the following statements is true?

- ❑ A. **Corticosteroids not only are ulcerogenic but also impair healing of preexisting ulcers**
- ❑ B. **The patient's hemoglobin concentration makes a significant GI bleed unlikely**
- ❑ C. **To exclude a diagnosis of ulcerated gastric cancer, gastric ulcers should be followed endoscopically until they are completely healed**
- ❑ D. **Patients with *H. pylori*–related gastric ulcers should be managed with antibiotics and a 4-week regimen of a high-dose proton pump inhibitor**

Key Concept/Objective: To understand the treatment of a bleeding gastric ulcer

Patients with gastric ulcers should be followed endoscopically until complete healing has been achieved so that an ulcerated gastric cancer is not missed. Corticosteroids, which block cyclooxygenase-2 (COX-2) but not COX-1, are not ulcerogenic when used alone, though they impair healing of preexisting ulcers. However, when corticosteroids are used in combination with NSAIDs, the risk of ulcer formation is much greater than when NSAIDs are used alone. In the first several hours after an episode of acute ulcer bleeding, the hemoglobin concentration will not completely reflect the severity of the blood loss until compensatory hemodilution occurs or until intravenous fluids such as isotonic saline are administered. Thus, the pulse rate and blood pressure in the supine and upright positions are better initial indicators of the extent of blood loss than are red cell counts. Gastric ulcer associated with *H. pylori* should be treated with antibiotics. Because they are larger than duodenal ulcers, gastric ulcers take longer to heal. Thus, after antibiotic administration, the patient should be treated with an acid antisecretory agent for an additional 4 to 8 weeks. *(Answer: C—To exclude a diagnosis of ulcerated gastric cancer, gastric ulcers should be followed endoscopically until they are completely healed)*

6. A 43-year-old woman presents to establish primary care. Her medical history is significant for an uncomplicated duodenal ulcer, which she experienced 18 months ago. At the time of diagnosis, she was treat-

ed with a clarithromycin-based regimen for *H. pylori*. She has since been asymptomatic.

For this patient, which of the following statements is true?

❑ A. **Given a success rate of only 90%, eradication of *H. pylori* should be confirmed after completion of a course of ulcer therapy**

❑ B. **Reinfection with *H. pylori* is common in the United States**

❑ C. **Patients who experience recurrence of ulcer symptoms during the first 2 years after therapy should be assessed by EGD, a urea breath test, or fecal antigen test**

❑ D. **The sensitivity of the urea breath test is unaffected by use of a proton pump inhibitor**

Key Concept/Objective: To understand the mechanism and diagnosis of treatment failure for eradication of H. pylori

After a patient has completed a course of ulcer therapy for an *H. pylori*–related uncomplicated duodenal ulcer, it is acceptable to follow the patient clinically without confirming eradication, because most compliant patients will be successfully cured of their *H. pylori* infection. Reinfection with *H. pylori* remains an uncommon event in the United States (approximately one reinfection per 100 patients a year). If symptoms of an *H. pylori*–related duodenal ulcer do not recur within 2 years after antimicrobial therapy, the patient is probably cured. Those in whom recurrent ulcer symptoms develop within 2 years after therapy should be assessed by endoscopy, a urea breath test, or fecal antigen test. Because proton pump inhibitors can suppress *H. pylori* without eradicating it, use of these drugs should be avoided for 2 weeks before the urea breath test is administered to minimize false negative results. *(Answer: C—Patients who experience recurrence of ulcer symptoms during the first 2 years after therapy should be assessed by EGD, a urea breath test, or fecal antigen test)*

For more information, see Feldman M: 4 Gastroenterology: II Peptic Ulcer Diseases. ACP Medicine Online (www.acpmedicine.com). Dale DC, Federman DD, Eds. WebMD Inc., New York, November 2004

Diarrheal Diseases

7. A 28-year-old man comes to your clinic complaining of diarrhea of 10 months' duration. He is a graduate student and is currently writing a thesis. He has been sexually active with men in the past but not during the past 2 years. He denies experiencing weight loss or other constitutional symptoms. He notes no blood in the stool. He has no medical history. He explains that he has not sought attention before now because the problem is intermittent, and he notes that he sometimes experiences constipation rather than diarrhea. You include irritable bowel syndrome in your differential diagnosis.

Which of the following descriptions is characteristic of irritable bowel syndrome?

❑ A. **Painless diarrhea that occurs during the day or night**

❑ B. **Abdominal pain with defecation and an altered bowel habit**

❑ C. **Painless, chronic watery diarrhea of moderate severity**

❑ D. **Diarrhea associated with postprandial flushing and a drop in blood pressure**

Key Concept/Objective: To know the characteristic clinical presentation of irritable bowel syndrome

Patients with chronic diarrhea in whom no other etiology is established are commonly diagnosed with irritable bowel syndrome or functional diarrhea. Irritable bowel syndrome is characterized chiefly by abdominal pain that is associated with altered bowel function, including constipation, diarrhea, or alternating diarrhea and constipation. A diagnosis of functional diarrhea is made when patients do not have prominent abdominal pain and

have no evidence of other specific causes of diarrhea. Obviously, these diagnoses are reliable only if a thorough evaluation has been done to exclude other causes of diarrhea. Nevertheless, there are certain clues to the diagnosis of irritable bowel syndrome or functional diarrhea that should be sought by the physician. Features that suggest a diagnosis of irritable bowel syndrome include a long history of diarrhea, dating back to adolescence or young adulthood; passage of mucus; and exacerbation of symptoms with stress. Historical points that argue against irritable bowel syndrome include recent onset of diarrhea, especially in older patients; nocturnal diarrhea; weight loss; blood in stools; voluminous stools (> 400 g/24 hr); blood tests indicating anemia, leukocytosis, or low serum albumin concentration; or a high erythrocyte sedimentation rate. *(Answer: B—Abdominal pain with defecation and an altered bowel habit)*

8. A 32-year-old woman presents as a walk-in patient in the emergency department. She complains of nausea and diarrhea that began early that evening. She reports that she ate a sandwich at a fast-food establishment for lunch, and she began experiencing symptoms several hours later. She denies seeing blood in the stool. She reports no similar experiences in the past; she has no recent travel history, nor has she had any contacts with sick persons. She was treated with a 3-day course of antibiotics for an upper urinary tract infection 2 months ago and is otherwise healthy.

Which organism is the most likely cause of this patient's acute diarrheal illness?

❑ A. ***Campylobacter jejuni***

❑ B. ***Salmonella enteritidis***

❑ C. ***Staphylococcus aureus***

❑ D. ***C. difficile***

Key Concept/Objective: To understand that diarrhea caused by preformed toxin occurs within hours of exposure

Most acute diarrheas (i.e., those lasting < 4 weeks) are caused by infections and are self-limiting. Most are caused by viruses (e.g., adenovirus, Norwalk agent, rotavirus), but some are caused by bacteria (e.g., *Campylobacter, Salmonella, Shigella, Escherichia coli*) and others by protozoa (e.g., *Giardia lamblia, Entamoeba histolytica*). One mechanism for acute diarrhea is ingestion of a preformed toxin. Several species of bacteria, such as *S. aureus, C. perfringens,* and *Bacillus cereus,* can produce toxins that produce so-called food poisoning (i.e., vomiting and diarrhea) within 4 hours of ingestion. In such cases, the bacteria do not need to establish an intraluminal infection; ingestion of the toxin alone can produce the disease. Symptoms subside after the toxin is cleared, usually by the next day; evidence of toxicity (e.g., fever) is minimal. *(Answer: C—*Staphylococcus aureus*)*

For more information, see Schiller LR: 4 Gastroenterology: III Diarrheal Diseases. ACP Medicine Online (www.acpmedicine.com). Dale DC, Federman DD, Eds. WebMD Inc., New York, April 2003

Inflammatory Bowel Disease

9. A 26-year-old man presents with intermittent crampy abdominal pain, diarrhea without noticeable blood, and weight loss of 15 lb over 10 months. The bowel symptoms, including the diarrhea, wake him from sleep. On a few occasions, he has had fevers, nausea, and vomiting. The patient is an architect, and he describes his work as being stressful; he resumed smoking cigarettes a year ago. His older brother has had similar symptoms but has not yet been evaluated. On examination, the patient is a slender man with normal vital signs. He has an oral aphthous ulcer and poorly localized lower abdominal to midabdominal tenderness without peritoneal signs. Anal and rectal examinations are normal, and a stool guaiac test is negative. Stool leukocytes are present. The hematocrit is 34%. Results of examination with flexible sigmoidoscopy are normal.

Which of the following is the most likely diagnosis for this patient?

❑ A. Irritable bowel syndrome
❑ B. Acute appendicitis
❑ C. Crohn disease
❑ D. Ulcerative colitis
❑ E. Colon cancer

Key Concept/Objective: To be able to distinguish inflammatory bowel disease from other disorders, and to be able to distinguish between Crohn disease and ulcerative colitis

The diagnosis of inflammatory bowel disease is suggested by the fact that the patient's symptoms developed over a number of months, that the patient has an oral aphthous ulcer, that fecal leukocytes are present, that the patient has experienced weight loss and has anemia, and by the possibility that the patient's brother has a similar problem. The presence of nocturnal symptoms and fecal leukocytes eliminates irritable bowel syndrome. The long course makes acute appendicitis unlikely, though either irritable bowel syndrome or acute appendicitis can occur in patients with inflammatory bowel disease. The history is not suggestive of colon cancer, especially given this patient's young age and in the absence of an inherited polyposis syndrome. The factors favoring a diagnosis of Crohn disease over that of ulcerative colitis at this stage in the evaluation include the association of smoking with the onset of symptoms. Crohn disease is strongly associated with smoking, but smoking decreases the risk of ulcerative colitis. In addition, the negative results on flexible sigmoidoscopy essentially eliminate ulcerative colitis from consideration. *(Answer: C—Crohn disease)*

10. A 33-year-old woman with Crohn disease presents with a flare of disease activity consisting of fever, right lower quadrant pain, weight loss of more than 10% of body weight, guaiac-positive diarrhea, and macrocytic anemia. Her disease is limited to the small intestine and terminal ileum. Her examination is significant for a temperature 100.2° F (37.9° C), active bowel sounds, and right lower quadrant tenderness.

Which of the following statements is true for this patient?

❑ A. The anemia is probably caused by folate deficiency
❑ B. Sulfasalazine is first-line therapy and will probably be sufficient to control her symptoms
❑ C. An aminosalicylate will be required to control this flare
❑ D. Corticosteroids will be necessary to control her symptoms
❑ E. She should be hospitalized and given infliximab

Key Concept/Objective: To understand the treatment of inflammatory bowel disease

This patient has moderate to severe Crohn disease, as judged on the basis of her fever, weight loss, abdominal pain without obstruction, and ability to continue oral intake. Sulfasalazine is unlikely to deliver much anti-inflammatory activity to the small bowel because sulfasalazine is poorly hydrolyzed into its component sulfa and active salicylate moieties until it comes into contact with colonic bacteria. Aminosalicylate would be helpful, but for symptoms of this severity, a corticosteroid will be necessary. Infliximab, an anti–tumor necrosis factor monoclonal antibody, is an option for treatment of severe Crohn disease in patients who are not responsive to salicylates, antibiotics, or steroids. Unless the small bowel mucosal disease is very extensive, the macrocytic anemia is most likely caused by a deficiency of vitamin B_{12}, which is absorbed in the terminal ileum. *(Answer: D—Corticosteroids will be necessary to control her symptoms)*

11. Two 28-year-old men with inflammatory colonic disease are seen in clinic; one has ulcerative colitis and the other has Crohn disease. Each is concerned about complications of his disease.

Which of the following is a correct assessment of these two patients?

❑ A. Each may have arthritis in both HLA-B27–related and non–HLA-B27–related distributions

❑ B. **Kidney stones can occur in each but are more common in patients who have ulcerative colitis**

❑ C. **Sclerosing cholangitis in a spectrum from mild to severe can occur in ulcerative colitis but not in Crohn disease**

❑ D. **Erythema nodosum and peripheral joint manifestations of colitis secondary to inflammatory bowel disease follow a course independent of the bowel disease and should be treated with NSAIDs**

❑ E. **These two men have toxic megacolon, which is a complication unique to ulcerative colitis**

Key Concept/Objective: To know the extraintestinal manifestations of inflammatory bowel disease

Inflammatory bowel disease is associated with peripheral joint arthritis and other conditions, such as erythema nodosum, that are not HLA-B27–associated and whose manifestations correlate with those of inflammatory bowel disease. NSAIDs worsen inflammatory bowel disease and can lead to bowel disease becoming refractory. Arthritis of the axial skeleton is HLA-B27–related and progresses independently of intestinal disease. Kidney stones are seen primarily in Crohn disease of the small intestine and are caused by increased oxalate absorption associated with malabsorption of intestinal fat and the binding of calcium to fatty acids. Cholangitis occurs in both ulcerative colitis and Crohn colitis. Toxic megacolon can occur in infectious colitis and Crohn disease as well as ulcerative colitis. *(Answer: A—Each may have arthritis in both HLA-B27–related and non–HLA-B27–related distributions)*

For more information, see Hanauer SB: 4 Gastroenterology: IV Inflammatory Bowel Disease. ACP Medicine Online (www.acpmedicine.com). Dale DC, Federman DD, Eds. WebMD Inc., New York, June 2001

Diseases of the Pancreas

12. A 64-year-old woman presents to the emergency department with abdominal pain, nausea, and vomiting of 3 days' duration. The pain is epigastric and radiates to her back. She takes no medications. The physical examination reveals a patient with mild obesity; the patient's temperature is 100.3° F (37.9° C), and epigastric tenderness is present. An abdominal CT scan with contrast shows pancreatitis with enhancement of the entire gland and a 5 cm collection of fluid next to the pancreas.

Which of the following is the most accurate diagnosis for this patient?

❑ A. **Interstitial pancreatitis with an acute fluid collection**

❑ B. **Interstitial pancreatitis with an uncomplicated pseudocyst**

❑ C. **Necrotizing pancreatitis with a peripancreatic phlegmon**

❑ D. **Interstitial pancreatitis with a pancreatic abscess**

Key Concept/Objective: To understand the diagnosis of acute pancreatitis

The definitions used to differentiate acute from chronic pancreatitis have changed recently, and more precise definitions were developed to describe the complications of acute pancreatitis. An acute fluid collection is defined as a collection of fluid occurring in or around the pancreas early in the course of acute pancreatitis. These collections are seen as areas of low attenuation without a visible capsule on CT. They are quite common in acute pancreatitis, occurring in 30% to 50% of cases. Many of these acute fluid collections resolve, but some may persist and develop a visible capsule, at which time they should be termed a pseudocyst. Pseudocysts are defined as collections of fluid surrounded by a fibrous capsule. It takes at least 4 to 6 weeks for an acute fluid collection to develop a capsule and become a pseudocyst. Pseudocysts may remain sterile or may become secondarily infected. Pancreatic necrosis is defined as an absence of enhancement of pancreatic parenchyma after the infusion of intravenous contrast on contrast-enhanced CT (CECT). Acute necro-

tizing pancreatitis is defined by the presence of necrosis on CECT; it is subclassified as either sterile necrosis or infected necrosis. Acute interstitial pancreatitis is defined by the absence of these CECT findings of necrosis. Finally, pancreatic abscess is defined as a circumscribed collection of pus containing little necrotic tissue. What was formerly called infected pseudocyst is now termed pancreatic abscess. The term phlegmon was abandoned, because no consensus could be reached as to its definition. *(Answer: A—Interstitial pancreatitis with an acute fluid collection)*

13. A 52-year-old man with a history of poorly controlled diabetes mellitus presents to the emergency department with severe abdominal pain of 36 hours' duration. He had a similar episode 4 months ago. Physical examination is significant for tachycardia, diminished bowel sounds, epigastric tenderness, and a papular rash on his knees. Laboratory studies are significant for the following: leukocytes, 15,000 cells/mm^3; blood glucose level, 450 mg/dl; amylase level, normal.

Which of the following is the most likely diagnosis for this patient?

- ❑ **A. Acute on chronic pancreatitis**
- ❑ **B. Gallstone pancreatitis**
- ❑ **C. Alcoholic pancreatitis**
- ❑ **D. Pancreatitis secondary to hypertriglyceridemia**

Key Concept/Objective: To be able to recognize hypertriglyceridemia as a cause of pancreatitis

Many factors have been implicated as causes of acute pancreatitis. Gallstones and alcohol abuse account for 70% to 80% of all cases of acute pancreatitis. Other etiologies include sphincter of Oddi dysfunction; benign and malignant strictures of the pancreatic duct; congenital anatomic abnormalities and genetic disorders; drugs; toxins; trauma; infections; and metabolic causes. Some cases are idiopathic. Metabolic causes of acute pancreatitis include hypertriglyceridemia and hypercalcemia. Serum triglycerides generally need to be in excess of 1,000 mg/dl to produce acute pancreatitis. This is most commonly seen in type V hyperlipoproteinemia and is usually associated with diabetes mellitus. Acute pancreatitis can itself raise triglyceride levels, but not to this degree. The diagnosis is usually confirmed with a combination of laboratory tests and imaging studies. Serum amylase measurement has long been the most widely used confirmatory laboratory test. At least 75% of all patients will have elevations in serum amylase at the time of initial evaluation. The serum amylase level may be normal in some patients with acute pancreatitis associated with alcohol use and in those with hyperlipidemic pancreatitis (marked elevations in the triglyceride level can interfere with the laboratory assay for amylase); the serum amylase level may be normal in patients with acute pancreatitis if the measurement is made several days after the onset of symptoms. Measurement of serum lipase is often used as an adjunct to or in place of serum amylase as a confirmatory test. The presence of a papular rash on this patient is consistent with eruptive xanthomas, supporting the diagnosis of pancreatitis secondary to hypertriglyceridemia. *(Answer: D—Pancreatitis secondary to hypertriglyceridemia)*

14. A 22-year-old man comes to your clinic for evaluation of chronic abdominal pain. The patient has been experiencing pain for 1 year. Initially, the pain was episodic, but lately it has become constant. It is felt in the epigastrium and radiates to the back. Sometimes the pain is accompanied by nausea and vomiting. The patient denies having diarrhea. Physical examination is unremarkable. An upper endoscopy and abdominal CT scan are unremarkable. You suspect chronic idiopathic pancreatitis.

Which of the following would be the most appropriate test to confirm the diagnosis?

- ❑ **A. Measurement of serum trypsinogen**
- ❑ **B. Measurement of serum amylase and lipase**
- ❑ **C Direct pancreatic function tests**
- ❑ **D. Abdominal ultrasound**

Key Concept/Objective: To understand the different tests for assessing pancreatic function

Diagnostic tests for chronic pancreatitis include those tests that detect functional abnormalities and those that detect abnormalities of pancreatic structure. Serum amylase or lipase levels may be elevated during acute exacerbations, but these elevations are usually modest and are neither routinely present nor diagnostic for chronic pancreatitis. A low serum trypsinogen level (< 20 ng/ml) is highly specific for chronic pancreatitis, but the trypsinogen level only drops to this level in advanced disease. The bentiromide test utilizes the measurement in urine of a metabolite that can only be produced by the action of pancreatic enzymes. The bentiromide test is no longer available in the United States. A 72-hour stool collection for fat is the gold standard to detect steatorrhea. Steatorrhea is only seen in far-advanced chronic pancreatitis. Fecal levels of elastase and chymotrypsin are reduced in more advanced cases of chronic pancreatitis. Direct pancreatic function tests involve placing a tube into the duodenum to collect pancreatic juice. This test directly measures pancreatic output of enzymes or bicarbonate after stimulation with a secretagogue. These tests are the most sensitive tests available and are able to detect chronic pancreatitis at an earlier stage than any other test. They are particularly useful in diagnosing those patients with small-duct chronic pancreatitis, in whom alternative diagnostic tests are likely to miss the diagnosis. Abdominal ultrasonography is most likely to detect advanced abnormalities of pancreatic structure and is diagnostic in only 60% of patients. *(Answer: C—Direct pancreatic function tests)*

15. A 38-year-old woman is being evaluated for abdominal pain, which has been present for 2 months. Her medical history and physical examination are unremarkable, and she takes no medications. An abdominal CT scan reveals a 5 cm cystic structure in the pancreas.

Which of the following is the most appropriate step to take next in the treatment of this patient?

- ❑ **A. Percutaneous drainage**
- ❑ **B. Endoscopic drainage**
- ❑ **C. Surgical resection**
- ❑ **D. Follow-up and repeat imaging in 6 weeks**

Key Concept/Objective: To be able to recognize mucinous cystic neoplasms

Besides the commonly seen pseudocysts, a number of other cystic lesions may occur in the pancreas, including true cysts and cystic neoplasms. Serous cystic neoplasms are benign, but mucin-producing cystic neoplasms may follow a more malignant course. Mucinous cystic neoplasms present as large cystic collections (cystadenomas and cystadenocarcinomas) and may be relatively asymptomatic. Most cystic neoplasms occur in middle-aged patients, particularly women. They are often mistaken for pseudocysts and inappropriately treated as such. These cystic neoplasms may follow an initially benign course, but when they undergo malignant degeneration, outcomes are as poor as in patients with standard adenocarcinoma. The presence of a cystic collection of the pancreas in a middle-aged (particularly female) patient without a previous history of pancreatitis should immediately suggest a cystic neoplasm, not a pseudocyst. The diagnosis of a cystic neoplasm requires histologic evidence of epithelial or neoplastic tissue in the cyst wall. When these collections are mistaken for pseudocysts, treatment involves drainage, and no tissue is obtained to allow differentiation of a cystic neoplasm from a pseudocyst. The therapy of choice for cystic neoplasms is surgical resection, not drainage. *(Answer: C—Surgical resection)*

16. A 62-year-old woman presents to the emergency department complaining of intense abdominal pain, nausea, and vomiting for the past 48 hours. On physical examination, the patient is visibly uncomfortable, with a low-grade fever, mild tachycardia, and normal blood pressure; her upper abdomen is markedly tender. Laboratory tests are remarkable for an amylase of 1150, bilirubin of 2.5, and creatinine of 2.3.

Which of the following is the most useful imaging test to determine whether this patient's pancreatitis is caused by gallstones?

- ❑ **A. Plain film**
- ❑ **B. Ultrasonography**

- ❑ C. CT scan
- ❑ D. Endoscopic retrograde cholangiopancreatography (ERCP)

Key Concept/Objective: To understand the role of abdominal ultrasonography in acute pancreatitis

Ultrasonography is recommended in the initial evaluation of all pancreatitis to rule out obstruction caused by gallstones. It is more sensitive than CT for the diagnosis of gallstone disease, though CT is usually better at demonstrating morphologic changes in the pancreas caused by inflammation. Findings on plain film (such as the colon cutoff sign; enhancement of perirenal fat caused by retroperitoneal inflammation that creates a halo around the left kidney; or an abnormal duodenal loop) can suggest the diagnosis of pancreatitis but do not reveal its cause. ERCP does not play a role in the diagnosis of pancreatitis but can be useful in its management. *(Answer: B—Ultrasonography)*

17. A 50-year-old man comes to your clinic complaining of intermittent upper abdominal pain that radiates to his back and worsens with meals. He has a long history of binge drinking. He notes that lately he has been losing weight and that his stools have been loose.

Which of the following should be the first test to determine whether this patient has chronic pancreatitis?

- ❑ A. Plain film
- ❑ B. Ultrasonography
- ❑ C. CT of the abdomen
- ❑ D. ERCP
- ❑ E. Secretin test

Key Concept/Objective: To know the stepwise approach to the diagnosis of chronic pancreatitis

The diagnosis of chronic pancreatitis can be made with an appropriate clinical history and demonstration of calcification of the pancreas on plain film. This should therefore be the first imaging test, though at most only 30% of patients with chronic pancreatitis will have this finding. If plain films are unrevealing, ultrasonography may demonstrate the characteristic findings of focal or diffuse enlargement of the pancreas, ductal irregularity and dilatation, and fluid collections adjacent to the gland. CT has a higher sensitivity than ultrasound (> 90%) and is the next step in diagnostic imaging. ERCP is the gold standard for diagnosing chronic pancreatitis on the basis of ductal abnormalities; the degree of ductal abnormalities correlates roughly with exocrine dysfunction. The secretin test, in which duodenal contents are sampled before and after secretin is administered intravenously, is probably the most sensitive direct assessment of pancreatic exocrine function, but because of improvement in imaging tests, the secretin test is used infrequently. *(Answer: A—Plain film)*

For more information, see Forsmark CE: 4 Gastroenterology: V Diseases of the Pancreas. ACP Medicine Online (www.acpmedicine.com). Dale DC, Federman DD, Eds. WebMD Inc., New York, October 2003

Gallstones and Biliary Tract Disease

18. A 15-year-old girl presents to the emergency department complaining of right upper quadrant pain. She has had two similar episodes in the past 3 months. The pain started 3 hours ago and increased rapidly. The pain is located in the epigastrium and radiates to the right shoulder. The patient is also complaining of nausea and vomiting. At presentation, she says the pain is starting to disappear. On physical examination, the patient has tenderness to palpation in the right upper quadrant. Laboratory testing shows a white cell count of 7,000, a hematocrit of 26%, and a normal platelet count. Her liver function test results are significant only for an indirect bilirubin of 2 mg/dl. Ultrasonography shows three stones in the gallbladder, no pericholecystic fluid, and no gallbladder wall edema. The common bile duct measures 4 mm.

Which of the following statements is the most accurate regarding this patient?

- ❑ **A. The patient should be started on antibiotic therapy; in 2 to 3 days, after this acute process resolves, a cholecystectomy should be performed**
- ❑ **B. The patient has acute viral hepatitis; the gallstones are an incidental finding**
- ❑ **C. If the patient undergoes a cholecystectomy, an analysis of the gallstones is likely to show black pigment stones**
- ❑ **D. An endoscopic retrograde cholangiopancreatography (ERCP) should be done, because it is likely that a stone has passed to the common bile duct and is now causing obstruction**

Key Concept/Objective: To understand the processes that lead to the formation of gallstones

Two principal types of stone, the cholesterol stone and the pigment stone, form in the gallbladder and biliary tract. The cholesterol stone is composed mainly of cholesterol (> 50% of the stone) and comprises multiple layers of cholesterol crystals and mucin glycoproteins. Mixed gallstones contain 20% to 50% cholesterol. The pigment stones contain a variety of organic and inorganic components, including calcium bilirubinate (40% to 50% of dry weight). Black pigment stones are most often seen in patients with cirrhosis or hemolytic anemia and are found predominantly in the gallbladder. This patient likely has biliary colic secondary to gallstones. Her laboratory results show evidence of hemolysis (low hematocrit, increased indirect bilirubin). Acute cholecystitis is unlikely in this clinical scenario because the pain is starting to disappear after 3 hours, there is no fever, and there is no evidence of leukocytosis on complete blood count. Also, ultrasonography did not show evidence of acute cholecystitis, such as the presence of pericholecystic fluid or edema of the gallbladder. Acute viral hepatitis can present as right upper quadrant pain; however, it is unlikely in this case because the pain is acute and is starting to resolve, and the only abnormal liver function test result is the indirect bilirubin value, suggesting hemolysis. An ERCP is not indicated because there is no evidence of obstruction or cholestasis, such as an elevation in the direct bilirubin level or the alkaline phosphatase level or a finding of a dilated common bile duct on ultrasound. *(Answer: C—If the patient undergoes a cholecystectomy, an analysis of the gallstones is likely to show black pigment stones)*

19. You are asked to consult regarding a 52-year-old man with fever who is in the surgical intensive care unit. The patient has been in the hospital for 6 weeks after being injured in a car accident. He had a cranial fracture and multiple rib fractures; three feet of his jejunum were surgically removed, and he has had multiple complications since then, including pneumonia, sinusitis, and coagulase-negative *Staphylococcus* bacteremia. All of these complications seem to have resolved with adequate treatment. Over the past 2 days, he has been having increasing fever. He is still intubated and on total parenteral nutrition. On physical examination, the patient's temperature is 102° F (38.9° C), his heart rate is 104 beats/min, and his blood pressure is 124/76 mm Hg. The patient has jaundice, and there is tenderness in the right upper quadrant. The examination is otherwise unchanged from previous notes in the chart. His complete blood count shows a white blood cell (WBC) count of 22,000 with left shift; the WBC count has been increasing over the past 2 days. Liver function testing shows a direct bilirubin level of 2.5 mg/dl and an alkaline phosphatase level of 415 mg/dl; these values were normal 3 days ago. An abdominal ultrasound done yesterday shows a thickened gallbladder wall with pericholecystic fluid and no sludge or stones. The chest x-ray is unchanged; blood cultures done yesterday are negative so far. The patient is receiving vancomycin for his *Staphylococcus* bacteremia. The primary team thinks that the ultrasound findings are not significant in this case, and they are looking for another source of fever.

Which of the following would be your recommendation?

- ❑ **A. Continue to follow cultures and wait for results before doing further workup**
- ❑ **B. Recommend cholescintigraphy (HIDA scan) to evaluate for acute cholecystitis; add antibiotics to cover gram-negative and anaerobic organisms**

❑ C. **Recommend that a repeat abdominal ultrasound be performed in 72 hours; continue current antibiotic regimen**

❑ D. **Recommend performing a CT scan to look for other sources of infection**

Key Concept/Objective: To understand the presentation of acute acalculous cholecystitis

Cholelithiasis is present in 90% to 95% of patients with acute cholecystitis, and most patients have had previous attacks of biliary colic. Acute cholecystitis may present as an acalculous cholecystitis in 5% to 10% of patients. It is predominantly noted in older men who are critically ill after major surgery, severe trauma, or extensive burn injury. This patient has fever, right upper quadrant pain, elevated bilirubin and alkaline phosphatase levels, and ultrasound findings suggestive of acute cholecystitis. Cholescintigraphy is the most accurate method of confirming the clinical diagnosis of acute cholecystitis (calculous or acalculous); this procedure involves the intravenous injection of technetium-99m–labeled hepatoiminodiacetic acid, which is selectively excreted into the biliary tree and enters the gallbladder. In the presence of cholecystitis, radiolabeled material enters the common bile duct but not the gallbladder. Because in this case the primary team does not think cholecystitis is an active problem, cholescintigraphy would be indicated to help confirm your presumptive diagnosis of acute acalculous cholecystitis; if confirmed, cholecystectomy would be recommended. Broad-spectrum antibiotic coverage is indicated in this patient, but there is still a need to find the etiology for his clinical deterioration. A CT scan would be appropriate only if the results of cholescintigraphy are negative. *(Answer: B—Recommend cholescintigraphy [HIDA scan] to evaluate for acute cholecystitis; add antibiotics to cover gram-negative and anaerobic organisms)*

20. A 54-year-old white man with a history of hypertension and diabetes presents to your clinic for follow-up after he was seen in a local emergency department with left flank pain. At that time, he had hematuria, and an ultrasound showed kidney stones. His liver function test results were normal. The report describes two stones in the left kidney. Also, as an incidental finding, three gallstones measuring 1 × 1 cm were seen; otherwise, the gallbladder was normal. The patient is concerned about the presence of these gallstones. On being asked about pain, he reports no episodes of pain except for the episode that caused him to visit the emergency department.

What would be your recommendation regarding the management of this patient's gallstones?

❑ A. **Recommend not having surgery and continue to monitor clinically**

❑ B. **Recommend cholecystectomy, because he has diabetes and he is at high risk for developing complications from acute cholecystitis in the future**

❑ C. **Recommend surgery, because he is at high risk for developing gallbladder cancer in the next few years**

❑ D. **Recommend oral ursodiol for dissolution of the stones**

Key Concept/Objective: To know the appropriate treatment of asymptomatic cholelithiasis

Most gallstones are asymptomatic and are an incidental finding on ultrasonography performed for other reasons. Silent gallstones seldom lead to problems. Cholecystectomy is generally not indicated. Exceptions may be made for patients at increased risk for gallbladder cancer. In this case, the pain was related to nephrolithiasis (hematuria, left-sided pain, left kidney stones), and the patient has been otherwise asymptomatic. He has no risk factors for gallbladder cancer. Oral dissolution therapy is usually unsuccessful and requires long-term treatment. On the basis of this information, prophylactic cholecystectomy is not indicated for this patient; observation is the appropriate management. *(Answer: A—Recommend not having surgery and continue to monitor clinically)*

21. A 35-year-old man comes in for evaluation because his wife thinks he looks yellow. He feels fine, his medical history is unremarkable, and he takes no medications. On review of systems, he has no weight loss, anorexia, fevers, chills, or abdominal pains. He has no personal or family history of gallbladder problems. Lately, he has noted dark urine and pale stools. On examination, the patient's vital signs are normal, but he is clearly jaundiced. His abdomen is nontender and free of organomegaly. Complete blood count and electrolyte and amylase levels are normal. An abdominal ultrasound shows multiple small gallstones in the gallbladder but none in the common bile duct. The common bile duct, however, is dilated.

Which of the following should be the next step in diagnosing this patient?

❑ A. **ERCP**

❑ B. **Transhepatic cholangiography**

❑ C. **CT**

❑ D. **Repeat ultrasound**

❑ E. **Cholescintigraphy**

Key Concept/Objective: To understand the role of different imaging modalities in evaluating cholestatic jaundice and their ability to detect common bile duct stones

This patient has posthepatic cholestasis. Although ultrasound can often detect dilatation of the common bile duct, it may detect only 50% of common bile duct stones. CT and cholescintigraphy have similar limitations. In this case, ERCP is the procedure of choice because it will provide not only direct visualization of the common bile duct but also an opportunity to intervene therapeutically. If ERCP cannot be performed, transhepatic cholangiography is an alternative method for visualizing the bile ducts. *(Answer: A—ERCP)*

22. A 49-year-old man presents with right upper quadrant abdominal pain that began 8 hours ago. The pain is constant and is associated with nausea, vomiting, and fever. Over the past few months, he has had intermittent episodes of similar pain, but those were less intense, resolved spontaneously within 1 or 2 hours, and were never associated with vomiting or fever. Results of physical examination are as follows: temperature, 101.3° F (38.5° C); blood pressure, 130/90 mm Hg; pulse, 90 beats/min; and respirations, 16 breaths/min. The patient looks tired and moderately uncomfortable. Bowel sounds are present, but he has right upper quadrant tenderness. There is no palpable liver or gallbladder. Laboratory results are remarkable for a white blood cell count of 14,000, with a left shift. Bilirubin, amylase, and alkaline phosphatase levels are normal.

Which of the following is the best diagnostic imaging test for this patient?

❑ A. **Oral cholecystogram**

❑ B. **HIDA scan**

❑ C. **Ultrasound**

❑ D. **CT scan**

❑ E. **Plain abdominal x-ray**

Key Concept/Objective: To understand the roles of various imaging modalities in the setting of acute cholecystitis

Ultrasound is the imaging test of choice. For detecting gallstones, it has a sensitivity of 88% to 90% and a specificity of 97% to 98%. It is noninvasive and readily available in most areas. If ultrasound results are equivocal, a HIDA scan can be performed to confirm the diagnosis of acute cholecystitis. HIDA scans are highly accurate, but they can be confounded by cirrhosis and can be misleading in patients who are fasting or who are receiving parenteral nutrition. CT is less sensitive than ultrasound. Oral cholecystograms are time-consuming. Because most gallstones are radiolucent, plain x-rays have limited usefulness. *(Answer: C—Ultrasound)*

23. The obese sister of the patient in Question 22 comes in the week after her brother's visit with severe epigastric right upper quadrant pain that has been unrelenting for 24 hours. She has fevers, rigors, nausea, and vomiting. Results of physical examination are as follows: temperature, 102.2° F (39° C); blood pressure, 120/65 mm Hg; pulse, 100 beats/min; and respirations, 18 breaths/min. The patient looks ill and slightly jaundiced. She is shivering beneath a pile of blankets. Bowel sounds are hypoactive. There is

marked right upper quadrant tenderness but no palpable liver or gallbladder. Laboratory results show a white blood cell count of 16,000 with a left shift. Bilirubin is 4.5, and alkaline phosphatase is 260. Her amylase level is normal.

Which of the following represents the diagnosis and best treatment for this patient?

- ❑ A. **Acute cholecystitis; treat with ampicillin-sulbactam**
- ❑ B. **Acute cholecystitis; treat with ceftriaxone**
- ❑ C. **Cholangitis; treat with ampicillin-sulbactam**
- ❑ D. **Cholangitis; treat with ceftriaxone**
- ❑ E. **None of the above**

Key Concept/Objective: To be able to recognize the characteristic signs and symptoms of cholangitis and to select the appropriate antibiotic to cover likely organisms

This patient has the classic triad of jaundice, right upper quadrant pain, and fever with rigors (Charcot triad), which suggests cholangitis. If she also had shock and mental status changes (Reynold pentad), her prognosis would be grave: mortality in such patients approaches 50%. In addition to antibiotics and supportive care, patients who are very ill should be considered for biliary tract decompression (percutaneous or surgical decompression, or decompression with ERCP). The organisms that most commonly cause cholangitis are *Escherichia coli, Klebsiella,* enterococci, and *Bacteroides fragilis.* Ceftriaxone is not recommended in this case because it does not cover enterococci and has been associated with the development of gallbladder sludge. *(Answer: C—Cholangitis; treat with ampicillin-sulbactam)*

24. A 75-year-old man presents with gradually worsening pruritus, jaundice, and vague right upper quadrant abdominal ache. He has a 30-year history of ulcerative colitis. On exam, he has normal vital signs, scleral icterus, and hepatomegaly. His abdominal ultrasound shows dilated intrahepatic and extrahepatic ducts but no evidence of stones. His bilirubin level is 10, alkaline phosphatase level is 400, and amylase level is normal. An abdominal CT scan finds no pancreatic masses or adenopathy.

The differential diagnosis for this patient should include which of the following?

- ❑ A. **Primary biliary cirrhosis**
- ❑ B. **Sclerosing cholangitis**
- ❑ C. **Carcinoma of the biliary tract**
- ❑ D. **Drug-induced cholestasis**
- ❑ E. **B and C**

Key Concept/Objective: To know that the differential diagnosis of cholestasis with ductal dilatation includes sclerosing cholangitis and ductal carcinoma

In this case, other possible diagnoses include a solitary common bile duct stone that escaped detection on ultrasound and CT, occult pancreatic carcinoma, bile duct stricture, and extrahepatic compression of the biliary tract. Although sclerosing cholangitis usually develops in younger men (aged 20 to 50 years), it is often associated with ulcerative colitis. About 60% of patients will also have a positive perinuclear antineutrophil cytoplasmic antibody (p-ANCA) test result. The hallmark finding on ERCP is segmental stenosis of the biliary tree. Primary biliary cirrhosis is an autoimmune disease that typically affects women. About 95% of patients have antimitochondrial antibodies. Both primary biliary cirrhosis and drug-induced cholestasis cause intrahepatic cholestasis without extrahepatic duct dilatation. *(Answer: E—B and C)*

For more information, see Ahmed A, Keeffe EB: 4 Gastroenterology: VI Gallstones and Biliary Tract Disease. ACP Medicine Online (www.acpmedicine.com). Dale DC, Federman DD, Eds. WebMD Inc., New York, December 2002

Gastrointestinal Bleeding

25. A 55-year-old man presents to the emergency department with a 2-day history of "coffee-ground emesis." On physical examination, the patient is noted to have tachycardia and orthostatic hypotension. Volume resuscitation with intravenous normal saline is initiated; a complete blood count, coagulation studies, and routine chemistries are done, and esophagogastroduodenoscopy (EGD) is planned for further evaluation and management.

Which of the following is the most common cause of upper GI bleeding?

- ❑ **A. Mallory-Weiss tear**
- ❑ **B. Variceal hemorrhage**
- ❑ **C. Dieulafoy lesion**
- ❑ **D. Peptic ulcer disease (PUD)**

Key Concept/Objective: To understand that PUD is the most common cause of upper GI bleeding

Upper GI bleeding is arbitrarily defined as hemorrhage from a source proximal to the ligament of Treitz. Hematemesis essentially always reflects upper GI bleeding. Stools may range from black (melena) to bright red (hematochezia), depending on rates of bleeding and intestinal transit. The most common cause of upper GI bleeding is PUD, accounting for 60% of cases found on emergency endoscopy. About 50% of cases will have a clean-based ulcer with a low probability of rebleeding, so that pharmacologic intervention is required. Adherent clots, visible vessels, or active bleeding portend less favorable outcomes unless endoscopic or surgical treatment is applied. Use of NSAIDs and *Helicobacter pylori* infection are the two most important risk factors; heavy alcohol ingestion and smoking are also associated with PUD bleeding risk. *(Answer: D—Peptic ulcer disease [PUD])*

26. A 39-year-old woman with a history of cirrhosis presents to the emergency department with massive hematemesis. Volume resuscitation with intravenous normal saline is initiated, and emergent EGD is planned for further evaluation and management. You are concerned about variceal bleeding.

Which of the following endoscopic interventions is considered first-line therapy in the management of esophageal varices?

- ❑ **A. Sclerotherapy**
- ❑ **B. Band ligation**
- ❑ **C. Thermal therapy**
- ❑ **D. Injection therapy**

Key Concept/Objective: To understand that band ligation is first-line therapy for the management of esophageal varices

With variceal bleeding, endoscopic treatment is used primarily for esophageal varices; the techniques include sclerotherapy and band ligation. Sclerotherapy utilizes a variety of sclerosants to induce variceal thrombosis, with sodium tetradecyl sulfate and ethanolamine oleate used most frequently. Complications include retrosternal chest pain, low-grade fever, ulceration (usually deep ulcers that heal within 3 weeks), dysphagia, delayed perforation (1 to 4 weeks later), and stricture formation. Complication rates vary from 19% to 35%. The popularity of sclerotherapy has diminished as a result of these complications. Intravariceal injections are more effective than paraesophageal injections in controlling bleeding. Band ligation is now considered the first-line endoscopic therapy for esophageal varices. The band ligator is readily attached to the distal end of the endoscope, which is advanced to the varix; the endoscopist then suctions the varix into the ligator cap and deploys a rubber band around the varix. This results in the plication of the varices and surrounding submucosal tissue, with fibrosis and eventual obliteration of varices. Comparative studies report better initial control of bleeding (91% versus 77%) and rebleeding rates (24% versus 47%) with band ligation than with sclerotherapy. Complications of banding include retrosternal chest pain, dysphagia from compromise of the esophageal lumen, band ulceration (usually superficial ulcers that heal within 2 weeks), overtube

injury, and perforation. Complication rates vary from 2% to 19%. *(Answer: B—Band ligation)*

For more information, see Rajan E, Ahlquist DA: 4 Gastroenterology: X Gastrointestinal Bleeding. ACP Medicine Online (www.acpmedicine.com). Dale DC, Federman DD, Eds. WebMD Inc., New York, July 2003

Malabsorption and Maldigestion

27. A 36-year-old man presents to your clinic complaining of fatigue. His fatigue started 3 or 4 months ago. His medical history is unremarkable. Review of systems is positive for occasional diarrhea, which the patient has been experiencing for several months, and for a 20-lb weight loss. Physical examination shows pallor. Occult blood is found on rectal examination. The rest of the examination is normal. Laboratory tests reveal iron deficiency anemia, and the patient tests positive on a qualitative fecal fat test. Results of an upper endoscopy and a colonoscopy are normal.

Which of the following tests would be most likely to provide helpful information in the workup of this patient?

❑ **A. Selenium-75–labeled homocholic acid-taurine (^{75}SeHCAT) absorption test**

❑ **B. Xylose absorption test**

❑ **C. Bentiromide test**

❑ **D. Tissue transglutaminase antibody**

Key Concept/Objective: To understand that gluten-sensitive enteropathy (GSE) is a cause of iron deficiency anemia

Patients with GSE may present with a variety of complaints, including weight loss, fatigue, abdominal cramps, distention, bloating, and diarrhea. Other presentations include iron deficiency anemia, osteoporosis, and easy bruising. In a patient in whom the suspicion of GSE is high, a positive tissue transglutaminase antibody test makes the diagnosis almost certain. Alternatively, the diagnosis might rest on small bowel biopsy findings. Another helpful test is the identification of an endomysial antibody. The presence of fecal fat is helpful in this patient because it confirms the suspicion of an underlying malabsorptive disorder. The xylose absorption test evaluates the absorptive surface area of the small bowel. The bentiromide test is a noninvasive test to evaluate for pancreatic exocrine insufficiency. All of these tests can, however, be helpful in the evaluation of a patient with malabsorption and diarrhea. On the basis of this patient's clinical presentation, the tissue transglutaminase antibody test is the one most likely to be helpful with the diagnosis. *(Answer: D—Tissue transglutaminase antibody)*

28. A 44-year-old woman with a history of GSE is evaluated for refractory disease. She was diagnosed with GSE 8 years ago. Her disease was initially well controlled with a gluten-free diet. Over the past few months, she has had persistent diarrhea and malabsorption that has not responded to her usual diet. Findings on physical examination are consistent with chronic malnutrition. An abdominal CT scan shows no masses or anatomic abnormalities that would account for her symptoms. An endoscopy is obtained, and small bowel biopsy shows villous atrophy and a layer of collagen underneath the enterocytes.

Which of the following is the most likely explanation for this patient's symptoms?

❑ **A. Poor adherence to gluten-exclusion diet**

❑ **B. Collagenous sprue**

❑ **C. Small bowel lymphoma**

❑ **D. Tropical sprue**

Key Concept/Objective: To know that collagenous sprue is a possible complication of gluten-sensitive enteropathy

Collagenous sprue is a rare, devastating disease in which there is a layer of collagen underneath the enterocytes of the small bowel. The origin of collagenous colitis is unknown, but it develops in approximately half the patients who have refractory celiac disease. The symptoms are severe and include obvious malabsorption. The diagnosis is made on the basis of the classic histologic picture of villous atrophy and subepithelial collagen deposition. Therapy for collagenous sprue is uncertain; some patients respond to steroids. Poor adherence to gluten-exclusion diet is common; however, it would not explain the histologic changes seen in this patient. Small bowel lymphoma can be a complication of GSE; however, there is no evidence of this disorder on the imaging studies and biopsy. Tropical sprue is a malabsorptive disorder that appears in certain areas of the world. The diagnosis is based on the history of travel to endemic areas and a biopsy showing villous atrophy and inflammatory cells. *(Answer: B—Collagenous sprue)*

29. A 60-year-old man is being evaluated in your clinic for diarrhea. He started having diarrhea 6 months ago. He has undergone extensive evaluation over the past 2 months. His stool studies were consistent with steatorrhea. A stool culture for bacterial organisms was negative, as were stool studies for the presence of ova and parasites. An abdominal CT scan was normal. The patient has had arthritis for 5 years. Review of systems is positive for weight loss and occasional fever over the past 3 months. On physical examination, the patient's temperature is 100.4° F (38° C). Skin hyperpigmentation and cervical lymphadenopathy are noted. You order an upper endoscopy. A small bowel biopsy shows villous atrophy and macrophages with sickleform particles. A periodic acid–Schiff (PAS) stain is positive.

Which of the following therapies is indicated for this patient?

- ❑ **A. Gluten-exclusion diet**
- ❑ **B. Steroids**
- ❑ **C. Trimethoprim-sulfamethoxazole (TMP-SMX)**
- ❑ **D. Cholestyramine**

Key Concept/Objective: To be able to recognize Whipple disease

The patient has clinical and laboratory findings consistent with the diagnosis of Whipple disease. This is a rare multisystem disease caused by infection with *Tropheryma whippelii*. Classically, the disease begins in a middle-aged man with a nondeforming arthritis that usually starts years before the onset of the intestinal symptoms. Arthralgias, diarrhea, abdominal pain, and weight loss are the cardinal manifestations of Whipple disease. Other complaints include fever, abdominal distention, lymphadenopathy, hyperpigmentation of the skin, and steatorrhea. The diagnosis rests on identifying the classic PAS-positive macrophages, which contain sickleform particles. The histologic lesion shows distended villi filled with the foamy, PAS-positive macrophages. Lymphatic dilatation is also present. A flat, villous surface can be seen in extreme cases. For treatment of Whipple disease, TMP-SMX is given for 1 year. Gluten-exclusion diet is indicated in cases of GSE. Prednisone has no role in the treatment of Whipple disease. Cholestyramine is a resin that binds bile acids and can be used in cases of diarrhea related to bile acid malabsorption. *(Answer: C—Trimethoprim-sulfamethoxazole [TMP-SMX])*

30. A 10-year-old boy is evaluated for edema. He developed unilateral left upper and lower extremity edema 1 year ago. On review of systems, abdominal swelling and occasional diarrhea are noted. The physical examination is remarkable for unilateral edema and abdominal shifting dullness to percussion. A complete blood count shows lymphopenia. The serum albumin level is low at 1 g/dl. Urinalysis shows no protein; liver function tests are within normal limits.

Which of the following would be the most likely finding on small bowel biopsy for this patient?

- ❑ **A. Dilated lymphatics with club-shaped villi**
- ❑ **B. Intense lymphocyte infiltration of the lamina propria**
- ❑ **C. Eosinophilic invasion of the crypts on the small intestine**
- ❑ **D. Lack of plasma cells**

Key Concept/Objective: To be able to recognize intestinal lymphangiectasia

This patient has classic findings of congenital intestinal lymphangiectasia. Intestinal lymphangiectasia is often a congenital condition in which deformed lymphatics impair the transport of chylomicrons from the enterocytes to the mesenteric lymph duct. The blockage of lymphatic drainage may result in chylous ascites. Protein-losing enteropathy and lymphopenia are prominent features. Modest steatorrhea is also present. In the congenital form of the disease, lymphedema of the legs or of one leg and one arm is seen. With endoscopic examination, white villi, white nodules, and submucosal elevations may be noted. The white appearance of the mucosa is undoubtedly caused by retained chylomicron triacylglycerol. Double-contrast barium x-ray examination shows smooth nodular protrusions and thick mucosal folds without ulceration. On histologic examination, dilated lymphatics with club-shaped villi are seen. Lymphocytic infiltration of the lamina propria can be found in other disorders, such as lymphomas and immunoproliferative disease of the small intestine. Eosinophilic invasion of the crypts on the small intestine can be found in eosinophilic gastroenteritis. Lack of plasma cells can be found in patients with hypogammaglobulinemic sprue. *(Answer: A—Dilated lymphatics with club-shaped villi)*

31. A 32-year-old woman presents for evaluation of a sensitive tongue, which she has been experiencing for 2 weeks. She describes loss of appetite, weight loss of 15 lb over 3 months, and frequent (four or five times a day) loose stools. She denies having bloody stools, risk factors for HIV infection, or a personal or family history of gastrointestinal disease. She does recall briefly taking ciprofloxacin for traveler's diarrhea while in Indonesia 18 months ago, which resolved with therapy. Review of systems is otherwise negative. Examination reveals normal conjunctiva; a swollen, tender tongue; a normal abdomen; and trace pedal edema. Laboratory tests show a hematocrit of 27, mild hypokalemia, and hypomagnesemia.

Which of the following pairs of interventions is most likely to help with this patient's condition?

- ❑ A. **Folate and niacin**
- ❑ B. **Iron sulfate and tetracycline**
- ❑ C. **Gluten-free diet and prednisone**
- ❑ D. **Folate and tetracycline**
- ❑ E. **Azathioprine and prednisone**

Key Concept/Objective: To be able to recognize the presentation and potential time course of tropical sprue and to understand the initial approach to therapy

Tropical sprue is a malabsorptive disease that occurs primarily in tropical locales among both residents and visitors. Its cause is unclear, but coliform bacteria have been selectively isolated from the jejunum of tropical sprue patients. The disease can occur while the patient is in the tropical locale, or it can present as late as 10 years after return. This patient spent time in Indonesia 18 months before presentation. Symptoms are generally much more apparent than in GSE and include prominent anorexia, weight loss, and diarrhea, as well as a high frequency of folate and vitamin B_{12} deficiencies with accompanying manifestations (macrocytic anemia, glossitis) and lower extremity edema. Folate should be administered as initial therapy; if the patient has had symptoms for a period longer than 4 months before the time of presentation, antibiotic therapy with tetracycline or a sulfonamide should be administered. Other than having glossitis, this patient has no evidence of niacin deficiency (pellagra). The patient's anemia could be that of iron deficiency, but in light of the normal conjunctiva and other physical findings, that is less likely. A gluten-free diet and, in some cases, prednisone are required for treatment of GSE. Azathioprine and prednisone may be the initial regimen for a patient with Crohn disease. *(Answer: D—Folate and tetracycline)*

32. A 64-year-old man presents to his primary care physician with a complaint of foul-smelling diarrhea, which he has had for the past 4 to 5 months. He has three or four stools a day, which he describes as oily in nature. He denies experiencing a change in the caliber of his stools, and he also denies having abdominal pain, melena, or blood per rectum. His appetite is still fairly good, but he has lost 10 lb over the past 2 months and is somewhat fatigued. His medical history is notable for hypertension, hyperlipi-

demia, type 2 diabetes with retinopathy and mild neuropathy, and gastroesophageal reflux disease. His medications include metformin, insulin, atenolol, simvastatin, aspirin, and omeprazole. The neurologic examination is notable only for mild stocking-glove neuropathy, and an S_4 is heard on cardiac examination. Laboratory tests reveal macrocytic anemia and mild hypoalbuminemia.

Which of the following is the most likely diagnosis for this patient?

❑ **A. Crohn disease**

❑ **B. Intestinal lymphoma**

❑ **C. Bacterial overgrowth syndrome**

❑ **D. Hemochromatosis**

❑ **E. Chronic pancreatitis**

Key Concept/Objective: To understand the precipitants for the bacterial overgrowth syndrome

This patient has a subacute to chronic presentation with steatorrhea and likely folate deficiency, vitamin B_{12} deficiency, or both. He has diabetes mellitus, which can cause stasis through autonomic neuropathy, which is not uncommon in a patient with other diabetic complications. Anything that causes intestinal stasis allows a proliferation of bacteria, which leads to changes in bile salt metabolism and impaired absorption, primarily of vitamin B_{12}. In addition, this patient is taking a proton pump inhibitor, which can both reduce motility and change the acid milieu of the proximal small bowel, often precipitating symptoms in a predisposed patient. Therapy usually entails repeated courses of antibiotics active against anaerobes. There is no convincing evidence for the effectiveness of any of the other choices presented. *(Answer: C—Bacterial overgrowth syndrome)*

33. A 38-year-old man with debilitating Crohn disease who is status post a 40 cm ileal resection presents for evaluation. He recounts progressive nonbloody diarrhea since his surgery 9 months ago, which is worse in the evening. He denies having abdominal pain, nausea or vomiting, fevers, chills, or sweats. He reports no recent travel, camping, or use of antibiotics. The exam is unrevealing. Chemistries show modest hypokalemia and a mild non–anion gap acidosis. Fecal fat quantitative analysis reveals minimal steatorrhea.

Which therapy is most likely to help this patient?

❑ **A. Cholestyramine**

❑ **B. Loperamide**

❑ **C. Tetracycline**

❑ **D. High-protein, low-fat diet**

❑ **E. Safflower oil before meals**

Key Concept/Objective: To understand the effects of ileal resection on absorption, and recognize the appropriate therapy to minimize these effects

Ileal involvement is a common component of Crohn disease (regional enteritis) and may result in a poorly functioning ileum or even require resection. With moderate resections (30 to 100 cm), as in this case, malabsorption of bile salts is significant and results in bile salts entering the colon. This can lead to a secretory diarrhea known as choleretic enteropathy, the causal mechanism of which is bile salt-induced chloride secretion. Cholestyramine reduces the distal delivery of bile salts, thus lessening the diarrhea, and would be the most appropriate therapy in this patient. With larger ileal resections (> 100 cm), steatorrhea predominates, and cholestyramine may actually exacerbate the diarrhea. Therapy for patients undergoing larger resections is similar to that for patients with short bowel syndrome and includes antimotility agents such as loperamide and steps to increase the proportion of medium-chain fatty acids, which do not require bile salts for absorption. Safflower oil may also be used preprandially to act via peptide YY to slow gastric emptying, but it would be less useful in bile salt-induced diarrhea. Tetracycline is used to treat the bacterial overgrowth syndrome. *(Answer: A—Cholestyramine)*

For more information, see Mansbach CM III: 4 Gastroenterology: XI Diseases Producing Malabsorption and Maldigestion. ACP Medicine Online (www.acpmedicine.com). Dale DC, Federman DD, Eds. WebMD Inc., New York, September 2003

Diverticulosis, Diverticulitis, and Appendicitis

34. A 54-year-old man presents with a 3-day history of left lower quadrant pain. He reports that his appetite has decreased and that he has been experiencing mild nausea. He denies having any significant change in bowel function, hematochezia, or melena. On examination, his temperature is 101.3° F (38.5° C) and his blood pressure is 145/84 mm Hg. He has significant tenderness in the left lower quadrant, with some mild local fullness. No rebound is appreciated. The white blood cell count is 13,400.

What is the most appropriate diagnostic test for this patient?

- ❑ A. **Barium enema**
- ❑ B. **Colonoscopy**
- ❑ C. **Abdominal CT**
- ❑ D. **Anoscopy**
- ❑ E. **Diagnostic laparotomy**

Key Concept/Objective: To understand appropriate diagnostic testing in presumptive diverticulitis

This patient presents with fairly severe clinical diverticulitis, and hospitalization is appropriate. Abdominal CT is the most useful test in this situation. It allows confirmation of the diagnosis as well as identification of complications. In this case, the possibility of abscess raised by the examination would be evaluated. Also, feasibility of percutaneous drainage would be determined. Colonoscopy is relatively contraindicated in cases of suspected diverticulitis because its use increases the risk of perforation. Barium enema is also not advisable, because its use increases the risk of peritoneal contamination if perforation is present. Water-soluble enema would be safer but would not provide the same degree of information as CT scanning. Most authorities would not recommend surgical intervention without initial diagnostic evaluation, because most patients do well without urgent surgery. Anoscopy would not be helpful; it is used primarily to evaluate very distal sources of GI bleeding. *(Answer: C—Abdominal CT)*

35. A 67-year-old woman presents to the office with 6 days of mild left-lower-quadrant cramping. She describes previous bouts of diverticulitis similar in character. She denies having fever, chills, nausea, or evidence of gastrointestinal bleeding. On examination, she is afebrile with mild left-lower-quadrant tenderness. A presumptive diagnosis of diverticulitis is made. She denies having any allergies to medication.

What is the most appropriate choice for antibiotic monotherapy?

- ❑ A. **Metronidazole**
- ❑ B. **Amoxicillin-clavulanate**
- ❑ C. **Cephalexin**
- ❑ D. **Clindamycin**
- ❑ E. **Azithromycin**

Key Concept/Objective: To understand appropriate antimicrobial choice in diverticulitis

This patient presents with mild diverticulitis. It is important to use an antibiotic that provides good anaerobic and gram-negative coverage, making amoxicillin-clavulanate a good choice. Metronidazole and clindamycin provide good anaerobic coverage but insufficient coverage against gram-negative rods. These two drugs are frequently used in combination with trimethoprim-sulfamethoxazole or quinolones (to cover gram-negative rods). Azithromycin and cephalexin provide inadequate coverage for both anaerobes and gram-negative rods. *(Answer: B—Amoxicillin-clavulanate)*

36. A 52-year-old man presents for follow-up after undergoing colonoscopy because he has a history of colon cancer. He was reassured to learn that no polyps or tumors were seen but was told that he has diverticulosis. He asks what the chances are that this will cause future difficulties.

What is the likelihood that a patient with asymptomatic diverticulosis will go on to develop diverticulitis?

- ❑ A. < 5%
- ❑ B. 10% to 25%
- ❑ C. 40% to 50%
- ❑ D. 70% to 80%
- ❑ E. > 90%

Key Concept/Objective: To understand the natural history of minimally symptomatic diverticulosis

Diverticulosis is common and is often discovered during evaluation for another problem (e.g., colon cancer). As more individuals undergo colon evaluation, more cases of asymptomatic diverticular disease will be identified. It is important to be able to educate patients on symptoms to watch for. It is also important to be able to inform them about the prognosis. Current data suggest that the likelihood of developing diverticulitis is 10% to 25%. An estimated 80% of patients with diverticulosis are completely asymptomatic. *(Answer: B—10% to 25%)*

37. Some months later, the patient in Question 36 comes to you for evaluation after experiencing two brief episodes of left-lower-quadrant cramping. He denies having any bleeding or severe symptoms. He has not required antibiotics or hospitalization. He is not particularly bothered by these symptoms but asks if there is anything he should be doing with respect to the diverticulosis.

Which of the following interventions would be most appropriate at this time?

- ❑ A. **Narcotic analgesic**
- ❑ B. **Anticholinergic agent**
- ❑ C. **Colonic resection**
- ❑ D. **Fiber supplementation**
- ❑ E. **Repeat colonoscopy**

Key Concept/Objective: To understand the management of mild diverticulosis

In patients with asymptomatic or minimally symptomatic diverticulosis, an increase in the amount of fiber consumed—as would occur through eating more fruits and vegetables—appears to reduce the risk of symptoms and complications. Bran has been shown to improve constipation but not pain. There is no evidence to support the use of narcotic or anticholinergic agents. This patient underwent colonoscopy within the past year, so repeat colonscopy would be very unlikely to offer any additional information. *(Answer: D—Fiber supplementation)*

For more information, see Harford WV: 4 Gastroenterology: XII Diverticulosis, Diverticulitis, and Appendicitis. ACP Medicine Online (www.acpmedicine.com). Dale DC, Federman DD, Eds. WebMD Inc., New York, April 2001

Enteral and Parenteral Nutritional Support

38. A 74-year-old man is transported to the emergency department by ambulance for evaluation of cough, dyspnea, and altered mental status. Upon arrival, the patient is noted to be minimally responsive. Results of physical examination are as follows: temperature, 102.1° F (38.9° C); heart rate, 116 beats/min; blood pressure, 94/62 mm Hg; respiratory rate, 34 breaths/min; and O_2 saturation, 72% on 100% O_2 with a nonrebreather mask. The patient is intubated in the emergency department, and mechanical ventilation

is initiated. Coarse rhonchi are noted bilaterally. A portable chest x-ray reveals good placement of the endotracheal tube and lobar consolidation of the right lower lobe. Laboratory data are obtained, including sputum Gram stain and culture and blood cultures. Empirical antimicrobial therapy is initiated, and the patient is admitted to the medical intensive care unit for further management. The intern on call inquires about the appropriateness of initiating nutritional support (enteral or parenteral feeds) at this time.

Which of the following statements regarding nutritional support is true?

- ❑ A. **Enteral nutrition is less likely to cause infection than parenteral nutrition**
- ❑ B. **Parenteral nutrition has consistently been shown to result in a decrease in mortality, compared with standard care**
- ❑ C. **The use of oral supplements in hospitalized elderly patients has been shown to be harmful**
- ❑ D. **Parenteral nutrition is the preferred mode of nutrition in cancer patients because of its lower incidence of infections**

Key Concept/Objective: To understand that enteral nutrition is less likely to cause infection than parenteral nutrition

Comparisons of enteral nutrition with parenteral nutrition have consistently shown fewer infectious complications with enteral nutrition. Elderly patients should receive supplemental feeding or enteral nutrition if they are incapable of eating adequately. A trial in 501 hospitalized elderly patients randomized to oral supplements or a ward diet showed that, irrespective of their initial nutritional status, the patients receiving oral supplements had lower mortality, better mobility, and a shorter hospital stay. The difference between ward diet and supplementation was even more pronounced in a secondary analysis of patients with weight loss. *(Answer: A—Enteral nutrition is less likely to cause infection than parenteral nutrition)*

39. A 32-year-old man with AIDS who is experiencing chronic diarrhea, anorexia, and wasting is referred for evaluation for nutritional support. Results of physical examination are as follows: temperature, 97.6° F (36.4° C); heart rate, 67 beats/min; blood pressure, 102/62 mm Hg; respiratory rate, 12 breaths/min; height, 70 in; and weight, 50 kg. The patient appears chronically ill; there is bitemporal wasting, and his hair is easily pluckable. The patient says he has friends with AIDS who are receiving "I.V. nutrition," and he would like to know if such therapy would benefit him.

Which of the following statements regarding home total parenteral nutrition (TPN) is true?

- ❑ A. **Evidence demonstrates improved survival and quality of life in patients with metastatic cancer who are receiving home TPN**
- ❑ B. **Evidence demonstrates improved survival and quality of life in patients with AIDS who are receiving home TPN**
- ❑ C. **Evidence demonstrates improved survival and quality of life in patients with short bowel from Crohn disease who are receiving home TPN**
- ❑ D. **No evidence supports the use of home TPN in any patient population**

Key Concept/Objective: To understand which patients clearly benefit from home TPN

Patients with intestinal failure from a short bowel, chronic bowel obstruction, radiation enteritis, or untreatable malabsorption can be nourished by TPN at home. Long-term success has been achieved with a tunneled silicone rubber catheter or an implanted reservoir. Premixed nutrients are infused overnight. The catheter is then disconnected and a heparin lock applied, leaving the patient free to attend to daily activities. Survival of patients with short bowel resulting from the treatment of Crohn disease or pseudo-obstruction is excellent. Home TPN increases quality-adjusted years of life in these patients and is cost-effective. On the other hand, mean survival in AIDS patients or those with metastatic cancer who receive home TPN is about 3 months. There is no evidence that home TPN prolongs

survival for these patients or enhances their quality of life. Trials are urgently required to justify the use of home TPN in patients with terminal cancer and AIDS. *(Answer: C—Evidence demonstrates improved survival and quality of life in patients with short bowel from Crohn disease who are receiving home TPN)*

For more information, see Jeejeebhoy KN: 4 Gastroenterology: XIII Enteral and Parenteral Nutritonal Support. ACP Medicine Online (www.acpmedicine.com). Dale DC, Federman DD, Eds. WebMD Inc., New York, January 2003

Gastrointestinal Motility Disorders

40. A 45-year-old man presents to your office complaining of nausea, early satiety, anorexia, and abdominal discomfort. His medical history is remarkable for a Roux-en-Y partial gastrectomy a few months ago. You suspect that the surgery has resulted in disruption of gastric motility.

Which of the following is most likely to relieve this patient's symptoms?

- ❑ **A. Metoclopramide, 10 to 20 mg up to four times a day**
- ❑ **B. Erythromycin lactobionate, 3 to 6 mg/kg every 8 hours**
- ❑ **C. Further resection of the gastric remnant**
- ❑ **D. Omeprazole, 20 mg two times a day**

Key Concept/Objective: To know the most effective treatment for a patient with upper gut stasis resulting from gastric surgery

This patient most likely has upper gut stasis caused by his gastric surgery. This is most commonly the result of uncoordinated phasic pressure waves in the Roux limb. The vagotomized gastric remnant may also contribute to the development of symptoms because of derangements in its relaxation and contraction. In general, pharmacologic agents are ineffective in relieving symptoms in these patients. Further resection of the gastric remnant gives symptomatic relief in approximately two thirds of patients. *(Answer: C—Further resection of the gastric remnant)*

41. A 25-year-old woman presents to your clinic complaining of lower abdominal pain and periods of constipation alternating with episodes of diarrhea. Her previous physician diagnosed her with an irritable bowel after an extensive evaluation. She takes a selective serotonin reuptake inhibitor for depression but has no other significant medical history.

Which of the following abnormalities is NOT present in patients with functional gastrointestinal disorders?

- ❑ **A. Histologic changes, such as loss of normal villi, can be seen in small bowel biopsy**
- ❑ **B. Abnormal gastrointestinal motility**
- ❑ **C. Heightened visceral sensation**
- ❑ **D. Psychosocial disturbance**

Key Concept/Objective: To be able to identify the common pathogenetic features of the functional gastrointestinal disorders

Functional gastrointestinal disorders are characterized by disturbances in motor or sensory function in the absence of any known mucosal, structural, biochemical, or metabolic abnormality. These disorders include irritable bowel syndrome, functional dysphagia, nonulcer dyspepsia, slow-transit constipation, and outlet obstruction to defecation. The shared common pathogenetic features of these disorders are abnormal motility, heightened visceral sensation, and psychosocial disturbance. The loss of villi, as demonstrated on small bowel biopsy, is evidence of a mucosal abnormality and should prompt consideration of another diagnosis, such as celiac sprue. *(Answer: A—Histologic changes, such as loss of normal villi, can be seen in small bowel biopsy)*

42. For the past several months, a 50-year-old man has been experiencing upper abdominal discomfort, nausea, and bloating; these symptoms are worse exclusively after eating. You diagnose the patient with dyspepsia.

Which of the following is NOT one of the alarm features associated with dyspepsia caused by ulcers or cancer?

❑ **A. Dysphagia**

❑ **B. Emesis**

❑ **C. Weight loss**

❑ **D. Bleeding**

Key Concept/Objective: To know the clinical findings associated with dyspepsia caused by ulcers or cancer

Dyspepsia refers to symptoms of nausea, vomiting, upper abdominal discomfort, bloating, anorexia, and early satiety that usually occurs in the postprandial period. When such symptoms occur in the absence of a gastric or duodenal ulcer, the condition is referred to as nonulcer dyspepsia. This condition affects approximately 20% of the population of the United States. Certain clinical features suggest that dyspepsia may be associated with mucosal diseases, such as ulcers or cancer. The presence of these features makes exclusion of these disorders imperative. These alarm features include dysphagia, bleeding, and weight loss. Emesis is a nonspecific symptom frequently present in patients with dyspepsia. It should be noted, however, that cancer may be present in patients with dyspepsia despite the absence of these symptoms. *(Answer: B—Emesis)*

43. A 64-year-old man with a long history of poorly controlled diabetes is diagnosed as having gastroparesis on the basis of his medical history and transit tests showing delayed gastric emptying. He is referred to you for long-term treatment.

Which of the following should NOT be included in your treatment strategy?

❑ **A. Correction of dehydration and electrolyte and nutritional deficiencies**

❑ **B. Prokinetic therapy with metoclopramide or erythromycin**

❑ **C. Vagotomy**

❑ **D. Antiemetics as needed**

Key Concept/Objective: To know the major modalities used in the treatment of gastroparesis

The major treatment approaches for the patient with a gastric or small bowel motility disorder include correction of fluid, electrolyte, and nutritional deficiencies; the use of prokinetic agents such as metoclopramide and erythromycin; the use of antiemetic agents for symptomatic relief; suppression of bacterial overgrowth (if present); decompression in severe cases; and surgical resection if the disorder is determined to be isolated to one discrete area of the gut. Vagotomy can actually cause gastroparesis and should be avoided. *(Answer: C—Vagotomy)*

For more information, see Camilleri M: 4 Gastroenterology: XIV Gastrointestinal Motility Disorders. ACP Medicine Online (www.acpmedicine.com). Dale DC, Federman DD, Eds. WebMD Inc., New York, October 2002

Liver and Pancreas Transplantation

44. A patient with known chronic hepatitis C and cirrhosis comes to your office wondering about liver transplantation. He read on the Internet that the waiting time for liver transplantation is long and that one should be included "early" to improve the chances of getting a timely transplantation. The patient stopped smoking over 20 years ago and does not drink alcohol. He is otherwise in good health.

Which of the following is NOT a contraindication for orthotopic liver transplantation?

- ❑ A. **Ongoing abuse of drugs or alcohol**
- ❑ B. **Significant cardiovascular or neurologic disease**
- ❑ C. **Infection with hepatitis B or C**
- ❑ D. **Extrahepatic malignancy**
- ❑ E. **Extensive portal and splanchnic venous thrombosis**

Key Concept/Objective: To know the contraindications for liver transplantation

Contraindications for liver transplanatation can be categorized into issues of abuse, underlying significant medical problems, malignancy, and technical limitations. Ongoing abuse of drugs or alcohol is one of the most frequent contraindications to transplantation. Patients with significant cardiovascular or neurologic disease cannot withstand the stress of transplantation. Although transplantation is often performed for hepatocellular carcinoma, extrahepatic malignancy is a contraindication. Extensive portal and splanchnic venous thrombosis prevents viable blood flow to the transplanted liver. Although patients with hepatitis B or C may require antiviral therapy before and after transplantation, having hepatitis B or C is not a contraindication. *(Answer: C—Infection with hepatitis B or C)*

45. A 40-year-old man with cirrhosis secondary to hepatitis B is being evaluated for orthotopic liver transplantation. He asks you what he should expect after his operation.

Which of the following statements is true regarding this patient?

- ❑ A. **There is a 1% to 2% chance of failure of his transplanted organ in the immediate postoperative period**
- ❑ B. **Although he may develop progressive jaundice over time, suggesting ductopenic rejection, this has little consequence**
- ❑ C. **His hepatitis B will most likely be cured after transplantation, so he will not need his antiviral medications anymore**
- ❑ D. **Infections are among the most serious complications after liver transplantation**
- ❑ E. **Thirty percent of patients taking cyclosporine or tacrolimus develop kidney failure within 10 years after transplantation**

Key Concept/Objective: To know the most common and serious complications after liver transplantation

From 5% to 10% of liver transplant patients experience immediate graft failure. Although ductopenic rejection is a more indolent process, it usually creates a need for retransplantation. Hepatitis B is not cured by transplantation and can even cause rapidly progressive liver disease after transplantation; however, aggressive antiviral therapy before and after transplantation has been associated with prolonged graft longevity. Approximately 10% of patients treated with the calcineurin inhibitors cyclosporine or tacrolimus develop renal failure after transplantation. Because of the strong immunosuppressive agents required, infections remain among the most serious complications, both short-term and long-term, after transplantation. *(Answer: D—Infections are among the most serious complications after liver transplantation)*

46. A 37-year-old woman with a history of cryptogenic cirrhosis who underwent orthotopic liver transplanation 1 year ago asks you to assume her posttransplantation care.

Which of the following is true regarding this patient?

- ❑ A. **She can expect to return to work, but it is unlikely that she will be able to tolerate vigorous activity**
- ❑ B. **The phenytoin she takes for her seizure disorder may result in an ele-**

vation in serum cyclosporine level, leading to a need for lower doses of cyclosporine

- ❑ C. Infection is the leading cause of death in the posttransplantation population
- ❑ D. Most transplant centers report 75% to 80% 5-year survival rates
- ❑ E. If she develops hyperlipidemia as a result of taking cyclosporine, she is unlikely to benefit from a change in immunosuppressive medications

Key Concept/Objective: To understand the long-term prognosis of liver transplant recipients, in terms of both mortality and functional status

Many posttransplantation patients not only return to work but are able to participate in such vigorous activities as marathon running. Phenytoin induces the cytochrome P-450 system, leading to decreased serum levels of cyclosporine. Age-related cardiovascular disease is the leading cause of death in posttransplantation patients. Many patients receiving cyclosporine develop hyperlipidemia; some can be helped by changing this medication to tacrolimus. Because of advances in immunosuppressive medications and surgical techniques, most transplant centers report 5-year survival rates of 75% to 80%. *(Answer: D—Most transplant centers report 75% to 80% 5-year survival rates)*

47. A 28-year-old patient with type 1 diabetes mellitus of 5 years' duration asks your opinion regarding pancreas transplantation. He is concerned that in spite of his best efforts, it is very likely that he will develop both microvascular and macrovascular complications.

Which of the following statements about pancreas transplantation is false?

- ❑ A. Recipients of pancreas transplantation usually have normal insulin levels after successful transplantation
- ❑ B. Pancreas transplantation can prevent or reduce nephropathy in diabetic patients with kidney transplants
- ❑ C. The graft pancreas is usually placed in the right lower quadrant, with vascular anastomoses to the common iliac artery and common iliac vein or portal vein
- ❑ D. Rejection is the leading cause of graft loss after transplantation
- ❑ E. A major difficulty with islet cell transplantation is that more than one pancreas is required to provide enough islets for the recipient to become euglycemic

Key Concept/Objective: To understand the metabolic benefits of pancreas transplantation and the complications associated with this type of transplantation

Pancreas transplantation has been shown to prevent or reduce the nephropathy that often develops in kidney grafts in diabetic patients. The favored placement of the graft is the right lower quadrant, with vascular anastomoses to the common iliac artery and the common iliac vein or portal vein; in simultaneous pancreas and kidney transplantations, the preferred placement is the left lower quadrant. Rejection is the leading cause of graft loss; vascular thrombosis is the leading nonimmunologic cause. Glucose tolerance tests are usually normal or near normal for pancreas transplant recipients. However, insulin levels are much higher than normal in these patients. *(Answer: A—Recipients of pancreas transplantation usually have normal insulin levels after successful transplantation)*

48. Three months after liver transplantation for chronic hepatitis C infection, a 45-year-old man develops biochemical abnormalities suggestive of cholestatic hepatitis.

Which of the following evaluation strategies is most important for this patient at this time?

- ❑ A. Cytomegalovirus (CMV) culture of the blood
- ❑ B. Hepatitis C virus (HCV) RNA levels

- ❑ **C. Endoscopic retrograde cholangiopancreatography (ERCP)**
- ❑ **D. Doppler ultrasonography to look for hepatic artery thrombosis**
- ❑ **E. Liver biopsy**

Key Concept/Objective: To understand the evaluation of liver dysfunction 1 month and longer after liver transplantation

It is important to use liver biopsy to determine the specific cause of allograft dysfunction that occurs more than 30 days after transplantation. Neither serum hepatic enzyme levels nor measures of viral load can be reliably used to determine the specific cause of allograft dysfunction occurring as cholestatic hepatitis. Because HCV hepatitis, CMV hepatitis, and transplant rejection differ histologically, liver biopsy is important. If the biopsy results suggest biliary tract disease, ERCP would be performed. Doppler studies would be performed if there were histoloic evidence of ischemia. *(Answer: E—Liver biopsy)*

49. A 38-year-old woman with long-standing insulin-dependent diabetes mellitus has complications of nephropathy, retinopathy, peripheral neuropathy, and mild gastroparesis. She has been missing more and more time from work as a nurse administrator. She asks you about being referred for simultaneous pancreas and kidney transplantation. Assuming she is a candidate, your patient asks about what she might expect if she undergoes the procedure.

Which of the following outcomes has been shown to occur following successful simultaneous pancreas and kidney transplantation?

- ❑ **A. Improvement in macrovascular disease**
- ❑ **B. Improvement in gastroparesis**
- ❑ **C. Improvement in retinopathy**
- ❑ **D. Lowered use of immunosuppressive agents because of normoglycemia**
- ❑ **E. Increased likelihood of returning to full-time work**

Key Concept/Objective: To understand outcomes associated with simultaneous pancreas and kidney transplantation

Well-controlled, prospective studies assessing the long-term benefits of improved glucose control have yet to be carried out. The studies that have been reported reveal no improvement for patients with macroangiopathy, retinopathy, and gastroparesis. Glucose control does occur but does not diminish the need for immunosuppressive agents. Quality of life improves, including the capacity to return to full-time or part-time work. *(Answer: E—Increased likelihood of returning to full-time work)*

For more information, see Carithers RL Jr, Perkins JD: 4 Gastroenterology: XV Liver and Pancreas Transplantation. ACP Medicine Online (www.acpmedicine.com). Dale DC, Federman DD, Eds. WebMD Inc., New York, November 2003

SECTION 5

HEMATOLOGY

Approach to Hematologic Disorders

1. A 43-year-old woman presents for the evaluation of bleeding gums. The patient reports that for the past 2 months, her gums have bled more easily when she brushes her teeth. Physical examination reveals palatal petechiae and scattered petechiae over the lower extremities bilaterally.

   Which of the following laboratory tests is most likely to identify the abnormality responsible for this patient's bleeding disorder?

   - ❏ **A. Prothrombin time (PT) and international normalized ratio (INR)**
   - ❏ **B. Complete blood count (CBC)**
   - ❏ **C. Partial thromboplastin time (PTT)**
   - ❏ **D. A mixing study**

   Key Concept/Objective: To understand that thrombocytopenia usually presents as petechial bleeding

   Bleeding occurs as a consequence of thrombocytopenia, deficiencies of coagulation factors, or both. Thrombocytopenia usually presents as petechial bleeding that is first observed in the lower extremities. Deficiencies in coagulation factor more often cause bleeding into the gastrointestinal tract or joints. Intracranial bleeding, however, can occur with a deficiency of platelets or coagulation factors and can be catastrophic. CBCs are routinely performed in most laboratories through the use of an electronic particle counter, which determines the total white blood cell and platelet counts and calculates the hematocrit and hemoglobin from the erythrocyte count and the dimensions of the red cells. For this patient, a CBC would likely disclose a decreased platelet count (thrombocytopenia). Impaired hepatic synthetic function and vitamin K deficiency would result in prolongation of the PT and INR. Coagulation factor deficiencies and coagulation factor inhibitors would result in prolongation of the PTT. A mixing study is obtained to differentiate between a coagulation factor deficiency and a coagulation factor inhibitor by mixing patient plasma with normal plasma in the laboratory. *(Answer: B—Complete blood count [CBC])*

2. A 53-year-old man presents with fatigue, weight loss, and a petechial rash. A CBC reveals anemia and thrombocytopenia, with a peripheral smear containing 20% blast cells. A bone marrow biopsy is performed, revealing acute myelogenous leukemia (AML). The patient is treated with cytarabine and daunorubicin induction chemotherapy.

   Which of the following blood cell lineages has the shortest blood half-life and is therefore most likely to become deficient as a result of this patient's chemotherapy treatment?

   - ❏ **A. Red blood cells (RBCs)**
   - ❏ **B. Platelets**
   - ❏ **C. Megakaryocytes**
   - ❏ **D. Neutrophils**

   Key Concept/Objective: To understand differences in the dynamics of erythrocytes, platelets, and leukocytes in the blood

There are important differences in the dynamics or kinetics of erythrocytes, platelets, and leukocytes in the blood. For instance, neutrophils have a blood half-life of only 6 to 8 hours; essentially, a new blood population of neutrophils is formed every 24 hours. Erythrocytes last the longest by far: the normal life span is about 100 days. These differences partially account for why neutrophils and their precursors are the predominant marrow cells, whereas in the blood, erythrocytes far outnumber neutrophils. Similarly, the short half-life and high turnover rate of neutrophils account for why neutropenia is the most frequent hematologic consequence when bone marrow is damaged by drugs or radiation. Transfusion of erythrocytes and platelets is feasible because of their relatively long life span, whereas the short life span of neutrophils has greatly impeded efforts to develop neutrophil transfusion therapy. *(Answer: D—Neutrophils)*

3. A 54-year-old man presents with fatigue, weakness, and dyspnea on exertion. Physical examination reveals conjunctival pallor, palatal petechiae, and splenomegaly. A CBC reveals profound anemia and thrombocytopenia. A bone marrow biopsy reveals agnogenic myeloid metaplasia (myelofibrosis). The patient's splenomegaly is attributed to increased production of blood cells in the spleen.

Which of the following terms indicates blood cell production outside the bone marrow in the spleen, liver, and other locations?

- ❑ A. Adjunctive hematopoiesis
- ❑ B. Remote hematopoiesis
- ❑ C. Accessory hematopoiesis
- ❑ D. Extramedullary hematopoiesis

Key Concept/Objective: To understand the nomenclature of hematopoiesis

Hematopoiesis begins in the fetal yolk sac and later occurs predominantly in the liver and the spleen. Recent studies demonstrate that islands of hematopoiesis develop in these tissues from hemangioblasts, which are the common progenitors for both hematopoietic and endothelial cells. These islands then involute as the marrow becomes the primary site for blood cell formation by the seventh month of fetal development. Barring serious damage, such as that which occurs with myelofibrosis or radiation injury, the bone marrow remains the site of blood cell formation throughout the rest of life. In childhood, there is active hematopoiesis in the marrow spaces of the central axial skeleton (i.e., the ribs, vertebrae, and pelvis) and the extremities, extending to the wrists, the ankles, and the calvaria. With normal growth and development, hematopoiesis gradually withdraws from the periphery. This change is reversible, however; distal marrow extension can result from intensive stimulation, as occurs with severe hemolytic anemias, long-term administration of hematopoietic growth factors, and hematologic malignancies. The term medullary hematopoiesis refers to the production of blood cells in the bone marrow; the term extramedullary hematopoiesis indicates blood cell production outside the marrow in the spleen, liver, and other locations. *(Answer: D—Extramedullary hematopoiesis)*

4. A 35-year-old woman with advanced HIV disease complicated by anemia is seen for routine follow-up. The patient is started on erythropoeitin to decrease the severity of her anemia and to provide symptomatic improvement.

Which of the following laboratory findings is the most easily monitored immediate effect of erythropoietin therapy?

- ❑ A. An increase in the reticulocyte count
- ❑ B. An increase in the mean corpuscular volume
- ❑ C. An increase in the hemoglobin level
- ❑ D. An increase in the mean corpuscular hemoglobin level

Key Concept/Objective: To understand that an increase in the reticulocyte count is the most easily monitored immediate effect of erythropoietin therapy

Erythropoietin is a glycosylated protein that modulates erythropoiesis by affecting several steps in red cell development. The peritubular interstitial cells located in the inner cortex and outer medulla of the kidney are the primary sites for erythropoietin production. Erythropoietin can be administered intravenously or subcutaneously for the treatment of anemia caused by inadequate endogenous production of erythropoietin. Treatment is maximally effective when the marrow has a generous supply of iron and other nutrients, such as cobalamin and folic acid. For patients with renal failure, who have very low erythropoietin levels, the starting dosage is 50 to 100 units subcutaneously three times a week. The most easily monitored immediate effect of increased endogenous or exogenous erythropoietin is an increase in the blood reticulocyte count. Normally, as red cell precursors mature, the cells extrude their nucleus at the normal blast stage. The resulting reticulocytes, identified by the supravital stain of their residual ribosomes, persist for about 3 days in the marrow and 1 day in the blood. Erythropoietin shortens the transit time through the marrow, leading to an increase in the number and proportion of blood reticulocytes within a few days. In some conditions, particularly chronic inflammatory diseases, the effectiveness of erythropoietin can be predicted from measurement of the serum erythropoietin level by immunoassay. It may be cost-effective to measure the level before initiating treatment in patients with anemia attributable to suppressed erythropoietin production, such as patients with HIV infection, cancer, and chronic inflammatory diseases. Several studies have shown that erythropoietin treatment decreases the severity of anemia and improves the quality of life for these patients. In patients with anemia caused by cancer and cancer chemotherapy, current guidelines recommend erythropoietin treatment if the hemoglobin level is less than 10 g/dl. *(Answer: A—An increase in the reticulocyte count)*

5. A 55-year-old man with type 1 diabetes undergoes dialysis three times a week for end-stage renal disease. You recently started him on erythropoietin injections for chronic anemia (hematocrit, 25%).

   Which of the following is the best test to determine whether this patient will respond to the erythropoietin treatment?

   - ❑ A. **Erythropoietin level**
   - ❑ B. **Hematocrit**
   - ❑ C. **Creatinine level**
   - ❑ D. **Reticulocyte count**
   - ❑ E. **Blood urea nitrogen**

   Key Concept/Objective: To understand the site of production, effect, and therapeutic monitoring of erythropoietin

   In many renal diseases, the kidneys fail to produce sufficient amounts of erythropoietin. Replacement of endogenous erythropoietin stimulates red cell precursors in the bone marrow to mature more quickly. If the patient has normal bone marrow, an elevated reticulocyte count should be seen several days after initiation of therapy. *(Answer: D—Reticulocyte count)*

6. A 34-year-old woman undergoes chemotherapy for advanced-stage breast cancer. As expected, she develops pancytopenia.

   Which cell line would you expect to be the last to recover in this patient?

   - ❑ A. **Eosinophils**
   - ❑ B. **Platelets**
   - ❑ C. **Basophils**
   - ❑ D. **Monocytes**
   - ❑ E. **RBCs**

   Key Concept/Objective: To understand the time needed for cell-line recovery after bone marrow damage

The proliferation and maturation of platelets take longer than those of either red blood cells (7 to 10 days) or white blood cells (10 to 14 days) and thus are the slowest to recover from an acute bone marrow injury, such as occurs with chemotherapy. *(Answer: B—Platelets)*

For more information, see Dale DC: 5 Hematology: I Approach to Hematologic Disorders. ACP Medicine Online (www.acpmedicine.com). Dale DC, Federman DD, Eds. WebMD Inc., New York, June 2003

Red Blood Cell Function and Disorders of Iron Metabolism

7. An 86-year-old man visits your clinic for routine follow-up. Upon questioning, the patient admits to worsening dyspnea on exertion and generalized fatigue. He denies having fever, chills, cough, dysuria, blood loss, or weight loss. Routine laboratory studies reveal a hemoglobin concentration of 8.0 g/dl, a hematocrit of 24%, and a mean cell volume of 70 fl. The patient denies eating nonfood substances but does admit to craving and eating large amounts of ice daily. The patient's stool is positive for occult blood by guaiac testing.

For this patient, which of the following statements regarding iron deficiency anemia is true?

- ❑ **A. In men and postmenopausal women, pica and a poor supply of dietary iron are the most common causes of iron deficiency anemia**
- ❑ **B. Pagophagia, or pica with ice, is a symptom that is believed to be specific for iron deficiency**
- ❑ **C. Measurement of the serum iron concentration is the most useful test in the detection of iron deficiency**
- ❑ **D. The preferred method of iron replacement for this patient is parenteral therapy**

Key Concept/Objective: To understand the historical components, laboratory diagnosis, and treatment of iron deficiency anemia

Blood loss is the most common cause of increased iron requirements that lead to iron deficiency. In men and postmenopausal women, iron deficiency is almost always the result of gastrointestinal blood loss. In older children, men, and postmenopausal women, a poor supply of dietary iron is almost never the only factor responsible for iron deficiency; therefore, other etiologic factors must be sought, especially blood loss. Pagophagia, or pica with ice, is thought to be a highly specific symptom of iron deficiency and disappears shortly after iron therapy is begun. Measurement of the serum ferritin concentration is the most useful test for the detection of iron deficiency, because serum ferritin concentrations decrease as body iron stores decline. A serum ferritin concentration below 12 mg/L is virtually diagnostic of absent iron stores. In contrast, a normal serum ferritin concentration [illegible] storage iron, because serum ferritin may be increased independently of body iron by infection, inflammation, liver disease, malignancy, and other conditions. Oral and parenteral replacement therapy yield similar results, but for almost all patients, oral iron therapy is the treatment of choice. Oral iron therapy is effective, safe, and inexpensive. *(Answer: B—Pagophagia, or pica with ice, is a symptom that is believed to be specific for iron deficiency)*

8. A 55-year-old white man with type 2 diabetes mellitus and dyslipidemia presents to your clinic for follow-up. He has been a patient of yours for 2 years. His diabetes has been well controlled for the past year. On review of systems, the patient states that his skin has become tan over the past several months. Routine laboratory studies show that the patient's alanine aminotransferase level is elevated today; there are no other liver function abnormalities. Physical examination confirms that the patient's skin is hyperpigmented with a bronze hue. You strongly suspect that this patient may have hereditary hemochromatosis.

For this patient, which of the following statements regarding HFE-associated hereditary hemochromatosis is true?

- ❑ **A. The classic tetrad of clinical signs associated with hemochromatosis is liver disease, diabetes mellitus, skin pigmentation, and gonadal failure**

❑ B. **Measurement of the serum iron level is usually recommended as initial phenotypic screening, followed by genotypic testing**

❑ C. **The treatment of choice for hemochromatosis is chelation therapy or intermittent phlebotomy for 2 or 3 months**

❑ D. **In patients with hemochromatosis and cirrhosis, the rates of development of hepatocellular carcinoma equal that of the standard population**

Key Concept/Objective: To know the clinical features of and appropriate therapy for HFE-associated hemochromatosis

In homozygotes who present with hereditary hemochromatosis in middle age or later, the classic tetrad of clinical signs is liver disease, diabetes mellitus, skin pigmentation, and gonadal failure. Measurement of serum transferrin saturation is usually recommended as the initial phenotypic screening determination. Although individual laboratories may have their own reference ranges, a persistent value of 45% or higher is often recommended as a threshold value for further investigation. The serum ferritin level is then used as a biochemical indicator of iron overload; in the absence of complicating factors, elevated concentrations suggest increased iron stores. Genetic testing should be considered in patients with abnormal elevations in transferrin saturation, serum ferritin, or both. The treatment of choice for hereditary hemochromatosis is phlebotomy to reduce the body iron to normal or near-normal levels and to maintain it in that range. The phlebotomy program should remove 500 ml of blood once weekly or, for heavily loaded patients, twice weekly, until the patient is iron deficient. In patients with hereditary hemochromatosis, prolonged treatment is often needed. For example, if the initial body iron burden is 25 g, complete removal of the iron burden with weekly phlebotomy may require therapy for 2 years or more. If phlebotomy therapy removes the iron load before diabetes mellitus or cirrhosis develops, the patient's life expectancy is normal. If cirrhosis develops, however, the risk of hepatocellular carcinoma is increased by more than 200-fold. *(Answer: A—The classic tetrad of clinical signs associated with hemochromatosis is liver disease, diabetes mellitus, skin pigmentation, and gonadal failure)*

For more information, see Brittenham GM: 5 Hematology: II Red Blood Cell Function and Disorders of Iron Metabolism. ACP Medicine Online (www.acpmedicine.com). Dale DC, Federman DD, Eds. WebMD Inc., New York, March 2004

Anemia: Production Defects

9. A 30-year-old African-American woman presents to your office with a chief complaint of weakness. She states that she has been feeling "run down" for several weeks now. Further questioning reveals that she is diffusely weak. She is without focal deficits. She has experienced dyspnea on exertion, and she has a new rash. Physical examination is notable for mild tachycardia, pale conjunctiva, petechiae on her mucus membranes and lower extremities, and an absence of hepatomegaly or splenomegaly. Results of a complete blood cell count (CBC) are as follows: hematocrit, 21%; white blood cell count (WBC), 1,200 cells/mm^3; and platelet count, 12,000 cells/mm^3. The results of a bone marrow biopsy with aspirate are consistent with aplastic anemia.

Which of the following statements regarding aplastic anemia is false?

❑ A. **Aplasia can be a prodrome to hairy-cell leukemia, acute lymphoblastic leukemia, or acute myeloblastic leukemia**

❑ B. **Viral infections remain one of the major causes of aplastic anemia**

❑ C. **Ionizing irradiation and chemotherapeutic drugs that can be used to treat malignant or immunologic disorders can cause aplastic anemia**

❑ D. **Approximately 20% of patients with hepatitis can experience aplastic anemia 2 to 3 weeks after they experience a typical case of acute hepatitis**

Key Concept/Objective: To understand the etiologies of aplastic anemia

Pancytopenia (i.e., anemia, neutropenia, and thrombocytopenia) and a finding of aplastic marrow on biopsy establish a working diagnosis of aplastic anemia. Aplastic anemia has a number of causes, although in many cases the exact cause cannot be determined. Ionizing irradiation and chemotherapeutic drugs used in the management of malignant and immunologic disorders have the capacity to destroy hematopoietic stem cells. With careful dosing and scheduling, recovery is expected. Certain drugs, such as chloramphenicol, produce marrow aplasia that is not dose dependent. Gold therapy and the inhalation of organic solvent vapors (e.g., benzene or glue) can also cause fatal marrow failure. In 2% to 10% of hepatitis patients, severe aplasia occurs 2 to 3 months after a seemingly typical case of acute disease. Often, the hepatitis has no obvious cause, and tests for hepatitis A, B, and C are negative. Aplasia can also be part of a prodrome to hairy-cell leukemia, acute lymphoblastic leukemia, or, in rare cases, acute myeloid leukemia, or it can develop in the course of myelodysplasia. Parvovirus infection is the cause of the transient aplastic crises that occur in patients who have severe hemolytic disorders. The marrow in patients with such disorders must compensate for the peripheral hemolysis by increasing its production up to sevenfold. Although parvovirus can affect all precursor cells, the red cell precursors are the most profoundly affected. Anemia causes fatigue and shortness of breath; thrombocytopenia causes petechiae, oral blood blisters, gingival bleeding, and hematuria, depending on the level of the platelet count. By far the major problem is the recurrent bacterial infections caused by the profound neutropenia. The diagnosis of aplastic anemia requires a marrow aspirate and biopsy, as well as a thorough history of drug exposures, infections, and especially symptoms suggesting viral illnesses and serologic test results for hepatitis, infectious mononucleosis, HIV, and parvovirus. Measurement of red cell CD59 is helpful in the diagnosis of paroxysmal nocturnal hemoglobinuria. *(Answer: D—Approximately 20% of patients with hepatitis can experience aplastic anemia 2 to 3 weeks after they experience a typical case of acute hepatitis)*

10. A 43-year-old white man presents to your clinic complaining of fatigue and paresthesias. He is a vegetarian and does not take a multivitamin. His examination reveals pallor, an absence of hepatosplenomegaly, normal muscle strength throughout, and loss of position sensation and vibratory sensation distally. A CBC reveals anemia, with a mean corpuscular volume (MCV) of 106 fl. His WBC, platelet count, and serum chemistries are normal. He has had no toxic exposures and is taking no medications.

Which of the following statements about megaloblastic anemia is false?

- ❑ A. **Absorption of cobalamin in the small intestine is dependent on proteins produced in the mouth and stomach**
- ❑ B. **Megaloblastic erythropoiesis is characterized by defective DNA synthesis and arrest at the G2 phase, with impaired maturation and a buildup of cells that do not synthesize DNA and that contain anomalous DNA**
- ❑ C. **In most patients with severe cobalamin deficiency, the neurologic examination is normal**
- ❑ D. **Cobalamin deficiency is treated with parenteral cobalamin therapy**

Key Concept/Objective: To understand the etiology, diagnosis, and treatment of pernicious anemia

Megaloblastic erythropoiesis is characterized by defective DNA synthesis and arrest at the G2 phase, with impaired maturation and a buildup of cells that do not synthesize DNA and that contain anomalous DNA. This condition leads to asynchronous maturation between the nucleus and cytoplasm. RNA production and protein synthesis continue; thus, larger cells, or megaloblasts, are produced. In addition to macrocytic and megaloblastic anemia, the patient with cobalamin deficiency may have weakness, lethargy, or dementia, as well as atrophy of the lingual papillae and glossitis. Neuropathy is the presenting feature in about 12% of patients with cobalamin (vitamin B_{12}) deficiency without concomitant anemia. Patients with severe cobalamin deficiency initially complain of paresthesia. The sense of touch and temperature sensitivity may be minimally impaired. Memory impairment and depression may be prominent. The disease may progress, involving the dorsal columns, causing ataxia and weakness. The physical examination reveals a broad-based gait, the Romberg sign, slowed reflexes, and a loss of sense of position and feeling of

vibration (especially when tested with a 256 Hz tuning fork). *(Answer: C—In most patients with severe cobalamin deficiency, the neurologic examination is normal)*

11. A 53-year-old woman is referred to your office by her gynecologist for management of anemia. She experienced menopause at 48 years of age and has had no further vaginal bleeding. Two years ago, her hematocrit was 36%. During her last office visit, her hematocrit was 29%, and her MCV was 107 fl. The patient is dependent on alcohol. She admits to drinking a pint of wine daily, and she engages in occasional binge drinking on weekends. She denies any other sources of blood loss or icterus. She is apparently only mildly symptomatic with some fatigue.

Which of the following statements regarding megaloblastic anemia caused by folic acid deficiency is false?

- ❑ A. **Serum folic acid levels more accurately reflect tissue stores than do red blood cell folic acid levels**
- ❑ B. **Folic acid deficiency can be differentiated from cobalamin deficiency by measuring methylmalonic acid and homocysteine levels; both are elevated in cobalamin deficiency, but only homocysteine is elevated in folic acid deficiency**
- ❑ C. **Megaloblastic anemia caused by folic acid deficiency can be masked by concurrent iron deficiency anemia, but hypersegmented polymorphonuclear cells (PMNs) should still be present on the peripheral smear**
- ❑ D. **Folinic acid can be used to treat patients with megaloblastosis and bone marrow suppression associated with the use of methotrexate**

Key Concept/Objective: To understand the diagnosis and treatment of megaloblastic anemia caused by folic acid deficiency

Patients with megaloblastic anemia who do not have glossitis, a family history of pernicious anemia, or the neurologic features described for cobalamin deficiency may have folic acid deficiency. Tests to determine folic acid deficiency vary in their accuracy. Serum folic acid levels are less reliable than red blood cell folic acid levels. A serum folic acid level of less than 2 ng/ml is consistent with folic acid deficiency, as is a red blood cell folic acid level of less than 150 ng/ml. Because the combination of folic acid and iron deficiency is common, full expression of megaloblastosis is often blocked, and the patient will have a dimorphic anemia rather than the easily identifiable macro-ovalocytosis. Hypersegmentation of PMNs persists. The serum folic acid level decreases within 2 weeks after dietary folic acid ingestion completely ceases. Therefore, many hospitalized patients have low serum folic acid levels without real tissue folic acid deprivation. In evaluating patients for folic acid deficiency, values for the levels of serum folic acid, serum cobalamin, and red blood cell folic acid must be obtained. The red blood cell folic acid level reflects tissue stores. When it is difficult but necessary to distinguish the megaloblastosis of cobalamin deficiency from that of folic acid deficiency, measurements of the serum methylmalonic acid and homocysteine levels are helpful. *(Answer: A—Serum folic acid levels more accurately reflect tissue stores than do red blood cell folic acid levels)*

12. A 47-year-old man with a 10-year history of type 2 diabetes presents for a routine physical examination. His diabetes is poorly controlled, and there is evidence of retinopathy and neuropathy. He is currently receiving maximum doses of oral glipizide and metformin. His ROS is negative for cardiorespiratory symptoms. His examination reveals a blood pressure of 148/92 mm Hg and retinal changes consistent with diabetic background retinopathy. He also has decreased sensation in his feet, as evidenced by his results on monofilament neuropathy testing. Laboratory studies reveal a hemoglobin A_{1C} level of 10.6%, a microalbumin excretion rate of 300 µg/min, and a serum creatinine level of 1.4 mg/dl. His CBC reveals normal levels of leukocytes and platelets and a hemoglobin level of 9.1 g/dl, with a mean cell volume of 85. Three follow-up examinations for the presence of fecal occult blood were negative. On repeat testing, the hemoglobin level is 9.4 g/dl; the serum iron level is 35 µg/dl; total iron-binding capacity is 230; and the ferritin level is 170 ng/L.

Which of the following is the most likely cause of this patient's anemia?

- ❑ **A. Bone marrow suppression**
- ❑ **B. Sequestration of iron in the reticuloendothelial system**
- ❑ **C. Lack of erythropoietin**
- ❑ **D. Inhibition of folate metabolism**
- ❑ **E. A hemolytic process**

Key Concept/Objective: To understand the mechanism by which chronic disease can cause anemia

Anemia of chronic disease is generally associated with conditions that release cytokines (tumor necrosis factor–α, interleukin-1, and other inflammatory cytokines). These cytokines decrease erythropoietin production, decrease the levels of iron released from the reticuloendothelial system, and increase serum ferritin levels. Administration of erythropoietin in pharmacologic doses corrects the anemia of chronic disease by compensating for the decreased production of erythropoietin. *(Answer: B—Sequestration of iron in the reticuloendothelial system)*

13. A 75-year-old man is brought to the clinic for evaluation of forgetfulness that has developed slowly over the past 6 months. His wife indicates that he has occasionally become lost while out shopping and several times a day demonstrates forgetfulness in the course of attempting to complete a task. He has a history of controlled hypertension and is receiving lisinopril, 10 mg daily. He denies using alcohol, and review of systems is otherwise negative. His examination reveals a well-groomed man who appears to be as old as his stated age. His vital signs are normal, as is the rest of his examination. His Folstein Mini-Mental State Examination score is 24/30, with deficits noted in short-term memory. Thyroid-stimulating hormone test results and serum chemistries are normal. His CBC reveals a hemoglobin of 11.8 g/dl, with normal leukocyte and platelet counts. The differential reveals several granulocytes with 5 nuclear segments.

What should be the next step in the treatment of this patient?

- ❑ **A. Order T_4 and T_3 resin uptake tests**
- ❑ **B. Start donepezil, 10 mg daily**
- ❑ **C. Refer for a neuropsychiatric evaluation**
- ❑ **D. Obtain an MRI of the brain**
- ❑ **E. Determine the vitamin B_{12} serum level**

Key Concept/Objective: To understand that neuropsychiatric symptoms may occur in patients with vitamin B_{12} deficiency before many of the typical hematologic changes of vitamin B_{12} deficiency occur

Memory impairment in the absence of hematologic changes can be a presenting symptom of vitamin B_{12} deficiency. Studies have shown that in 20% to 30% of patients who are deficient in vitamin B_{12}, anemia and macrocytosis are absent. A diagnosis of vitamin B_{12} deficiency should be entertained in patients with neurologic disturbances in the absence of anemia and macrocytosis. The indications for vitamin B_{12} deficiency have broadened to include nonspecific forms of cerebral dysfunction. The finding of hypersegmented neutrophils remains a sensitive indicator of vitamin B_{12} deficiency. *(Answer: E—Determine the vitamin B_{12} serum level)*

14. A 27-year-old African-American man presents to the hospital with increased fatigue, which he has been experiencing for the past several months. He has been treated for sickle cell anemia in the past and has received many blood transfusions. He has been hospitalized multiple times in the past for apparent crises. He currently has no fever, and his general ROS is negative. On physical examination, his vital signs are normal. His cardiothoracic examination is normal, as is his extremity examination. His abdominal examination reveals diffuse tenderness without guarding or organomegaly. Laboratory studies reveal a hemoglobin level of 8.0 g/dl, with a mean cell volume of 90 and a reticulocyte count of 0.8%. Hemoglobin electrophoresis reveals 96% hemoglobin A and 4% hemoglobin A_2. Serum chemistries reveal an LDH level of 600.

What should be the next step in the treatment of this patient?

❑ A. CT scan of the abdomen

❑ B. Bone marrow aspiration and biopsy

❑ C. Direct Coombs test

❑ D. Serum folate level test

❑ E. Administration of 2 units of packed RBCs

Key Concept/Objective: To understand the importance of a bone marrow examination in evaluating anemia of unclear etiology

A bone marrow examination is necessary to identify several of the different types of anemia associated with impaired production of RBCs. This patient presents with a history of sickle cell disease, but his current clinical symptoms are not consistent with either a hemolytic crisis (low reticulocyte count) or a pain crisis. An aplastic crisis should be entertained but is not likely, given his normal WBC and platelet counts. Although parvovirus B19 infection should be considered because it can produce pure red cell aplasia in patients with sickle cell anemia, the normal results on hemoglobin electrophoresis rule out sickle cell disease in this patient. Therefore, the specific diagnosis of his anemia is in doubt. *(Answer: B—Bone marrow aspiration and biopsy)*

15. A previously healthy 66-year-old man presents with a 1-month history of increasing fatigue and easy bruising. He is on no medications and consumes no alcohol. He has been retired for the past 2 years from an accounting job. His examination reveals mild pallor of the palpebral conjunctiva, brisk carotid upstrokes, and a grade 2/6 systolic ejection murmur at the left sternal border, without radiation. His abdominal examination is normal. Examination of his extremities reveals many ecchymoses in various stages of healing and a few nonpalpable petechaie on his lower extremities. A CBC reveals a WBC count of 2.4, with 20% PMNs; hemoglobin of 9.7 g/dl; a reticulocyte count of 0.5%; and a platelet count of 20,000. Bone marrow aspiration and biopsy reveal 25% normal cellularity. A diagnosis of aplastic anemia is made.

Which of the following statements is true regarding this patient's prognosis?

❑ A. Prognosis is relatively good, with a 70% rate of spontaneous remission within 1 year

❑ B. Prognosis is poor, with a 70% mortality within 1 year

❑ C. A complete cure can be expected with immunosuppressive treatment

❑ D. Allogeneic bone marrow transplantation is associated with an 80% 5-year survival rate

Key Concept/Objective: To understand the poor prognosis for patients with severe aplastic anemia

Severe aplastic anemia is defined by a bone marrow cellularity of less than 25% normal or a cellularity of less than 50% normal with fewer than 30% hematopoeitic cells and low peripheral cell lines. The likelihood of spontaneous remission is very low, and mortality within 1 year is 70%. For mild cases, supportive treatment with blood product replacement and hematopoietic growth factor treatment is indicated; in severe cases, either immunosuppresive treatment—which would not be curative—or bone marrow transplantation may be indicated. The 5-year survival rate after bone marrow transplantation is excellent in patients younger than 49 years (86%) but drops to 54% in patients older than 60 years. *(Answer: B—Prognosis is poor, with a 70% mortality within 1 year)*

16. A 30-year-old woman presents for evaluation. Over the past month, she has been experiencing increasing dyspnea with exertion. She has otherwise been in good health and has no known cardiorespiratory problems. She has been consuming three or four alcoholic drinks an evening for the past 6 years. She is on no medications. In giving her family history, she reports having a sibling with anemia. Her examination reveals normal vital signs and mild pallor in the conjunctiva. Her cardiorespiratory examination is normal. A CBC reveals a WBC count of 3.5×10^3, a platelet count of 144,000, and a hemoglobin level of 8.4 g/dl, with a mean cell volume of 84 and a reticulocyte count of 0.8%.

What would be the most likely finding on this bone marrow examination?

❑ A. **Ringed sideroblasts and ineffective erythropoiesis**

❑ B. **Hypercellularity of RBC precursors**

❑ C. **Hypocellularity of the marrow blood-forming elements**

❑ D. **Normal cellularity**

❑ E. **Marrow fibrosis**

Key Concept/Objective: To understand the acquired form of sideroblastic anemia

Sideroblastic anemias are a heterogeneous group of disorders characterized by anemia and the presence of ringed sideroblasts in the marrow. There are hereditary forms and acquired forms, which are further subdivided into benign and malignant variants. Abnormalities of heme synthesis are the usual causes. Iron enters the RBC precursor but cannot be incorporated and accumulates to form ringed sideroblasts. The diagnosis is established by the presence of reticulcytopenia and ringed sideroblasts in the bone marrow. Cytogenetic studies of the bone marrow may reveal changes seen in myelodysplastic syndromes. Alcohol abuse can cause a reversible form of sideroblastic anemia, and stopping alcohol is an important aspect of patient care. *(Answer: A—Ringed sideroblasts and ineffective erythropoiesis)*

For more information, see Schrier SL: 5 Hematology: III Anemia: Production Defects. ACP Medicine Online (www.acpmedicine.com). Dale DC, Federman DD, Eds. WebMD Inc., New York, June 2004

Hemoglobinopathies and Hemolytic Anemia

17. A 31-year-old woman presents to you for follow-up after a visit to the emergency department 1 week ago. The patient went to the emergency department because of severe right upper quadrant pain of 2 days' duration. An abdominal CT was normal—there was no evidence of biliary disease, nephrolithiasis, or pelvic disease. The patient was sent home that day with minimal pain control. She now states that her abdominal pain has persisted and is unimproved. She also states that she now has bloody urine in the morning and that she has developed severe lower extremity swelling and abdominal distention. Physical examination is significant for marked ascites, tender hepatomegaly, and 3+ bilateral lower extremity pitting edema. You order magnetic resonance imaging of the abdomen, which reveals the presence of a hepatic vein thrombosis.

Which of the following statements regarding paroxysmal nocturnal hemoglobinuria (PNH) is true?

❑ A. **PNH is the result of a mutation that causes a deficiency of a membrane-anchoring protein, which in turn results in an inability to properly modulate complement attack**

❑ B. **PNH causes anemia but has no effect on other cell lines**

❑ C. **PNH can cause thromboses in unusual sites, such as in the mesenteric or hepatic vein; however, lower extremity thromboses and associated pulmonary emboli are not seen**

❑ D. **The diagnosis of PNH is a diagnosis of exclusion because there are no specific tests available for PNH**

Key Concept/Objective: To know the clinical characteristics of PNH

The mutation associated with PNH results in a deficiency of the membrane-anchoring protein phosphatidylinositol glycan class A. Normal human erythrocytes, and probably platelets and neutrophils, modulate complement attack by at least three glycosylphosphatidylinositol (GPI) membrane-bound proteins: DAF (CD55), C8-binding protein (C8BP), and MIRL (CD59). Because the defective synthesis of GPI affects all hematopoietic cells, patients with PNH may have variable degrees of anemia, neutropenia, or thrombocytopenia, or they may have complete bone marrow failure. Recurrent venous occlusions lead to pulmonary embolism and hepatic and mesenteric vein thrombosis, possibly result-

ing from the release of procoagulant microparticles derived from platelets. Diagnosis is made by specific tests based on fluorescence-activated cell sorter analysis using antibodies that quantitatively assess DAF (CD55) and particularly MIRL (CD59) on the erythrocyte or on the leukocyte surface. *(Answer: A—PNH is the result of a mutation that causes a deficiency of a membrane-anchoring protein, which in turn results in an inability to properly modulate complement attack)*

18. A 48-year-old black man presents to the emergency department for evaluation of severe fatigue. He has been HIV positive for several years. He reports that his last known CD4+ T cell count was "around 100." The patient is receiving drugs for prophylaxis against *Pneumocystis carinii* pneumonia (PCP). He was in his usual state of moderate health until 2 days ago. His only complaints are severe fatigue and some dyspnea on exertion. He denies having fever, chills, cough, abdominal pain, or dysuria. He states that his doctor recently changed his "PCP pill" because of a persistent rash. A chest x-ray is within normal limits. Laboratory values are remarkable for a hematocrit of 22% and a urinalysis that shows 4+ blood and 0–2 RBCs.

Which of the following statements regarding glucose-6-phosphate dehydrogenase (G6PD) deficiency is true?

- ❑ A. **G6PD is an enzyme that catalyzes the conversion of adenosine diphosphate (ADP) to adenosine triphosphate (ATP), a powerful reducing agent**
- ❑ B. **G6PD deficiency is very rare in the United States**
- ❑ C. **G6PD deficiency occurs with equal frequency in males and females**
- ❑ D. **Potential users of dapsone should be screened for G6PD deficiency**

Key Concept/Objective: To understand the function of G6PD and the epidemiology of G6PD deficiency

G6PD is the first enzyme in the pentose phosphate pathway, or hexose monophosphate shunt. It catalyzes the conversion of the oxidized form of nicotinamide-adenine dinucleotide phosphate (NADP$^+$) to the reduced form (NADPH), which is a powerful reducing agent. NADPH is a cofactor for glutathione reductase and thus plays a role in protecting the cell against oxidative attack. G6PD deficiency is one of the most common disorders in the world; approximately 10% of male blacks in the United States are affected. The gene for G6PD is on the X chromosome at band q28; males carry only one gene for this enzyme, so those males that are affected by the disorder are hemizygous. Females are affected much less frequently because they would have to carry two defective G6PD genes to show clinical disease of the same severity as that in males. Dapsone, which is capable of inducing oxidant-type hemolysis, has increasingly come into use as prophylaxis for PCP in patients infected with HIV. Therefore, it is important to screen potential users of dapsone for G6PD deficiency with the standard enzymatic tests. *(Answer: D—Potential users of dapsone should be screened for G6PD deficiency)*

19. A 25-year-old black man comes for a routine office visit. You have followed the patient for many years for his sickle cell disease. The patient takes very good care of himself and has only required hospital admission four times in the past 5 years. Two of these admissions occurred in the past 6 months. You feel that the patient's clinical course is worsening. He has recently required the addition of narcotics to his home regimen of nonsteroidal anti-inflammatory drug therapy. The patient states that he now has moderately severe pain in long bones two to three times monthly. He has also developed worsening left hip pain over the past month.

Which of the following statements regarding sickle cell disease is true?

- ❑ A. **In patients with homozygous sickle cell disease, roughly 50% of total hemoglobin is hemoglobin S**
- ❑ B. **Risk factors that predispose to painful crises include a hemoglobin level greater than 8.5 g/dl, pregnancy, cold weather, and a high reticulocyte count**

- ❑ C. **The most definitive test for the diagnosis of sickle cell anemia is the sodium metabisulfite test**
- ❑ D. **Hydroxyurea has never been shown to be of benefit in the therapy of sickle cell disease**

Key Concept/Objective: To know the clinical features of sickle cell disease

Sickle cell disease develops in persons who are homozygous for the sickle gene (*HbSS*), in whom 70% to 98% of hemoglobin is of the S type. About 0.2% of African Americans have sickle cell anemia. Risk factors that predispose to painful crises include a hemoglobin level greater than 8.5 g/dl, pregnancy, cold weather, and a high reticulocyte count. Conversely, the low hematocrit in sickle cell anemia reduces blood viscosity and is protective. The most definitive tests for sickle cell anemia are hemoglobin electrophoresis or high-performance liquid chromatography, which indicate the relative percentages of HbS and HbF. Hydroxyurea produces an increase in F reticulocyte and HbF levels. In a phase III trial, patients treated with hydroxyurea (starting dosage, 15 mg/kg/day) had fewer painful crises, fewer admissions for crisis, and fewer episodes of acute chest syndrome and required fewer transfusions than patients given a placebo. There was no effect on stroke; however, after 8 years of follow-up, mortality was reduced by 40%. *(Answer: B—Risk factors that predispose to painful crises include a hemoglobin level greater than 8.5 g/dl, pregnancy, cold weather, and a high reticulocyte count)*

20. A 47-year-old woman presents to your office with a complaint of severe fatigue, weakness, and dyspnea on exertion. She has had these symptoms for 2 days. The patient denies having fever, chills, weight changes, or dysuria. Her medical history is significant for pernicious anemia and hypothyroidism. Results of thyroid studies were within normal limits 1 week ago. Her physical examination is positive for mild icterus and hepatosplenomegaly. CBC is normal, with the exception of a hematocrit of 21%. Her hematocrit was 36% 3 months ago. Liver function tests show the total bilirubin level to be 4.6 mg/dl and the indirect bilirubin level to be 4.2 mg/dl. Other results are within normal limits. A direct Coombs test is positive.

Which of the following statements regarding autoimmune hemolytic anemia is true?

- ❑ A. **Autoimmune hemolytic anemia typically results in intravascular hemolysis**
- ❑ B. **Autoimmune hemolytic anemia may be idiopathic or secondary to disorders such as systemic lupus erythematosus, chronic lymphocytic leukemia (CLL), HIV infection, or hepatitis C infection**
- ❑ C. **Most patients with autoimmune hemolytic anemia are cured with steroid therapy**
- ❑ D. **Splenectomy is curative for those patients who do not respond to simple steroid therapy**

Key Concept/Objective: To understand the clinical features and chronic nature of autoimmune hemolytic anemia

Intravascular hemolysis in autoimmune hemolytic anemia is rare and indicates that an extremely rapid rate of erythrocyte destruction is occurring or that the extravascular removal mechanisms have been overwhelmed. Erythrocytes sensitized to IgG alone are usually removed in the spleen, whereas RBCs sensitized to IgG plus complement or to complement alone are generally destroyed in the liver, because hepatic Kupffer cells carry receptors specific for complement component C3b. Both an idiopathic variety of autoimmune hemolytic anemia and a variety that occurs secondary to other disorders have been described. Such primary disorders include systemic lupus erythematosus, non-Hodgkin lymphoma (especially chronic lymphocytic leukemia), Hodgkin disease, cancer, myeloma, dermoid cyst, HIV infection, angioimmunoblastic lymphadenopathy with dysproteinemia, hepatitis C infection, and chronic ulcerative colitis. Approximately 20% of patients remain well indefinitely after steroid therapy, but the majority suffer from a chronic, treacherous disease that can produce sudden relapses with abrupt anemia. If the cortico-

steroid dose required for long-term therapy produces significant morbidity, one can proceed empirically either to splenectomy or to the use of immunosuppressive agents. Splenectomy rarely results in extended remission but is valuable as a prednisone-sparing measure. *(Answer: B—Autoimmune hemolytic anemia may be idiopathic or secondary to disorders such as systemic lupus erythematosus, chronic lymphocytic leukemia [CLL], HIV infection, or hepatitis C infection)*

21. A 19-year-old African-American man comes to establish primary care. He knows that both of his parents are carriers of sickle cell anemia. He also knows that one of the parents has a second hemoglobin defect. He has never experienced pain crises.

Which of the following compound heterozygote states, if present, would make the patient susceptible to symptoms such as pain crises and avascular necrosis?

- ❑ A. **HbS/HbC**
- ❑ B. **HbS/HbE**
- ❑ C. **HbS/α-thalassemia**
- ❑ D. **HbS/α^+-thalassemia**
- ❑ E. **HbS/α^0-thalassemia**

Key Concept/Objective: To understand the mechanisms of sickling and the protective role of globin chains

Certain physiologic stresses make deoxygenated HbS more likely to polymerize and precipitate, forming a gel-like substance. Known stressors are a low pH, an increase in the level of intracorpuscular hemoglobin (MCHC), a high concentration of HbS, a low concentration of HbF, and slow transit time. Patients with α^+-thalassemia traits produce enough α^A-globin chains to maintain an HbA concentration greater than 25%, thus decreasing the amount of HbS. Patients with α-thalassemia tend to have lower levels of MCHC and, thus, decreased concentrations of HbS. HbE is an unstable hemoglobin in which lysine is substituted for glutamic acid in position 26 of the α-globin chain. Heterozygous patients are asymptomatic. Homozygous patients present with a clinical picture similar to that of patients with α^+-thalassemia. Similarly, patients with HbS/HbE have a clinical picture similar to that of patients with HbS/α^+-thalassemia. In patients with HbS/HbC, 50% of the hemoglobin is HbS. Although HbS/HbC disease is less severe than HbSS disease, patients with HbS/HbC frequently tend to have avascular necrosis of the femoral head. Patients with α^0-thalassemia have a very low concentration of HbA; in these patients, HbS constitutes more than 50% of the intracorpuscular hemoglobin. In extreme cases, the clinical picture of α^0-thalassemia is identical to that of HbSS. As HbS decreases, the clinical picture comes to resemble that of patients with HbS/HbC disease. *(Answer: E—HbS/α^0-thalassemia)*

22. A 38-year-old African-American man is admitted to the hospital with congestive heart failure (CHF) of new onset. He is noted to have a blood pressure of 210/140 mm Hg. Therapy with intravenous furosemide, intravenous nitroglycerin, and oral angiotensin-converting enzymes controls his symptoms and blood pressure over the next 48 hours. On the third day, a 10% drop of his hematocrit is noted. Laboratory data show the following: Hb, 11 g/dl (admission Hb, 14.5 g/dl); Hct, 35% (admission Hct, 45%); total bilirubin, 3.5 mg/dl (indirect, 2.8 mg/dl); LDH, 550 mg/dl; haptoglobin level, undetectable.

Which of the following tests is most likely to establish the diagnosis?

- ❑ A. **A test for immune hemolysis (i.e., direct Coombs test, indirect Coombs test, or both)**
- ❑ B. **A test for membrane fragility (i.e., sucrose lysis test)**
- ❑ C. **A test for red cell enzyme deficiency (e.g., pyruvate kinase assay)**
- ❑ D. **Hemoglobin electrophoresis**

Key Concept/Objective: To understand hemolysis secondary to use of oxidating agents (furosemide and nitroglycerin) and the timing of the G6PD assay

This patient experienced an episode of acute hemolysis after being hospitalized. It is likely that this is a case of drug-induced hemolysis. There are several mechanisms by which drugs can induce hemolysis; two well-recognized mechanisms are immunologic mediation (e.g., hemolysis caused by penicillin and methyldopa) and an increase in oxidative stress on red cells. Oxidative stress can occur as a result of hemoglobins becoming unstable or through a decrease in reduction capacity (as would result from G6PD deficiency). Penicillins and cephalosporins produce immune hemolysis by acting as a hapten in the red cell membrane. The protein/drug complex elicits an immune response. An IgG antibody is generated that acts against the drug-red cell complex. In such patients, the direct Coombs test is positive, but the indirect Coombs test is negative. Other drugs induce hemolysis by altering a membrane antigen. IgG autoantibodies that cross-react with the native antigen are produced. The direct Coombs test is also positive in this form of drug reaction. Methyldopa is the classic example of this form of interaction, although other drugs such as procainamide and diclofenac have been clearly implicated. Diclofenac can produce massive hemolysis with concomitant disseminated intravascular coagulation and shock. Sucrose lysis is still used to screen for membrane fragility. The most common disorder associated with this abnormality is paroxysmal nocturnal hemoglobinuria (PNH). The lack of associated cytopenias, the acuteness of the onset of symptoms, and the lack of history of venous thrombosis (especially thrombosis at unusual sites such as the inferior vena cava or the portal mesenteric system or thrombosis that produces Budd-Chiari syndrome) makes PNH an unlikely cause of this patient's symptoms. Some unstable hemoglobins, such as HbE, are susceptible to hemolysis from oxidative stress. This patient was exposed to both furosemide (a drug with a sulfa moiety) and nitroglycerin. This hemoglobinopathy is diagnosed by hemoglobin electrophoresis. However, this disease is seen almost exclusively in individuals from Southeast Asia (Cambodia, Thailand, and Vietnam). The most likely diagnosis in this case is G6PD deficiency. This enzymopathy affects 10% of the world population. It is commonly seen in African Americans. The red cell becomes hemolyzed when exposed to an oxidative stress. Older red cells are more susceptible to hemolysis because levels of G6PD decrease as red cells age. The results of the G6PD assay should be interpreted carefully. On occasion, the results of the G6PD assay will be normal in patients with G6PD deficiency; this occurs when the assay detects G6PD in very young cells (reticulocytes) that are being released as a result of the brisk hemolysis. *(Answer: D—Hemoglobin electrophoresis)*

23. A 17-year-old African-American woman is referred to you from the blood bank for evaluation of microcytic anemia detected at the time of screening for blood donation. She is unaware of this problem. She has no symptoms of fatigue or dyspnea. Her menstrual period appears to be normal in frequency and volume of blood loss. There is no history of GI bleeding. She has not been pregnant before. Her physical examination is unremarkable. Her laboratory values are as follows: Hb, 10.5 g/dl; Hct, 32%; MCV, 61; WBC, 7,500 with normal differential; platelet count, 235,000; peripheral smear shows hypochromia and microcytosis; red cell count, 5 million cells/mm^3; Hb electrophoresis: HbA, 97%; HbA_2, 2%; HbF, < 1%.

What is the most likely diagnosis for this patient?

- ❑ **A. Iron deficiency anemia**
- ❑ **B. α-Thalassemia minor**
- ❑ **C. Heterozygous α-thalassemia-1**
- ❑ **D. Hemoglobin H disease**
- ❑ **E. Homozygous α-thalassemia-2**

Key Concept/Objective: To understand the interpretation of the red cell count in patients with anemia, the results of hemoglobin electrophoresis in patients with thalassemia, and differences in genotype among the thalassemias

Microcytic and hypochromic anemia is common in clinical practice. The most likely cause is iron deficiency anemia, especially in women of childbearing age. In iron deficiency anemia, the production of red cells is deficient. Thus, the red cell count tends to be low when anemia is present. This patient has a normal red cell count and mild to moderate anemia. This combination should suggest a problem in red cell production. Both α- and β-tha-

lassemia can present as an asymptomatic microcytic/hypochromic anemia. In β-thalassemia, there is a decrease in production of β-globin chains. The α-globin chains are produced in normal amounts and combine with other globin chains. As such, HbA_2 production is increased. This change in hemoglobin patterns enables the diagnosis of β-thalassemia to be made through use of hemoglobin electrophoresis. With α-thalassemias, the hemoglobin electrophoresis pattern is normal. This globin chain is under control of two different loci with a total of four alleles. The absence of both the α-globin gene and the β-globin gene causes hemoglobin Barts syndrome during fetal life. This hemoglobinopathy results in children being born with hydrops fetalis. When three alleles are missing, the patient develops HbH disease. This disease is seen exclusively in patients of Mediterranean origin and is characterized clinically by chronic hemolysis and the presence of splenomegaly. All three features are absent in this patient. Of the two remaining possibilities, we can conclude that the patient has α-thalassemia-2 because of the ethnic origin. This disease is characterized by homozygous inheritance (--α/-- α) and is seen exclusively in African Americans. The heterozygous patient of this genotype (--α/α α) is the silent carrier. On the other hand, patients with α-thalassemia-1 have lost two α-chain genes in one chromosome (-- --/α α). This genotype is seen almost exclusively in Asians. *(Answer: E—Homozygous α-thalassemia-2)*

For more information, see Schrier SL: 5 Hematology: IV Hemoglobinopathies and Hemolytic Anemias. ACP Medicine Online (www.acpmedicine.com). Dale DC, Federman DD, Eds. WebMD Inc., New York, April 2004

The Polycythemias

24. A 60-year-old man presents with complaints of headache, light-headedness, blurry vision, and fatigue; these symptoms have been increasing over the past month. He reports that he has felt weak and has not had much energy. He also reports generalized itching, which usually occurs after he takes a hot shower. Physical examination reveals facial plethora. His spleen is palpable 2 cm below the left costophrenic angle. Laboratory results reveal the following: Hb, 18; Hct, 61; platelets, 500,000; leukocytes, 17,000.

Which of the following is the most appropriate diagnosis for this patient?

- ❑ A. Gaisböck syndrome (relative polycythemia)
- ❑ B. Pickwickian syndrome
- ❑ C. Polycythemia vera
- ❑ D. Acute myeloid leukemia
- ❑ E. Chronic myeloid leukemia

Key Concept/Objective: To understand the clinical characteristics of polycythemia vera and primary polycythemia and differentiate these characteristics from those of other types of polycythemia

Polycythemia vera is an acquired myeloproliferative disorder that is characterized by overproduction of all three hematopoietic cell lines with predominant elevation in red cell counts. This overproduction is independent of erythropoietin. Facial plethora is characteristic of all patients with polycythemia vera. Polycythemia vera is slightly more common in men than in women and is most frequently diagnosed in persons between 60 and 75 years of age. Patients commonly complain of pruritus, especially after a hot bath. Splenomegaly is also common. Gaisböck syndrome, also known as relative polycythemia, is usually found in men from 45 to 55 years of age; they are most often obese, hypertensive men who may also be heavy smokers. Pickwickian syndrome, or obesity-hypoventilation syndrome, is characterized by obesity with hypoxemia and hypercapnia; some patients experience nocturnal obstructive sleep apnea and daytime hypersomnolence. Although polycythemia vera and chronic myeloid leukemia are both classified as myeloproliferative disorders, the dominant features of chronic myeloid leukemia are dramatic leukocytosis, the presence of the Philadelphia chromosome, and certain evolution to acute myeloid leukemia. *(Answer: C—Polycythemia vera)*

25. A 62-year-old woman presents with a history of intermittent headache and vertigo. She finds it hard to concentrate. On questioning, she also complains of tinnitus. She has lost 10 lb over the past 6 months and frequently feels tired. She also complains of excessive sweating. On physical examination, she has facial plethora, her temperature is normal, her blood pressure is 130/80 mm Hg, and her heart rate is 90 beats/min. There is a soft systolic murmur at the lower sternal border, the lungs are clear on auscultation, and the spleen can be palpated 6 cm below the left costal margin. Laboratory evaluation reveals the following: Hct, 60%; WBC, 15,000/mm^3; platelets, 400,000/mm^3; oxygen saturation, 98%.

What is the most appropriate initial treatment for this patient?

- ❑ **A. Allogeneic stem cell transplantation**
- ❑ **B. Phlebotomy**
- ❑ **C. Hydroxyurea**
- ❑ **D. Anagrelide**

Key Concept/Objective: To recognize phlebotomy as a frequently used treatment for polycythemia

This patient has signs and symptoms characteristic of polycythemia vera; initial treatment might include phlebotomy, although no consensus has emerged about the best treatment approach. If phlebotomy is chosen as a treatment option, it should be continued at the rate of once or twice a week until the target hematocrit value of less than 45% is achieved. The patient must be instructed not to take multivitamins that contain iron. Modest iron deficiency is a desirable consequence of phlebotomy, as it helps maintain the hematocrit in the desired range. Most patients who are initially treated with phlebotomy alone will eventually require myelosuppressive therapy. Hydroxyurea is generally used for patients older than 70 years or for those who have previously had a thrombotic event or who require high-maintenance phlebotomy. Anagrelide is very expensive and has a number of side effects; it is useful in patients with polycythemia vera who require a supplemental agent for optimal control of thrombocytosis. Allogeneic stem cell transplantation is a highly investigational approach; only a few patients with polycythemia vera have undergone myeloablative therapy and allogeneic bone marrow transplantion. *(Answer: B—Phlebotomy)*

26. A 75-year-old man presents complaining of headache and memory difficulties. He has lost 10 lb since his last office visit 6 months ago. He smoked cigarettes for 40 years but was successful in quitting 10 years ago. He has a history of deep vein thrombosis in his left leg, which was successfully treated by medication. His blood pressure is 135/85 mm Hg, and his temperature is 101° F (38.3° C). He complains of feeling flushed and of sweating. His laboratory values are as follows: Hct, 60%; WBC, 15,000/mm^3; platelets, 400,000/mm^3; serum erythropoietin, 0.5 U/L.

What is the most appropriate treatment for this patient?

- ❑ **A. Phlebotomy**
- ❑ **B. Phlebotomy and hydroxyurea**
- ❑ **C. Hydroxyurea**
- ❑ **D. Anagrelide**

Key Concept/Objective: To understand that patients with polycythemia vera who are older than 70 years should be treated with a myelosuppressive agent such as hydroxyurea in combination with phlebotomy

The elevated hematocrit level, reduced serum erythropoietin level, headache, fever, memory difficulties, and weight loss seen in this patient are characteristic of polycythemia vera. Although there is not an overall consensus on treatment of polycythemia vera, phlebotomy is frequently used as an initial treatment. Because this patient is older than 70 years and has previously had a thrombotic event, a myelosuppressive agent such as hydroxyurea should be used in addition to phlebotomy. This combination of hydroxyurea and phlebotomy has been demonstrated to be an effective therapeutic regimen in controlling the hematocrit in most patients with polycythemia vera and in lowering the risk of thrombosis that occurs with use of phlebotomy alone. When hydroxyurea is used, complete blood

counts should be frequently monitored to avoid excessive myelosuppression. Patients may experience painful leg ulcers. Two reports have shown an increased risk of acute myeloid leukemia in patients taking hydroxyurea, although it remains controversial whether the use of hydroxyurea increases the risk of acute myeloid leukemia. *(Answer: B—Phlebotomy and hydroxyurea)*

27. A 45-year-old man presents with weakness and shortness of breath. He complains of a headache, fatigue, light-headedness, and ringing in his ears. He smokes three packs of cigarettes a day and has smoked for 30 years. He is 5 ft 8 in tall and weighs 280 lb. On physical examination, his complexion is ruddy. His blood pressure is 140/85 mm Hg. There is a history of heart disease in his family. He has been treated for hypertension for the past 10 years with a therapeutic regimen consisting of an antihypertensive agent and a diuretic. Laboratory reports reveal the following: Hct, 57%; red cell mass, 34 ml/kg; low-normal plasma volume; oxygen saturation, 97%.

Which of the following is the most likely diagnosis for this patient?

- ❑ **A. Gaisböck syndrome (relative polycythemia)**
- ❑ **B. Pickwickian syndrome**
- ❑ **C. Polycythemia vera**
- ❑ **D. Acute myeloid leukemia**
- ❑ **E. Chronic myeloid leukemia**

Key Concept/Objective: To recognize that middle-aged, obese, hypertensive men who are heavy smokers and who are being treated with diuretics may have Gaisböck syndrome even if their hematocrit levels are lower than 60%

The red cell mass of less than 36 ml/kg, reduced oxygen levels, and low-normal plasma volume seen in this patient suggest a diagnosis of Gaisböck syndrome. Gaisböck syndrome, or relative polycythemia, is often seen at an earlier age (45 to 55 years) than polycythemia vera. In the male population in the United States, 5% to 7% have Gaisböck syndrome. Those affected are usually middle-aged, obese, hypertensive men who may also be heavy smokers. Smoking-induced elevations in the level of carboxyhemoglobin or hypoxemia may play a role in the development of Gaisböck syndrome. Long-term exposure to carbon monoxide results in chronically high levels of carboxyhemoglobin. Carbon monoxide binds to hemoglobin with an affinity many times greater than oxygen, decreasing the quantity of hemoglobin available for oxygen transport. Thus, long-term carbon monoxide exposure in cigarette and cigar smokers may cause polycythemia. In this patient, diuretic use for treatment of hypertension may also have exacerbated the deficit in plasma volume. Before treatment with phlebotomy, patients may be taken off diuretics and encouraged to lose weight and stop smoking. *(Answer: A—Gaisböck syndrome [relative polycythemia])*

For more information, see Broudy VC: 5 Hematology: V The Polycythemias. ACP Medicine Online (www.acpmedicine.com). Dale DC, Federman DD, Eds. WebMD Inc., New York, August 2004

Nonmalignant Disorders of Leukocytes

28. A 21-year-old man presents to the emergency department for evaluation of pain and fever. One week ago, the patient was involved in a head-on motor vehicle accident; he was not wearing a seat belt. At that time, the patient underwent an emergent resection of his spleen. The patient states that for the past 2 days, he has been experiencing swelling and redness of his incision site, as well as fever. On physical examination, the patient's temperature is 102° F (38.9° C). Diffuse swelling and induration is noted at his incision site, and diffuse erythema surrounds the incision. Laboratory values are remarkable for a white blood cell (WBC) count of 26,000/mm^3 and a differential with 50% neutrophils and 22% band forms.

Which of the following statements regarding neutrophilia is true?

- ❑ A. **Neutrophilia is usually defined as a neutrophil count greater than 1,000/mm³**
- ❑ B. **Thrombocytosis is commonly associated with splenectomy, but splenectomy has no association with neutrophilia**
- ❑ C. **Serious bacterial infections are usually associated with changes in the number of circulating neutrophils, as well as the presence of younger cells, but they are not associated with changes in neutrophil morphology**
- ❑ D. **With serious bacterial infections, characteristic morphologic changes of the neutrophils include increased numbers of band forms and increased numbers of cells with Dohle bodies and toxic granulations**

Key Concept/Objective: To know the definition and morphologic characteristics of neutrophilia

Neutrophilia, or granulocytosis, is usually defined as a neutrophil count greater than 10,000/mm³. Neutrophilia most often occurs secondary to inflammation, stress, or corticosteroid therapy. Neutrophilia is also associated with splenectomy. Serious bacterial infections and chronic inflammation are usually associated with changes in both the number of circulating neutrophils and their morphology. Characteristic changes include increased numbers of young cells (bands), increased numbers of cells with residual endoplasmic reticulum (Dohle bodies), and increased numbers of cells with more prominent primary granules (toxic granulation). These changes are probably caused by the endogenous production of granulocyte colony-stimulating factor or granulocyte-macrophage colony-stimulating factor and are also seen with the administration of these growth factors. *(Answer: D—With serious bacterial infections, characteristic morphologic changes of the neutrophils include increased numbers of band forms and increased numbers of cells with Dohle bodies and toxic granulations)*

29. A 61-year-old woman visits your clinic for a follow-up visit. She has been coming to you for several weeks with complaints of diffuse rash, intermittent fevers, persistent cough, and dyspnea. Laboratory results were significant only for a WBC count of 15,000/mm³ with 40% eosinophils. You have completed an extensive workup for underlying allergy, connective tissue disease, malignancy, and parasitic infection, with negative results. A bone marrow biopsy revealed hypercellular marrow with eosinophils constituting 50% of the marrow elements. Your working diagnosis is hypereosinophilic syndrome (HES).

Which of the following statements regarding HES and eosinophilia is true?

- ❑ A. **The criteria used to diagnose HES are an unexplained eosinophil count of greater than 1,500/mm³ for longer than 6 months and signs or symptoms of infiltration of eosinophils into tissues**
- ❑ B. **The term HES is often used for patients with chronic eosinophilia resulting from parasitic infection**
- ❑ C. **[illegible] count greater than [illegible]**
- ❑ D. **Long-term corticosteroid therapy is the only available therapy for HES**

Key Concept/Objective: To understand HES

Evaluation of the patient with eosinophilia (i.e., a patient with an eosinophil count greater than 700/mm³) is difficult because the causes of this disorder are multiple and diverse. The term HES is often used for patients with chronic eosinophilia of unknown cause. The criteria used to diagnose HES are an unexplained eosinophil count of greater than 1,500/mm³ for longer than 6 months and signs or symptoms of infiltration of eosinophils into tissues. If symptoms involving the lungs or the heart are present, prednisone at a dosage of 1 mg/kg/day should be given for 2 weeks, followed by 1 mg/kg every other day for 3 months or longer. If this treatment fails or if an alternative is necessary to avoid steroid side effects, hydroxyurea at a dosage of 0.5 to 1.5 g/day should be given to lower the WBC count to less than 10,000/mm³ and the eosinophil count to less than 5,000/mm³. Studies suggest that treatment with imatinib mesylate is effective. Alternative agents include interferon alfa, cyclosporine, and etoposide. *(Answer: A—The criteria used to diagnose HES are an unexplained eosinophil count of greater than 1,500/mm³ for longer than 6 months and signs or symptoms of infiltration of eosinophils into tissues)*

30. A 52-year-old man presents to your office for his yearly physical examination. He is completely asymptomatic and is tolerating his single blood pressure medication well. On review of systems, the patient states that for several weeks, he has had severe pruritus after showering and that lately his face has been feeling "flushed." He has no history of food allergy or other allergy. Physical examination is significant only for facial plethora and moderate nontender splenomegaly. CBC reveals a WBC of 13,000/mm³ with 6% basophils, a hematocrit of 60%, and a platelet count of 640,000/mm³. Hemoglobin oxygen saturation on room air is 98% with a normal respiratory rate. The serum erythropoietin level is low.

Which of the following statements regarding basophils or basophilia is true?

- ❑ A. **Thrombocytosis is commonly associated with splenectomy, but splenectomy has no association with basophilia**
- ❑ B. **Basophilia is defined as a basophil count greater than 500/mm³**
- ❑ C. **Basophilia is seen in myeloproliferative disorders (MPDs) such as chronic myelogenous leukemia (CML), polycythemia vera (PV), and myeloid metaplasia, as well as in some hemolytic anemias and Hodgkin disease**
- ❑ D. **Granules in the basophil do not contain histamine**

Key Concept/Objective: To understand basophil physiology and the clinical significance of basophilia

Basophilia (i.e., a basophil count of greater than 150/mm³) is seen in MPDs such as CML, PV, and myeloid metaplasia; after splenectomy; in some hemolytic anemias; and in Hodgkin disease. The basophil count can also be increased in patients with ulcerative colitis or varicella infection. Although basophils and mast cells are involved in immediate hypersensitivity reactions and basophils are often seen in areas of contact dermatitis, basophilia is not seen in patients with these disorders. Most, if not all, of the circulating histamine in the body is synthesized by the basophil and stored in its granules. Degranulation causes the release of histamine, which mediates many immediate hypersensitivity effects and which, because it is a potent eosinophil chemoattractant, draws eosinophils to the site of degranulation. Other substances that are released on basophil degranulation include additional eosinophil chemotactic factors and a variety of arachidonic acid metabolites, the most important of which is leukotriene C_4. *(Answer: C—Basophilia is seen in myeloproliferative disorders [MPDs] such as chronic myelogenous leukemia [CML], polycythemia vera [PV], and myeloid metaplasia, as well as in some hemolytic anemias and Hodgkin disease)*

31. You are asked to consult on a case involving a 26-year-old man who developed leukocytosis after a motorcycle accident 3 days ago. The patient has multiple fractures of the pelvis and lower extremities, extensive soft-tissue injury, and aspiration pneumonia. His leukocyte count was 35,000 on admission and has subsequently ranged up to 50,000. Currently, the patient is sedated and is on a ventilator. He is being treated with I.V. antibiotics. Physical examination is remarkable for right lower lateral consolidation, ecchymoses of the lower extremities, and the absence of hepatosplenomegaly. Laboratory values are as follows: hemoglobin, 9.5 g/dl; platelets, 140,000/mm³; WBC, 55,000/mm³, with 95% neutrophils and bands. No myelocytes or metamyelocytes are noted, and there is no elevation of the basophil or eosinophil count. The leukocyte alkaline phosphatase (LAP) score is 140 µm/L.

Which of the following cannot be the cause of this patient's elevated neutrophil count?

- ❑ A. **Sepsis**
- ❑ B. **Hemorrhage**
- ❑ C. **Tissue injury**
- ❑ D. **CML**
- ❑ E. **Cytokine release**

Key Concept/Objective: To understand the causes of the leukemoid reaction and distinguish them from malignant causes

The term leukemoid reaction is used to describe a profound leukocytosis (generally defined as a leukocyte count exceeding 25,000 to 30,000/mm³) that is not leukemic in eti-

ology. Leukemoid reactions are the response of normal bone marrow to cytokine release by lymphocytes, macrophages, and other cells in response to infection or trauma. In a leukemoid reaction, the circulating neutrophils are usually mature and are not clonally derived. The major differential diagnosis is with regard to CML. Leukemoid reactions should also be distinguished from leukoerythroblastic reactions: the presence of immature white cells and nucleated red cells in the peripheral blood irrespective of the total leukocyte count. Although less common than leukemoid reactions in adults, leukoerythroblastosis reflects serious marrow stimulation or dysfunction and should prompt bone marrow aspiration and biopsy, unless it occurs in association with severe hemolytic anemia, sepsis in a patient with hyposplenism, or massive trauma. In such patients, trauma, hemorrhage, and infection all will contribute to a potent cytokine release and marrow stimulation. The absence of splenomegaly, leukocyte precursors (myelocytes, metamyelocytes), basophilia, or eosinophilia all point away from CML, and the elevated LAP score confirms the diagnosis of a leukemoid reaction. *(Answer: D—CML)*

32. On routine examination, a 45-year-old man is found to have a neutrophil count of 1,100/mm³. He feels well, takes no medications, and has no history of infection. His medical records reveal a persistent, asymptomatic neutropenia of 1,000 to 1,800 neutrophils/mm³ over the past 10 years.

Which of the following ethnicities would help explain this patient's low leukocyte count?

- ❑ **A. Native American**
- ❑ **B. Ashkenazi Jew**
- ❑ **C. Yemenite Jew**
- ❑ **D. Hmong**
- ❑ **E. Inuit**

Key Concept/Objective: To be able to recognize constitutional causes of neutropenia in certain populations

Neutropenia is present when the peripheral neutrophil count is less than 1,000 to 2,000 cells/mm³. The normal range in Africans, African Americans, and Yemenite Jews is lower. In these populations, neutrophil counts of 1,500/mm³ are common, and neutrophil counts as low as 100/mm³ are probably normal. Evaluation should focus on a history of unusual infections, medications, or toxic exposures. If these factors are absent and if previous asymptomatic neutropenia can be documented, no further evaluation or special precautions are needed. *(Answer: C—Yemenite Jew)*

33. A 59-year-old woman with severe, progressive rheumatoid arthritis is found to have a neutrophil count of 1,200/mm³ on routine hematologic testing. She takes methotrexate and prednisone for her rheumatoid arthritis. In addition to rheumatoid nodules and rheumatoid joint deformities, moderate splenomegaly is noted on physical examination.

Which of the following would not be contributing to this patient's neutropenia?

- ❑ **A. Methotrexate**
- ❑ **B. Corticosteroids**
- ❑ **C. Antineutrophil antibodies**
- ❑ **D. Felty syndrome**
- ❑ **E. Large granular lymphocyte syndrome**

Key Concept/Objective: To understand the various causes of neutropenia in rheumatoid arthritis

With the exception of prednisone, each of the listed factors can lead to neutropenia in patients with rheumatoid arthritis. Methotrexate (as well as gold, penicillamine, and other disease-modifying agents) can cause severe leukopenia and neutropenia and require CBC monitoring during therapy. Prednisone and other corticosteroids, however, do not lower the neutrophil count. Indeed, the neutrophil count rises acutely after corticosteroid

administration, owing to demargination. Felty syndrome is the triad of rheumatoid arthritis, splenomegaly, and neutropenia and frequently includes hepatomegaly, lymphadenopathy, fever, weight loss, anemia, and thrombocytopenia. Leg ulcers and hyperpigmentation may also be seen. This syndrome develops late in the course of chronic, seropositive rheumatoid arthritis, often after the inflammatory arthritis has resolved. Recurrent infections with gram-positive organisms can be a serious clinical problem, and infections do not always correlate with the severity of neutropenia. Large granular lymphocyte syndrome is a clonal expansion of $CD2^+$, $CD3^+$, $CD8^+$, $CD16^+$, and $CD57^+$ cells and is frequently associated with rheumatoid arthritis. Patients present with neutropenia, infections, and possibly splenomegaly and may be misdiagnosed as having Felty syndrome. Unlike patients with Felty syndrome, however, these patients present at an older age. Their neutropenia may develop within months of the onset of arthritis and is usually associated with a normal or elevated blood leukocyte (mostly lymphocytes) count. The clonal expansion may evolve into a lymphocytic leukemia. Peripheral blood smear shows increased numbers of large granular lymphocytes with abundant pale cytoplasm and prominent azurophilic granules. *(Answer: B—Corticosteroids)*

34. A 56-year-old man has felt unwell for 6 months. He complains of cough, exertional shortness of breath, paroxysmal nocturnal dyspnea, diarrhea, low-grade fever, and weight loss. He takes no medications and has not traveled outside the United States. On examination, his blood pressure is 110/50 mm Hg; his pulse is 96 beats/min and irregular; his respiration rate is 20; and his temperature is 99.3° F (37.4° C). Fine rales are present in the lower two thirds of the lung fields. The jugular venous pressure is estimated to be 15 cm, and a large V wave is present. A 3/6 holosystolic murmur is noted at the apex. A distinct S_3 gallop is audible; 2+ pitting edema is present in the ankles. Chemistry panel is normal, but the CBC reveals a WBC of 22,000, of which 60% are eosinophils. Electrocardiogram shows atrial fibrillation. Chest x-ray shows interstitial and alveolar edema and Kerley B lines. Echocardiogram reveals mitral regurgitation and features suggesting a restrictive cardiomyopathy. Multiple stool samples are negative for ova and parasites.

Which of the following is the most likely diagnosis for this patient?

- ❏ A. **Asthma**
- ❏ B. **Parasitic infestation**
- ❏ C. **Eosinophilic leukemia**
- ❏ D. **Hypersensitivity pneumonitis**
- ❏ E. **Hypereosinophilic syndrome**

Key Concept/Objective: To understand the diagnosis of hypereosinophilic syndrome

Hypereosinophilic syndrome consists of a chronic, unexplained eosinophilia without obvious cause (such causes would include parasitic infections, drug reactions, allergic reactions, hypersensitivity reactions, lymphoproliferative disorders, connective tissue disorders, and hematologic malignancies). The condition may be caused by excessive IL-5 production by a T cell clone. Eosinophils are found in the involved tissues and are thought to cause damage by the local deposition of toxic eosinophil products such as eosinophil major basic protein. Manifestations are multisystemic: fever, rash, cough and dyspnea, diarrhea, congestive heart failure, and peripheral neuropathy. The most severe complications involve the heart and CNS. Careful evaluation is necessary to exclude other causes of eosinophilia. Endomyocardial fibrosis (Löffler endocarditis) is a cardiac manifestation of hypereosinophilic syndrome. Eosinophilic deposits may lead to direct injury of the endocardium, followed by platelet thrombi and fibrosis. The cardiac apices can become obliterated, creating a characteristic finding on echocardiography. The mitral and tricuspid valves are affected by the same fibrotic process, resulting in valvular regurgitation. *(Answer: E—Hypereosinophilic syndrome)*

For more information, see Dale DC: 5 Hematology: VII Nonmalignant Disorders of Leukocytes. ACP Medicine Online (www.acpmedicine.com). Dale DC, Federman DD, Eds. WebMD Inc., New York, April 2004

Transfusion Therapy

35. A 57-year-old diabetic man presents to your office for presurgical evaluation for total hip replacement. After a thorough history and physical examination, you ask the patient if he has any questions. He says that the orthopedic surgeon told him that there was a possibility he will need blood products during or after the surgery, and the patient is concerned about the risks of contracting a contagious disease from blood products.

Which of the following statements about the risk of infection associated with transfusion is true?

- ❑ **A. Risk of transfusion-associated hepatitis A is higher in pooled products such as factor concentrates than in single-donor products**
- ❑ **B. Postdonation screening to identify donors likely to transmit blood-borne infections has produced the biggest decrease in the risk of transfusion-transmitted disease**
- ❑ **C. Directed donation offers a small but significant reduction in the risk of transfusion-associated infections**
- ❑ **D. Currently, there is no postdonation test available for West Nile virus**

Key Concept/Objective: To understand the screening process used to reduce transmission of infectious diseases through transfusion of blood products

Available prevalence data show that the risk of infectious disease from directed donors is no different from that of first-time donors. Predonation donor screening to identify clinical and lifestyle characteristics associated with higher incidences of infection has produced the biggest decrease in the risk of transfusion-transmitted disease. Postdonation testing is essential in identifying donors likely to transmit blood-borne infections who are missed in the initial screening process. Because the viremic phase of hepatitis A lasts about 17 days in humans before signs and symptoms develop, hepatitis A transmission from single-donor products is extremely rare. Pooled products, such as factor concentrates, however, carry a substantially higher risk. Transmission of West Nile virus by blood products has led to new donor questions to eliminate donors at risk for this disease. A nucleic acid–based test for all donated units was introduced in June 2003. *(Answer: A—Risk of transfusion-associated hepatitis A is higher in pooled products such as factor concentrates than in single-donor products)*

36. A 49-year-old woman is admitted to the hospital with newly diagnosed severe anemia. Her hemoglobin level is 7 g/dl, and she has shortness of breath and fatigue. She denies any obvious source of blood loss, such as menorrhagia or rectal bleeding. On examination, the patient is pale. She is tachycardic, with a pulse of 110 beats/min. Her blood pressure is 105/62 mm Hg. Rectal examination shows heme-positive brown stool. Before you leave the room to write your orders, you explain the risks and benefits of blood product transfusion.

Which of the following statements about blood components is true?

- ❑ **A. Whole blood transfusion would be preferable to red cell transfusion in this patient**
- ❑ **B. Leukocyte reduction reduces febrile transfusion reactions**
- ❑ **C. Cryoprecipitate consists of albumin and platelets**
- ❑ **D. Single-donor platelet transfusions carry a higher risk of blood-borne infection than platelet concentrates**

Key Concept/Objective: To understand the components of whole blood

Except for some autologous blood programs that use whole blood rather than packed red cells, use of whole blood has now been almost completely supplanted by therapy employing specific blood components. To prevent transfusion reactions or to delay alloimmunization, red cells are further processed by leukocyte reduction or washing to remove plasma proteins. Current filter technology reduces white cell counts to less than 5×10^6 cells per unit, a concentration that is sufficient to reduce febrile transfusion reactions and

delay alloimmunization and platelet refractoriness. With single-donor platelet therapy, there is a reduction in the risk of blood-borne infection and antigen exposure, because the product is from one donor rather than four to six; disadvantages are a longer collection time, greater cost, and often limited supply. Fresh frozen plasma (FFP) that is frozen within 8 hours of collection contains all the procoagulants at normal plasma concentrations. Cryoprecipitate consists of the cryoproteins recovered from FFP when it is rapidly frozen and then allowed to thaw at 2° to 6° C. These cryoproteins include fibrinogen, factor VIII, von Willebrand factor, factor XIII, and fibronectin. *(Answer: B—Leukocyte reduction reduces febrile transfusion reactions)*

37. A 58-year-old man with acute myelogenous leukemia received chemotherapy 10 days ago. He now presents to the emergency department with severe fatigue and shortness of breath. He has had no fever. Results of complete blood count are as follows: white cell count, 800/µl; hemoglobin level, 7.5 g/dl; platelet count, 43,000/µl.

Which of the following statements regarding indications for transfusion of blood products is true?

❑ A. In patients with acute blood loss, the first treatment goal is transfusion of packed red blood cells

❑ B. Platelet transfusions are contraindicated in autoimmune thrombocytopenia

❑ C. The prevalence of bleeding increases significantly below a threshold of about 10,000 platelets/µl in otherwise asymptomatic patients

❑ D. In chronically anemic patients, red cell 2,3-diphosphoglycerate production is decreased to maximize the red blood cells' oxygen affinity

Key Concept/Objective: To know the indications for transfusion of blood products

The decision whether to use red cells depends on the etiology and duration of the anemia, the rate of change of the anemia, and assessment of the patient's ability to compensate for the diminished capacity to carry oxygen that results from the decrease in red cell mass. Restoration of intravascular volume, usually with crystalloid, ensures adequate perfusion of peripheral tissue and is the first treatment goal for a patient with acute blood loss. In general, the decision to transfuse platelets rests on the answers to two questions: (1) Is the thrombocytopenia the result of underproduction or increased consumption of platelets? and (2) Do the existing platelets function normally? Thrombocytopenia can result from decreased production caused by marrow hypoplasia or from increased consumption caused by conditions such as idiopathic thrombocytopenic purpura (ITP). Studies have shown that the prevalence of bleeding increases significantly below a threshold of about 10,000 platelets/µl in otherwise asymptomatic patients. Transfusion is appropriate in a bleeding patient whose platelet count is adequate but whose platelets are nonfunctional as a result of medications such as aspirin or nonsteroidal anti-inflammatory drugs or as a result of bypass surgery. Proper investigation of the causes of thrombocytopenia will identify clinical situations in which platelets should be withheld because they contribute to evolution of the illness. These disorders include thrombotic microangiopathies such as thrombotic thrombocytopenic purpura, hemolytic-uremic syndrome, and the HELLP syndrome (hemolysis, elevated liver enzymes, and a low platelet count). Platelet transfusions will not help patients with autoimmune thrombocytopenia (e.g., ITP), but they also will not harm them. *(Answer: C—The prevalence of bleeding increases significantly below a threshold of about 10,000 platelets/µl in otherwise asymptomatic patients)*

38. A 33-year-old white man presents with an exacerbation of Crohn disease, which is manifested by bright-red blood from the rectum; abdominal pain; and anemia. You begin therapy for exacerbation of Crohn disease, and you also order the transfusion of 2 units of red blood cells. Approximately 30 minutes after the first unit of red cells is begun, the nurse calls and says the patient has a fever and "doesn't feel well."

Which of the following statements regarding transfusion complications is true?

❑ A. Immediate hemolytic reactions are the result of an anamnestic response to an antigen to which the recipient is already sensitized

❑ B. **Delayed hemolytic reactions occur during primary sensitization and can be as severe as immediate hemolytic reactions**

❑ C. **Until the cause of the hemolytic transfusion reaction is identified, the patient may only receive type O red cells or AB plasma**

❑ D. **Fever without signs of hemolysis can be managed with acetaminophen; no further laboratory workup is necessary**

Key Concept/Objective: To understand the potential complications of transfusions

Hemolytic transfusion reactions are classified as immediate or delayed, depending on their pathophysiology. Immediate hemolytic reactions are the result of a preexisting antibody in the recipient that was not detected during pretransfusion testing. Delayed hemolytic reactions are the result of an anamnestic response to an antigen to which the recipient is already sensitized. Clinical evidence of hemolysis is likely to be more severe in immediate hemolytic reactions and may include back pain, pain along the vein into which the blood is being transfused, changes in vital signs, evidence of acute renal failure, and signs of developing disseminated intravascular coagulation. Until the antibody causing the immune hemolysis is identified, only type O red cells and AB plasma should be used. Febrile reactions are characterized by the development of fever during transfusion or within 5 hours after transfusion. The differential diagnosis for a patient undergoing a nonhemolytic febrile transfusion reaction should always include unrecognized sepsis. When febrile reaction is suspected, immediate management consists of discontinuing the transfusion, obtaining appropriate cultures, and returning the product to the blood bank. *(Answer: C—Until the cause of the hemolytic transfusion reaction is identified, the patient may only receive type O red cells or AB plasma)*

39. A 65-year-old man presents to you for preoperative workup before undergoing aortic valve replacement for aortic regurgitation (indicated because of progressive left ventricular dysfunction, as revealed on echocardiogram) and coronary artery bypass surgery. He is interested in autologous blood donation. He has had chronic stable angina for the past 2 years, which is brought on by maximal exertion; his angina has remained unchanged for 1 year. For the past 2 days he has had increased urgency for urination and dysuria. On physical examination, he has a 2/4 diastolic murmur and suprapubic tenderness; otherwise, his examination is normal.

What absolute contraindication to autologous blood donation does this man have?

❑ A. **Angina**

❑ B. **Aortic regurgitation**

❑ C. **Active bacterial infection**

❑ D. **Age older than 60 years**

Key Concept/Objective: To know the absolute contraindications to autologous blood donation

This patient appears to have a UTI, so he cannot donate blood until that is resolved. Active bacterial infection is one of the three absolute contraindications to autologous blood donation; the other two are tight aortic stenosis and unstable angina. Although this man's stable angina might temper one's willingness to recommend autologous blood donation (especially because the risk of disease transmission in donated blood is low enough to make potential clerical error in the transfusion of autologous blood more of a concern), it is not an absolute contraindication, nor is aortic regurgitation or his age. *(Answer: C—Active bacterial infection)*

40. A 25-year-old woman who is 28 weeks pregnant is brought to the emergency department after an automobile collision. She complains of abdominal pain; her blood pressure is 85/60; and her pulse is 130. Normal fetal heart activity is found on fetal monitoring. Abdominal ultrasound reveals free fluid in the peritoneum.

Which of the following is the appropriate transfusion therapy for this patient?

❑ A. Whole blood

❑ B. Packed red cells

❑ C. Irradiated red cells

❑ D. Leukocyte-reduced red cells

Key Concept/Objective: To know the appropriate choice for transfusion of red cells in a pregnant woman

This question highlights the concern about transmission of cytomegalovirus (CMV) during pregnancy. Whole blood, packed red cells, and irradiated red cells all carry the risk of CMV transmission. Blood from a CMV-negative donor is another choice, but because the prevalence of CMV infection varies widely from region to region in the United States, it is not always available. Use of cellular blood components that contain fewer than 5 × 10⁶ leukocytes is effective in preventing the transmission of CMV. *(Answer: D—Leukocyte-reduced red cells)*

41. A 22-year-old man with hemophilia A is going to have impacted molars extracted. He has a history of prolonged bleeding after minor surgeries.

Which of the following is the most appropriate transfusion therapy for this patient during his dental procedure?

❑ A. Cryoprecipitate

❑ B. Factor VIII concentrate

❑ C. Fresh frozen plasma

❑ D. Platelets

Key Concept/Objective: To know the most appropriate transfusion support therapy for a patient with hemophilia A who is undergoing surgery in which there is a possibility of major bleeding

Factor VIII concentrate is the most appropriate of the choices because its means of preparation minimizes the risk of transmission of blood-borne infections to recipients. Cryoprecipitate is another option, but because it relies on the pooling of blood products from multiple donors, the risk of infection with blood-borne pathogens is much increased. Fresh frozen plasma does contain factor VIII, but only in low concentrations so that a much greater transfusion volume would be required. Platelet transfusion does not help to correct the underlying disorder. *(Answer: B—Factor VIII concentrate)*

42. ***Which of the following patients absolutely requires platelet transfusion?***

❑ A. A patient who has been taking aspirin for a headache and who is now scheduled for emergent evacuation of his subdural hemorrhage; platelet count, 100,000/μl

❑ B. A patient with idiopathic thrombocytopenia; platelet count, 10,000/μl

❑ C. A patient with thrombotic thrombocytopenic purpura; platelet count, 9,000/μl

❑ D. A patient with end-stage liver disease who is complaining of easy bruising; platelet count, 50,000/μl

Key Concept/Objective: To know the indications for platelet transfusion

Although a platelet count of 100,000/μl is adequate for major surgery, because of this patient's use of aspirin, those platelets are nonfunctional, and so platelet transfusion would be required. Although the platelet count of a patient with idiopathic thrombocytopenia is very close to the "trigger level" for platelet transfusion for an asymptomatic patient (< 10,000/μl), platelet transfusion is not absolutely required, especially owing to the fact that the platelets in these patients tend to function very well. Platelet transfusion is contraindicated in patients with thrombotic thrombocytopenic purpura; in such patients,

plasmapheresis with fresh frozen plasma is indicated. In a patient with end-stage liver disease who has a platelet count of 50,000/µl, mild bleeding (easy bruising) is not an indication for platelet transfusion. *(Answer: A—A patient who has been taking aspirin for a headache and who is now scheduled for emergent evacuation of his subdural hemorrhage; platelet count, 100,000/µl)*

43. A 63-year-old multiparous woman is receiving packed red cells to treat symptomatic anemia after hip replacement surgery. Fifteen minutes into the transfusion, she has rigors. On physical examination, she appears anxious and diaphoretic; her temperature is 102.2° F (39° C); the rest of her examination is normal.

What is the first step in the diagnosis and management of this transfusion reaction?

- ❑ **A. Administer acetaminophen or meperidine for symptomatic relief**
- ❑ **B. Draw blood for culturing**
- ❑ **C. Stop the transfusion**
- ❑ **D. Send the untransfused blood back to the blood bank for analysis**

Key Concept/Objective: To understand the management of febrile transfusion reactions

The most important first step in managing febrile transfusion reactions is to stop the infusion immediately. Because bacterial infection can be a complication of transfusion or surgery, drawing blood for culturing is indicated but would not be the first step. Acetaminophen or, if the rigors are particularly severe, meperidine is helpful in the management of febrile transfusion reaction but should be preceded by discontinuance of the infusion. Sending the untransfused blood back to the blood bank is important so that the blood bank can obtain cultures from the product and verify that there have not been any errors in its production. *(Answer: C—Stop the transfusion)*

For more information, see Churchill WH: 5 Hematology: X Transfusion Therapy. ACP Medicine Online (www.acpmedicine.com). Dale DC, Federman DD, Eds. WebMD Inc., New York, October 2004

Hematopoietic Cell Transplantation

44. A 42-year-old white woman presented 2 months ago with menorrhagia. She was noted to be pancytopenic on initial laboratory evaluation. After an exhaustive workup, a diagnosis of aplastic anemia was made. The patient is being considered for hematopoietic cell transplantation.

Which of the following statements regarding hematopoietic cell transplantation is false?

- ❑ **A. Hematopoietic stem cells for transplantation may derive from bone marrow, peripheral blood, or umbilical cord blood**
- ❑ **B. Syngeneic transplantations come from identical twins; identical twins are the best possible donors of stem cells**
- ❑ **C. In allogeneic transplantations, if two persons do not share the same HLA antigens, B cells taken from one person will react vigorously to the mismatched HLA molecules on the surface of the cells from the other person**
- ❑ **D. When compared with allogeneic transplantation, autologous transplantation has the advantage of avoiding graft versus host disease (GVHD) and associated complications**

Key Concept/Objective: To understand the different types of hematopoietic stem cell transplantations

Hematopoietic stem cell transplantation can be categorized according to the relation between the donor and the recipient and according to the anatomic source of the stem cell. Hematopoietic stem cells for transplantation may derive from bone marrow, peripheral blood, or umbilical cord blood and may be harvested from a syngeneic, allogeneic, or

autologous donor. Identical twins are the best possible donors of stem cells. When syngeneic donors are used, neither graft rejection nor GVHD will develop in the recipient. Only about one in 100 patients undergoing transplantation will have an identical twin. Allogeneic transplantation, which involves a related or unrelated donor, is more complicated than syngeneic or autologous transplantation because of immunologic differences between donor and host. With allogeneic hematopoietic cell transplantation, in which the immune system of the patient is provided by the graft, the clinical concerns are not only with the prevention of graft rejection by host cells surviving the pretransplant preparative regimen but also with the prevention of donor cells from causing immune-mediated injury to the patient (i.e., GVHD). Immunologic reactivity between donor and host is largely mediated by immunocompetent cells that react with HLAs, which are encoded by genes of the major histocompatibility complex. HLA molecules display both exogenous peptides (for example, from an infecting virus) and endogenous peptides, presenting them to T cells, an important step in the initiation of an immune response. If two persons do not share the same HLA antigens, T cells taken from one person will react vigorously to the mismatched HLA molecules on the surface of the cells from the other. These are reactions against so-called major HLA determinants. When compared with allogeneic transplantation, autologous transplantation has the advantage of avoiding GVHD and associated complications; disadvantages are that the autologous cells lack the antitumor effect of an infusion of allogeneic leukocytes (the so-called graft versus tumor effect) and may contain viable tumor cells. *(Answer: C—In allogeneic transplantations, if two persons do not share the same HLA antigens, B cells taken from one person will react vigorously to the mismatched HLA molecules on the surface of the cells from the other person)*

45. A 20-year-old African-American patient with sickle cell disease was recently evaluated for hematopoietic stem cell transplantation by his hematologist. He comes in to see you and is excited about the possibilities of cure but is concerned about possible complications of transplantations.

Which of the following statements regarding transplant complications is true?

- ❑ A. **Late toxicity (occurring weeks to months after transplantation) is usually the result of the preparative regimen and can include nausea, vomiting, skin rash, mucositis, and alopecia**
- ❑ B. **Graft failure that occurs after autologous transplantation can result from marrow damage before harvesting, during ex vivo treatment, during storage, after exposure to myelotoxic agents, or as a result of infections with cytomegalovirus (CMV) or human herpesvirus type 6 (HHV-6)**
- ❑ C. **Treatment of graft failure requires the use of higher doses of myelosuppressive agents**
- ❑ D. **Veno-occlusive disease of the liver usually occurs after the first year and only rarely occurs in the subacute setting**

Key Concept/Objective: To understand the complications of hematopoietic stem cell transplantation

Pretransplant preparative regimens are associated with a substantial array of toxicities, which vary considerably depending on the specific regimen used. For example, after the standard cyclophosphamide–total body irradiation regimen, nausea, vomiting, and mild skin erythema develop immediately in almost all patients. Oral mucositis inevitably develops about 5 to 7 days after transplantation and usually requires narcotic analgesia. By 10 days after transplantation, complete alopecia and profound granulocytopenia have developed in most patients. Veno-occlusive disease of the liver (also referred to as sinusoidal obstruction syndrome) is a serious complication of high-dose chemoradiotherapy; it develops in approximately 10% to 20% of patients. Veno-occlusive disease of the liver, characterized by the development of ascites, tender hepatomegaly, jaundice, and fluid retention, may occur at any time during the first month after transplantation; the peak incidence occurs at around day 16. Approximately 30% of patients who develop veno-occlusive disease of the liver die as a result of the disease, with progressive hepatic failure leading to a terminal hepatorenal syndrome. Although complete and sustained engraftment is the gen-

eral rule after transplantation, in some cases marrow function does not return; in other cases, after temporary engraftment, marrow function is lost. Graft failure after autologous transplantation can result from marrow damage before harvesting, during ex vivo treatment, during storage, or after exposure to myelotoxic agents after transplantation. Infections with CMV or HHV-6 may also result in poor marrow function. Graft failure after allogeneic transplantation may be the result of immunologically mediated graft rejection and is more common after conditioning regimens that are less immunosuppressive, in recipients of T cell–depleted marrow, and in recipients of HLA-mismatched marrow. The treatment of graft failure begins with removal of all potentially myelosuppressive agents. *(Answer: B—Graft failure that occurs after autologous transplantation can result from marrow damage before harvesting, during ex vivo treatment, during storage, after exposure to myelotoxic agents, or as a result of infections with cytomegalovirus [CMV] or human herpesvirus type 6 [HHV-6])*

46. A 49-year-old woman is admitted to the hospital for weight loss, fatigue, and night sweats. A CBC ordered in the emergency department revealed anemia, thrombocytosis, and pronounced leukocytosis with a relatively normal differential consistent with a myeloproliferative disorder. You are concerned that her symptoms may be caused by a hematologic malignancy.

Which of the following statements regarding hematopoietic stem cell transplantation for malignant disease is false?

- ❑ **A. Hematopoietic stem cell transplantation is first-line therapy for chronic lymphocytic leukemia (CLL) and has a cure rate of 80%**
- ❑ **B. The best results with allogeneic transplantation for acute myeloid leukemia (AML) are obtained in patients undergoing transplantation in first remission**
- ❑ **C. Allogeneic transplantation can cure 15% to 20% of patients with acute lymphocytic leukemia (ALL) who fail induction therapy or in whom chemotherapy-resistant disease develops**
- ❑ **D. In CML, the best results from allogeneic transplants are obtained in patients who receive transplants within 1 year of diagnosis**

Key Concept/Objective: To know the indications for hematopoietic stem cell transplantation in malignant diseases

Allogeneic marrow transplantation cures 15% to 20% of patients with AML who fail induction therapy; indeed, it is the only form of therapy that can cure such patients. Thus, all patients 55 years of age or younger with newly diagnosed AML should have their HLA type determined, as should their families, soon after diagnosis to enable transplantation for those who fail induction therapy. The best results with allogeneic transplantation for AML are obtained in patients undergoing transplantation in first remission, in whom a cure rate of 40% to 70% is reported. As with AML, allogeneic transplantation can cure 15% to 20% of patients with ALL who fail induction therapy or in whom chemotherapy-resistant disease develops; thus, these patients are candidates for the procedure. Allogeneic and syngeneic marrow transplantations are the only forms of therapy known to cure CML. Time from diagnosis influences the outcome of transplantation during the chronic phase. The best results are obtained in patients who receive transplants within 1 year of diagnosis; progressively worse results are seen the longer the procedure is delayed. Use of marrow transplantation in CLL has received only limited attention, probably because of the indolent nature of the disease and its propensity to occur in older patients. *(Answer: A—Hematopoietic stem cell transplantation is first-line therapy for chronic lymphoctic leukemia [CLL] and has a cure rate of 80%)*

47. You are called to see a 26-year-old man in the hematology-oncology service because of fever and a low WBC count. He recently underwent induction chemotherapy for acute myelogenous leukemia. Yesterday, his absolute neutrophil count (ANC) was 500/mm^3, and today it is 100/mm^3. He has been anemic and thrombocytopenic but has not required transfusion. This morning, he developed a fever of 103.1° F (39.5° F). He has no focal central nervous sytem, respiratory, gastrointestinal, or urinary complaints other than severe stomatitis, caused by the chemotherapy. A careful physical examination fails to reveal any source of infection. Chest x-ray, blood and urine cultures, and a repeat complete blood count are ordered.

Which of the following would you recommend for this patient at this time?

- ❑ A. No treatment until culture results are known
- ❑ B. Lumbar puncture
- ❑ C. Intravenous gentamicin and piperacillin
- ❑ D. Oral ciprofloxacin
- ❑ E. Administration of granulocyte colony-stimulating factor (G-CSF) and granulocyte-macrophage colony-stimulating factor (GM-CSF)

Key Concept/Objective: To know the indications for empirical treatment of febrile neutropenia and the best antibiotic combination

Febrile neutropenia (ANC < 500/mm^3) is an urgent indication for careful history and physical examination, expedient collection of cultures, expedient use of radiography (e.g., chest x-ray), and initiation of empirical antibiotics. In febrile neutropenic patients, the most common sources of infection are the lungs, the genitourinary system, the GI tract, the oropharynx, and the skin. Initially, the infecting organisms are the usual flora or are infecting agents commonly found at the anatomic site of infection. However, in patients with recurrent infections or those who require prolonged courses of antibiotics, unusual organisms can be responsible for the infection. Frequently, the usual signs and symptoms of infection are attenuated or absent in these patients because of the absence of the inflammatory responses to infection. In the neutropenic patient, minor infections that might otherwise have been well localized can become serious disseminated infections very quickly. Management includes careful evaluation of the oropharynx, skin, lungs, GI tract, and genitourinary tract for subtle signs of infection. Cultures and a chest x-ray are obtained, and empirical antibiotics are started. Clinicians can select traditional combinations of a β-lactam antibiotic active against *Pseudomonas* (e.g., piperacillin) and an aminoglycoside (e.g., gentamicin or tobramycin). Although colony-stimulating factors may be considered for adjunctive use in selected high-risk, severely ill neutropenic patients, they are not indicated in most febrile neutropenic patients. *(Answer: C—Intravenous gentamicin and piperacillin)*

48. A 23-year-old woman underwent allogeneic bone marrow transplantation for acute myelogenous leukemia. On day 11, she began to complain of right upper quadrant pain, and her weight began to climb. On examination, peripheral edema and tender hepatomegaly were appreciated. Skin examination was unremarkable. Laboratory testing revealed a bilirubin level of 2.4 mg/dl and an alanine aminotransferase level of 146 U/L. Over the next several days, she developed increasing abdominal girth, and her bilirubin level increased to 12 mg/dl.

What is the most likely diagnosis for this patient?

- ❑ A. Graft versus host disease (GVHD)
- ❑ B. Acute hepatitis A infection
- ❑ C. Acute cytomegalovirus infection
- ❑ D. Graft rejection
- ❑ E. Veno-occlusive disease of the liver

Key Concept/Objective: To recognize veno-occlusive disease as a potential complication of hematopoietic stem cell transplantation

This patient presents with typical findings of veno-occlusive disease, including ascites, hepatomegaly, jaundice, and fluid retention. Veno-occlusive disease typically occurs in the first few weeks after transplantation. Pathologically, there is cytotoxic injury to the hepatic venulae and sinusoidal endothelium, resulting in vascular blockage (the clinical picture is similar to that of Budd-Chiari syndrome). There is a high mortality, and research continues in the fields of treatment and prevention. Other possible causes include GVHD, viral hepatitis, drug reaction, sepsis, heart failure, and tumor invasion. However, acute ascites and fluid retention are more typical of veno-occlusive disease. *(Answer: E—Veno-occlusive disease of the liver)*

49. A 42-year-old man presents with fatigue and progressive left upper quadrant pain. On examination, the spleen is palpable. CBC reveals a hematocrit of 32% and a WBC count of 97,000/mm^3. Bone marrow biopsy reveals hyperplasia of the granulocytic series, and the cytogenetic analysis confirms the presence of the Philadelphia chromosome. A diagnosis of chronic myeloid leukemia (CML) is made.

What is the most appropriate step to take next for this patient?

- ❑ **A. Search for HLA-matched sibling**
- ❑ **B. Initiate busulfan therapy**
- ❑ **C. Initiate interferon-alfa therapy**
- ❑ **D. Initiate hydroxyurea therapy**
- ❑ **E. Leukapheresis**

Key Concept/Objective: To understand the role of allogeneic transplantation in chronic myelogenous leukemia

If an appropriate HLA-matched sibling can be found, most experts would recommend allogeneic transplantation as initial therapy for a person younger than 50 years who is diagnosed with CML. In older patients, therapy with interferon alfa or hydroxyurea may be more appropriate. Therefore, the search for potential donors is the critical first step. Leukapheresis is only infrequently used (primarily in chronic lymphocyte leukemia) when white cell counts are extremely elevated and there are acute CNS symptoms. *(Answer: A—Search for HLA-matched sibling)*

50. ***What is the chance that the sister of the patient in Question 48 will be an HLA match?***

- ❑ **A. 0%**
- ❑ **B. 10%**
- ❑ **C. 25%**
- ❑ **D. 50%**
- ❑ **E. 75%**

Key Concept/Objective: To know the odds of finding an appropriate donor in a transplant candidate

The genes that encode HLA class I and II antigens are tightly linked and are typically inherited together. Therefore, there is a one-in-four chance of inheriting the identical haplotype of a sibling. *(Answer: C—25%)*

51. An 18-year-old woman underwent allogeneic bone marrow transplantation for Hodgkin disease that had failed to respond to [illegible] acute GVHD.

Which of the following is not typically associated with GVHD?

- ❑ **A. Abdominal pain**
- ❑ **B. Acute renal failure**
- ❑ **C. Maculopapular rash**
- ❑ **D. Diarrhea**
- ❑ **E. Elevation of hepatic transaminase levels**

Key Concept/Objective: To understand the clinical presentation of acute GVHD

GVHD is quite common in patients receiving allogeneic transplants. The most common manifestation is that of a maculopapular rash, frequently involving the palms and soles. The second most common organ affected is the liver. Symptoms of liver involvement typically include an elevation in levels of transaminase, alkaline phosphatase, and conjugated bilirubin; these changes are the result of damage to the small bile ducts. GI symptoms

include diarrhea, anorexia, and crampy abdominal pain. Efforts to prevent GVHD include the use of immunosuppressive agents in the early posttransplantation period. GVHD is most frequently treated with glucocorticoids. *(Answer: B—Acute renal failure)*

52. A 43-year-old man with CML is being evaluated for allogeneic bone marrow transplantation. On questioning, he states that in the past, he had an allergic rash to trimethoprim-sulfamethoxazole.

What would be the most appropriate regimen for* Pneumocystis carinii *prophylaxis for this patient?

- ❑ **A. Dapsone**
- ❑ **B. Atovaquone**
- ❑ **C. Attempted desensitization to sulfa before transplantation**
- ❑ **D. Intravenous pentamidine**
- ❑ **E. Aerosolized pentamidine**

Key Concept/Objective: To appreciate the superiority of sulfa in preventing P. carinii *infection in the transplant patient*

***P. carinii* once caused pneumonia in up to 10% of transplant patients. The risk of this complication is nearly eliminated through the use of appropriate prophylaxis. Trimethoprim-sulfamethoxazole given 1 week before transplantation and then twice weekly after engraftment is very effective. The other agents listed as choices are all active against *Pneumocystis*, but trimethoprim-sulfamethoxazole is the most effective. Efforts should be made to desensitize the patient to sulfa. If these efforts are unsuccessful, dapsone is typically used.** *(Answer: C—Attempted desensitization to sulfa before transplantation)*

For more information, see Appelbaum FR: 5 Hematology: XI Hematopoietic Cell Transplantation. ACP Medicine Online (www.acpmedicine.com). Dale DC, Federman DD, Eds. WebMD Inc., New York, April 2004

Hemostasis and Its Regulation

53. A newborn develops significant bleeding from the circumcision site. The family history indicates that one cousin has a bleeding disorder. The patient's platelet count and morphology are normal; however, the bleeding time is very prolonged. A platelet function assay-100 (PFA-100) is abnormal; prothrombin time (PT) and partial thromboplastin time (PTT) are normal. Platelet aggregometry shows poor aggregation.

Which of the following molecules is most likely to be deficient in this newborn?

- ❑ **A. von Willebrand factor**
- ❑ **B. Glycoprotein (GP) Ib-IX-V**
- ❑ **C. GPIIb-IIIa**
- ❑ **D. Tissue plasminogen activator**

Key Concept/Objective: To understand the mechanisms of platelet activation

Platelets are activated at the site of vascular injury to form a plug to stop bleeding. Platelet activation involves four distinct processes: adhesion, aggregation, secretion, and procoagulant activity. Platelet adhesion is primarily mediated by the binding of GPIb-IX-V complex to von Willebrand protein. Aggregation involves binding of fibrinogen to the platelet fibrinogen receptor GPIIb-IIIa. Congenital deficiency of GPIIb-IIIa or fibrinogen leads to Glanzmann thrombasthenia and afibrinogenemia. The GPIIb-IIIa fibrinogen pathway is the final common course for platelet aggregation. Platelet protein secretion occurs after platelet stimulation, with the release of granules containing serotonin and adenosine diphosphate (ADP), which stimulate and recruit more platelets. Platelet procoagulation involves the assembly of the enzyme complexes in the clotting cascade on the platelet surface. Tissue plasminogen activator is a fibrinolytic factor; its deficiency causes a hypercoagulable state. *(Answer: C—GPIIb-IIIa)*

54. A 42-year-old man with advanced AIDS presents to a walk-in clinic complaining of leg pain that started 4 days ago. The patient has no history of deep vein thrombosis (DVT) and no family history of DVT. He denies experiencing any recent trauma, fractures, or surgeries. On physical examination, the patient looks chronically ill. His left leg has moderate edema and tenderness to palpation. Compression ultrasonography shows a proximal DVT. His platelet count, PT, and PTT are within normal limits.

Which of the following is the most likely cause of this patient's hypercoagulable state?

- ❑ **A. Antiphospholipid syndrome**
- ❑ **B. Decreased levels of free protein S**
- ❑ **C. Decreased levels of factor XIII**
- ❑ **D. Congenital protein S deficiency**

Key Concept/Objectives: To understand the mechanisms for acquired protein S deficiency

Antithrombin III, protein C, and protein S are important components of the control mechanisms that modulate coagulation. Protein S circulates in two forms: a free form, in which it is active as an anticoagulant; and a bound, inactive form, in which it is complexed to C4b-binding protein of the complement system. C4b-binding protein acts as an acute phase reactant. The resultant increase in inflammatory state reduces the activity of free protein S, enhancing the likelihood of thrombosis. In this patient, advanced HIV disease is causing an inflammatory state in which the levels of free functional protein S are decreased. Antiphospholipid syndrome can be a cause of a hypercoagulable state; commonly seen laboratory abnormalities are thrombocytopenia and a prolonged PTT secondary to the presence of an inhibitor. Factor XIII deficiency causes a bleeding disorder. *(Answer: B—Decreased levels of free protein S)*

55. A 37-year-old woman was scheduled to undergo elective cholecystectomy. As part of her preoperative evaluation, her surgeon ordered an assessment of bleeding time, which showed that bleeding time was prolonged. The patient has now been referred to you for evaluation. She remembers having one episode of moderate bleeding after a tooth extraction a few years ago. Her father had a history of mild to moderate bleeding after surgical procedures. Her physical examination is unremarkable, and her platelet count is normal.

Which of the following tests would be appropriate for the initial evaluation of this patient?

- ❑ **A. Thrombin time**
- ❑ **B. Assessment of factor VII levels**
- ❑ **C. Assessment of factor XIII levels**
- ❑ **D. PFA-100**

Key Concept/Objective: To understand the uses of different coagulation tests

This patient has a prolonged bleeding time and a history of a previous bleeding episode. She also has a family history of a mild bleeding disorder. Von Willebrand disease is the most likely etiology. The testing of bleeding time primarily measures platelet function. A prolonged bleeding time with a platelet count over 100,000/µl suggests impaired platelet function. The bleeding time is difficult to standardize, and a normal bleeding time does not predict the safety of a surgical procedure. Bleeding time should not be used as a general screening test in a preoperative setting. Although once used commonly for screening of platelet disorders, bleeding time has been replaced by the PFA-100. PFA-100 is a newly developed automated test of platelet function. Citrated blood from the patient is aspirated onto a membrane coated with collagen and epinephrine or collagen and ADP in which a central aperture is made. The time it takes for blood flow through the membrane to stop is denoted as the closure time and is a measure of platelet function. The closure time is prolonged in patients with von Willebrand disease or other platelet functional defects. PFA-100 should be considered the first-line test for platelet function disorders. Thrombin time is used to test for abnormalities of the conversion of fibrinogen to fibrin. Thrombin time is prolonged in patients with severe liver disease and DIC and those undergoing heparin therapy. Factor VII levels are measured in patients who have a prolonged PT; it is a test of

the extrinsic system. Factor XIII is the only clotting factor whose activity is not assessed in PT or PTT; a deficiency should be suspected in an infant who experiences bleeding after circumcision or in an adult with unexplained bleeding. *(Answer: D—PFA-100)*

56. A 25-year-old man comes to your clinic for follow-up after being discharged from a local hospital, where he presented with a DVT. He did not have any previous episodes of DVT, and he denied having any obvious precipitating factor. He says his older brother was diagnosed with a DVT 1 year ago. At the hospital, the patient was started on heparin and warfarin as an inpatient; he was discharged on warfarin, with instructions to take it for 6 months. The discharge summary from the hospital contains some laboratory information from blood obtained at the moment of discharge. His PTT was slightly prolonged; his INR was 2.2; his protein C levels were decreased at 70% of normal; and his protein S levels were decreased at 40% of normal.

On the basis of this information, which of the following is the most likely diagnosis for this patient?

- ❑ **A. No diagnosis can be made on the basis of this information**
- ❑ **B. Antiphospholipid syndrome**
- ❑ **C. Protein S deficiency**
- ❑ **D. Combined protein S and protein C deficiencies**

Key Concept/Objective: To understand the appropriate timing of tests for inhibitors of hemostasis

This patient is a young man with a DVT and a family history of DVT. He likely has a hereditary condition causing a hypercoagulable state. Levels of protein C and protein S were obtained to assess for the possibility of an occult hypercoagulable state. Levels of protein C and protein S can be obtained by functional and immunologic methods. Because protein C and protein S are vitamin K dependent, their measurement can be problematic in patients taking warfarin. It is best to measure protein C or protein S when the patient has been off warfarin for 3 to 4 weeks. The low values seen in this patient could be explained by the use of warfarin; in addition, the formation of a clot will per se cause a decrease in both protein C and protein S levels. A prolonged PTT can be caused by a clotting factor deficiency or an inhibitor. Antiphospholipid syndrome can cause an inhibitor that can be associated with a hypercoagulable state. A mixing study will still show the PTT to be prolonged if an inhibitor is present. The most likely explanation of the slightly prolonged PTT in this patient is the patient's receiving heparin as an inpatient, just before the blood sample was obtained. *(Answer: A—No diagnosis can be made on the basis of this information)*

For more information, see Leung LLK: 5 Hematology: XII Hemostasis and its Regulation. ACP Medicine Online (www.acpmedicine.com). Dale DC, Federman DD, Eds. WebMD Inc., New York, June 2003

Hemorrhagic Disorders

57. A 25-year-old woman presents for routine examination. She has been well, but she has a long history of having heavier menstrual periods than other women she knows. This has not caused her any major problems. On review of systems, she notes a history of easy bleeding after dental work. Physical examination is normal except for petechiae on her shins. Results of coagulation studies are normal; her hematocrit is 32, with a platelet count of 56,000/µl. Your differential diagnosis includes idiopathic thrombocytopenic purpura (ITP).

Which of the following statements about ITP is false?

- ❑ **A. ITP is associated with splenomegaly**
- ❑ **B. ITP is associated with HIV infection, acute viral illnesses, and some autoimmune diseases**
- ❑ **C. Patients with platelet counts over 50,000/µl do not routinely require treatment**
- ❑ **D. Treatment is indicated for patients with platelet counts below 20,000 to 30,000/µl or for those whose platelet count is less than 50,000/µl**

and who have risk factors for bleeding (including hypertension, peptic ulcer disease, or a vigorous lifestyle)

❑ **E. The disorder is relatively benign; the most common cause of death in adult patients with this disorder is intracranial bleeding**

Key Concept/Objective: To be familiar with the presentation, course, associations, and platelet levels requiring treatment in cases of ITP

The presentation of ITP as a chronic illness with a mild bleeding diathesis is not uncommon in adults. Women are affected more frequently than men. In most adult patients (90%), ITP will follow a course characterized by chronic thrombocytopenia; in most children, platelet counts will return to normal within 3 months. ITP is infrequently associated with splenomegaly. In patients with this finding, other causes of thrombocytopenia, such as hypersplenism associated with liver disease, should be considered. Other diagnoses to be considered in patients with ITP and splenomegaly are lymphoma and systemic lupus erythematosus (SLE). Although most cases of ITP are idiopathic, it is well known that ITP can be associated with a number of underlying conditions, including HIV, viral illnesses (e.g., Epstein-Barr virus [EBV] infection), and autoimmune disease, most notably SLE. In adults, in contrast to children, ITP can present as a smoldering disease. Therapy is recommended for asymptomatic patients whose platelet counts are persistently lower than 20,000 to 30,000/µl and for patients with significant bleeding complications. Although in most patients ITP follows a relatively benign course, serious bleeding complications are occasionally seen. Of these bleeding complications, intracranial bleeding is the most dreaded because it is commonly fatal. Intracranial bleeding is more commonly seen when the platelet count drops below 10,000/µl; other risk factors include advanced age and concomitant medical illness. *(Answer: A—ITP is associated with splenomegaly)*

58. A 33-year-old woman is admitted to the hospital with altered mental status. Her physician calls you for consultation; he is concerned that the patient may have thrombotic thrombocytopenic purpura (TTP). He notes that she has anemia, thrombocytopenia, and a high fever and that she is disoriented. He asks your opinion regarding certain laboratory tests he has sent.

Which of the following findings is NOT consistent with a diagnosis of TTP?

❑ **A. Schistocytes and helmet cells seen on blood smear**

❑ **B. A positive direct Coombs test**

❑ **C. Normal results on coagulation testing**

❑ **D. An elevated serum LDH level**

❑ **E. Neutrophilic leukocytosis**

Key Concept/Objective: To be able to recognize the laboratory abnormalities associated with TTP

Patients with TTP typically present with the following pentad of signs and symptoms: (1) thrombocytopenia; (2) microangiopathic hemolytic anemia with schistocytes and helmet cells; (3) renal dysfunction, which is usually mild; (4) fever, which can be very high; and (5) neurologic symptoms, including seizures and a clouded sensorium. TTP is not associated with a positive direct Coombs test; hemolysis is not immune mediated. This finding should make one consider autoimmune hemolytic anemias (such as those associated with Evan syndrome and SLE, both of which should be considered in the differential diagnosis). The other findings are consistent with TTP and are helpful in establishing the diagnosis and differentiating it from other causes of anemia and thrombocytopenia (such as disseminated intravascular coagulation). Prompt plasmapheresis should be instituted in patients with TTP. *(Answer: B—A positive direct Coombs test)*

59. A dentist wishes to learn more about von Willebrand disease (vWD); he recently had a patient who has the disorder suffer excessive bleeding after dental work. In your discussion, you outline several key facts about vWD, including how these patients may require treatment before dental procedures and other surgeries.

Which of the following statements is true about vWD?

- ❑ A. **Results of coagulation studies are normal in patients with vWD**
- ❑ B. **Patients with vWD have thrombocytopenia**
- ❑ C. **Most cases are the result of impaired function of von Willebrand factor (vWF)**
- ❑ D. **An abnormal result on the ristocetin-induced platelet aggregation test is consistent with abnormal function of the patient's vWF (type 2 vWD)**
- ❑ E. **It affects very few people**

Key Concept/Objective: To know some common facts about vWD

vWD is the most common hereditary bleeding disorder. It may be the result of low levels of vWF (type I vWD, which accounts for 75% of cases); qualitative defects in vWF function (type II vWD), which can be determined by use of the ristocetin-induced platelet aggregation test; or a severe or total deficiency of vWF (type 3 vWD, the least common form). vWF acts as a carrier molecule for factor VIII and is important in the stability and half-life of factor VIII; therefore, vWD is associated with a prolonged activated partial thromboplastin time. The disorders of platelet function associated with vWD are not associated with decreases in platelet count. *(Answer: D—An abnormal result on the ristocetin-induced platelet aggregation test is consistent with abnormal function of the patient's vWF [type 2 vWD])*

60. A 7-year-old boy with advanced pancreatic adenocarcinoma is diagnosed with Trousseau syndrome (chronic disseminated intravascular coagulation [DIC] secondary to malignancy). Approximately 2 months ago, he was found to have a deep vein thrombosis (DVT).

Which of the following is seen in cases of chronic (compensated) DIC?

- ❑ A. **Thrombocytopenia**
- ❑ B. **Elevated coagulation studies**
- ❑ C. **Elevated D-dimer level**
- ❑ D. **Predisposition toward bleeding rather than thrombosis**

Key Concept/Objective: To be familiar with the common laboratory and clinical findings of chronic (compensated) DIC

Trousseau syndrome is a chronic form of DIC. When onset of DIC is slow, as is seen in some patients with cancer, compensation can occur. In these patients, a procoagulant state exists, and the patient has a predisposition for arterial and venous thrombosis (unlike in the acute forms of DIC, in which bleeding predominates). The typical laboratory abnormalities associated with acute DIC (thrombocytopenia, elevations in levels of coagulation factors, microangiopathic hemolytic anemia, decreased fibrinogen levels, and elevated D-dimer levels) are usually not present in patients with the chronic form; the exception to this is an elevated D-dimer level. Therapy is directed at the underlying disease. This patient with Trousseau syndrome and DVT should receive subcutaneous heparin if its use is not contraindicated. *(Answer: C—Elevated D-dimer level)*

For more information, see Leung LLK: 5 Hematology: XIII Hemorrhagic Disorders. ACP Medicine Online (www.acpmedicine.com). Dale DC, Federman DD, Eds. WebMD Inc., New York, January 2002

Thrombotic Disorders

61. A 38-year-old woman develops a deep vein thrombosis (DVT) in her left leg during a cross-country car trip. She is treated with heparin for 3 days, and she is started on warfarin. She is discharged from the hospital with an international normalized ratio (INR) of 2.5. Three days later, she presents with severe pain

in her left hand. Examination reveals an infarction of the third digit, with severe pain, purpura, and erythema. Her INR is 2.4. She has been compliant with regard to her medication regimen.

Which of the following is most consistent with this patient's disease process?

- ❑ **A. Protein S deficiency**
- ❑ **B. Protein C deficiency**
- ❑ **C. Hyperhomocysteinemia**
- ❑ **D. Antithrombin III (AT-III) deficiency**

Key Concept/Objective: To understand the diagnosis of protein C deficiency

Protein C deficiency results in a loss of ability to inactivate factor VIIa and factor Va, two major cofactors that regulate the clotting cascade. Warfarin lowers protein C levels as well as the levels of all the vitamin K-dependent clotting factors. Because the half-lives of factor Xa and prothrombin are longer than that of protein C, initiation of warfarin therapy can induce a paradoxical state of hypercoagulability. This patient likely has a heterozygous protein C deficiency that was uncovered when she was treated with warfarin. In patients in whom protein C deficiency is suspected, heparin and warfarin should be initiated concomitantly. Heparin therapy is initially started on an inpatient basis; warfarin is indicated for outpatient treatment. Another rare complication of warfarin therapy is skin necrosis, which can be severe. *(Answer: B—Protein C deficiency)*

62. A 58-year-old man with type 2 diabetes mellitus, hypertension, and coronary artery disease presents to your clinic for pain and swelling of his left leg. He states that his symptoms have been progressively worsening for 3 days and that he has now developed pain with ambulation. He denies having fever, shortness of breath, palpitations, or rash, but he adds that he was admitted to the hospital 10 days ago for chest pain. He states that he was treated with "medicine" and was told that he had had a small heart attack. On physical examination, the circumference of his left calf is 49 cm; the circumference of his right calf is 45 cm. The Homan sign is negative. On review of laboratory data, the complete blood count (CBC) is normal except for the platelet count, which is 60,000/µl. In the past, his CBC has been normal. Doppler ultrasound reveals a left superficial femoral DVT.

Which of the following statements regarding this patient is true?

- ❑ **A. Heparin-induced thrombocytopenia (HIT) is not likely in this patient because he developed symptoms more than 5 days after treatment was initiated**
- ❑ **B. DVT is the most common event leading to the diagnosis of HIT**
- ❑ **C. Diagnosis of HIT should be made by heparin-induced platelet aggregation assay because of the high sensitivity of this test**
- ❑ **D. The patient can be safely treated with warfarin and low-molecular-weight heparin because of the low immunogenicity of this type of heparin**

Key Concept/Objective: To understand heparin-induced thrombocytopenia

HIT is a relatively frequent drug reaction that can potentially cause life-threatening arterial and venous thrombosis. HIT typically develops 5 to 10 days after initiation of therapy; it can, however, develop up to 2½ weeks afterward. In patients who received heparin within the previous 100 days and are being retreated, the onset can be rapid—within hours after starting heparin. HIT is generally defined as a platelet count below 150×10^9 or a drop in the platelet count by more than 50% of the pretreatment peak. Venous thrombosis is more common than arterial thrombosis; DVT is the most common event leading to diagnosis of HIT. Diagnosis of HIT should be based on history and clinical findings; treatment should be initiated before laboratory confirmation. The most widely used assay in the diagnosis of HIT is heparin-induced platelet aggregation; however, this test has a low sensitivity. Treatment of HIT involves discontinuing all forms of heparin, including the use of heparin in flushes of subcutaneous lines. Various anticoagulants have been approved, including danaparoid, hirudin, lepirudin, and argatroban. Low-molecular-weight heparin

is not safe to use in patients with HIT because of its high cross-reactivity with standard heparin. *(Answer: B—DVT is the most common event leading to the diagnosis of HIT)*

63. A 24-year-old woman presents with a 1-day history of pain and swelling in her right leg. She had a DVT once before, when she was receiving oral contraceptives; she now takes no medications. On physical examination, the circumference of her right leg is increased. Ultrasound reveals a DVT in her thigh.

Which of the following tests would be helpful in the acute setting to determine the cause of her suspected hypercoagulable state?

- ❑ **A. Protein S level**
- ❑ **B. Protein C level**
- ❑ **C. Factor V Leiden**
- ❑ **D. AT-III level**

Key Concept/Objective: To understand the implications of timing on the workup of a hypercoagulable state

In this young woman with a history of DVTs, a hypercoagulable state should be suspected. In acute thrombosis, many clotting factor inhibitors are consumed, and therefore, an assessment of the levels of these inhibitors would not be useful. If plasma levels are high, it would be possible to argue that the patient does not have a hereditary deficiency; levels could be low secondary to the acute event or to an inherited cause. Some of the coagulation cascade inhibitors that are consumed immediately after a clotting event are protein C, protein S, and AT-III. Factor V Leiden mutations can be tested at any time. *(Answer: C—Factor V Leiden)*

64. A 44-year-old white woman presents with pain and swelling in her left lower extremity. Ultrasound reveals a left superficial femoral DVT. In the past, she experienced one other episode of DVT, for which she underwent treatment with warfarin for 6 months. She takes no medications except oral contraceptive pills. Her family history is significant in that, last year, a younger sister was diagnosed as having DVT.

Which of the following statements is true regarding the treatment of this patient?

- ❑ **A. She should again be treated with warfarin for 6 months**
- ❑ **B. She should avoid the use of oral contraceptives**
- ❑ **C. She should be tested for factor V Leiden after her anticoagulation therapy is terminated**
- ❑ **D. All family members need to be screened for factor V Leiden**

Key Concept/Objective: To understand the management of factor V Leiden mutations

Factor V Leiden, now considered the most common hereditary hypercoagulable state, is a defect caused by a mutated form of factor V that is resistant to the anticoagulation effects of activated protein C. In patients with thrombophilia, its prevalence is as high as 20% to 50%. The clinical manifestations are similar to other anticoagulant deficiencies and consist mainly of venous thrombosis. Management of factor V Leiden is also similar to that of other hypercoagulable states; warfarin is the mainstay of therapy. Patients with a first episode of thrombosis should undergo anticoagulation therapy for a period of 6 months. Patients with recurrent thromboses require lifelong therapy. Although the lifetime relative risk of thrombosis for patients with this deficiency is comparatively lower than that associated with protein C, protein S, and AT-III deficiencies, there is a synergistic relationship with the use of oral contraceptives. As such, women with factor V Leiden should avoid the use of oral contraceptives. Routine screening of family members is not warranted and is not cost-efficient. *(Answer: B—She should avoid the use of oral contraceptives)*

65. An 18-year-old man presented to the emergency department with complaints of shortness of breath. He reported that the symptoms came on suddenly 2 days ago and that they had been progressively worsening. He complained of left-sided chest pain that occurred when he took a deep breath; the pain did not radiate, nor was it associated with nausea, vomiting, or diaphoresis. He stated that he had had a bicycle accident 1 week earlier but that otherwise he had been doing well. On examination, the patient was tachypneic and tachycardic; his heart rate was 110 beats/min. With the patient receiving 2 L of oxygen by nasal cannula, the oxygen saturation was 94%. Physical examination revealed some crackles in the left base but was otherwise unremarkable. CBC and blood chemistries were within normal limits, and a chest x-ray was normal. Arterial blood gas measurements were made; the arterial oxygen tension (P_aO_2) was 60 mm Hg on room air. Ventilation-perfusion scanning showed a large right lower lobe perfusion defect, which was interpreted as indicating a high probability of pulmonary embolism. The patient underwent anticoagulation therapy for 6 months. At follow-up, with the patient off medication, a hypercoagulable workup is performed. Laboratory results are all within normal limits except for the AT-III level, which is low.

Which of the following statements regarding AT-III deficiency is false?

❑ **A. AT-III deficiency can be inherited or acquired**

❑ **B. AT-III inactivates factor Xa and thrombin**

❑ **C. AT-III deficiency causes severe arterial thrombosis**

❑ **D. For patients with AT-III deficiency, the risk of thrombosis increases with age**

Key Concept/Objective: To understand AT-III deficiency

AT-III deficiency is an autosomal dominant trait that affects nearly 1 in 2,000 people. There are two types of AT-III deficiency: inherited and acquired. The inherited form has two subsets: quantitative deficiency and qualitative deficiency. In some cases, AT-III deficiency may be acquired, as with disseminated intravascular coagulation or severe liver disease or through the administration of I.V. heparin. AT-III normally inactivates factor Xa and thrombin; patients with AT-III deficiency show evidence of continuous factor X activation and thrombin generation. The typical presentation of AT-III deficiency is similar to that of other hypercoagulable states. There is no evidence that AT-III deficiency increases the risk of arterial thrombosis. The two hypercoagulable states more closely related to arterial thrombosis are the antiphospholipid syndrome and hyperhomocystinemia. *(Answer: C—AT-III deficiency causes severe arterial thrombosis)*

66. A 26-year-old man presents with new-onset left lower extremity swelling and pain of 6 hours' duration. He takes no medications and has no history of trauma, immobilization, or prior thrombosis. His family history is remarkable for two "blood clots" in his mother. Compression ultrasonography confirms occlusive thrombus in the left superficial femoral vein.

Which of the following is the most appropriate sequence of interventions for this patient?

❑ **A. Start heparin and warfarin immediately, send tests for the hypercoagulable state before warfarin reaches therapeutic levels, and discontinue heparin after the international normalized ratio (INR) reaches therapeutic levels**

❑ **B. Send tests for the hypercoagulable state, then start heparin and warfarin concurrently, and discontinue heparin after 5 days' overlap**

❑ **C. Send tests for the hypercoagulable state, then start heparin and warfarin concurrently, and discontinue heparin when the INR reaches therapeutic levels**

❑ **D. Start heparin and warfarin immediately, discontinue heparin after 5 days' overlap, and evaluate for the hypercoagulable state after warfarin therapy is completed**

❑ **E. Evaluate for the hypercoagulable state, but no anticoagulation is indicated for superficial thrombophlebitis**

Key Concept/Objective: To understand the timing of workup and duration of therapy for patients presenting with a new DVT

A 26-year-old man presenting with new-onset thrombosis and a positive family history is highly suspicious for a hereditary hypercoagulable state and should be worked up for this. Because the levels of protein C and antithrombin III can be diminished in the setting of acute thrombosis and because heparin and warfarin also alter these levels, the optimal time for the workup is after the patient has completed therapy. Exceptions to this rule include the antiphospholipid antibody syndrome, in which early diagnosis can affect therapy and disorders for which specific genotypic tests are available (e.g., factor V Leiden), which will be accurate at any time. Because the INR (prothrombin time) is heavily dependent on factor VII, which has a short half-life, it rises fairly quickly after warfarin is begun. However, therapeutic anticoagulation may take several days longer because of the persistence of factor X and prothrombin. Overlapping heparin and warfarin by 5 days is thought to limit the risk of propagation of thrombus caused by delayed therapeutic anticoagulation. The confusingly named superficial femoral vein is in fact in the deep system and warrants therapy. *(Answer: D—Start heparin and warfarin immediately, discontinue heparin after 5 days' overlap, and evaluate for the hypercoagulable state after warfarin therapy is completed)*

67. A 58-year-old woman is 2 days' status post–total hip replacement. She has been receiving subcutaneous heparin as prophylaxis for DVT. You are asked to see the patient to evaluate new-onset dyspnea. On examination, the patient is tachypneic, tachycardic, and diaphoretic. She is agitated and complains of substernal chest pain. Chest examination reveals few bibasilar crackles. Cardiac, abdominal, and extremity examinations are normal except for her surgical wounds, which seem to be healing well. Laboratory results are as follows: pH, 7.47; P_aCO_2, 31; PO_2, 65; WBC, 11,500; Hb, 11.2; HCT, 33; platelets, 54,000/µl; prothrombin time, 14 sec; INR, 1.1; PTT, 44 sec (normal, 24–32; therapeutic range for heparin, 60–80); and chemistry panel, within normal limits. ECG reveals a 2 mm ST depression in leads II, III, and aVf; and chest x-ray is normal.

Which of the following is the best course of action for this patient at this point?

- ❑ A. **Bolus with I.V. heparin; begin heparin infusion; and arrange for urgent coronary angiography**
- ❑ B. **Bolus with I.V. heparin; begin heparin infusion; and arrange for urgent ventilation-perfusion scan**
- ❑ C. **Switch to low-molecular-weight heparin (LMWH) subcutaneously while arranging further diagnostic testing**
- ❑ D. **Stop all heparin, and bolus with I.V. methylprednisolone and diphenhydramine for allergic reaction to heparin**
- ❑ E. **Stop all heparin, and anticoagulate with hirudin while arranging further diagnostic testing**

Key Concept/Objective: To understand heparin-induced thrombocytopenia and its therapy

This patient is status post-hip surgery and has been receiving heparin for 2 days. She now presents with a clinical scenario that suggests pulmonary embolism or myocardial ischemia, or both, as well as a platelet count of 54,000/µl. In this setting, one should be highly suspicious of heparin-induced thrombocytopenia, which can present with venous or arterial thrombosis. While the next diagnostic test is a matter of clinical judgment, the crucial first step is discontinuing all heparin, including I.V. flushes, and initiating anticoagulation with hirudin (a potent thrombin inhibitor derived from medicinal leeches). Other alternatives would be lepirudin or danaparoid. LMWH, unfortunately, is not considered safe in the setting of heparin-induced thrombocytopenia and would not be a good alternative in this setting. *(Answer: E—Stop all heparin, and anticoagulate with hirudin while arranging further diagnostic testing)*

68. A 68-year-old man presents with new onset of right-sided DVT without apparent risk factors. Therapy is initiated, and the possibility of underlying cancer is raised. You are consulted regarding appropriate evaluation for occult malignancy.

What would you recommend for this patient?

- ❑ A. **Careful history, physical examination, routine blood counts and chemistries, chest x-ray (CXR), fecal occult blood testing (FOBT), and prostate-specific antigen (PSA); if these are not revealing, no further evaluation is necessary**
- ❑ B. **Careful history, physical examination, routine blood counts and chemistries, CXR, FOBT, and PSA; if these are not revealing, proceed with colonoscopy**
- ❑ C. **Careful history, physical examination, routine blood counts and chemistries, CXR, FOBT, and PSA; if these are not revealing, proceed with CT scan of the chest, abdomen, and pelvis**
- ❑ D. **Careful history, physical examination, routine blood counts and chemistries, CXR, FOBT, and PSA; if these are not revealing, proceed with bone scan**

Key Concept/Objective: To understand the malignancy workup in a patient presenting with new-onset DVT

There is a documented association between malignancy and thrombosis; in a recent prospective trial, patients with idiopathic DVT had an 8% incidence of diagnosis of cancer in the following 2 years, with an odds ratio of 2.3. However, it has never been shown that an exhaustive workup for malignancy is cost-effective or beneficial. On the basis of a recent large cohort study, it has been recommended that the evaluation of idiopathic DVT be limited to a careful history, physical examination, CXR, routine blood counts and chemistries, FOBT, and possibly PSA in men and pelvic ultrasound in women. Further studies should be directed by this initial evaluation; if it is unrevealing, then additional tests will not likely help and may produce substantial psychological stress in the patient. *(Answer: A—Careful history, physical examination, routine blood counts and chemistries, chest x-ray [CXR], fecal occult blood testing [FOBT], and prostate-specific antigen [PSA]; if these are not revealing, no further evaluation is necessary)*

For more information, see Leung LLK: 5 Hematology: XIV Thrombotic Disorders. ACP Medicine Online (www.acpmedicine.com). Dale DC, Federman DD, Eds. WebMD Inc., New York, January 2005

SECTION 6

IMMUNOLOGY/ALLERGY

Innate Immunity

1. A 58-year-old white man presents with weight loss, night sweats, and dyspnea. On examination, the patient appears chronically ill and is pale. Laboratory testing reveals leukocytosis, anemia, and thrombocytopenia. A bone marrow biopsy with aspirate is performed, and a diagnosis of acute myelogenous leukemia is confirmed. In counseling the patient about chemotherapy, you inform him that he is going to be at increased risk for infections and that a major source of infection will be his own gastrointestinal tract.

Which of the following statements regarding the innate immune system and the epithelial barrier in the GI tract is false?

- ❑ **A. Lectins found in secretions bind sugars on pathogens and activate the lectin pathway of complement activation**
- ❑ **B. Granulocytes marginate in small blood vessels throughout much of the barrier tissues and are available for rapid recruitment to a possible site of infection**
- ❑ **C. Mucus itself is a protective barrier that traps organisms and debris**
- ❑ **D. Secretions on the epithelial barrier concentrate complement in such a way that the concentration of complement in secretions is higher than the concentration in plasma**
- ❑ **E. Monocytes are present in secretions and in most tissues, where they phagocytose unwanted microbes**

Key Concept/Objective: To understand the basic principles of the innate immune system

The innate immune system is particularly active at the interface between the environment and the surfaces of the body that are lined with epithelial cells—namely, the skin and the GI, genitourinary, and sinopulmonary tracts. Intact physical barriers are critically important for preventing infections. In addition to the epithelial barrier itself, the fluids in these tracts contain mucus, natural antibodies (IgG and IgA), a complement system, and lectins. The complement system in secretions is present at about 10% to 20% of the concentration found in plasma. The lectins in these secretions bind sugars on pathogens and thereby activate the lectin pathway of complement activation. Granulocytes marginate in small blood vessels throughout much of these barrier tissues and are available for rapid recruitment to a possible site of infection. Monocytes/macrophages are also present in secretions and in most tissues, where they phagocytose unwanted microbes. Mucus itself is a protective film that traps organisms and debris; it also contains antibacterial substances. *(Answer: D—Secretions on the epithelial barrier concentrate complement in such a way that the concentration of complement in secretions is higher than the concentration in plasma)*

2. A 26-year-old female patient has had recurrent infections with pyogenic organisms. She has a follow-up appointment with you today to discuss her options. You remember that complement is a major mechanism by which the innate immune system can act and that certain complement deficiencies can cause disease.

Which of the following statements regarding the complement cascade is false?

- ❑ **A. The alternative pathway requires antibodies for initiation**

❑ B. The three complement pathways are the classical pathway, the alternative pathway, and the lectin pathway

❑ C. The membrane attack complex (MAC) allows perforation via channel or pore formation into the foreign membrane

❑ D. C3 degradation occurs spontaneously all the time, and C3 fragments bind to host cells and foreign cells; however, regulatory proteins on host cells protect cells by inactivating such fragments

Key Concept/Objective: To understand the complement system and its pathways

The complement system lies at the interface between innate and acquired immunity. As a key component of innate immunity, it promotes the inflammatory response and attacks and destroys foreign substances. Inherited deficiencies of components in the activating cascade predispose to infectious diseases, primarily of a pyogenic type; surprisingly, such deficiencies also predispose to autoimmunity, especially systemic lupus erythematosus (SLE). The early part of the complement system is divided into three branches: the antibody-initiated classical pathway; the antibody-independent (i.e., innate) alternative pathway; and the more recently described lectin pathway. Although each branch is triggered differently, all share the common goal of depositing clusters of C3b on a target. This deposition results in the assembly of a common lytic mechanism called the MAC or C5b-9. The alternative pathway is an ancient pathway of innate immunity. Unlike the classical pathway, the alternative pathway does not require antibody for initiation. Rather, the natural breakdown (low-grade turnover) of plasma C3 via spontaneous cleavage of a highly reactive thioester bond allows such C3 to attach to any nearby host or foreign surface. Regulatory proteins on host cells protect cells by inactivating such fragments. However, foreign membranes usually do not possess such inhibitors, so amplification (the feedback loop of the alternative pathway) becomes engaged. As a further assault against a pathogen, the alternative pathway assembles the MAC. In this case, the C5 convertase (C3bBbC3bP) cleaves C5 to C5b. This promotes assembly of C6 + C7 + C8 and multiple C9s to allow perforation (channel or pore formation) into the foreign membrane. *(Answer: A—The alternative pathway requires antibodies for initiation)*

3. A 32-year-old African-American woman with systemic lupus erythematosus (SLE) presents to your office for an examination. Her disease course has been complicated by hemolytic anemia, renal disease, synovitis, and rash. Her current regimen consists of low-dose prednisone. During her visit, she says she has done some research on the Internet and wants to know if her SLE is caused by a problem with complement.

Which of the following statements regarding complement is false?

❑ A. Almost all inherited complement deficiencies are inherited as autosomal dominant traits

❑ B. Immune complexes can lodge in blood vessel walls and activate complement to produce synovitis, vasculitis, dermatitis, and glomerulonephritis

❑ C. A deficiency of complement regulatory proteins usually causes excessive activation

❑ D. Deficiencies of early components (e.g., C1q, C1r/C1s, C4, and C2) predispose to SLE, whereas deficiencies of C3, MBL, or MAC components lead to recurrent bacterial infections

Key Concept/Objective: To understand the basic principles of complement and disease states

The pathophysiology of many inflammatory diseases involves the synthesis of autoantibodies and the presence of excessive quantities of immune complexes. If immune complexes lodge in blood vessel walls, they may activate complement to produce synovitis, vasculitis, dermatitis, and glomerulonephritis. Similarly, a powerful complement barrage may follow ischemia-reperfusion injury as the alternative pathway elicits C3b deposition on the damaged tissue, which is regarded as foreign. Complement component deficiencies,

although rare, predispose to autoimmune diseases (e.g., SLE) and bacterial infections. Deficiencies of complement regulatory proteins allow for excessive activation. These conditions are usually inherited as autosomal codominant traits (i.e., recessive), with the exception of C1-Inh (autosomal dominant) and properdin (X-linked). Deficiencies of early components (e.g., C1q, C1r/C1s, C4, and C2) predispose to SLE, whereas deficiency of C3, MBL, or MAC components leads to recurrent bacterial infections. *(Answer: A—Almost all inherited complement deficiencies are inherited as autosomal dominant traits)*

For more information, see Atkinson JP, Liszewski MK: 6 Immunology/Allergy: II Innate Immunity. ACP Medicine Online (www.acpmedicine.com). Dale DC, Federman DD, Eds. WebMD Inc., New York, June 2004

Histocompatibility Antigens/Immune Response Genes

4. A 43-year-old man comes for a routine follow-up. Several months ago, the patient presented for evaluation of weight loss, rash, and iron-deficiency anemia. You diagnosed him as having celiac disease. The patient states he is doing well on his gluten-free diet. He has gained 10 lb since his last visit 2 months ago. Today his anemia is also seen to have improved. You remember that celiac disease results from immune dysregulation, and you are stimulated to learn more about adaptive immunity.

Which of the following statements regarding the antigens of the major histocompatibility complex (MHC) is false?

- ❑ A. **There are two structural types of MHC molecules, called class I and class II**
- ❑ B. **Clonally determined antigen receptors on B cells recognize and bind to specific peptide-MHC complexes**
- ❑ C. **MHC molecules act by binding peptide fragments of antigens that have been processed in specialized antigen-presenting cells**
- ❑ D. **Class II antigens are encoded by the HLA-D region**

Key Concept/Objective: To understand MHC molecules

There are two structural types of MHC molecules, called class I and class II. The molecules of both classes are active in antigen recognition and help focus immune defenses during invasions from the microbial world. They are also engaged in the communication that occurs between cells during the immune response. MHC molecules act by binding peptide fragments of antigens that have been processed in specialized antigen-presenting cells. Clonally determined antigen receptors on T cells then recognize and bind to specific peptide-MHC complexes, setting into motion the appropriate immune response. Class II antigens are encoded by the HLA-D region, which is divided into at least three subregions: HLA-DP, HLA-DQ, and HLA-DR. Class I heavy chains are the gene products of three MHC loci, designated HLA-A, HLA-B, and HLA-C. *(Answer: B—Clonally determined antigen receptors on B cells recognize and bind to specific peptide-MHC complexes)*

5. A 22-year-old man presents to establish primary care. He has been healthy most of his life, but he does have type 1 diabetes mellitus, which he reports has been under very good control. He informs you that when last measured, his hemoglobin A_{1C} value was 5.2%. He has no history of retinopathy or neuropathy, and he states that he saw his ophthalmologist 6 weeks ago. The patient has had protein in his urine, and he takes an angiotensin-converting enzyme (ACE) inhibitor. He asks you, "What causes type 1 diabetes?" You explain that the underlying problem is that his body has mistaken its own pancreatic molecules for foreign molecules. Later that day, you decide to read further on adaptive immunity.

Which of the following statements regarding antigen processing and presentation is false?

- ❑ A. **Class I molecules are expressed on virtually all tissues and are important in the recognition of virally infected cells**
- ❑ B. **Class II molecules are expressed on a limited variety of cells known as antigen-presenting cells**

- ❑ C. **MHC molecules first bind peptide fragments after the MHC molecules reach the cell surface**
- ❑ D. **Exogenous proteins are taken up by endosomes or lysosomes, where they are catabolized; their peptides are then bound to MHC class II molecules**

Key Concept/Objective: To understand the processing of foreign proteins and their relationship to the MHC system

The breakdown of protein molecules into peptide fragments is an important part of the process by which antigens are presented to T cells and other immune effector cells. MHC molecules come to the cell surface with peptides already bound. Proteins are first degraded internally, and the peptide fragments are bound to MHC class I and MHC class II molecules within the cell. Class I molecules are expressed on virtually all tissues. Virally infected cells are recognized principally by class I-restricted T cells, usually those with a cytotoxic function. In contrast, class II-directed T cells are restricted to antigen-presenting cells of the immune system (i.e., B cells, macrophages, dendritic cells, or Langerhans cells) that are principally concerned with defense against external infectious agents. Exogenous and endogenous antigens reach the cell surface by different pathways. Exogenous proteins are taken up into endosomes or lysosomes, where they are catabolized. Peptides from exogenous proteins are generally bound to MHC class II molecules, and the class II–peptide complexes are then brought to the surface for presentation to T cells. Peptides from endogenous proteins (e.g., secretory proteins or products of viral infection) appear to be complexed in the endoplasmic reticulum to MHC class I molecules. *(Answer: C—MHC molecules first bind peptide fragments after the MHC molecules reach the cell surface)*

6. A 23-year-old primigravida who is known to be Rh-negative is told by her obstetrician that she needs a medication to prevent complications (i.e., erythroblastosis fetalis) of her next pregnancy. She wonders why she should be using this medication.

Which of the following immunologic responses is prevented by the use of anti–Rh-positive antibodies (RhoGAM)?

- ❑ A. **Primary immune response to antigen**
- ❑ B. **Secondary immune response (anamnestic or booster response)**
- ❑ C. **Somatic hypermutation**
- ❑ D. **Class switch recombination**

Key Concept/Objective: To understand the genesis and prevention of the secondary immune response

If an antigen is encountered a second time, a secondary response (also called an anamnestic or booster response) occurs because of the existence of memory B cells. Administration of RhoGAM to the mother at the time of delivery prevents the fetal red blood cells, which are Rh positive, from generating a primary response in the Rh-negative mother, thus decreasing significantly the possibility of an anamnestic response in future pregnancies. Both IgM and IgG titers rise exponentially, without the lag phase seen in the primary response. Whereas the peak IgM level during the secondary response may be the same as, or slightly higher than, the peak IgM level during the primary response, the IgG peak level during the secondary response is much greater and lasts longer than the peak level during the primary response. This variation in response is an apt illustration of immunologic memory and is caused by a proliferation of antigen-specific B cells and helper T cells during the primary response. The primary immune response characterizes the first exposure to antigen and is largely IgM mediated; later production of IgG is not as great in magnitude or duration as that produced during the secondary response. Somatic hypermutation, class switch recombination, and immunoglobulin class switching are all mechanisms involved in producing the appropriate immunoglobulin with the highest antigen specificity. *(Answer: B—Secondary immune response [anamnestic or booster response])*

7. A 48-year-old woman with severe rheumatoid arthritis (RA) is advised by a rheumatologist to consider a novel antibody, because her arthritis is not responding to therapy with methotrexate. She asks you about this new medication.

Of the following, which is the therapeutic target of approved engineered human monoclonal antibodies in the management of RA?

- ❑ A. **Interleukin-6 (IL-6)**
- ❑ B. **IL-10**
- ❑ C. **Tumor necrosis factor–α (TNF-α)**
- ❑ D. **IL-1**

Key Concept/Objective: To understand the clinical application of engineered monoclonal antibodies

Humanized monoclonal antibodies to TNF-α have been used successfully in the treatment of Crohn disease and RA. These monoclonal antibodies are indicated for patients with moderate to severe RA that is not responsive to methotrexate or for patients in whom methotrexate toxicity has occurred. IL-1 is a proinfammatory cytokine implicated in the pathogenesis of RA. There is an FDA-approved IL-1 receptor antagonist, but it is not a monoclonal antibody. Monoclonal antibodies against IL-6 have been used in clinical trials, but they failed to demonstrate clinical benefit and are not approved for use at this time. IL-10 is an endogenous inhibitor of IL-1, TNF-α, and interferon gamma; attempts at using IL-10 in the treatment of RA failed. Clinical therapeutics utilizing monoclonal antibodies will expand with the emergence of new understanding of the underlying pathophysiology of various disease processes. *(Answer: C—Tumor necrosis factor–α [TNF-α])*

For more information, see Carpenter CB, Terhorst CP: 6 Immunology/Allergy: V Adaptive Immunity: Histocompatibility Antigens and Immune Response Genes. ACP Medicine Online (www.acpmedicine.com). Dale DC, Federman DD, Eds. WebMD Inc., New York, July 2004

Immunogenetics of Disease

8. A 42-year-old white man presents to primary care clinic complaining of fatigue. Physical examination is significant for splenomegaly. Laboratory data reveal a leukocytosis with 3% blasts and numerous immature cells of the granulocytic lineage, and a low leukocyte alkaline phosphatase (LAP) level. Cytogenetic analysis reveals the Philadelphia chromosome [t(9;22)], and a diagnosis of chronic myelogenous leukemia (CML) is made. Subsequently, the patient seeks evaluation for allogeneic stem cell transplantation. During your discussion with him, you explain the importance of human leukocyte antigen (HLA) matching of donor and recipient to reduce the incidence of graft-versus-host disease.

Which cluster of highly polymorphic genes encodes these cell surface markers?

- ❑ A. **The cytokine cluster loci**
- ❑ B. **The major histocompatibility complex (MHC)**
- ❑ C. **The cytokine histocompatibility complex**
- ❑ D. **The chemokine histocompatibility cluster**

Key Concept/Objective: To understand that MHC encodes HLA

The MHC—so called because of its prominent role in rejection of allogeneic tissue—is a primary barrier to transplantation of solid organ, tissue, and hematopoietic stem cells. This closely linked cluster of highly polymorphic genes, grouped on the short arm of chromosome 6, encodes cell surface molecules (e.g., HLA). The normal role of the MHC is presentation of endogenous and exogenous peptide antigen fragments to T lymphocytes, thereby initiating an immune response against the molecule (or pathogenic organism) from which the peptide was derived. The extreme variability of molecular structure in the MHC antigens permits a wide range of different peptides to be presented by autologous human antigen-presenting cells, although individual subjects may have a specific repertoire of

MHC antigens that do not present certain antigens effectively. The focused immunogenicity of MHC molecules and the variability of these molecules among individuals render them prominent targets for the immune response in the context of solid organ and bone marrow transplantation. In cases in which live allogeneic cells are the target of the immune response, the apparent target is the nonself MHC molecule itself. Freedom from rejection and, in the case of bone marrow transplantation, graft-versus-host disease is improved with HLA matching of donor and recipient. *(Answer: B—The major histocompatibility complex [MHC])*

9. A 72-year-old woman with emphysema presents for evaluation for possible lung transplantation. Laboratory evaluation for cytokine polymorphism of the transforming growth factor (TGF) gene, considered as homozygosity for TGF-α, is associated with graft fibrosis in 93% of lung transplant recipients. TGF-α has two well-studied dimorphic positions within the leader sequence of the gene whose variants are found in concert with one another.

What designation is given to variants at polymorphic positions that display this relationship?

- ❑ A. Hardy-Weinberg equilibrium
- ❑ B. Allelic equilibrium
- ❑ C. Linkage disequilibrium
- ❑ D. Allelic disequilibrium

Key Concept/Objective: To understand the relationships between polymorphic nucleotide positions in or near an expressed gene on the same chromosome with regards to whether they occur in populations independently of one another

There can be multiple polymorphic nucleotide positions in or near an expressed gene on the same chromosome. In such cases, it is desirable to know whether specific variants at each of the polymorphic positions are independent of the variants at the other positions. If examination of a population shows that the variants at the different positions occur independently of one another, the system is said to be in Hardy-Weinberg equilibrium. If certain variants at one of the positions are statistically associated with specific variants at another of the linked positions, the system is said to exhibit linkage disequilibrium. Hardy-Weinberg equilibrium can be reestablished over many generations through recombination events. The closer the polymorphic loci are to each other on the chromosome, the less likelihood there is of a recombination, and the specific alleles at the two linked loci are more likely to be inherited en bloc as a haplotype. *(Answer: C—Linkage disequilibrium)*

10. A clinical investigator studying the genetic predisposition of individuals with a family history of diabetes mellitus to develop clinical diabetes discovers a novel genetic polymorphism in a cohort of such patients.

Which of the following describes a mutation whose frequency becomes established in more than 1% to 2% of the population?

- ❑ A. A haplotype
- ❑ B. An allele
- ❑ C. A unique polymorphism
- ❑ D. A single nucleotide polymorphism

Key Concept/Objective: To understand that genetic polymorphisms with a frequency of more than 1% to 2% are alleles

The fundamental basis of genetic polymorphism in a population is variation of the nucleotide sequence of DNA at homologous locations in the genome. These differences in sequence can result from mutations involving a single nucleotide or deletions or insertions of variable numbers of contiguous nucleotides. Each of these variants presumably occurred in a single ancestor in the distant past. Most new mutations are extinguished through random genetic drift and never become established in the population at any significant frequency. When the gene frequency of a mutation becomes established at more than 1% to

2%, it is often given the appellation of allele. If there are two polymorphic positions within a gene, each of which has two alleles, a given individual will have up to four definable alleles. These are inherited as two parental haplotypes, each of which carries one allele from each of the two loci. Extensive population studies permit sophisticated maximum-likelihood estimates of haplotype frequencies within the population. The ability to deduce haplotypes provides a much higher degree of specificity to the analysis of genetic polymorphism, because the haplotype more accurately defines a larger inherited region of DNA. *(Answer: B—An allele)*

For more information, see Milford EL, Carpenter CB: 6 Immunology/Allergy: VII Immunogenetics of Disease. ACP Medicine Online (www.acpmedicine.com). Dale DC, Federman DD, Eds. WebMD Inc., New York, March 2003

Immunologic Tolerance and Autoimmunity

11. A 24-year-old black woman comes to your office complaining of bilateral hand pain, a painful mouth, and a rash on her face that is particularly bothersome when she is exposed to the sun. She has had these symptoms for 6 weeks. Her examination is remarkable for patchy alopecia and multiple mouth ulcers; the musculoskeletal examination is normal. The patient tests positive for both ANA and anti–double-stranded DNA. You make a diagnosis of systemic lupus erythematous, a disease in which autoimmunity is known to play a central role.

Which of the following is NOT a possible mechanism of tolerance?

- ❑ A. **Clonal deletion in the thymus**
- ❑ B. **Failure of T cells bearing low-affinity receptors to recognize antigens in the periphery**
- ❑ C. **Sequestration of an antigen from the immune system as a result of anatomic barriers**
- ❑ D. **Acquisition of anergy after ligation of the T cell receptor complex in the absence of costimulation**
- ❑ E. **T cells in the thymus with high affinity for a self-antigen undergo positive selection**

Key Concept/Objective: To know the mechanisms of tolerance

Immature lymphocytes are more susceptible to induction of tolerance. Tolerance can be induced in immature lymphocytes either centrally (thymus for T cells, bone marrow for B cells) or in the periphery. If a T cell has a high affinity for a self-antigen in the thymus, it can undergo negative selection with activation-induced death (apoptosis). Positive selection in the thymus occurs when T cells bearing receptors with a moderate affinity for self-antigens receive survival and maturation signals and are exported to the periphery. Normally, these cells do not cause autoimmune phenomena because of peripheral tolerance. The most common mechanism of peripheral tolerance is the failure of T cells bearing low-affinity receptors to recognize an antigen. T cells bearing receptors with high affinity for an antigen can remain in an inactivated state if that antigen is sequestered from the immune effector cells. Apoptosis is also a mechanism of peripheral tolerance. A third mechanism of peripheral tolerance involves the acquisition of anergy after ligation with the T cell receptor complex. The most extensively characterized mechanism of anergy induction occurs when the T cell receptor is ligated in the absence of costimulation. Another mechanism of tolerance is T cell-mediated suppression, in which regulatory T cells actively inhibit an immune response to an antigen. *(Answer: E—T cells in the thymus with high affinity for a self-antigen undergo positive selection)*

12. You are asked to see a 34-year-old pregnant woman in the emergency department who is experiencing shortness of breath. She has pulmonary edema, and an echocardiogram shows mitral stenosis. She is from South America. When asked, she says that many years ago, she had an illness with rash, fever, and joint pain that kept her in bed for a few weeks. On the basis of this history, you make a presumptive diagnosis of rheumatic mitral stenosis.

Which of the following constitutes the best immunologic causative mechanism of rheumatic fever?

- ❑ **A. Direct bacterial infection of the heart**
- ❑ **B. Antistreptocococcal antibodies cross-reacting with myocardial antigens**
- ❑ **C. Toxins released by group A Streptococcus that cause valvular damage**
- ❑ **D. Pathogenic autoantibodies directed against the endocardium of heart valves**

Key Concept/Objective: To understand the mechanism of molecular mimicry

In rare cases, the normal immune response to a specific microbial peptide can trigger immunity to a related self-peptide, a phenomenon known as molecular mimicry. This mechanism has been described in rheumatic heart disease and Lyme disease. In the case of rheumatic heart disease, antistreptococcal antibodies cross-react with myocardial antigens. The specific peptides have not been identified. Pathogenic autoantibodies have been clearly associated with myasthenia gravis, pemphigus, and a number of endocrinopathies but not rheumatic fever. *(Answer: B—Antistreptocococcal antibodies cross-reacting with myocardial antigens)*

For more information, see Anderson P: 6 Immunology/Allergy: IX Immunologic Tolerance and Autoimmunity. ACP Medicine Online (www.acpmedicine.com). Dale DC, Federman DD, Eds. WebMD Inc., New York, November 2002

Allergic Response

13. A 35-year-old woman with a history of asthma and atopic dermatitis presents to your office for follow-up. She was recently hospitalized for community-acquired pneumonia complicated by an acute exacerbation of her asthma.

Which of the following statements most accurately describes the T cell response to allergenic peptides in an atopic patient?

- ❑ **A. In the T_{H2} response, T cells form interleukin-4 (IL-4), IL-5, and IL-13, thereby directing the production of allergen-specific antibodies**
- ❑ **B. In the T_{H1} response, T cells produce interferon gamma (IFN-γ), thereby inducing T cell differentiation**
- ❑ **C. In the T_{HO} response, T cells produce IL-12 and IL-18, thereby causing differentiation from T_{HO} cells to T_{H1} cells**
- ❑ **D. In the T_H response, naive helper T cells differentiate into mature T lymphocytes, producing IgG1 and IgG4 antibodies**

Key Concept/Objective: To recognize T cell response in an atopic host

The pathophysiologic response to allergenic peptides such as bacterial DNA sequences differs in a normal person from an atopic patient. Bacterial DNA sequences have immunostimulatory regions containing deoxycytidine-phosphate-deoxyguanosine (CpG) repeats. CpG repeats are recognized as foreign by pattern recognition receptors called Toll-like receptor-9 (TLR-9) on antigen-presenting cells. These CpG repeats stimulate macrophages and dendritic cells to secrete inflammatory cytokines, including IL-12 and IL-18. These cytokines then induce T cells and natural-killer (NK) cells to produce IFN-γ, a cytokine known to promote nonallergic, protective responses. This pattern of response by helper T cells is termed a TH1 response, because it is associated with the differentiation of naive T helper (T_{HO}) lymphocytes into mature T_{H1} lymphocytes. Similarly, the T helper cells of persons without atopy respond to presentation of potentially allergenic peptides by producing IFN-γ and directing the production of allergen-specific IgG1 and IgG4 antibodies.

In contrast, T helper cells of atopic persons respond to processed aeroallergens by forming IL-4, IL-5, and IL-13 and by directing the production of allergen-specific IgE antibod-

ies. This type of T helper cell response is termed a T_{H2} response. IL-4 and IL-13 share a number of functions, which are mediated through the IL-4Rα/IL-13Rα heterodimer. However, only IL-4 is able to induce the differentiation of T_{H0} cells to T_{H2} cells and to antagonize the differentiation of T_{H0} cells to T_{H1} cells, resulting in IgE-mediated allergic inflammation. In contrast, both IL-12 and IFN-γ induce the differentiation to T_{H1} cells; T_{H2} cell differentiation is inhibited by IFN-γ. Differentiation to T_{H1} cells results in cell-mediated immunity and inflammation. Therefore, the differentiation of T_{H0} cells to either T_{H1} cells or T_{H2} cells appears to be the crucial event that determines which type of immune response will follow. *(Answer: A—In the T_{H2} response, T cells form interleukin-4 [IL-4], IL-5, and IL-13, thereby directing the production of allergen-specific antibodies)*

14. A 28-year-old graduate student with a history of chronic allergic rhinitis and asthma presents to your clinic. His symptoms, which are continuous, have been somewhat refractory to the therapies you have tried thus far. He recently ran across a proposed new drug therapy for asthma while reading a scientific journal. The name of this drug is omalizumab, and he asks you to explain how it works.

Which of the following responses is the most accurate answer to this patient's question?

- ❑ **A. Omalizumab is a monoclonal antibody that is directed against the tumor necrosis factor (TNF) receptor; it inhibits the action of TNF**
- ❑ **B. Omalizumab is a monoclonal antibody directed against the Fcε portion of IgE; it inhibits activation of mast cells**
- ❑ **C. Omalizumab is a monoclonal antibody directed against the IL-5 receptor; it inhibits eosinophil development**
- ❑ **D. Omalizumab is a cyclic polypeptide immunosuppressant that suppresses inflammation**

Key Concept/Objective: To understand the mechanism of action of omalizumab, a promising new therapeutic agent directed against allergic response

Clearly, treatment that interferes with IgE activation of mast cells and basophils may be beneficial. Omalizumab, a recombinant, humanized monoclonal antibody directed against the Fcε portion of IgE, has recently been developed. Important features of this anti-IgE molecule are (1) it does not bind IgE already attached to FcεRI and, therefore, does not cause anaphylaxis; (2) it does not activate complement; and (3) it has a much longer half-life than IgE. In phase III trials, omalizumab was administered by subcutaneous injections given every 2 or 4 weeks to patients with allergic rhinitis or with allergic asthma of varying severity. All studies showed dramatic reductions in free IgE levels that were dependent on omalizumab dose as well as baseline IgE levels. The posttreatment level of free IgE directly correlated with reduced symptom scores, reduced use of rescue medication, and improved quality of life. For asthma, significant reductions in asthma exacerbations, in hospitalizations for asthma, and in the dose of inhaled or oral steroids were also found. As levels of serum IgE decreased, so did surface expression of FcåRI on basophils. *(Answer: B—Omalizumab is a monoclonal antibody directed against the Fcε portion of IgE; it inhibits activation of mast cells)*

15. An 18-year-old woman is brought to the emergency department after a bee sting. She is flushed and in mild respiratory distress. She is afebrile. Her heart rate is 110 beats/min; her blood pressure is 80/40 mm Hg; and her respiratory rate is 28 breaths/min. As you prepare to initiate supportive therapy and empirical treatment for anaphylaxis, the nurse, who has drawn blood, asks what tests you would like to order.

Which of the following serum markers, if elevated, most consistently suggests anaphylaxis as the cause of hypotension?

- ❑ **A. Histamine**
- ❑ **B. Chymase**
- ❑ **C. Cathepsin G**
- ❑ **D. Tryptase**

Key Concept/Objective: To know a serum marker that identifies anaphylaxis as a cause of hypotension

Peak plasma levels of histamine occur 5 minutes after insect-sting-induced anaphylaxis begins and decline to baseline within 20 minutes. Because they are relatively transient, these histamine elevations in plasma are difficult to utilize for the clinical determination of anaphylaxis as a cause of hypotension. However, tryptase diffuses into, and is removed from, the circulation more slowly than histamine. Tryptase levels peak in the circulation 15 minutes to 2 hours after mast cell degranulation and decline with a half-life of about 2 hours. Peak levels during insect-sting–induced anaphylaxis correlate closely to the drop in mean arterial blood pressure, which is an important measure of clinical severity. For that reason, serum or plasma tryptase levels have recently been recognized as a clinically useful marker for the diagnosis of systemic anaphylaxis. *(Answer: D—Tryptase)*

16. A 42-year-old woman presents to your clinic complaining of continuing allergic rhinitis. A biopsy of her nasal mucosa would almost certainly reveal eosinophils. There are several mechanisms that lead to the preferential accumulation of eosinophils, rather than neutrophils, at sites of allergic inflammation.

Of the following mediators and receptors, which is specifically involved with eosinophil chemotaxis?

- ❑ **A. Leukotriene C4 (LTC4)**
- ❑ **B. CCR3 chemokine receptor**
- ❑ **C. Very late antigen–4 (VLA-4)**
- ❑ **D. All of the above**

Key Concept/Objective: To understand the different receptors and mediators involved in the preferential accumulation of eosinophils as compared with neutrophils

Receptors for complement (C3a and C5a); the lipid mediators platelet-activating factor (PAF), LTC4, and LTB4; and numerous cytokines and chemokines bind to and activate eosinophils. Chemokines of the C-C family play an important chemotactic role for eosinophils. Chemokines of this family have the same receptors. A particular C-C chemokine receptor, CCR3, is found abundantly on eosinophils but not on neutrophils. CCR3 binds at least four chemokines that play crucial roles in the homing of eosinophils to epithelial tissues and that activate eosinophils to release mediators. Another mechanism, which leads to preferential accumulation of eosinophils rather than neutrophils at sites of allergic inflammation, relates to differences in expression of surface adhesion molecules. Eosinophils and neutrophils share several selectins and integrins that initiate rolling of circulating cells along the endothelium, as well as the subsequent firm adhesion, diapedesis, and transmigration of these cells through the vessel wall. However, eosinophils—but not neutrophils—express an integrin, VLA-4, whose ligand on endothelial cells (VCAM-1) is upregulated by IL-4 and IL-13, cytokines that are present during T_{H2} responses. *(Answer: D—All of the above)*

For more information, see Daffern PJ, Schwartz LB: 6 Immunology/Allergy: X Allergic Response. ACP Medicine Online (www.acpmedicine.com). Dale DC, Federman DD, Eds. WebMD Inc., New York, February 2003

Diagnostic and Therapeutic Principles in Allergy

17. A 28-year-old man presents to your clinic for evaluation of allergies. He has a long history consistent with allergic rhinoconjunctivitis but also experiences urticarial lesions when he eats certain types of food. He also occasionally has back pain from a recent sports injury. His medications include loratadine and low-dose corticosteroids, which were prescribed by his primary care doctor, as well as ibuprofen and a daily baby aspirin. You decide to perform skin testing on the patient.

Which of the following interventions should you recommend before performing epicutaneous testing?

- ❑ **A. The patient should discontinue all medications 1 week before testing**
- ❑ **B. The patient should discontinue loratadine and steroids 3 days before testing**

❑ C. **The patient should discontinue loratadine 1 week before testing**

❑ D. **The patient should discontinue loratadine, steroids, and ibuprofen 1 week before testing**

Key Concept/Objective: To understand the use and preparation of skin tests

Of the two most common tests for allergy, skin testing and serologic testing, the former is the more rapid and sensitive. The premise for allergy testing is the interaction of an allergen with specific IgE that is either mast cell-bound or basophil-bound. To elicit a positive reaction, degranulation of mast cells or basophils must occur and histamine must be released. Therefore, medications that inhibit histamine release and activity must be discontinued before testing. These medications mainly include antihistamines; however, other medications, such as tricyclic antidepressants, may have some antihistaminic activity as well. Most antihistamines need to be discontinued 1 week before testing; however, diphenhydramine and chlorpheniramine can be discontinued 3 days before testing. Medications such as corticosteroids do not inhibit the immediate-phase response of antihistamines and therefore can be continued. Aspirin and ibuprofen have no effect on degranulation and histamine release. *(Answer: C—The patient should discontinue loratadine 1 week before testing)*

18. A 35-year-old man comes to your office with symptoms of nasal congestion and itchy eyes and throat. He has been experiencing such symptoms for several years. Symptoms are present throughout the year, and he is able to enjoy outdoor activities without worsening of the symptoms. He owns a cat, which does not sleep in the same room with him. You order allergy skin testing and receive a report indicating a positive response to dust mites and cat dander.

Which of the following therapeutic interventions is the most effective for this patient's symptoms?

❑ A. **Antihistamines**

❑ B. **Removal of the allergen from the patient's environment**

❑ C. **Leukotriene receptor antagonists**

❑ D. **Cromolyn sodium**

Key Concept/Objective: To understand the importance of environmental control of atopic disease

Despite the advances in medications and pharmacologic therapy for allergic illnesses, the most effective therapeutic intervention is still removal of the offending agent or allergen from the patient's environment. This includes appropriate linens for mattresses and pillows, adequate cleaning, and lowering the ambient humidity in the house to minimize mold spores. Pets should be removed from the house or kept out of the room at all times. Patients sensitive to pollen should try to minimize the amount of time spent outdoors during those times of the year when the specific pollen is prevalent. *(Answer: B—Removal of the allergen from the patient's environment)*

For more information, see Grayson MH, Korenblat P: 6 Immunology/Allergy: XI Diagnostic and Therapeutic Principles in Allergy. ACP Medicine Online (www.acpmedicine.com). Dale DC, Federman DD, Eds. WebMD Inc., New York, September 2002

Allergic Rhinitis, Conjunctivitis, and Sinusitis

19. A 20-year-old woman comes to your office in early spring with complaints of nasal congestion, runny nose, and paroxysms of sneezing. She has been experiencing these symptoms for 10 days. She denies having fever, cough, myalgias, or malaise. She states that she typically experiences bouts of similar symptoms in September and October. Her medical history includes mild intermittent asthma since childhood. On examination, she has dark rings under her eyes but no sinus tenderness. The nasal mucosa appears pale and swollen, and there is clear rhinorrhea.

Which of the following statements regarding this patient's condition is false?

- ❑ A. **Nasal smear is likely to show a preponderance of eosinophils**
- ❑ B. **Her symptoms are the result of the IgE-mediated release of substances such as histamine that increase epithelial permeability**
- ❑ C. **Treatment of the condition can result in improvement of coexisting asthma in certain patients**
- ❑ D. **Although daily nasal steroid sprays can alleviate symptoms, they are generally not recommended because of the risk of rhinitis medicamentosa**
- ❑ E. **Immunotherapy can be employed in patients whose symptoms persist despite the avoidance of triggers and the use of pharmacotherapy**

Key Concept/Objective: To understand the diagnosis and treatment of allergic rhinitis

Allergic rhinitis is the most common atopic disorder in children and adults in the United States. The airborne allergens responsible for the condition may be seasonal (such as pollen, grass, and mold) or perennial (such as dust mites, pet dander, and insects). In genetically predisposed persons, the antigens crosslink IgE molecules that are attached to mast cells and basophils, resulting in the release of mediators such as histamine that cause increased epithelial permeability, vasodilatation, and stimulation of a parasympathetic reflex. In addition to the common nasal symptoms, patients may display dark circles under their eyes ("allergic shiners") and a nasal crease caused by continual upward rubbing of the tip of the nose (the "allergic salute"). Nasal smear often shows a preponderance of eosinophils (in infectious rhinitis, neutrophils predominate). In patients with coexisting asthma, control of allergic rhinitis may improve asthma control. The three arms of treatment of allergic rhinitis include trigger avoidance, pharmacotherapy (with antihistamines, decongestants, and nasal steroids), and, in certain cases, immunotherapy. The daily use of inhaled corticosteroids is the most effective therapy. Their use is not generally associated with systemic side effects. Long-term use of nasal decongestants should be avoided because this can result in rhinitis medicamentosa: an overuse syndrome in which symptoms are perpetuated. *(Answer: D—Although daily nasal steroid sprays can alleviate symptoms, they are generally not recommended because of the risk of rhinitis medicamentosa)*

20. A 45-year-old man with a history of seasonal allergic rhinitis presents with complaints of itching, tearing, and mild burning of both eyes. He has had these symptoms for several days. He has not had any vision changes or systemic symptoms. He reports that the ocular symptoms began in association with nasal congestion and rhinorrhea, a pattern he has experienced in the past. You suspect that he has allergic conjunctivitis.

Which of the following statements regarding the diagnosis and treatment of allergic conjunctivitis is false?

- ❑ A. **Bilateral involvement, although not universal, helps to distinguish the condition from acute infectious conjunctivitis**
- ❑ B. **The presence of another atopic disorder such as allergic rhinitis, asthma, or atopic dermatitis (eczema) is present in approximately three fourths of patients with ocular allergy**
- ❑ C. **Corticosteroid eyedrops are the most effective treatment and are generally given as first-line agents**
- ❑ D. **Patients with viral or bacterial conjunctivitis are more likely to complain of pain and to display matting of the eyelids and purulent ocular discharge**

Key Concept/Objective: To understand the diagnosis and treatment of allergic conjunctivitis

Allergic conjunctivitis is the ocular counterpart of allergic rhinitis. A majority of patients with this condition (approximately 70%) have another atopic condition, such as asthma, eczema, or allergic rhinitis. Symptoms usually include bilateral itching, tearing, and burning of the eyes. Findings on examination include conjunctival injection and periocular edema and erythema. If the patient has had direct hand-to-eye contact with an allergen

such as pet dander, there may be unilateral involvement. The differential diagnosis includes viral or bacterial conjunctivitis: patients with infectious conjunctivitis more often have mucopurulent discharge with matting of eyelids, deeply red conjunctivae, and less bothersome itching than patients with allergic conjunctivitis. The first-line treatment consists of over-the-counter eyedrops containing a combination of antihistamine and decongestant (e.g., antazoline and naphazoline). Other treatments include selective H_1 receptor antihistamine drops and, in severe or refractory cases, ophthalmic glucocorticoid preparations. Steroid eyedrops should be given only in consultation with an ophthalmologist because long-term use of these agents is associated with an increased risk of cataracts, glaucoma, and secondary ocular infection. *(Answer: C—Corticosteroid eyedrops are the most effective treatment and are generally given as first-line agents)*

21. An 18-year-old man comes to clinic complaining of nasal stuffiness, left-sided maxillary tooth pain, and postnasal drip. He has had these symptoms for more than 2 months. After the first 2 weeks of symptoms, he was seen in a walk-in clinic and given a 5-day course of antibiotics, but his symptoms did not improve significantly. He has not had fever or chills but complains that he wakes up with a sore throat on most days; the throat pain tends to get better as the day goes on. On examination, he is afebrile, with mild tenderness to palpation over the left maxilla and left forehead. His posterior oropharynx is slightly erythematous, with yellowish drainage present, but there is no tonsillar exudate. Examination of the nares reveals hyperemic mucosa and mucopurulent discharge.

Which of the following statements regarding this patient's condition is true?

- ❑ **A. Chronic sinusitis can be defined as sinus inflammation that persists for more than 3 weeks**
- ❑ **B. Sinus radiographs are the procedure of choice for evaluating patients suspected of having chronic sinusitis**
- ❑ **C. It is likely that anaerobic bacteria are the primary pathogens responsible for this patient's condition**
- ❑ **D. Nasal culture has sufficient sensitivity and specificity to guide further antimicrobial therapy**
- ❑ **E. In patients with medically resistant chronic sinusitis, further workup for conditions such as cystic fibrosis, structural abnormality, or fungal infection is appropriate**

Key Concept/Objective: To understand the approach to chronic sinusitis

Rhinosinusitis can be classified as acute or chronic. Acute rhinosinusitis is defined as sinusitis that persists for more than 8 weeks in adults and for more than 12 weeks in children. Chronic sinusitis is defined as sinusitis that persists from 8 to 12 weeks or as documented sinus inflammation that persists for more than 4 weeks after initiation of appropriate medical therapy. This patient has findings consistent with chronic sinusitis, which may occur after acute sinusitis if mucopus is not sufficiently evacuated. Patients often have unilateral nasal congestion and discharge, purulent postnasal secretions, fetid breath, and facial pain. Although it was previously thought that anaerobic organisms were responsible for chronic sinusitis, it has recently been shown that aerobes are likely the primary pathogens. Chronic inflammation, rather than infection, may be the most important etiologic factor in many patients. Alhough nasal culture does not adequately reflect the bacterial pathogens that may play a role in sinusitis, microscopic examination of nasal secretions may help in diagnosis; for instance, sheets of polymorphonuclear leukocytes and bacteria suggest sinusitis, whereas predominance of eosinophils suggests allergic rhinitis. The diagnostic value of plain films (which may demonstrate mucosal thickening, air-fluid levels, or opacification) is controversial; currently, limited coronal computed tomography of the paranasal sinuses is considered the radiographic test of choice. Whereas cost was once prohibitive, costs are roughly comparable between the two imaging techniques at present. CT may additionally give useful anatomic detail that radiographs cannot and can better rule out the possibility of an anatomic abnormality that has predisposed the patient to chronic obstruction of sinus drainage. Other important considerations in a patient who has failed to respond to appropriate therapy include cystic fibrosis (especially in a younger patient with recurrent or chronic sinusitis), infection with an atyp-

ical organism such as a fungus, and Wegener granulomatosis. *(Answer: E—In patients with medically resistant chronic sinusitis, further workup for conditions such as cystic fibrosis, structural abnormality, or fungal infection is appropriate)*

For more information, see Slavin RG: 6 Immunology/Allergy: XII Allergic Rhinitis, Conjunctivitis, and Sinusitis. ACP Medicine Online (www.acpmedicine.com). Dale DC, Federman DD, Eds. WebMD Inc., New York, January 2005

Urticaria, Angioedema, and Anaphylaxis

22. A 43-year-old woman comes to your clinic complaining of nonhealing hives. She says that she started having hives 6 weeks ago. The hives are mildly pruritic. When asked, she says that each individual hive lasts for 2 or 3 days. Physical examination reveals multiple urticarial papules that do not blanch on diascopy. You ask the patient to come back to your clinic after 3 days, and you confirm that some of the lesions are still present.

On the basis of this patient's history and physical examination, what would be the next step in the workup?

- ❑ **A. Administer thyroid function tests**
- ❑ **B. Perform an abdominal CT scan to rule out an intra-abdominal malignancy**
- ❑ **C. Check sinus films, hepatitis serology, and stool studies for ova and parasites**
- ❑ **D. Perform a biopsy of one of the lesions**

Key Concept/Objective: To understand the indication for biopsy in cases of urticaria

Urticaria is a very common disorder, and an etiology cannot be found in the majority of cases. The patient described here has urticarial lesions, each of which persists for more than 24 hours. Generalized urticarial lesions that persist for longer than 24 hours, produce a burning sensation, or are not very pruritic may be a manifestation of vasculitis. Lesions associated with rheumatic illness usually do not blanch on diascopy and may result in ecchymosis and eventually hyperpigmentation. A biopsy should be performed on any urticaria that lasts more than 24 hours, is only mildly pruritic or nonpruritic, is associated with vesicles or bullae, or does not respond to appropriate therapy. The subtleties of the histologic variances demand interpretation by a dermatopathologist. Approximately 5% to 10% of patients with chronic urticaria have been reported to have antithyroid antibodies, but there is only anecdotal evidence that treating these patients with thyroid hormone leads to a significant improvement. Lymphomas and carcinomas may promote urticaria, but urticaria in patients with neoplasms is usually coincidental. In most cases the malignancy is known, and current evidence does not warrant routinely subjecting patients with unexplained urticaria to an exhaustive evaluation for an occult neoplasm. Urticaria has been associated with several different infections, but extensive searches for infections as the cause of urticaria are consistently unsuccessful. *(Answer: D—Perform a biopsy of one of the lesions)*

23. A 34-year-old man presents to your clinic complaining of a recurrent, extremely pruritic rash on his trunk and back. The rash started a few months ago. The rash comes and goes; the patient thinks it appears when he exercises or eats spicy foods. Physical examination reveals multiple 2 to 3 mm scattered papular wheals surrounded by large, erythematous flares.

Which of the following is a likely diagnosis for this patient?

- ❑ **A. Cholinergic urticaria**
- ❑ **B. Pressure urticaria**
- ❑ **C. Idiopathic urticaria**
- ❑ **D. Aquagenic urticaria**

Key Concept/Objective: To understand the different forms of urticaria

There are several forms of physical urticaria with distinct clinical presentations. Papular urticaria consists of 4 to 8 mm wheals, often grouped in clusters and especially appearing in areas of exposed skin. Papular urticaria is very pruritic; it is usually caused by insect bites. Delayed pressure urticaria results from localized, continuous pressure (4 to 6 hours). The lesions of cold urticaria develop 5 to 30 minutes after exposure to cold, and cold urticaria can be caused by wind, water, and contact. Solar urticaria is a rare idiopathic disorder in which erythema heralds a pruritic wheal that appears within 5 minutes of exposure to a specific wavelength of light and dissipates within 15 minutes to 3 hours after onset. Aquagenic urticaria appears 2 to 30 minutes after water immersion, regardless of water temperature. The lesions of cholinergic urticaria are highly distinctive: they consist of 2 to 3 mm scattered papular wheals surrounded by large, erythematous flares. These lesions are extremely pruritic; they may affect the entire body but often spare the palms, soles, and axilla. Precipitating stimuli include exercise, warm temperature, ingestion of hot or spicy foods, and possibly emotional stress. The condition often remits within several years but can last for more than 30 years. The diagnosis can be made by provocation with exercise or a hot bath. *(Answer: A—Cholinergic urticaria)*

24. While traveling in an airplane, a flight attendant asks you to evaluate a 44-year-old woman who has sudden onset or urticaria, flushing, pruritus, shortness of breath, nausea, and vomiting. You learn that she has a history of allergy to peanuts and that she may have eaten some without knowing it. On physical examination, the patient is alert and is in moderate respiratory distress. Her blood pressure is 90/50 mm Hg, and her heart rate 120 beats/min. She has diffuse inspiratory and expiratory wheezing, and she is experiencing diffuse urticaria.

What is the most appropriate treatment for this patient?

- ❑ A. **Administer oxygen and start I.V. steroids and I.V. fluids; the flight can be continued**
- ❑ B. **Start an I.V., inject 1 mg of epinephrine I.V., and give I.V. steroids, I.V. fluids, and oxygen; the flight can be continued**
- ❑ C. **Administer oxygen and epinephrine subcutaneously or intramuscularly, give I.V. antihistamines and I.V. fluids, start steroids, and ask the pilot to land and transport the patient to an emergency care facility**
- ❑ D. **Give oral antihistamines and oral prednisone and continue to watch the patient for further clinical deterioration**

Key Concept/Objective: To understand the appropriate treatment of anaphylaxis

Anaphylaxis is an explosive, massive activation of mast cells, with release of their inflammatory mediators to the skin, respiratory tract, and circulatory system. The classic symptoms of anaphylaxis include flushing, urticaria, angioedema, pruritus, bronchospasm, and abdominal cramping with nausea, vomiting, and diarrhea. Hypotension and shock can result from intravascular volume loss, vasodilation, and myocardial dysfunction. The essential steps in the treatment of anaphylaxis are prevention, recognition, prompt therapy, and early transport to an emergency care facility. Anaphylaxis can rarely be overtreated. Treatment must be expeditious and appropriate. Supplemental oxygen should be given, and aqueous epinephrine (1:1,000) should be administered subcutaneously or intramuscularly. The epinephrine dose is 0.2 to 0.5 mg in adults and 0.01 mg/kg in children. If the patient is in cardiopulmonary arrest, epinephrine (1:10,000) should be administered intravenously in a dose of 0.1 to 1 mg in adults and 0.001 to 0.002 mg in children. Intravenous H_1 antihistamines and H_2 antihistamines should be given. Once the reaction is under control, systemic corticosteroids may be administered, and the patient should be transferred to an emergency care facility. *(Answer: C—Administer oxygen and epinephrine subcutaneously or intramuscularly, give I.V. antihistamines and I.V. fluids, start steroids, and ask the pilot to land and transport the patient to an emergency care facility)*

For more information, see Beltrani VS: 6 Immunology/Allergy: XIII Urticaria, Angioedema, and Anaphylaxis. ACP Medicine Online (www.acpmedicine.com). Dale DC, Federman DD, Eds. WebMD Inc., New York, February 2003

Drug Allergies

25. A 50-year-old woman is admitted to the hospital with a history of subjective fever of 2 weeks' duration. The patient underwent mitral valve replacement surgery 5 years ago; in addition, she once experienced an allergic reaction to penicillin, which she describes as a rash that occurred a few minutes after she received a single dose of I.V. penicillin. Physical examination is remarkable for the presence of a diastolic and systolic murmur in the mitral area. Transthoracic echocardiography shows a vegetation in the mitral valve. Blood cultures show penicillin-sensitive viridans streptococci.

On the basis of this patient's history of penicillin allergy, which of the following would be the most appropriate course of action?

- ❑ **A. Start a cephalosporin**
- ❑ **B. Administer a penicillin skin test before starting antibiotics**
- ❑ **C. Start a different β-lactam, such as imipenem**
- ❑ **D. Start vancomycin**

Key Concept/Objective: To understand the management of penicillin allergy

Penicillin is among the most common causes of immunologic drug reactions. Most deaths from penicillin allergies occur in patients who have no history of penicillin allergy. Nonimmunologic rashes are frequently seen with ampicillin or amoxicillin in patients who have concomitant viral infections, chronic lymphocytic leukemia, or hyperuricemia, as well as in those taking allopurinol. These rashes are typically nonpruritic and are not associated with an increased risk of future intolerance of penicillin antibiotics. Most immunologic reactions to penicillins are directed against β-lactam core determinants and are IgE dependent. Patients who have suffered IgE-mediated penicillin reactions tend to lose their sensitivity over time if penicillin is avoided. By 5 years after an immediate reaction, 50% of patients have negative skin tests. Skin testing with a major determinant preparation and penicillin G identifies 90% to 93% of patients at risk for immediate reaction to penicillin. Not everyone with a history of a reaction to penicillin should undergo skin testing, but it is important to perform such tests in patients who have a history of anaphylaxis or urticaria associated with penicillin use. Patients who have had maculopapular or morbilliform skin rashes are not at higher risk for immediate skin reaction, but skin testing may be considered because studies have demonstrated that patient histories can be unreliable. Cephalosporins and penicillin share a similar bicyclic β-lactam structure; patients with a history of penicillin allergy are more likely than the general population to have a reaction. Carbapenems (imipenem) and carbacephems can have significant cross-reactivity with penicillin. Vancomycin would not be indicated in this patient if a skin test can be obtained; if the skin test is positive, desensitization to penicillin can be performed. *(Answer: B—Administer a penicillin skin test before starting antibiotics)*

26. A 33-year-old man is admitted to the hospital with fever, knee pain, and swelling. Physical examination is remarkable for fever and a swollen, red, painful right knee. Arthrocentesis shows gram-positive cocci in clusters and 150,000 white blood cells. The patient is started on vancomycin. After a few minutes, you are called to see the patient, who is complaining of flushing and back pain. His blood pressure is 90/60 mm Hg, and he has a diffuse erythematous macular rash on his trunk, abdomen, and legs.

Which of the following would be the most appropriate course of action for this patient?

- ❑ **A. Administer 0.3 mg of epinephrine I.M., 50 mg of diphenhydramine I.V., and 125 mg of methylprednisolone I.V.**
- ❑ **B. Discontinue vancomycin; await culture results and sensitivities before restarting antibiotics**
- ❑ **C. Slow down the vancomycin infusion rate and premedicate with diphenhydramine**
- ❑ **D. Obtain a vancomycin skin test**

Key Concept/Objective: To be able to recognize the red-man syndrome

This patient has the characteristic clinical presentation of the vancomycin-related red-man syndrome, which is characterized by hypotension, flushing, erythema, pruritus, urticaria, and pain or muscle spasms of the chest and back. The syndrome is caused by non–IgE-mediated histamine release that is more likely with rapid infusion rates (> 10 mg/min). Tolerance of readministration is promoted by reduction of the infusion rate and pretreatment with H_1 (but not H_2) antihistamines. Anaphylaxis is treated with epinephrine, H_1 and H_2 blockers, and steroids. However, this patient's clinical picture is more suggestive of the red-man syndrome. The patient has septic arthritis, so antibiotics are indicated and cannot be stopped at this time. Rarer IgE-mediated reactions to vancomycin can be identified by skin tests if the clinical picture suggests an IgE-mediated mechanism. *(Answer: C—Slow down the vancomycin infusion rate and premedicate with diphenhydramine)*

27. A 45-year-old man with a history of diabetes and hypertension comes to the emergency department with chest pain. He is found to have a myocardial infarction with ST segment depression. After 4 days in the hospital, the patient has recurrent chest pain; ECG changes are consistent with further ischemia. His cardiologist schedules cardiac catheterization; however, the patient says that 10 years ago, when he had an abdominal CT scan, he had a bad reaction to intravenous contrast.

Which of the following would be the most appropriate approach in the management of this patient?

- ❑ **A. Proceed with the catheterization; premedicate with corticosteroids and antihistamines; use nonionic contrast**
- ❑ **B. Perform a contrast media radioallergosorbent test (RAST)**
- ❑ **C. Continue with medical management**
- ❑ **D. Obtain a contrast media skin test**

Key Concept/Objective: To understand the management of patients who are allergic to contrast media

Radiographic contrast media cause non–IgE-mediated anaphylactoid reactions that involve direct mast cell and perhaps complement activation. A previous anaphylactoid reaction to contrast at any time in a patient's history is predictive of persistently increased risk of a repeated anaphylactoid reaction, even though the patient may have tolerated contrast without a reaction in the interim. The use of nonionic contrast media and medication pretreatment can reduce the risk of reaction. One commonly used pretreatment regimen consists of corticosteroids, antihistamines, and oral adrenergic agents. This patient has a clear indication for cardiac catheterization and should undergo the procedure after premedication. Skin tests, RAST, and test dosing are not helpful in predicting a reaction. *(Answer: A—Proceed with the catheterization; premedicate with corticosteroids and antihistamines; use nonionic contrast)*

28. A 34-year-old woman with AIDS is admitted to the hospital with altered mental status. During workup, she is found to test positive on a Venereal Disease Research Laboratory (VDRL) test and to have elevated levels of white cells in her cerebrospinal fluid. The patient is diagnosed with neurosyphilis. Her sister reports that 15 years ago, the patient had an allergic reaction to penicillin; she describes this reaction as involving lip swelling, hives that appeared all over the patient's body, shortness of breath, low blood pressure, and diarrhea. These symptoms occurred 10 minutes after receiving a penicillin shot.

Which of the following would be the most appropriate course of action for this patient?

- ❑ **A. Premedicate with corticosteroids and antihistamines; start penicillin**
- ❑ **B. Start ceftriaxone**
- ❑ **C. Do not start penicillin; consider erythromycin**
- ❑ **D. Consult an allergist for desensitization**

Key Concept/Objective: To understand the indications for desensitization

This patient had a life-threatening reaction to penicillin in the past; however, she currently has an infection that is best treated with penicillin. If the probability of a drug allergy is high and drug administration is essential, one may consider desensitization, in which the

drug is administered in increasing doses in small increments. Because of the risk of adverse reactions, only experienced physicians should perform desensitization. Once desensitization is achieved, the drug must be continued or desensitization will be lost; the patient would then require repeated desensitization before readministration. Pretreatment with antihistamines and corticosteroids is not reliable for preventing IgE-mediated anaphylaxis. Patients with a history of penicillin allergy are more likely than the general population to have a reaction, which can be severe. Cephalosporins and erythromycin are not appropriate treatment options for neurosyphilis. *(Answer: D—Consult an allergist for desensitization)*

For more information, see Dykewicz MS, Gray H: 6 Immunology/Allergy: XIV Drug Allergies. ACP Medicine Online (www.acpmedicine.com). Dale DC, Federman DD, Eds. WebMD Inc., New York, August 2003

Allergic Reactions to Hymenoptera

29. Allergic reactions to insect stings can be either local or systemic. They result primarily from the stings of insects of the Hymenoptera order, which includes bees, wasps, and imported fire ants. In the United States, at least 40 deaths occur each year as a result of insect stings.

Which of the following statements is false?

- ❑ **A. A person who has suffered a number of uneventful stings in the past has no risk of a significant allergic reaction to future stings**
- ❑ **B. Although almost 20% of adults demonstrate allergic antibodies to Hymenoptera venom, only 3% of adults and 1% of children suffer from anaphylaxis as the result of being stung**
- ❑ **C. Fatalities from systemic allergic reactions are more common in people older than 45 years**
- ❑ **D. A person's risk of anaphylaxis varies in accordance with reactions to previous stings and with results of venom skin tests and radioallergosorbent tests (RASTs) for specific IgE antibodies**

Key Concept/Objective: To understand important epidemiologic aspects of allergic reactions to Hymenoptera stings

Insect stings, which usually cause only minor local injury to the victim, can cause both local and systemic allergic reactions. Such reactions can occur in patients of all ages and may be preceded by a number of uneventful stings. Systemic (anaphylactic) reactions to Hymenoptera stings occur in approximately 1% of children and 3% of adults. An estimated 10% of adults may experience large local reactions that consist of prolonged swelling at the site of envenomation. Fatal anaphylactic reactions can occur at any age but are more common in adults older than 45 years. Half of the persons who experience a fatal reaction has no history of allergy to insect stings. RAST can detect venom-specific IgE antibodies in the bloodstream of patients with Hymenoptera allergy, although these antibodies are also found in a large number of adults (17% to 26% of the adult population) who have no history of allergic reactions. *(Answer: A—A person who has suffered a number of uneventful stings in the past has no risk of a significant allergic reaction to future stings)*

30. A patient who in the past suffered from anaphylaxis after a bee sting has recently moved from New York to the southeastern United States. She is concerned about increased exposure to stinging insects in this part of the country and asks your advice.

Which one of the following statements might you include in a discussion with this patient regarding the distribution and behavior of various families of Hymenoptera?

- ❑ **A. Africanized honeybees ("killer bees") are present in the southeastern United States and pose a larger threat in terms of anaphylaxis because the antigen in their venom is unique and is more potent than that found in typical honeybees and bumblebees**

- ❑ B. **Yellow jackets are relatively docile and tend to stay away from human beings, and they thus pose little threat to this patient**
- ❑ C. **Imported fire ants have increasingly become a problem in the southeast but do not tend to cause allergic reactions, because they cause injury only by biting, not stinging**
- ❑ D. **Paper wasps, which often build open nests under windowsills or eaves, have the ability to sting multiple times**

Key Concept/Objective: To know general aspects about the behavior of Hymenoptera to appropriately counsel a patient regarding avoidance

A basic familiarity with the families of the Hymenoptera order can help the clinician to establish the cause of an allergic reaction and to educate patients regarding avoidance. Many insects are more abundant in warmer climates, such as those in the southeastern United States; if this patient spends a significant amount of time outdoors, she may be at increased risk of exposure to stinging insects. The three most important families of Hymenoptera in terms of allergic reactions are the bees (including honeybees and bumblebees), the vespids (including yellow jackets, hornets, and wasps), and imported fire ants. Honeybees are relatively docile and usually do not sting unless provoked. Often, exposure occurs as a result of gardening or stepping on a bee with a bare foot. Africanized honeybees ("killer bees") are present in the southern United States; they have a tendency to swarm with little provocation and to sting in large numbers. Their venom is identical to that of the common honeybee, and an individual sting is no more potent. Unlike honeybees, vespids, such as yellow jackets and wasps, can sting multiple times. Yellow jackets scavenge food and are often found around picnics and garbage cans. They are aggressive and will sting without provocation: thus, allergic persons should be on the lookout for yellow jackets in the appropriate settings. Paper wasps are abundant in the southeastern United States and along the Gulf Coast; they build nests under overhangs. Imported fire ants have become an increasing hazard; their sting induces a unique sterile pustule that is readily recognized. *(Answer: D—Paper wasps, which often build open nests under windowsills or eaves, have the ability to sting multiple times)*

31. A mother and her 14-year-old son are in your office. Several months ago, the boy was stung by a wasp. He subsequently developed severe swelling at the site of envenomation; the swelling increased over 24 hours and persisted for several days. He did not, however, develop generalized urticaria, dyspnea, dysphonia, or weakness. The mother is concerned about the possibility of his having a life-threatening reaction to stings and wants to know what to look for and what tests can be done to determine his risk.

Which of the following statements is false?

- ❑ A. **Involvement of the pulmonary and circulatory systems distinguishes a systemic allergic reaction from a severe localized cutaneous reaction**
- ❑ B. **RAST must be interpreted in light of the patient's allergic history because venom-specific IgE antibodies may be present in patients who have never demonstrated an allergic reaction to stings**
- ❑ C. **RAST is less sensitive than skin testing, and up to 15% to 20% of patients with a documented anaphylactic reaction and positive skin-test results may have undetectable levels of venom-specific IgE antibodies**
- ❑ D. **The degree of reaction to a venom skin test (as measured by the size of the wheal and flare) closely correlates with the severity of a patient's allergic reaction to stings**

Key Concept/Objective: To be able to use clinical and laboratory information to diagnose allergic reactions to Hymenoptera stings

Allergic reactions to stings are IgE mediated and may be local or systemic. Local reactions are late-phase reactions consisting of swelling at the site of the sting: they may be massive and cause considerable pain. Systemic reactions, although sometimes localized to the skin (especially in children, who may develop only generalized urticaria), may also involve the pulmonary, circulatory, and gastrointestinal systems and are a medical emergency. Skin

testing and RAST can help establish the diagnosis of allergy in a patient with a history that suggests the patient is at risk. Skin testing is more sensitive for detecting allergy (up to 20% of patients with a positive skin test and documented allergic reaction to a sting may not have detectable IgE with RAST), but the size of the wheal and flare reaction has absolutely no relation to the severity of the allergic response to a sting. RAST should not be performed as a screening test in patients without an appropriate clinical history, because adults who never develop allergic reactions may demonstrate venom-specific IgE antibodies. *(Answer: D—The degree of reaction to a venom skin test [as measured by the size of the wheal and flare] closely correlates with the severity of a patient's allergic reaction to stings)*

32. A 25-year-old woman with a history of eczema presents to the emergency department 2 hours after being stung by a bee while gardening. Initially, swelling occurred at the site of the sting; this was followed by a diffuse urticarial eruption, dyspnea, wheezing, and dizziness. At the triage station, she is awake but somewhat lethargic. She is using accessory muscles to breathe. Her blood pressure is 94/32 mm Hg, and her heart rate is 112 beats/min.

Which of the following statements concerning this patient is false?

- ❑ **A. Epinephrine is the initial drug of choice for anaphylactic reactions and may be lifesaving**
- ❑ **B. If the patient demonstrates initial improvement after treatment, it is safe to discharge her home after observing her for 2 to 4 hours**
- ❑ **C. Corticosteroids such as hydrocortisone are appropriate to administer, although their ability to prevent late-phase reactions is debated**
- ❑ **D. Before discharge, the patient should be instructed on the use of self-administered epinephrine**

Key Concept/Objective: To understand the acute treatment of anaphylaxis

Anaphylactic reactions to insect stings must be recognized promptly and treated urgently; failure to do so can result in patient mortality. Patients with evidence of laryngeal edema, bronchospasm, or hypotension should receive intravenous or intramuscular epinephrine without delay because it has the potential to reverse these effects. Milder reactions can be treated with subcutaneous epinephrine. It should be noted that patients taking beta blockers may be resistant to the effects of epinephrine in this setting. Other supportive measures include continuous pulse oximetry, administration of intravenous fluids, and frequent monitoring of vital signs. Additional pharmacologic adjuncts include H_1 and H_2 receptor antagonists, such as diphenhydramine and ranitidine; pressors, such as dopamine; and corticosteroids. There is conflicting evidence on the ability of steroids to prevent late-phase reactions, but their relatively low risk-to-benefit ratio warrants their use in most cases. In some cases, anaphylaxis is prolonged or recurrent for 6 to 24 hours and may require intensive medical care. Patients with moderate to severe systemic allergic reactions should be admitted to the hospital for observation, even if they are initially stabilized. All patients who have suffered an anaphylactic reaction should be prescribed an epinephrine autoinjector and educated on its use. *(Answer: B—If the patient demonstrates initial improvement after treatment, it is safe to discharge her home after observing her for 2 to 4 hours)*

33. A 32-year-old woman whose medical history includes an anaphylactic reaction to a yellow jacket sting would like to know if there are any measures she can take to decrease her risk of anaphylaxis in the event of a future insect sting. You recommend immunotherapy.

Which of the following statements best supports your recommendation of immunotherapy for this patient?

- ❑ **A. Children and adults with a history of large local reactions to stings are at relatively high risk for developing anaphylaxis, and venom immunotherapy in these patients is required**
- ❑ **B. Although standard venom immunotherapy is generally well tolerated, it is only 40% to 50% effective in completely preventing systemic allergic reactions to stings**

- ❑ C. **In a patient who has had a single anaphylactic reaction to a sting and whose skin test is positive, immunotherapy is indicated**
- ❑ D. **In a patient receiving immunotherapy, the skin test usually becomes negative within the first 4 to 6 months; failure to do so may indicate a lack of response to the treatment**

Key Concept/Objective: To understand the indications for and typical outcomes of venom immunotherapy

Patients with anaphylactic reactions to Hymenoptera stings should be educated about the risk of future reactions and about avoiding exposure. These patients should also understand the need for an epinephrine kit, and in most cases they should be evaluated by an allergist. The indications for venom immunotherapy are a history of a systemic allergic reaction to a sting and a positive venom skin test. In patients with these indications, the risk of anaphylaxis after subsequent stings approaches 50%. On the other hand, children and adults with a history of large local reactions have only a 10% chance of developing anaphylaxis after subsequent stings; in these patients, immunotherapy is an option (which many patients choose) but is not required. Standard immunotherapy is quite effective; it completely prevents subsequent systemic allergic reactions in 85% to 98% of patients. In the initial weeks of treatment, patients may develop a systemic allergic reaction, which is usually mild. Skin-test results generally remain unchanged during the first 2 to 3 years of treatment but usually decline after 4 to 6 years. The risk of life-threatening systemic allergic reactions occurring after 5 years of immunotherapy is low. Currently, it is recommended that immunotherapy be continued for an indefinite period. *(Answer: C—In a patient who has had a single anaphylactic reaction to a sting and whose skin test is positive, immunotherapy is indicated)*

For more information, see Golden DBK: 6 Immunology/Allergy: XV Allergic Reactions to Hymenoptera. ACP Medicine Online (www.acpmedicine.com). Dale DC, Federman DD, Eds. WebMD Inc., New York, October 2002

Food Allergies

34. A 36-year-old man is being evaluated for diarrhea. The patient has a 3-month history of diarrhea, postprandial nausea and vomiting, and weight loss. There is no specific food that he can relate to his symptoms. A complete blood count reveals anemia and eosinophilia. His serum IgE level is increased. Small bowel biopsy reveals eosinophilic infiltration without vasculitis.

Which of the following is the most likely diagnosis for this patient?

- ❑ A. **Oral allergy syndrome**
- ❑ B. **Churg-Strauss syndrome**
- ❑ C. **Eosinophilic gastroenteropathy**
- ❑ D. **Immediate gastrointestinal hypersensitivity**

Key Concept/Objective: To be able to recognize allergic eosinophilic gastroenteropathy

Allergic eosinophilic gastroenteropathy is a disorder characterized by infiltration of the gastric or intestinal walls with eosinophils; absence of vasculitis; and, frequently, peripheral blood eosinophilia. The symptoms include postprandial nausea and vomiting, abdominal pain, diarrhea, and, occasionally, steatorrhea. Young infants have failure to thrive, and adults have weight loss. There appears to be a subset of patients with allergic eosinophilic gastroenteritis who have symptoms secondary to food. These patients generally have the mucosal form of this disease, with IgE-staining cells in jejunal tissue, elevated IgE in duodenal fluids, atopic disease, elevated serum IgE concentrations, positive prick skin tests to a variety of foods and inhalants, peripheral blood eosinophilia, iron deficiency anemia, and hypoalbuminemia. The diagnosis of eosinophilic gastroenteropathy is based on an appropriate history and a GI biopsy demonstrating a characteristic eosinophilic infiltration. The oral allergy syndrome is a form of contact urticaria that is confined almost exclusively to the oropharynx and rarely involves other target organs. Patients with immediate GI hypersensi-

tivity present with GI symptoms after the ingestion of a specific food. Churg-Strauss syndrome is a form of small-vessel vasculitis; patients present with asthma, sinusitis, and eosinophilia. It can have GI manifestations as well. *(Answer: C—Eosinophilic gastroenteropathy)*

35. A 3-year-old boy is brought to your office by his mother, who relates that her son was diagnosed as having peanut hypersensitivity 1 year ago. He developed urticaria and nasal congestion after ingestion of peanuts. Since then, he has had two more episodes of hypersensitivity, with similar symptoms. His mother asks about treatment.

Which of the following is the most appropriate treatment for this patient?

❑ **A. Long-term use of antihistamines**

❑ **B. Immunotherapy**

❑ **C. Elimination diet**

❑ **D. Ketotifen**

Key Concept/Objective: To understand the management of food allergy

The only proven therapy for food allergy is the strict elimination of that food from the patient's diet. Elimination diets should be supervised, because they may lead to malnutrition or eating disorders, especially if they involve the elimination of a large number of foods or are utilized for extended periods of time. Studies have shown that symptomatic food sensitivity generally is lost over time, except for sensitivity to peanuts, tree nuts, and seafood. Symptomatic food sensitivity is usually very specific; patients rarely react to more than one member of a botanical family or animal species. Consequently, clinicians should confirm that patients are not unnecessarily limiting their diet for fear of allergic reactions. Except in the case of patients who are at risk for life-threatening reactions to minuscule amounts of peanuts, immunotherapy is not useful in food allergies. The importance of prompt administration of epinephrine when symptoms of systemic reactions to foods develop cannot be overemphasized. *(Answer: C—Elimination diet)*

36. A 30-year-old woman presents with shortness of breath, angioedema, urticaria, and hypotension after eating shellfish. She is successfully treated with epinephrine, intravenous fluids, and antihistamines. She has a history of asthma and hypertension. She takes lisinopril and inhaled beclomethasone. Radioallergosorbent testing reveals the presence of shellfish-specific IgE.

Which of the following statements regarding this patient's condition is the most accurate?

❑ **A. She had a type III hypersensitivity reaction**

❑ **B. This allergy is likely to disappear in a few years**

❑ **C. She should avoid other highly allergenic foods, such as peanuts and tree nuts, as well as shellfish**

❑ **D. She is at high risk for developing a more severe anaphylactic reaction in the future if she ingests shellfish**

Key Concept/Objective: To know the risk factors for severe anaphylactic reactions

Risk factors for severe anaphylaxis include the following: (1) a history of a previous anaphylactic reaction; (2) a history of asthma, especially if the asthma is poorly controlled; (3) allergy to peanuts, nuts, fish, or shellfish; (4) current treatment with beta blockers or angiotensin-converting enzyme (ACE) inhibitors; and, possibly, (5) female sex. This patient had a type I, or IgE-mediated, hypersensitivity reaction. A type III reaction is antigen-antibody complex mediated. Allergies to foods such as tree nuts, fish, and seafood are generally not outgrown, regardless of the age at which they develop. Persons with these allergies are likely to retain their allergic sensitivity throughout their lifetime. *(Answer: D—She is at high risk for developing a more severe anaphylactic reaction in the future if she ingests shellfish)*

For more information, see Burks AW: 6 Immunology/Allergy: XVI Food Allergies. ACP Medicine Online (www.acpmedicine.com). Dale DC, Federman DD, Eds. WebMD Inc., New York, September 2003

SECTION 7

INFECTIOUS DISEASE

Infections Due to Gram-Positive Cocci

1. A 43-year-old man presents to the emergency department with fever, cough, and shortness of breath. He has no chronic medical illnesses. He was in his usual state of health until 2 days ago, when he developed fatigue and anorexia. During the previous night, he developed fever of 103° F (39.4° C), a shaking chill, and copious, thick sputum production. He denies having nausea, emesis, diarrhea, or rash or having come into contact with anyone who was sick. He has smoked one pack of cigarettes a day for the past 25 years. On physical examination, the patient's temperature is found to be 102.4° F (39.1° C). Rales are heard in the left posterior midlung field, with associated egophony and increased palpable fremitus. Chest x-ray reveals consolidation of the left lower lobe. Sputum Gram stain reveals gram-positive diplococci. The patient's white blood cell count is 25,000/mm^3, with a marked left shift.

Which of the following statements regarding pneumococcal pneumonia is true?

- ❑ **A. Pneumococcal pneumonia accounts for up to 90% of community-acquired pneumonias**
- ❑ **B. Pneumococcal pneumonia typically causes significant tissue necrosis, resulting in prominent fibrosis**
- ❑ **C. In patients with pneumococcal pneumonia, a bronchopneumonic pattern is radiographically more common than lobar consolidation**
- ❑ **D. This patient's fever and marked leukocytosis reflect an unfavorable host response to his infection**

Key Concept/Objective: To know the important clinical features of pneumococcal pneumonia

The classic physical and radiographic findings of lobar consolidation may be absent in patients with pneumococcal pneumonia. In fact, a bronchopneumonic pattern is radiographically more common than lobar consolidation. Dehydration may minimize pulmonary findings, and underlying chronic lung disease may predispose to patchy areas of pulmonary infiltration. The pneumococcus accounts for up to 40% of community-acquired pneumonias, causing or contributing to 40,000 deaths annually. Because pneumococci only rarely produce significant tissue necrosis, healing is usually complete and residual fibrosis is minimal. Interestingly, a lack of febrile response and a normal or low white blood cell count are readily measurable factors that are associated with worse outcome. Thus, although white blood cell counts of 25,000 to 30,000/mm^3 with a left shift may be alarming, they indicate a favorable host response to infection. *(Answer: C—In patients with pneumococcal pneumonia, a bronchopneumonic pattern is radiographically more common than lobar consolidation)*

2. A 71-year-old man presents to your office for evaluation of fever and cough. His illnesses include hypertension with chronic renal disease; diabetes; and ischemic cardiomyopathy. He was in his usual state of health until yesterday morning, when he awoke with fatigue and dizziness. In addition, his wife told him he was not "acting right." Later that day, he developed cough with minimal sputum and fever. Currently, his temperature is 101° F (38.3° C). Marked orthostasis is noted, and the patient's respiratory rate is 30 breaths/min. On the basis of his vital signs, you admit him to the hospital for additional studies and therapy. In the hospital, rales are noted bilaterally in his lung bases. Chest x-ray reveals bronchopneumonic infiltrate in the right middle lobe. Laboratory testing reveals a leukocytosis with left shift and a worsening of his chronic renal failure. Blood cultures are positive for gram-positive cocci.

Which of the following statements regarding the treatment and prevention of pneumococcal disease is true?

- ❑ A. **Pneumococci often display plasmid-mediated penicillinase production, requiring the addition of a β-lactamase inhibitor to penicillin therapy**
- ❑ B. **Typically, penicillin-nonsusceptible pneumococci are also resistant to both third-generation cephalosporins and the newer fluoroquinolones**
- ❑ C. **The pneumococcal vaccine is often associated with serious and distressing reactions, such as fever or severe local reactions**
- ❑ D. **The pneumococcal vaccine is recommended for healthy adults older than 65 years and for patients with chronic medical illnesses**

Key Concept/Objective: To understand the prevention and treatment of pneumococcal disease

Pneumococci do not produce plasmid-mediated penicillinase, but they can develop chromosomal mutations that confer resistance to penicillin by altering the affinity of the penicillin-binding proteins in their cell walls. Pneumococci that are resistant to penicillin are often resistant to other antimicrobial drugs. First- and second-generation cephalosporins are generally ineffective against these organisms, but third-generation cephalosporins (particularly ceftriaxone and cefotaxime) and carbapenems are usually active. Whereas many pneumococci have become resistant to the older fluoroquinolones, such as ciprofloxacin, newer agents in this class, such as levofloxacin, sparfloxacin, gatifloxacin, and moxifloxacin, are generally active against penicillin-resistant pneumococci. The pneumococcal vaccine is recommended for healthy adults older than 65 years and for patients with chronic cardiopulmonary disease, functional or anatomic asplenia (including sickle cell disease), Hodgkin disease, multiple myeloma, cirrhosis, alcoholism, renal failure, cerebrospinal fluid leaks, immunosuppression, or HIV infection. *(Answer: D—The pneumococcal vaccine is recommended for healthy adults older than 65 years and for patients with chronic medical illnesses)*

3. A 47-year-old woman is in the hospital waiting to undergo a gastric bypass procedure. A central venous line is placed in the subclavian position for vascular access. Her procedure is completed without complication. On the fifth day after her procedure, she develops a fever of 103.5° F (39.7° C). On physical examination, the patient's postoperative wounds are normal. Her lung fields are clear to auscultation, and she denies having any abdominal pain, dysuria, or cough. Urinalysis is negative for pyuria. Sputum Gram stain reveals normal flora. Blood cultures grow gram-positive cocci in clusters.

Which of the following statements regarding Staphylococcus aureus ***bacteremia is true?***

- ❑ A. **In recent years, community-acquired methicillin-resistant *S. aureus* (MRSA) infections have decreased in prevalence throughout the United States.**
- ❑ B. **Patients with community-acquired *S. aureus* bacteremias are more likely to have endocarditis and secondary metastatic infections than patients with nosocomial infections**
- ❑ C. **All patients with *S. aureus* bacteremia should be treated for a minimum of 7 days with parenteral intravenous antibiotic therapy**
- ❑ D. **When compared with monotherapy, combination antibiotic therapy reduces long-term mortality in patients with *S. aureus* bacteremia and endocarditis**

Key Concept/Objective: To understand the important clinical features of S. aureus *bacteremia*

Patients with community-acquired bacteremias are more likely to have endocarditis and secondary metastatic infections than patients with nosocomial infections, who are more likely to have an evident portal of entry and severe underlying diseases. In recent years, community-acquired MRSA infections have increased in prevalence in many

regions of the United States, Japan, and Southeast Asia. Controlled trials are necessary to determine the safety and efficacy of short-term therapy for staphylococcal bacteremia. It may therefore be prudent to treat patients with staphylococcal bacteremia as though they have endocarditis. I.V. antibiotic therapy should, in any case, be continued for at least 10 to 15 days. Because of the high mortality associated with staphylococcal bacteremia and endocarditis, combination therapies utilizing nafcillin or vancomicin with gentamycin or rifampin are being studied. Thus far, combination therapy appears to reduce the duration of bacteremia but not to change the long-term mortality. *(Answer: B—Patients with community-acquired* S. aureus *bacteremias are more likely to have endocarditis and secondary metastatic infections than patients with nosocomial infections)*

4. A 37-year-old woman underwent elective laparoscopic cholecystectomy without complications. On postoperative day 3, the patient developed fever. At that time, chest x-ray and urinalysis were unremarkable. A careful inspection of previous I.V. access sites revealed no induration or erythema. Because of some persistent right-upper-quadrant pain, the patient's primary physician ordered a CT with contrast of the abdomen and pelvis on postoperative day 6. This study revealed a 5 × 7 cm fluid collection in the right upper quadrant. It is now day 7. You have been asked to evaluate the patient. You request a drainage procedure by interventional radiology, which reveals straw-colored fluid with gram-positive cocci in clusters on Gram stain. Culture of the fluid reveals methicillin MRSA.

Which of the following statements regarding MRSA is true?

- ❑ **A. MRSA is strictly a nosocomial pathogen confined to hospitals and other long-term care facilities**
- ❑ **B. MRSA is more virulent than methicillin-susceptible *S. aureus***
- ❑ **C. Vancomycin is less effective than nafcillin for isolates sensitive to both agents**
- ❑ **D. There is no reported resistance to vancomycin for *S. aureus***

Key Concept/Objective: To know the important clinical concepts of treatment for MRSA infection

Vancomycin is less effective than nafcillin for strains sensitive to both agents. The virulence and clinical manifestations of MRSA are no different from those of methicillin-susceptible *S. aureus*; compared with methicillin-sensitive strains, however, a higher percentage of MRSA strains may possess the toxins toxic-shock syndrome toxin–1 (TSST-1), enterotoxins, and the Panton-Valentine leukocidin. With the increase in use of vancomycin, strains of *S. aureus* with reduced susceptibility to vancomycin have begun to appear. Daptomycin and linezolid have excellent activity against vancomycin-intermediate and vancomycin-resistant *Staphylococcus*. *(Answer: C—Vancomycin is less effective than nafcillin for isolates sensitive to both agents)*

5. A 34-year-old African-American woman presents to the emergency department complaining of fever, chills, pain in the right upper quadrant, and productive cough with blood-tinged sputum. She reports that she recently had a cold and that about 2 days ago she had a severe chill lasting about 20 minutes. Subsequently, she developed a temperature of 105° F (40.5° C), cough, and pain in her right side. She reports that initially she was able to control the fever with antipyretics, but now the fever will not subside with medications. She reports that she has sickle cell anemia and that she smokes two packs of cigarettes daily. On examination, she appears toxic; her temperature is 104.8° F (40.4° C); and upon auscultation, fine rales are noted in the right lower lung field. Chest x-ray shows a bronchopneumonic pattern in the right lower lung field. Sputum Gram stain reveals many polymorphonuclear leukocytes and abundant lancet-shaped gram-positive diplococci.

For this patient, which of the following statements is false?

- ❑ **A. The virulence of this infectious agent is related to surface protein A and penicillinase production**
- ❑ **B. This patient's smoking history is the strongest independent risk factor for invasive disease**

❑ C. The case-fatality rate for this infection is 5% to 12%; bacteremia is the most common extrathoracic complication, increasing the case-fatality rate to 20%

❑ D. This patient should be treated with ceftriaxone or cefotaxime until the results of susceptibility testing are available

❑ E. A vaccine is available for the infectious agent causing this patient's illness and should be recommended

Key Concept/Objective: To understand the pathogenesis, diagnosis, and treatment of pneumococcal infections

The pneumococcal polysaccharide capsule is crucial to virulence. The capsule allows the bacteria to resist phagocytosis by leukocytes. Although the polysaccharide capsule is the critical factor in determining the virulence of the pneumococci, several proteins, including surface protein A, contribute to the pathogenesis of pneumococcal infections. Pneumococcal infections typically occur after a viral respiratory infection. Patients present with severe rigor or chill and pleurisy. Chest x-rays display findings of lobar consolidation or bronchopneumonic involvement. The key to diagnosis is Gram stain of a sputum smear, which typically reveals many polymorphonuclear leukocytes and abundant lancet-shaped gram-positive diplococci. Pneumococci display penicillin resistance, the mechanism of which is chromosomal mutation, not penicillinase production. Cigarette smoking is the strongest independent risk factor for invasive pneumococcal disease in immunocompetent adults who are not elderly. Other patients at increased risk are those with cirrhosis, sickle cell anemia, chronic lung disease, or cancer. Pneumococci cause or contribute to 40,000 deaths annually; the overall case-fatality rate of this pneumonia is 5% to 12%. Bacteremia is an adverse prognostic sign and increases the case-fatality rate to 20%: a rate that has not changed over the past 40 years. First- and second-generation cephalosporins are generally ineffective against these organisms, but third-generation cephalosporins, particularly ceftriaxone and cefotaxime, are usually active. Until the results of susceptibility testing are available, it may be advisable to add vancomycin to this regimen for life-threatening pneumococcal infections. A vaccine containing 23 pneumococcal types is available and should be given to adults older than 65 years and patients with chronic cardiopulmonary disease, asplenia or splenic dysfunction, sickle cell disease, immunosuppression, or renal failure. The efficacy of this vaccine varies among patients. *(Answer: A—The virulence of this infectious agent is related to surface protein A and penicillinase production)*

6. A 16-year-old male adolescent presents to the emergency department with chest pain, dyspnea, fever, and pain in several joints. He was treated for streptococcal pharyngitis 2 weeks ago with an injection. His sore throat seemed to improve, but over the past 4 days, he has developed fever and dyspnea, and his chest pain has worsened. On examination, he has a temperature of 101° F (38.3° C), he is tachypneic, and he has a pericardial friction rub. Chest x-ray shows early evidence of congestive heart failure, electrocardiogram shows a first-degree heart block, and the laboratory results show an elevated erythrocyte sedimentation rate (ESR).

For this patient, which of the following statements is true?

❑ A. Bacterial culture of the infectious agent responsible for this patient's symptoms is likely to show alpha hemolysis and no inhibition with bacitracin

❑ B. In this patient, the pathogenesis of the infectious agent is by the elaboration of exotoxin

❑ C. This patient's symptoms fulfill four major Jones criteria

❑ D. This patient should be given antibiotics for prophylaxis against recurrent infections

❑ E. The class of infectious agent responsible for this patient's symptoms is also the leading cause of subacute bacterial endocarditis

Key Concept/Objective: To understand the pathogenesis, diagnosis, and treatment of streptococcal infections

Patients with a history of acute rheumatic fever are particularly susceptible to recurrent attacks. Consequently, they should receive continuous prophylaxis for at least 5 years. Prophylaxis can be discontinued when patients who are at low risk of recurrence reach adulthood. Acute rheumatic fever is strictly a sequela of streptococcal pharyngitis and usually begins 1 to 3 weeks after a group A streptococcal infection. Streptococci are gram-positive organisms; although they can appear in pairs, they more commonly appear in chains of varying length. Streptococcal infections can cause disease through direct invasion (e.g., upper respiratory tract infections, pneumonia, wound infections, lymphadenitis, necrotizing fasciitis), elaboration of exotoxins (e.g., streptococcal toxic-shock syndrome, scarlet fever), and host immune response reactions (e.g., acute rheumatic fever, acute glomerulonephritis). Acute rheumatic fever is caused by group A streptococci, which produce α-hemolysis and are inhibited by low concentrations of bacitracin. Group A streptococci cause acute rheumatic fever through a host immune response that causes tissue damage. Elaboration of exotoxins is responsible for scarlet fever and toxic-shock syndrome. The Jones criteria are clinical findings used in making the diagnosis of acute rheumatic fever and consist of either two major criteria or one major and two minor criteria. The major criteria are carditis, polyarthritis, chorea, subcutaneous nodules, and erythema marginatum. The minor criteria are fever, arthralgias, and inflammation, as demonstrated by an elevated ESR. The leading cause of subacute bacterial endocarditis is viridans streptococci. *(Answer: D—This patient should be given antibiotics for prophylaxis against recurrent infections)*

7. A 72-year-old man presents with fever and chills of 2 days' duration. He denies having any respiratory or gastrointestinal symptoms but reports some frequency in urination. He states that he has poorly controlled diabetes and a history of prostate surgery. He takes a daily dose of trimethoprim-sulfamethoxazole for prophylaxis against urinary tract infections. On physical examination, the patient appears ill. His temperature is 101.3° F (38.5° C). He has tenderness in the suprapubic region and has bilateral costovertebral tenderness. After admission, urine culture grows *Enterococcus*.

Which of the following statements regarding this patient is false?

- ❑ **A. The infectious agent that is causing this patient's symptoms is uniformly resistant to penicillin**
- ❑ **B. The type of infection seen in this patient is most common in persons with underlying genitourinary disease and in the elderly**
- ❑ **C. Changing resistance patterns will necessitate changes in antibiotic therapy for this patient's enterococcal infection**
- ❑ **D. The infectious agent responsible for this patient's symptoms is morphologically and immunologically similar to *Streptococcus***
- ❑ **E. Vancomycin is the drug of choice for treatment of this patient's enterococcal infection**

Key Concept/Objective: To understand the pathogenesis, diagnosis, and treatment of enterococcal infections

Traditionally, ampicillin has been the drug of choice for enterococcal urinary tract infections. Recently, vancomycin-resistant enterococci have been recognized as nosocomial pathogens. Enterococci are morphologically and immunologically similar to group D streptococci, but unlike streptococci, they are uniformly penicillin-resistant. They have unique penicillin-binding proteins that permit cell wall synthesis to proceed even in the presence of β-lactam antibiotics. Enterococcal infections are most common in persons with underlying genitourinary or gastrointestinal disease, in the elderly, and in debilitated persons. The primary reason that enterococci have emerged as major pathogens is that these organisms are resistant to many antibiotics. Changing resistance patterns will necessitate changes in antibiotic therapy for patients with enterococcal infections. *(Answer: E—Vancomycin is the drug of choice for treatment of this patient's enterococcal infection)*

8. A 33-year-old woman who is a known intravenous drug abuser and who is HIV positive presents with fever and chills. She has been injecting in her right femoral vein and reports a red swollen mass in the area. She has been hospitalized multiple times in the past for infections as a result of her intravenous drug abuse. On examination, the patient appears toxic and has a temperature of 105° F (40.5° C). She has a large, tender, erythematous mass in the right groin. Gram stain shows gram-positive cocci in grape-like clusters.

Which of the following statements regarding this patient's condition is true?

- ❑ **A. The virulence of this bacteria is related to the fact that teichoic acid is a component of its cell wall**
- ❑ **B. The incidence of serious infection from this bacteria is decreasing because of the availability of powerful antibiotics**
- ❑ **C. This patient is at high risk for osteomyelitis, endocarditis, meningitis, and pneumonia**
- ❑ **D. This patient should be treated with oral antibiotics for 14 days**
- ❑ **E. Surgical drainage of the right groin mass should not be performed until the bacteremia resolves**

Key Concept/Objective: To understand the pathogenesis, diagnosis, and treatment of staphylococcal infections

Hematogenous spread of staphylococci is among the principal causes of septic arthritis, osteomyelitis, aseptic meningitis, and pneumonia. Patients with community-acquired bacteremias are most likely to have endocarditis and secondary metastatic infections; half of such patients are intravenous drug abusers. *Staphylococcus aureus* can cause skin and soft tissue infections, bone and joint infections, respiratory infections (including pneumonia), and bacteremia. Teichoic acid is a carbohydrate antigen in the cell wall of staphylococci. Antibodies to teichoic acid can be detected in normal human serum. Teichoic acid has no established role in virulence, and antibodies to this antigen are not protective. For serious staphylococcal infections, parenteral antibiotics are mandatory and are generally administered for 4 to 6 weeks. Unlike other gram-positive cocci, the incidence of serious staphylococcal infection increased after the introduction of antibiotics. *(Answer: C—This patient is at high risk for osteomyelitis, endocarditis, meningitis, and pneumonia)*

9. An 84-year-old woman who resides in a nursing home presents for evaluation of fever of unknown origin. Two weeks ago, she was transferred to the nursing home after undergoing 3 months of inpatient treatment for a cerebrovascular accident. After readmission, bacterial cultures grow MRSA.

What is the most appropriate antibiotic choice for this patient?

- ❑ **A. Ceftriaxone**
- ❑ **B. Vancomycin**
- ❑ **C. Linezolid**
- ❑ **D. Erythromycin**
- ❑ **E. Cefuroxime**

Key Concept/Objective: To understand the pathogenesis, diagnosis, and treatment of MRSA infections

Vancomycin is the drug of choice for MRSA infections; its results are comparable to those achieved with β-lactam antibiotic treatment of infections caused by methicillin-sensitive strains. MRSA is a growing problem. It first appeared as nosocomial pathogens in university hospitals, but it now also occurs in long-term care facilities. The virulence and clinical manifestations of MRSA are no different from those of methicillin-susceptible species. Linezolid is also active against MRSA, but until more experience is available, it should probably be reserved for infections in which vancomycin is ineffective or unsuitable. Most MRSA strains are resistant to penicillin, cephalosporins, erythromycins, and chloramphenicol. Even if the organisms appear to be sensitive to

cephalosporins in disk diffusion testing, cephalosporins should not be relied upon in cases involving MRSA. *(Answer: B—Vancomycin)*

10. A 70-year-old man is evaluated in the emergency department for fever, confusion, and a stiff neck. His medical history is notable for Hodgkin lymphoma (20 years ago), diet-controlled diabetes mellitus, and hypertension. His only medication is lisinopril, 5 mg daily, and he has no known allergies. Routine laboratory tests, including blood cultures, are obtained, and a lumbar puncture is performed. A Gram stain of the cerebrospinal fluid indicates *Streptococcus pneumoniae* infection.

Which of the following choices represents the most appropriate empirical antibiotic therapy (pending final culture and sensitivity results)?

- ❑ **A. High-dose trimethoprim-sulfamethoxazole**
- ❑ **B. Ceftazidime**
- ❑ **C. Ceftriaxone**
- ❑ **D. Ceftriaxone plus vancomycin**
- ❑ **E. Rifampin**

Key Concept/Objective: To know the appropriate empirical antibiotic management of suspected Streptococcus pneumoniae *meningitis*

Pneumococcal resistance to penicillin is an increasing problem and is seen with a greater frequency among patients who have been using antibiotics, children younger than 6 years, and adults older than 65 years. Higher doses of penicillin or cephalosporins may be adequate for pneumonia or upper respiratory infections caused by penicillin-nonsusceptible pneumococci. For life-threatening infections such as meningitis caused by *S. pneumoniae*, however, most authorities would recommend adding vancomycin to either ceftriaxone or cefotaxime until susceptibility data are available. If the organism is proven to be susceptible, the vancomycin may be discontinued. *(Answer: D—Ceftriaxone plus vancomycin)*

11. ***Which of the following statements regarding pneumococcal infection in persons infected with HIV is true?***

- ❑ **A. Pneumococcal infection typically occurs only in HIV-infected persons with $CD4^+$ T cell counts < 50 cells/µl**
- ❑ **B. The mortality rate of pneumococcal pneumonia is two to three times greater among HIV-infected persons than among non–HIV-infected persons**
- ❑ **C. The incidence of pneumococcal infection is significantly increased among HIV-infected persons**
- ❑ **D. The pneumococcal serotypes causing infection among HIV-infected persons are significantly different from those among non–HIV-infected persons**
- ❑ **E. Relapse of pneumococcal pneumonia is very rare**

Key Concept/Objective: To know the similarities and differences in pneumococcal infections between HIV-positive persons and HIV-negative persons

The pneumococcus is the leading cause of invasive bacterial respiratory tract infection in HIV-positive persons. The clinical features, causative serotypes, antimicrobial-resistance patterns, and mortality rates of pneumococcal infection in HIV-seropositive patients are similar to those in HIV-seronegative patients. However, unusual extrapulmonary manifestations and late relapses can occur in those infected with HIV. *(Answer: C—The incidence of pneumococcal infection is significantly increased among HIV-infected persons)*

12. A 68-year-old man is evaluated for symptoms of fever, weight loss, and dyspnea on exertion. Physical examination reveals a new diastolic murmur and stigmata of peripheral emboli. He is admitted to the

hospital for further evaluation and management of endocarditis. A cardiac echocardiogram shows a 1 cm aortic valve vegetation, and two of two blood cultures subsequently grow *Streptococcus bovis* that is susceptible to penicillin.

After appropriate management of this patient's endocarditis, the patient should undergo which of the following?

- ❑ **A. Glucose tolerance test**
- ❑ **B. Chest radiograph to screen for lung cancer**
- ❑ **C. Upper endoscopy**
- ❑ **D. Colonoscopy**
- ❑ **E. No specific further evaluation is warranted**

Key Concept/Objective: To understand the association between Streptococcus bovis *and colon carcinoma*

The patient in this case has *Streptococcus bovis* bacteremia with endocarditis. There is a strong association between *S. bovis* and carcinoma of the colon, and any patient with documented *S. bovis* bacteremia should be evaluated specifically for the possibility of colon carcinoma. *(Answer: D—Colonoscopy)*

13. ***Which of the following statements about pneumococcal resistance to penicillin is true?***

- ❑ **A. Penicillin resistance is usually mediated by a plasmid-encoded β-lactamase**
- ❑ **B. The frequency of penicillin resistance is significantly higher among HIV-infected patients than among others**
- ❑ **C. Penicillin resistance is usually mediated by a chromosomally mediated β-lactamase**
- ❑ **D. Most penicillin-resistant pneumococci are also vancomycin-resistant**
- ❑ **E. Penicillin resistance is mediated by altered penicillin-binding proteins**

Key Concept/Objective: To understand the mechanism of penicillin resistance in Streptococcus pneumoniae

Penicillin resistance among pneumococci is becoming increasingly common. The usual mechanism of resistance is alteration of penicillin-binding proteins, not production of either plasmid or chromosomal β-lactamase. Penicillin resistance is commonly associated with resistance to other classes of antibiotics, further complicating treatment of such infections. The prevalence of penicillin-resistant pneumococci appears to be higher in patients taking antibiotics, children younger than 6 years, and adults older than 65 years. *(Answer: E—Penicillin resistance is mediated by altered penicillin-binding proteins)*

For more information, see Stevens DL: 7 Infectious Disease: I Infections Due to Gram-Positive Cocci. ACP Medicine Online (www.acpmedicine.com). Dale DC, Federman DD, Eds. WebMD Inc., New York, September 2004

Infections Due to Mycobacteria

14. A young woman presents to your office and states that her roommate has just been diagnosed with active tuberculosis. She is concerned about her own health. She recently had a fever, a nonproductive cough, and pleuritic chest pain. A chest x-ray shows no infiltrate, but there is a moderate-sized left pleural effusion.

Which of the following statements is true regarding this patient?

- ❑ **A. If this patient has become infected, the most likely initial site of infection is the lung apices**

❑ B. This patient should be tested for HIV

❑ C. A test with purified protein derivative (PPD) should have 10 mm of induration to be considered positive

❑ D. If this patient does have tuberculous pleuritis, the diagnosis can be reliably made on the basis of an acid-fast smear of pleural fluid

❑ E. This patient's presentation is very common for patients with primary tuberculosis infection

Key Concept/Objective: To understand the epidemiology and possible features of primary tuberculosis infection

This patient is a close contact of a person known to have active tuberculosis, so 5 mm of induration would be a positive result on PPD testing. Tuberculosis is transmitted by inhalation of a tubercle bacillus into the pulmonary alveoli. Initial infection usually occurs in the lower lung fields, not the apices, because of gravity and the greater ventilation of the lung bases. Reactivation (in an immunocompetent host) tends to occur in the apices because the bacillus has a propensity to disseminate to areas of higher Po_2. About 90% of patients with primary tuberculosis infection are asymptomatic. Thus, pleuritis is fairly uncommon, as are the three other potential manifestations of symptomatic primary infection (atypical pneumonia, extrapulmonary tuberculosis, and direct progression to upper lobe disease). Patients who are HIV positive, who are immunologically suppressed, or who are in some way debilitated are at increased risk for symptomatic primary infection. Thus, this patient should be tested for HIV. Patients with tuberculous pleuritis present with a high fever, cough, and pleuritic chest pain. Only one third of patients will have a positive result on acid-fast smear of the pleural fluid; for two thirds of patients, noncaseating granulomas will be found on pleural biopsy. *(Answer: B—This patient should be tested for HIV)*

15. A 27-year-old man known to have HIV presents to the emergency department with fever, mild shortness of breath, and a productive cough with streaky hemoptysis. Recent records show his $CD4^+$ T cell count to be 150 cells/µl. He is not receiving antiretroviral medication. A chest x-ray shows bilateral lower lobe consolidation. Results of acid-fast staining of the first sputum sample obtained are positive.

Which of the following statements is accurate?

❑ A. Because this patient is immunocompromised and has lower lobe disease, he most likely has a primary tuberculosis infection

❑ B. The infection should quickly improve if antiretroviral therapy is initiated

❑ C. Plans to initiate highly active antiretroviral therapy (HAART) do not affect the choice of antituberculous chemotherapy regimen

❑ D. Because the patient has HIV, he should receive an empirical four-drug regimen regardless of the rate of isoniazid resistance in his community

❑ E. This patient very likely has tuberculous involvement of one or more extrapulmonary sites

Key Concept/Objective: To understand the ways in which reactivation tuberculosis in a patient with HIV differs from that in an immunocompetent patient

Symptomatic tuberculosis in a patient with HIV is usually caused by reactivation of latent infection, just as in the immunocompetent population. When tuberculosis occurs early in the course of HIV infection, before severe immunosuppression has occurred, the clinical and radiographic features resemble tuberculosis in patients who are HIV negative. With more advanced immunosuppression, *M. tuberculosis* tends to produce infections that are more widespread, severe, and unusual than conventional tuberculosis. The chest x-ray is normal in 10% to 15% of patients with HIV; the chest x-ray may simply show intrathoracic adenopathy. When infiltrates occur, lower lobe consolidation of

diffuse infiltrates are much more common than upper lobe abnormalities. Up to 70% of symptomatic patients with AIDS have tuberculous involvement of one or more extrapulmonary sites.

If this patient does not begin antiretroviral therapy, he can be treated in the same way as a patient with tuberculosis who is not infected with HIV. He should initially receive a three-drug regimen unless the rate of isoniazid resistance in his community is greater than 4%. Rifampin is contraindicated in patients receiving protease inhibitors or nonnucleoside reverse transcriptase inhibitors (NNRTIs). This is because rifampin activates the hepatic cytochrome CYP450 enzyme system, thus reducing levels of protease inhibitors and NNRTIs. Without rifampin, an initial regimen of four drugs is required. Because of immune reconstitution, this patient's tuberculosis infection may worsen on initiation of antiretroviral therapy. *(Answer: E—This patient very likely has tuberculous involvement of one or more extrapulmonary sites)*

16. A 54-year-old man with fairly severe chronic obstructive pulmonary disease (COPD) presents to the emergency department with increased shortness of breath (i.e., shortness of breath that is worse than his baseline), fever, and mildly productive cough. His symptoms have been progressing for about 2 months. His chest x-ray shows apical pulmonary infiltrates. He has had no previous tuberculosis exposure. Gram stain and culture of sputum are negative for routine bacteria. Infection with either atypical mycobacteria or tuberculosis is considered.

Which statement is true regarding the diagnosis and management of this patient?

❑ **A. Isolation of one colony of atypical mycobacteria from one of four sputum specimens would prove the existence of active infection**

❑ **B. Regimens for the treatment of all atypical mycobacteria should include isoniazid or rifampin**

❑ **C. If the patient has an atypical mycobacterial infection, presence of a cavity on chest x-ray would be diagnostic of *Mycobacterium kansasii* infection**

❑ **D. Surgery may have a role in the management of atypical mycobacterial disease**

❑ **E. Patients infected with nontuberculous bacteria would have a negative result on PPD testing**

Key Concept/Objective: To understand basic concepts of the diagnosis and treatment of atypical myobacterial pulmonary disease

In a presumably immunocompetent patient, diagnosis of atypical mycobacterial pulmonary infection is difficult because the mycobacteria are ubiquitous in the environment and could simply be contaminants. Risk factors for the development of such an infection are preexisting lung disease (including COPD), cancer, cystic fibrosis, and bronchiectasis. In a patient who is not infected with HIV, a diagnosis of atypical mycobacterial disease requires evidence of disease on chest imaging in addition to the repeated isolation of multiple colonies of the same strain. Different atypical mycobacteria are sensitive to different antibiotics. For example, *M. kansasii* responds well to regimens containing rifampin, ethambutol, and isoniazid, and *M. avium* intracellulare complex (MAC) is most sensitive to the macrolides azithromycin and clarithromycin. Cavitary disease is not specific to *M. kansasii*, because it can occur with MAC infection or infections with other atypical mycobacteria. Partial lung resection may have a role in the treatment of patients who do not respond to therapy, especially if they appear to have localized disease. It is important to note that persons can become sensitized by nontuberculous mycobacteria, and this can lead to a positive result on PPD testing. *(Answer: D—Surgery may have a role in the management of atypical mycobacterial disease)*

17. A 72-year-old woman with a history of tuberculosis presents to your clinic with fever, headache, weight loss, cough, dyspnea, and dysuria of 2 months' duration. Her examination is remarkable for coarse breath sounds. The neurologic examination is normal. Chest x-ray shows a miliary reticulonodular pattern. Laboratory results are remarkable for an elevated alkaline phosphatase level.

Which of the following statements is true regarding this patient's presentation?

- ❑ **A. Her presentation is typical of tuberculous meningitis**
- ❑ **B. Because there is evidence of pulmonary involvement, the diagnosis can be reliably made with an acid-fast sputum stain**
- ❑ **C. An acid-fast stain of the urine can be helpful in determining whether renal tuberculosis is present**
- ❑ **D. Liver biopsy can confirm a diagnosis of miliary tuberculosis**
- ❑ **E. Clinical response to appropriate chemotherapy for miliary tuberculosis is generally rapid and dramatic**

Key Concept/Objective: To understand the presentation of miliary tuberculosis and some organ-specific manifestations of tuberculosis

Although the lungs are the portal of entry of tuberculosis, it is truly a disseminated disease. After a few weeks multiplying in the lungs, bacilli invade lymphatics, spread to regional lymph nodes, and then reach the bloodstream. It is not uncommon for patients with miliary tuberculosis to have a history of tuberculosis, but it is not the norm. Virtually all of those patients who have a history of tuberculosis and who develop an extrapulmonary manifestation were inadequately treated initially.

Tuberculous meningitis is the most rapidly progressive form of tuberculosis. Without therapy, the illness progresses from headache, fever, and meningismus to cranial nerve palsies or other focal deficits, alterations of sensorium, seizures, coma, and eventually death. Renal tuberculosis generally presents with symptoms and signs of UTI, such as hematuria, dysuria, and pyuria. However, asymptomatic sterile pyuria occurs in up to 20% of patients with tuberculosis. Acid-fast staining of the urine should not be performed because of the significant likelihood that nonpathogenic mycobacteria exist in the urine. Instead, three first-morning urine specimens should be submitted for analysis; positive cultures will be obtained in at least 90% of patients with renal tuberculosis. Acid-fast sputum staining is positive in only 30% of patients with miliary tuberculosis, despite the presence of pulmonary infiltrates. Bronchoscopy with biopsy can establish the diagnosis in 70% of patients with an abnormal chest x-ray. Liver biopsy is especially helpful, revealing granulomas in 60% of patients. However, these granulomas are often noncaseating and nonspecific. Clinical improvement is often very slow, with fever persisting for 1 to 3 weeks. Despite therapy, mortality is 5% to 35%. *(Answer: D—Liver biopsy can confirm a diagnosis of miliary tuberculosis)*

18. A 55-year-old businessman is brought to the clinic for an evaluation of personality change. His wife describes several weeks of lassitude, fatigue, malaise, low-grade fever, headache, and irritability. In the past few days, he has become intermittently confused. Results of physical examination are as follows: temperature, 100.6° F (38.1° C); heart rate, 78 beats/min; blood pressure, 145/90 mm Hg. The patient is confused and scores 22/30 on the Folstein Mini-Mental State Examination. Mild meningismus and a left cranial nerve VI palsy are noted. Chest x-ray is negative except for an old Ghon complex. Results of cerebrospinal fluid examination are as follows: opening pressure, 160 mm Hg; glucose, 45 mg/dl; protein, 140 mg/dl; 250 cells/mm^3 (75% lymphocytes). Gram stain and rapid tests for fungal and bacterial antigens are negative.

Which of the following is the most likely diagnosis for this patient?

- ❑ **A. Bacterial meningitis**
- ❑ **B. Brain tumor**
- ❑ **C. Fungal meningitis**
- ❑ **D. Viral meningitis**
- ❑ **E. Tuberculous meningitis**

Key Concept/Objective: To be able to recognize tuberculous meningitis

Although uncommon in HIV-seronegative patients, this is one of the most serious and rapidly progressive forms of tuberculosis. Adults characteristically experience an indo-

lent phase of headache, malaise, low-grade fever, and personality changes. After several weeks, more characteristic CNS signs and symptoms develop, including meningismus, cranial nerve palsies, seizures, and signs of increased intracranial pressure (vomiting, altered consciousness, severe headache). Some patients present with a rapidly progressive picture resembling bacterial meningitis. Only a minority will have a clinical history of prior tuberculosis. An early CSF examination is critical to accurate diagnosis. Characteristic findings include lowered CSF glucose (hypoglycorrhachia), elevated CSF protein, and a lymphocytic pleocytosis. A high index of suspicion is needed to make the diagnosis, because mycobacterial CSF cultures are positive in no more than 75% of cases, and acid-fast smears are positive in only 25% of cases. A number of biochemical, immunologic, and molecular biologic tests are currently available, but none has yet emerged as the gold standard. At times, a clinical diagnosis depends on response to antituberculous therapy. *(Answer: E—Tuberculous meningitis)*

19. A 32-year-old resident of the state penitentiary is found to test positive on a purified protein derivative skin test (PPD), with 10 mm of induration. One year ago, his PPD was negative. He is asymptomatic, and his chest x-ray is negative.

Which of the following would you recommend at this time?

- ❑ A. No therapy; follow chest x-rays yearly
- ❑ B. Induced sputum cultures; treat only if positive
- ❑ C. Daily isoniazid (INH) for 6 months
- ❑ D. Daily INH for 12 months
- ❑ E. Daily therapy with pyrazinamide and rifampin for 2 months

Key Concept/Objective: To understand the indications for INH prophylaxis

The decision to initiate chemoprophylactic therapy depends on several variables: the patient's age, HIV status, strength of PPD reaction, socioeconomic status, and risk factors for the development of active tuberculosis. HIV-seropositive patients with a PPD of 5 mm or greater should receive 9 to 12 months of INH chemoprophylaxis. Patients younger than 35 years with a recent PPD conversion of 10 mm or greater and patients older than 35 years with a 15 mm PPD conversion are candidates for chemoprophylaxis. Several other factors lower the threshold for chemoprophylaxis, including recent exposure, an abnormal chest x-ray consistent with old TB, and membership in high-incidence population groups (e.g., prisoners, immigrants, medically underserved populations). INH chemoprophylaxis is no longer administered for 1 year; therapy for 6 to 9 months achieves the best balance between reducing the risk of active TB and minimizing the risk of hepatitis. Rifampin and pyrazinamide for 2 months can be substituted for INH chemoprophylaxis in patients who are unable to take INH or in whom INH resistance is suspected. *(Answer: C—Daily isoniazid [INH] for 6 months)*

20. A 48-year-old physician from New York City develops fever, night sweats, cough, weight loss, and malaise. Chest x-ray reveals an infiltrate in the posterior-apical segment of the right upper lobe. CT scan of the lesion reveals cavitation. Sputum examination reveals acid-fast bacteria. Cultures are pending.

Which of the following treatment options would you institute for this patient at this time?

- ❑ A. Await cultures and sensitivity testing before instituting therapy
- ❑ B. INH and rifampin
- ❑ C. INH, rifampin, and ethambutol
- ❑ D. INH, rifampin, ethambutol, and pyrazinamide
- ❑ E. INH, rifampin, ethambutol, pyrazinamide, and streptomycin

Key Concept/Objective: To understand the treatment of active tuberculosis

This patient has a clinical syndrome very suggestive of tuberculosis. He is smear-positive, and treatment should be initiated immediately, pending the results of mycobacterial culture and antimicrobial sensitivity. He should be hospitalized and placed in a negative-pressure isolation room for induction of chemotherapy until his symptoms improve and he becomes smear-negative. The United States Public Health Service recommends initiation of therapy with INH, rifampin, ethambutol, and pyrazinamide unless the INH-resistance rate in the community is low (< 4%), in which case ethambutol can be withheld. Treatment is continued for 2 months. In drug-sensitive cases, treatment is then changed to INH and rifampin for an additional 4 months (until sputum cultures have been negative for at least 3 months). *(Answer: D—INH, rifampin, ethambutol, and pyrazinamide)*

21. A 27-year-old HIV-seropositive Haitian man develops cough, fever, and weight loss. Chest x-ray reveals a cavitary lesion in the left upper lobe. Sputum culture is found to be smear-positive and, subsequently, culture-positive for *Mycobacterium tuberculosis*. He is hospitalized and placed in isolation. Medications include zidovudine, lamivudine, and indinavir, as well as trimethoprim-sulfamethoxazole.

Which of the following drugs is contraindicated in this patient?

- ❑ A. Rifampin
- ❑ B. Ethambutol
- ❑ C. Isoniazid
- ❑ D. Streptomycin
- ❑ E. Pyrazinamide

Key Concept/Objective: To know the major drug interactions between antiretroviral and antituberculosis drugs

Rifampin is contraindicated in patients receiving protease inhibitors (PIs). It is also contraindicated in patients taking nonnucleoside reverse transcriptase inhibitors (NNRTIs) such as nevirapine, delavirdine, and efavirenz. Rifampin is a potent inductor of the cytochrome P-450 enzyme system, and reduced levels of both the PIs and NNRTIs can result from coadministration. Conversely, PIs can raise rifampin concentrations to potentially toxic levels. The other four drugs listed may be used to treat HIV-seropositive patients with tuberculosis. Rifabutin (in lower than usual doses) is also used in place of rifampin. *(Answer: A—Rifampin)*

22. A 32-year-old I.V. drug abuser has been HIV-seropositive for 3 years. He has had several courses of antiretroviral therapy but has been intermittently noncompliant with treatment. He is admitted to the hospital with fevers, chills, night sweats, severe diarrhea, and weight loss. He has no cough. Chest x-ray reveals fibrotic changes at the bases but no infiltrates. Results of physical examination are as follows: temperature, 101.3° F (38.5° C); blood pressure, 108/50 mm Hg; heart rate, 94 beats/min; respiratory rate, 18 breaths/min. Generalized lymphadenopathy and hepatosplenomegaly are present. No skin lesions are noted.

Which of the following cultures is most likely to reveal the diagnosis for this patient?

- ❑ A. Sputum
- ❑ B. Blood
- ❑ C. Bone marrow
- ❑ D. Lymph node
- ❑ E. Stool

Key Concept/Objective: To be able to recognize Mycobacterium avium *complex infection in AIDS*

***M. avium* complex infection is a frequent opportunistic infection in AIDS patients with low CD4$^+$ T cell counts. Patients present with a disseminated infection, and symptoms**

can be protean. Systemic symptoms (fever, sweats, weight loss) are common. Diarrhea and malabsorption may overshadow pulmonary symptoms. Hepatosplenomegaly may be present. Aggressive culturing may be necessary to make the diagnosis. The organism may be recovered from blood, bone marrow, lymph nodes, stool, and many other sites. Blood culture using special media has the highest yield and should be the first diagnostic test. Bacteremia may be intermittent, so repeat cultures on subsequent days may be necessary to make the diagnosis. *(Answer: B—Blood)*

For more information, see Simon HB: 7 Infectious Disease: II Infections Due to Mycobacteria. ACP Medicine Online (www.acpmedicine.com). Dale DC, Federman DD, Eds. WebMD Inc., New York, February 2002

Infections Due to Neisseria

23. A 21-year-old man is brought to the emergency department of your hospital by the emergency medical service. The patient has altered mental status, fever, and rash. He is critically ill and requires endotracheal intubation by the resident in the emergency department. The patient is then transferred to the medical intensive care unit. The patient is started on a third-generation cephalosporin. Lumbar puncture shows purulent fluid with gram-negative cocci in pairs. You are asked to give recommendations regarding the use of prophylactic antibiotics for *Neisseria meningitidis* in people who have been near the patient.

Which of the following people should receive prophylactic antibiotics?

- ❑ **A. The patients who were seen in the emergency department on the same day**
- ❑ **B. The resident who performed the endotracheal intubation in the emergency department**
- ❑ **C. The paramedics who brought the patient to the emergency department**
- ❑ **D. The persons who attended the restaurant where the patient had lunch the previous day**

Key Concept/Objective: To know the indications for postexposure prophylaxis in persons in contact with a patient with N. meningitidis *meningitis*

Although outbreaks account for only 2% to 3% of all cases of meningococcal disease in the United States, prevention of the spread of the disease carries high priority. The risk of invasive disease in family members of persons with invasive meningococcal disease is increased by a factor of 400 to 800. Prophylaxis is recommended for close contacts of infected persons. Close contacts are defined as household members, day care center contacts, and anyone directly exposed to the patient's oral secretions (as might occur through kissing, via mouth-to-mouth resuscitation, during endotracheal intubation, or during endotracheal tube management by health care workers not wearing appropriate masks). The likelihood of contracting invasive disease from close contacts is highest in the first few days after exposure. Prophylaxis should therefore be administered within 24 hours after identification of the index case; it is unlikely to be of value if given 14 days or longer after onset of illness in the index case. The patients seen in the emergency department on the same day, the paramedics who brought the patient to the emergency department, and the persons who were in the same restaurant are not considered close contacts and do not need prophylaxis with antibiotics. *(Answer: B—The resident who performed the endotracheal intubation in the emergency department)*

24. You live in a town with a population of 80,000 people. Last year, one case of meningitis caused by *N. meningitidis* was reported, and one case was reported 2 months ago. As part of a community initiative, you are asked to give recommendations regarding the use of vaccines against *N. meningitidis* in your town.

Vaccination is warranted for which of the following groups of people?

- ❑ **A. Military recruits at a nearby base**

❑ **B. Patients with HIV infection**

❑ **C. People older than 2 years living in your town, because of the recent outbreak**

❑ **D. Every child younger than 2 years**

Key Concept/Objective: To know the indications for vaccination against N. meningitidis

A quadrivalent polysaccharide vaccine for protection against *N. meningitidis* serogroups A, C, Y, and W-135 is currently available. Vaccination is recommended for persons at increased risk, for prospective travelers, and for the control of outbreaks. Persons at increased risk include military recruits and persons with terminal complement pathway deficiencies or functional or anatomic asplenia. Vaccination is recommended for travelers to areas endemic for invasive meningococcal disease, including parts of sub-Saharan Africa during peak periods of disease incidence. Vaccination may be considered as a means of controlling outbreaks caused by serogroups covered by the vaccine. The Advisory Committee on Immunization Practices (ACIP) recommends that mass vaccination of persons 2 years of age or older be considered when three cases of serogroup C meningococcal disease occur within a 3-month period in a community or organization with an incidence of 10 cases per 100,000 or greater. Routine vaccination of infants is not recommended because of the poor immune response to the vaccine in this age group. *(Answer: A—Military recruits at a nearby base)*

25. A 21-year-old woman comes to your office complaining of fever, joint pain, and a rash; she has had these symptoms for the past 4 days. Her last menstrual period was 1 week ago. On physical examination, the patient has signs of arthritis in her left knee and right wrist, and there is tenderness and erythema on her tendon sheaths in both ankles. She also has a few pustules on her hands and knees. She recently traveled to Hawaii, where she had unprotected sex with a new partner. You order a ligase chain reaction test of her urine; the results are positive for *N. gonorrhoeae* and negative for *Chlamydia*. You make a diagnosis of disseminated gonococcal infection.

What is the antibiotic agent of choice for this patient?

❑ **A. Penicillin**

❑ **B. Tetracycline**

❑ **C. Ceftriaxone**

❑ **D. Ciprofloxacin**

Key Concept/Objective: To know the patterns of N. gonorrhoeae *resistance in different geographic areas*

***N. gonorrhoeae* has multiple means of resistance to antibiotics. Plasmid-mediated mechanisms confer resistance to penicillin by encoding altered penicillin-binding proteins. Resistance to tetracycline is mediated by chromosomal mechanisms. Resistance to fluoroquinolones is conferred by production of an altered DNA gyrase, to which these antibiotics are unable to bind. According to the CDC's 2002 Sexually Transmitted Disease Treatment Guidelines, 14% of the gonococcal isolates in Hawaii exhibit resistance to fluoroquinolones. Patients in whom physicians should consider the possibility of quinolone-resistant *N. gonorrhoeae* include those in whom treatment with fluoroquinolone therapy has failed, those who have traveled to Hawaii or Southeast Asia, or those who reside in California, where recent data indicate an increasing prevalence of fluoroquinolone-resistant *N. gonorrhoeae*. In 2000, 25% of *N. gonorrhoeae* isolates were resistant to penicillin, tetracycline, or both. Ciprofloxacin remains effective in the other geographic areas of the United States. Cefixime and ceftriaxone continue to have excellent activity against *N. gonorrhoeae*.** *(Answer: C—Ceftriaxone)*

For more information, see Marrazzo JM: 7 Infectious Disease: III Infections Due to Neisseria. ACP Medicine Online (www.acpmedicine.com). Dale DC, Federman DD, Eds. WebMD Inc., New York, January 2003

Anaerobic Infections

26. A 72-year-old woman presents to clinic with diarrhea of 7 days' duration. She was hospitalized briefly 1 month ago for community-acquired pneumonia, for which she was treated successfully with ceftriaxone. She describes having frequent watery stools that are greenish in color and are associated with abdominal cramping. She denies having fever, nausea, or vomiting. Examination reveals slight lower abdominal tenderness without peritoneal signs. Initial laboratory evaluation of stool is significant for the presence of fecal leukocytes. *Clostridium difficile*–associated diarrhea (CDAD) is suspected.

Which of the following statements regarding the diagnosis and treatment of CDAD is false?

- ❑ **A. The risk of developing CDAD after antibiotic treatment is highest with the use of cephalosporins, clindamycin, and amoxicillin**
- ❑ **B. Patient-to-patient spread in the hospital setting is a clinically significant mode of transmission**
- ❑ **C. For the detection of *C. difficile* enterotoxin in stool, enzyme-linked immunosorbent assay (ELISA) has a sensitivity approaching 95% when used with multiple samples**
- ❑ **D. Treatment with oral metronidazole and loperamide is indicated if the results of toxin assay are positive**
- ❑ **E. Use of intravenous metronidazole and vancomycin is an appropriate alternative if oral agents are not tolerated**

Key Concept/Objective: To be able to recognize CDAD and to understand its management

C. difficile **is the major etiologic agent of antibiotic-associated diarrhea and is capable of causing a spectrum of clinical syndromes, ranging from asymptomatic carriage to toxic megacolon. *C. difficile* is part of the normal fecal flora of humans, and about 80% of people acquire it in infancy. Adult carriers can spread the organism to others in the hospital setting, and medical personnel likely contribute to this spread through inadequate hand washing. Individuals who acquire the organism in the hospital setting have a higher risk of developing CDAD than asymptomatic carriers; this is possibly related to the development of antitoxin antibodies in the carriers.**

The patient described has findings typical of CDAD, including loose, watery stools and abdominal cramping. The diarrhea may begin several days to several weeks after treatment with antibiotics. Hospital stay longer than 15 days and the use of cephalosporins are factors that have been associated with positive results on *C. difficile* toxin assays in patients who experience diarrhea after the use of antibiotics. Clindamycin and amoxicillin are also commonly associated with the development of CDAD. A cytotoxin tissue-culture assay has traditionally been used to demonstrate the presence of the organism's enterotoxins, but newer enzyme-linked immunoassays have recently been employed. The sensitivity of such assays for detecting toxin in patients with pseudomembranous colitis is over 95%. Treatment consists of cessation of the offending antibiotic (if still being administered) and initiation of oral metronidazole or, alternatively, vancomycin. Intravenous therapy is appropriate if oral therapy is not tolerated. Antimotility agents are generally contraindicated, as they may predispose to the development of toxic megacolon. *(Answer: D—Treatment with oral metronidazole and loperamide is indicated if the results of toxin assay are positive)*

27. A 29-year-old construction worker presents to the emergency department with a puncture wound on his left foot, which he suffered when he stepped on a board with protruding nails at a job site. The wound appears to be contaminated with dirt. The patient reports that he received all immunizations as a child and was last given a tetanus booster in high school at 16 years of age. He is otherwise healthy.

Which of the following is the most appropriate choice for tetanus prophylaxis in this patient?

- ❑ **A. Tetanus immune globulin (TIG) administered intravenously**
- ❑ **B. Adult tetanus and diphtheroid toxoid (Td) given intramuscularly**
- ❑ **C. Td and TIG**

❑ D. **Diphtheria and tetanus toxoid combined with pertussis vaccine (DTP)**

❑ E. **Vigorous cleansing of the wound and oral administration of an antibiotic with activity against anaerobes (e.g., amoxicillin-clavulanate) for 3 days**

Key Concept/Objective: To understand the indications for and appropriate use of tetanus prophylaxis

Tetanus is a life-threatening infection caused by the spore-forming anaerobic bacteria *C. tetani*. The organism exists throughout the world in soil and feces and produces a potent neurotoxin that induces intense muscle spasm. Tetanus is rare in industrialized nations because of widespread active immunization with tetanus toxoid. Immunization is recommended for all infants (in the form of DTP or diphtheria-tetanus-acellular pertussis vaccine) at ages 2, 4, 6, and 18 months and again at 4 to 5 years of age. A booster dose of the Td vaccine is recommended at 16 years of age. Immunization with tetanus toxoid does not confer lifelong immunity, and booster doses are recommended every decade thereafter.

There are well-established guidelines for the prevention of tetanus after wounds are sustained. The need for tetanus toxoid or TIG depends on the nature of the wound and the patient's immunization status. TIG, which confers short-term passive immunity, is reserved for cases in which the following criteria are met: (1) the patient has received fewer than three doses of tetanus toxoid or the patient's immunization status is unknown, and (2) the injury is not a clean, minor wound (e.g., there is contamination with dirt, or the injury is a puncture wound or is an avulsion injury). If a patient's immunity is insufficient or the patient's immune status is unknown but the wound is minor, tetanus toxoid alone (in the form of Td) provides sufficient protection. Patients who have received more than three doses of tetanus toxoid previously, as this patient has, and who have a contaminated wound or a puncture wound will require Td if the last booster was given more than 5 years ago; patients who have received three doses of tetanus toxoid previously and who have a clean, minor wound will require Td if the last booster was given more than 10 years ago. Wound cleansing is an important component of management, but routine use of antibiotics has no role in tetanus prophylaxis. *(Answer: B—Adult tetanus and diphtheroid toxoid [Td] given intramuscularly)*

28. An elderly man with complaints of weakness and shortness of breath is brought to the emergency department by his neighbor. He awoke that morning with nausea, vomiting, and abdominal cramping, and several hours later he began to experience blurred vision and weakness in his arms. The neighbor reports that the patient appeared well yesterday. The patient lives alone; he cooks and cleans for himself. He is known to consume home-canned vegetables, which he grows in a garden during the spring months. Within 3 hours of arriving at the emergency department, he is intubated for respiratory failure. You suspect food-borne botulism.

Which of the following statements regarding this patient's condition is false?

❑ A. **His neurologic symptoms are caused by irreversible binding of toxin to presynaptic nerve endings, which prevents the release of acetylcholine**

❑ B. **Diagnosis can be established by demonstration of toxin in serum or stool specimens**

❑ C. **Clinical disease is caused by ingestion of spores, which germinate and allow colonization of the intestinal tract with toxin-producing organisms**

❑ D. **Antitoxin is only effective in neutralizing toxin before it binds to cholinergic synapses and therefore must be administered promptly**

Key Concept/Objective: To understand the pathogenesis and management of food-borne botulism

Botulism is caused by the spore-forming anaerobe *C. botulinum*, which produces the potent botulinum neurotoxin. There are three major forms of illness caused by *C. botulinum*: food-borne botulism, wound botulism, and infantile botulism. Food-borne bot-

ulism, which this patient has, is an intoxication (i.e., toxin is directly ingested). Spores of the organism may contaminate foods such as home-processed canned goods; these spores subsequently germinate into organisms that produce the neurotoxin. The toxin is heat labile, but if food is heated insufficiently, the intact toxin will be ingested and can be absorbed from the gastrointestinal tract. The toxin binds to peripheral cholinergic synapses and induces weakness, which progresses to flaccid paralysis. Infant botulism is an infection caused by the ingestion of spores (typically in honey), which replicate in the GI tract and produce toxin. Wound botulism is caused by direct inoculation of a wound with the organisms or its spores; heroin use is an important predisposing factor.

Proper recognition and diagnosis of this relatively rare illness can be difficult without a high index of suspicion: the presentation can resemble Guillain-Barré syndrome, myasthenia gravis, or stroke. Analysis of serum, stool, and suspected contaminated food is useful for confirming the diagnosis of botulism.

Antitoxin is administered early in the course of illness in an attempt to neutralize the toxin before it has bound to the cholinergic synapses. Hypersensitivity reactions to the equine-derived product are a serious adverse effect. Treatment is otherwise largely supportive and often includes mechanical ventilation, infection control, and nutritional support. *(Answer: C—Clinical disease is caused by ingestion of spores, which germinate and allow colonization of the intestinal tract with toxin-producing organisms)*

29. A 50-year-old man with type 2 diabetes, hypertension, and peripheral vascular disease is admitted to the hospital 2 days after injuring his right leg. While mowing the grass, he was struck in the calf by a rock, which resulted in a deep puncture wound. On the day of admission, he noted the rather abrupt onset of pain in the area of the wound, followed by the development of localized edema and the discharge of a thin, bloody fluid. On examination, he appears ill. His vital signs are as follows: temperature, 100.4° F (38° C); heart rate, 112 beats/min; blood pressure, 102/44 mm Hg; respiratory rate, 18 breaths/min. The right leg appears markedly swollen in the area around the wound; the skin of the lower leg is pale and cool, and there is slight crepitus over the calf muscle. Radiographs of the leg reveal gas formation in the surrounding soft tissue.

Which of the following statements is false regarding this patient's condition?

- ❑ **A. Gram stain of wound exudate is likely to demonstrate large gram-positive rods and a paucity of inflammatory cells**
- ❑ **B. The most appropriate initial antibiotic therapy consists of intravenous clindamycin and high-dose penicillin G**
- ❑ **C. Urgent surgical debridement is indicated, and amputation may be necessary**
- ❑ **D. Initial treatment should be guided by the results of anaerobic culture**
- ❑ **E. With adequate treatment, the mortality is 10% to 25%**

Key Concept/Objective: To be able to recognize clostridial myonecrosis and to understand the need for prompt treatment

Clostridial myonecrosis (gas gangrene, clostridial myositis) is a rapidly progressive but relatively rare infection that occurs in deep necrotic wounds. Infection is usually caused by *C. perfringens*. It often occurs after trauma. It can also occur in the setting of necrotic bowel; after surgery involving the biliary tract; and in association with vascular insufficiency, as in this patient. The incubation period is short, usually ranging from 1 to 3 days. After inoculation of a wound with spores (which are ubiquitous in the environment), replicative organisms are generated. These organisms elaborate several toxins, including α-toxin. α-Toxin lyses myofibrils and allows for rapid invasion and destruction of surrounding healthy tissue. Typical features of severe infection include pain and swelling at the wound site, pallor, tachycardia, and diaphoresis. Progression to hypotension, acute renal failure, shock, and death occur in the absence of definitive treatment. Radiographs often reveal gas formation, for which the infection receives its common name. Gram stain may demonstrate the pathogenic *Clostridia* species and mixed anaerobic flora; a typical finding is the absence of a prominent inflammatory

response. If meticulously collected, anaerobic cultures will often grow *C. perfringens*, but given the rapid clinical course, these cultures serve no useful purpose in guiding initial therapy. Prompt surgical debridement of necrotic tissue is the mainstay of therapy. Adjuvant antibiotic therapy with high-dose penicillin G has been routinely recommended; studies have demonstrated that combination therapy with clindamycin appears superior to penicillin alone. Despite adequate medical and surgical management, there remains significant morbidity and mortality associated with clostridial myonecrosis. *(Answer: D—Initial treatment should be guided by the results of anaerobic culture)*

30. You are treating a 75-year-old woman for severe community-acquired pneumonia with ceftriaxone and azithromycin. By hospital day 6, she has improved markedly with respect to her pulmonary status but has developed frequent watery diarrhea with cramping abdominal pain. You suspect *C. difficile* colitis, and stool toxin tests confirm this.

Which of the following is the most cost-effective initial treatment for this patient's condition?

- ❑ **A. I.V. vancomycin**
- ❑ **B. Oral vancomycin**
- ❑ **C. I.V. metronidazole**
- ❑ **D. Oral metronidazole**
- ❑ **E. Oral bacitracin**

Key Concept/Objective: To know the most cost-effective therapy for C. difficile *colitis*

Metronidazole and vancomycin are equally effective as initial therapy for *C. difficile* colitis. Metronidazole is considerably less expensive, however, and the oral route is preferable over the I.V. route when the patient can tolerate oral therapy. Bacitracin is as effective as vancomycin and metronidazole in treating the symptoms of *C. difficile* colitis but is not as effective as these two agents in eradicating the organism. *(Answer: D—Oral metronidazole)*

31. A 46-year-old woman presents to the emergency department complaining of facial spasms and muscle stiffness. Five days ago, while working with barbed wire on her ranch, she sustained a deep puncture wound of the left thenar eminence. This morning during breakfast, she experienced difficulty opening her mouth and felt pain with swallowing; this has progressed to stiffness and pain in her back, neck, thighs, and abdomen. On examination, the patient's face is held in a stiff grimace. Any sudden stimulus produces tonic muscle contractions.

Which of the following therapies will best treat this patient's muscle spasms?

- ❑ **A. Penicillin G, 10 million units/day I.V.**
- ❑ **B. Diazepam**
- ❑ **C. Tetanus antitoxin (immune globulin)**
- ❑ **D. Propranolol**
- ❑ **E. Tetanus toxoid**

Key Concept/Objective: To know the symptomatic management of patients who present with tetanospasm

The use of muscle relaxants is essential to the control of muscle spasms and rigidity, and diazepam is the drug of choice because it acts rapidly as a muscle relaxant and produces a sedative effect without inducing depression. The value of antimicrobial agents in the treatment of tetanus is doubtful; the only beneficial effects of antibiotics would be to eradicate from the wound vegetative cells of *C. tetani* that could produce additional toxin. Tetanus antitoxin binds circulating toxin, but its administration does not alter those manifestations of tetanus already evident. Propranolol can be useful in treating sympathetic overactivity (hypertension, tachycardia, sweating) but not muscle spasm. Tetanus toxoid must be administered after an episode of tetanus because clinical

tetanus does not establish natural immunity, but tetanus toxoid will not control tetanospasm once it is established. *(Answer: B—Diazepam)*

32. ***Metronidazole is effective as monotherapy for which of the following infections?***

- ❑ A. ***Bacteroides fragilis*** **brain abscess**
- ❑ B. **Vincent angina (trench mouth)**
- ❑ C. **Mixed intra-abdominal infections**
- ❑ D. **Lung abscess caused by *Actinomyces***

Key Concept/Objective: To know the antimicrobial activity of metronidazole

Metronidazole is the drug of choice for *B. fragilis* brain abscess because of its excellent penetration into the central nervous system and its virtually universal activity against *Bacteroides* species. Some *Actinomyces, Propionibacterium acnes,* and microaerophilic streptococci are resistant, however, as are facultative anaerobes. Thus, the addition of a second antimicrobial agent is indicated for mixed facultative-anaerobic infections, such as intra-abdominal or pulmonary infections. Metronidazole or penicillin very effectively treats Vincent angina or trench mouth, but the mainstay of therapy is surgery initially. *(Answer: A—*Bacteroides fragilis *brain abscess)*

33. A 52-year-old man with a history of alcoholism presents with a complaint of recurring fever, malaise, and cough with occasional hemoptysis. He has had these symptoms for the past 3 months. On physical examination, the patient appears chronically ill, and he has a low-grade fever of 100.8° F (38.2° C). On the posterior chest wall there is a sinus tract draining fluid with a few sulfur granules. Chest x-ray shows a pleural-based cavitary lesion in the superior segment of the right lower lobe that appears to correspond with the fistulous tract. A smear of the fluid from the sinus tract shows slender, branching, gram-positive filamentous organisms.

What is the appropriate treatment of this patient's infection?

- ❑ A. **Penicillin G, 10 to 20 million units/day I.V. for 2 weeks**
- ❑ B. **Penicillin G, 10 to 20 million units/day I.V. for 6 weeks**
- ❑ C. **Resection of the cavitary lesion, followed by penicillin G, 10 to 20 million units/day I.V. for 6 weeks**
- ❑ D. **Penicillin G, 10 to 20 million units/day I.V. for 2 weeks, followed by oral therapy for 3 to 6 weeks**
- ❑ E. **Penicillin G, 10 to 20 million units/day I.V. for 2 weeks, followed by oral therapy for 3 to 6 months**

Key Concept/Objective: To know the appropriate course of therapy for Actinomyces infection

Antibiotics are the mainstay of therapy for *Actinomyces* infections, and penicillin is the drug of choice. Daily doses of 10 to 20 million units are usually administered intravenously for a period of 2 to 4 weeks, followed by oral therapy for 3 to 6 months. These prolonged treatment schedules are designed to prevent recurrent infection. Resection does not play a role in the management of actinomycotic lung abscess. Tetracycline is the drug of choice for those patients allergic to penicillin; clindamycin, ceftriaxone, and ciprofloxacin have also been used with success. *(Answer: E—Penicillin G, 10 to 20 million units/day I.V. for 2 weeks, followed by oral therapy for 3 to 6 months)*

34. A 65-year-old man with poorly controlled diabetes underwent transurethral resection of the prostate 2 days ago. Today he presents with a complaint of scrotal pain. On physical examination, the patient is somnolent but arousable. His temperature is 101.7° F (38.7° C), his blood pressure is 100/70 mm Hg, and his pulse is 120 beats/min. His scrotum is markedly swollen, erythematous, and exquisitely tender.

What is the best step to take next in the treatment of this patient?

- ❑ A. **Immediate institution of broad-spectrum antibiotics**

❑ B. Immediate institution of broad-spectrum antibiotics and hyperbaric oxygen therapy

❑ C. Immediate surgical exploration and resection without regard to reconstruction

❑ D. Immediate surgical exploration and resection with caution with regard to future reconstruction

Key Concept/Objective: To be able to recognize and treat Fournier gangrene

Fournier gangrene is a form of necrotizing fasciitis occurring in the male genitals. It is a life-threatening infection with mortality ranging from 13% to 22%. Predisposing factors include diabetes mellitus, local trauma, paraphimosis, periurethral extravasation of urine, perirectal or perianal infections, and surgery in the area. When the clinical situation is suspected, surgery should be performed urgently to define the nature and extent of the infectious process, with resection of the involved tissue. Antibiotics are an important adjunct to surgery. Because anaerobes play a prominent role in this diseases pathogenesis, empirical therapy should be directed toward them, usually with a combination of ampicillin, clindamycin, and gentamicin. Hyperbaric oxygen therapy is sometimes advocated along with surgery and antibiotics, but data supporting its efficacy are lacking, and its precise role in treating serious soft tissue anaerobic infections remains to be defined. *(Answer: C—Immediate surgical exploration and resection without regard to reconstruction)*

For more information, see Simon HB: 7 Infectious Disease: V Anaerobic Infections. ACP Medicine Online (www.acpmedicine.com). Dale DC, Federman DD, Eds. WebMD Inc., New York, January 2002

Syphilis and Nonvenereal Treponematoses

35. Syphilis in its various manifestations has been recognized for many centuries. After the introduction of penicillin in the 1940s, there was a steady decline in incidence of the disease in the United States. In the late 1980s, there occurred a surge in the incidence of primary and secondary syphilis. The incidence of new cases peaked around 1990; since then, the number of new cases has declined and is currently at historically low levels. The Centers for Disease Control and Prevention has recently initiated a program to eliminate syphilis in the United States.

Which of the following statements regarding the epidemiology of syphilis is false?

❑ A. Although vertical transmission occurs, sexual contact remains the primary mode of transmission of the disease

❑ B. In the United States, transmissible syphilis is primarily concentrated in a few geographic regions in the Southeast

❑ C. The resurgence of new cases of syphilis in the late 1980s has been linked to the epidemic use of crack cocaine and the exchange of sex for drugs

❑ D. White and minority populations are affected with equal frequency

❑ E. Incidence rates are higher in inner-city populations than in rural ones

Key Concept/Objective: To understand the epidemiology of syphilis

Disease caused by the spirochete *Treponema pallidum* has been recognized for centuries. With advances in drug therapy and diagnostic methods, the control and, possibly, the eradication of syphilis in the United States have become realistic goals. The goals of the CDC's program are to reduce primary and secondary syphilis cases to fewer than 1,000 cases in a given year and to increase the number of syphilis-free counties to 90% or greater by the year 2005. Syphilis is transmitted through sexual contact primarily, with few cases associated with nonsexual exposure. The highest rates of infection occur in inner-city populations with lower socioeconomic status and are largely confined in the

southeastern United States. Minorities are affected to a much higher degree than whites (25:1 in some studies). The high rates of new syphilis cases among inner-city populations in the late 1980s and early 1990s has been linked strongly to the epidemic use of crack cocaine. *(Answer: D—White and minority populations are affected with equal frequency)*

36. Infection with *T. pallidum* typically progresses through well-described stages if left untreated.

Which of the following findings would NOT be consistent with the secondary stage of syphilis?

- ❑ **A. Diffuse, painless lymphadenopathy and patchy alopecia**
- ❑ **B. A hyperpigmented maculopapular rash involving the trunk, extremities, palms, and soles**
- ❑ **C. Signs and symptoms of meningitis (fever, stiff neck, photophobia) accompanied by abnormalities of the cerebrospinal fluid**
- ❑ **D. A single indurated and nontender ulcerative genital lesion accompanied by nonsuppurative regional lymphadenopathy**
- ❑ **E. Raised, moist, nontender plaques in intertriginous areas and on mucosal surfaces, the swabbing of which reveals spirochetes on darkfield microscopy**

Key Concept/Objective: To know the distinguishing features of secondary syphilis

Once *T. pallidum* has penetrated the epithelium, typically through sexual contact, the organism replicates locally and in regional lymph nodes. The characteristic lesion of primary syphilis is the chancre, an indurated, painless ulcer that can be up to 1 to 2 cm in size. Without treatment, the chancre typically resolves in 2 to 8 weeks; in a majority of cases, the chancre is not present by the time signs and symptoms of dissemination (secondary syphilis) develop. The clinical findings of secondary syphilis are varied but often include fever, malaise, diffuse lymphadenopathy, patchy alopecia, and a characteristic maculopapular rash, which involves the palms and soles. Condylomata lata, which are moist, indurated plaques (not truly ulcers) that occur primarily in intertriginous areas, are typically seen in patients with secondary syphilis. They are teeming with organisms and are highly infectious. Although symptomatic parenchymal neurosyphilis is commonly associated with late-stage (tertiary) syphilis, up to 40% of patients with secondary disease have involvement of the CNS, manifested clinically as meningitis. A positive CSF–Venereal Disease Research Laboratory (CSF-VDRL) test result confirms neurosyphilis in this setting, but the sensitivity ranges only from 30% to 70%. *(Answer: D—A single indurated and nontender ulcerative genital lesion accompanied by nonsuppurative regional lymphadenopathy)*

37. A 32-year-old man presents to the health department to establish primary care. He has not seen a physician since childhood and reports no chronic medical problems. On review of systems, he relates that approximately 1 year ago he developed an illness consisting of fever, "swollen glands," and a diffuse rash, which involved the palms. The illness resolved after a few weeks, and he did not seek medical care. Over the past 2 years, he has had several sexual partners, and he states he has not routinely used condoms. He currently feels well and has no complaints.

For this patient, which of the following findings would be most consistent with latent syphilis infection?

- ❑ **A. Diffuse, painless lymphadenopathy and a faint, widespread macular rash**
- ❑ **B. A rapid plasma reagin (RPR) titer of 1:32 and negative results on fluorescent treponemal antibody-absorption (FTA-ABS) testing**
- ❑ **C. An RPR titer of 1:16 and positive results on FTA-ABS testing**
- ❑ **D. An RPR titer of 1:256 and positive results on FTA-ABS testing**
- ❑ **E. Negative results on RPR and FTA-ABS testing**

Key Concept/Objective: To know the clinical and laboratory findings of latent syphilis

Latency refers to the period after resolution of secondary disease during which there are no signs or symptoms of disease: thus, by definition, there are no clinical findings to suggest active infection. Results of serologic testing, however, will usually remain positive. Because of the immune response to the infection, levels of nontreponemal titers (e.g., RPR) typically fall to low to moderate levels (often 1:1 to 1:16). Treponemal-specific tests (e.g., FTA-ABS), which confirm the diagnosis of syphilis in people with a positive RPR, remain positive. During the first few years of latency (early latency), there is a higher chance of recurrence of the symptoms of secondary syphilis, which are typically accompanied by a rise in nontreponemal serologic titers such as RPR. A high-titer RPR (e.g., 1:256) coupled with a positive FTA-ABS would generally suggest such a recurrence of active disease. A positive RPR accompanied by a negative FTA-ABS is not consistent with latent syphilis infection but instead indicates false positivity of the RPR. In 1% to 2% of the general population, nontreponemal serologic tests may be falsely reactive; false reactive results occur more frequently in patients with collagen vascular diseases (e.g., systemic lupus erythematosus), pregnant women, and the elderly. Negative results on RPR and FTA-ABS testing suggest the absence of infection in an untreated individual. *(Answer: C—An RPR titer of 1:16 and positive results on FTA-ABS testing)*

38. A 30-year-old woman with a history of pelvic inflammatory disease has recently tested positive for HIV. On a follow-up visit, she expresses concern about the possibility of other sexually transmitted diseases. As part of her initial workup, you recommend that she undergo testing for syphilis.

Which of the following statements regarding coinfection with HIV and syphilis is false?

- ❑ **A. Early-stage syphilis has been demonstrated to enhance the transmission of HIV**
- ❑ **B. Some studies have shown that the progression of early-stage syphilis to neurosyphilis is accelerated in HIV-infected individuals, compared with patients who are not infected with HIV**
- ❑ **C. Single-dose penicillin therapy for early syphilis is just as likely to be effective in a patient infected with both HIV and syphilis as in a patient infected with syphilis alone**
- ❑ **D. There is a higher incidence of false positive results on nontreponemal serologic testing in HIV-infected individuals, compared with those not infected with HIV**
- ❑ **E. CNS involvement is common in HIV patients with syphilis**

Key Concept/Objective: To understand the relationship between HIV and syphilis and the impact each of these diseases may have on the other

Syphilis and HIV are both sexually transmitted diseases, and risk behaviors that contribute to the transmission of syphilis are clearly associated with transmission of HIV. Thus, coinfection is common. Each disease has been shown to have an important impact on the course of the other. Primary syphilis enhances the transmission of HIV, probably because of the increased ability of the HIV virus to enter a sexual partner at the site of a genital ulcer (chancre). Since the beginning of the HIV epidemic, multiple reports have suggested that syphilis may follow an accelerated course in HIV-infected individuals and that it has a propensity to involve the CNS in such patients. It has repeatedly been demonstrated that single-dose penicillin therapy for early symptomatic syphilis is more likely to fail in an HIV-infected patient than in a patient with syphilis alone. HIV-infected patients have higher rates of false positive nontreponemal serologic test results. *(Answer: C—Single-dose penicillin therapy for early syphilis is just as likely to be effective in a patient infected with both HIV and syphilis as in a patient infected with syphilis alone)*

For more information, see Augenbraun M: 7 Infectious Disease: VI Syphilis and the Nonvenereal Treponematoses. ACP Medicine Online (www.acpmedicine.com). Dale DC, Federman DD, Eds. WebMD Inc., New York, April 2002

E. coli and Other Enteric Gram-Negative Bacilli

39. *Escherichia coli* is a facultative anaerobe that colonizes the human intestine. At least six pathotypes have been identified that can cause diarrhea, urinary tract infections (UTIs), and nosocomial illness.

Which of the following does NOT contribute to the pathogenicity of the various* E. coli *strains?

- ❑ **A. Production of Shiga toxin**
- ❑ **B. Direct binding of enterocytes and destruction of microvilli**
- ❑ **C. Production of catalase**
- ❑ **D. Production of coagulase**
- ❑ **E. Production of heat-labile enterotoxins**

Key Concept/Objective: To understand the pathogenic mechanisms of E. coli

Several distinct pathotypes of *E. coli* are known to induce a wide range of disease. Among the common virulence factors shared by all pathotypes of *E. coli* is the catalase enzyme, which helps protect the organism from host respiratory burst defenses by reducing hydrogen peroxide to water and oxygen. The enterotoxigenic pathotypes of *E. coli* also produce heat-labile and heat-stable enterotoxins that bind to intestinal cells and cause the efflux of chloride, sodium, and water into the intestinal lumen, resulting in diarrhea. The enterohemorrhagic pathotypes (among which serotype O157:H7 is the most important) cause diarrhea by binding to the apical surface of enterocytes, which results in destruction of microvilli (described histologically as the attaching and effacing effect). In addition, these enterohemorrhagic strains share with *Shigella* the ability to release Shiga toxin, which induces cell death and is responsible for the serious systemic complications of infection with these strains, including hemolytic-uremic syndrome (HUS). Coagulase production is not a significant means of pathogenesis for *E. coli*. *(Answer: D—Production of coagulase)*

40. A 24-year-old man presents to clinic after recently returning from a weeklong trip to Mexico. On the day of his return, he developed watery, nonbloody diarrhea that has persisted for 3 days. He reports passing up to 10 diarrheal stools a day but denies having significant pain or fever. Examination reveals a soft, nondistended abdomen with active bowel sounds that is mildly and diffusely tender. You suspect turista, or traveler's diarrhea.

Which of the following statements regarding this patient's illness is false?

- ❑ **A. It is likely that the causative agent is an enterotoxigenic strain of *E. coli***
- ❑ **B. Person-to-person transmission is a significant means of spread of the agent**
- ❑ **C. Examination of stool is unlikely to reveal blood and fecal leukocytes**
- ❑ **D. Treatment with an oral fluoroquinolone and an antimotility agent may reduce the duration of symptoms**
- ❑ **E. Disease is usually self-limited and often lasts fewer than 5 days**

Key Concept/Objective: To be able to recognize and appropriately treat diarrhea caused by enterotoxigenic E. coli

Enterotoxigenic strains of *E. coli* (ETEC) are a frequent cause of watery diarrhea in children living in developing nations and in travelers to these regions (hence the name traveler's diarrhea, or turista). The disease is spread by ingestion of food or water contaminated with the bacteria. Because a large inoculum is required to cause disease, person-to-person spread of the illness is uncommon. Diarrhea is caused primarily by the effects of the bacteria's enterotoxin, which is similar to cholera toxin in its ability to induce a secretory diarrhea. The organism does not directly invade the intestinal mucosa or cause extensive inflammatory changes. Thus, diarrhea is typically nonbloody, and examination of stool does not reveal fecal leukocytes. Patients typically

present with watery diarrhea and do not have fever or severe cramps. In travelers, the disease is generally self-limited, but the course can be shortened with the use of any of several regimens of antibiotics and antimotility agents (e.g., ciprofloxacin and loperamide for 3 days). Adequate fluid replacement in patients with diarrhea is the mainstay of therapy. Prevention can be accomplished most effectively in travelers by avoiding contaminated foods in endemic areas (including raw fruits and vegetables) and water that is not bottled. *(Answer: B—Person-to-person transmission is a significant means of spread of the agent)*

41. A 75-year-old man who lives alone is brought to the emergency department by his daughter because of diarrhea and lethargy. He was well until 4 days ago, when he developed severe abdominal cramps and watery diarrhea. The diarrhea persisted despite the use of loperamide and subsequently became bloody. His daughter reports that over the past 24 hours, he has produced little urine and has become progressively lethargic and intermittently confused. On examination, the patient appears dehydrated and is oriented to person and place only. The abdomen is soft but diffusely tender to palpation. Results of laboratory studies include the following: hematocrit, 23%; platelet count, 55,000/µl; white blood cell count, 15,000/µl; blood urea nitrogen, 60 mg/dl; serum creatinine, 3.9 mg/dl. Examination of the stool reveals blood and numerous fecal leukocytes; review of the peripheral blood smear demonstrates schistocytes.

Which of the following statements regarding this patient's diarrheal illness and its complications is false?

- ❑ **A. Systemic effects are the result of bacterial production of a toxin that damages endothelial cells**
- ❑ **B. The pathogenic organism causes disease in outbreaks associated with contaminated food, including undercooked beef**
- ❑ **C. A relatively small inoculum is required to cause disease, increasing the likelihood of person-to-person spread in facilities such as day care centers and nursing homes**
- ❑ **D. Early treatment with antibiotics and antimotility agents has been shown to reduce the rate of the development of life-threatening complications, especially in young children and the elderly**
- ❑ **E. Diagnosis can be established in most cases by stool culture using specific indicator plates**

Key Concept/Objective: To understand disease caused by enterohemorrhagic E. coli *(EHEC) and possible sequelae, including HUS*

This patient has diarrhea caused by EHEC and has developed HUS, a life-threatening complication of the infection manifested by acute renal failure, hemolytic anemia, and thrombocytopenia. Serotype O157:H7 is the most important serotype of this group of *E. coli* and has caused the largest and most frequent outbreaks. Consumption of undercooked beef has been most commonly associated with recent outbreaks of disease. Person-to-person spread is a significant problem, resulting in large outbreaks in settings such as day care centers, nursing homes, swimming pools, and water parks. This bacteria causes inflammatory diarrhea both by directly binding to enterocytes and by producing Shiga toxin. Patients typically present with severe abdominal cramping and diarrhea that progresses from watery to bloody. Young children and the elderly are particularly susceptible to the development of HUS. The primary means by which EHEC causes HUS is thought to be through the effects of Shiga toxin, which damages vulnerable endothelial cells in the renal microvasculature, inducing coagulation and microangiopathic hemolytic anemia. Recent studies have suggested that treatment with antibiotics and antimotility agents is actually associated with an increased risk of developing HUS, especially in children. Thus, it is important to identify serotype O157:H7 in patients with the appropriate clinical picture; careful monitoring and supportive care is warranted in these patients. If requested, identification of the causative organism can be accomplished in most laboratories because this serotype ferments sorbitol slowly (unlike most other *E. coli* strains), allowing its identification on specific indicator plates. *(Answer: D—Early treatment with antibiotics and anti-*

motility agents has been shown to reduce the rate of the development of life-threatening complications, especially in young children and the elderly)

42. You are called to see one of your clinic patients, a previously healthy 31-year-old woman, in the emergency department. She presented with dysuria and urinary frequency of 2 days' duration; these symptoms were followed by the development of fever and left flank pain. She denies having nausea and vomiting, and she has been taking liberal amounts of fluid. Initial urinalysis showed 10 to 25 red cells and more than 50 white cells per high-power field, and Gram stain of a spun urine sample demonstrated short, plump gram-negative rods. The emergency department physician has administered initial intravenous fluids and antibiotics for presumed acute pyelonephritis caused by *E. coli.*

After an initial period of observation in the emergency department, which of the following is the most appropriate course of action?

- ❑ **A. Admit the patient to the hospital and treat with intravenous ampicillin**
- ❑ **B. Admit the patient to the hospital and treat with intravenous piperacillin-tazobactam**
- ❑ **C. Discharge the patient after giving her a prescription for oral ciprofloxacin and scheduling a follow-up visit in clinic within 2 days**
- ❑ **D. Discharge the patient after giving her a prescription for oral trimethoprim-sulfamethoxazole and scheduling a follow-up visit in clinic within 2 days**
- ❑ **E. Discharge the patient after giving her a prescription for oral trimethoprim-sulfamethoxazole and scheduling a follow-up visit in clinic in 3 weeks**

Key Concept/Objective: To understand the treatment of acute uncomplicated pyelonephritis caused by E. coli

E. coli **is the most common cause of UTI in otherwise healthy patients, and it is also an important pathogen in patients with chronic indwelling catheters and abnormal urinary tract anatomy and in those who are immunocompromised. This patient has acute uncomplicated pyelonephritis that is likely caused by** ***E. coli.*** **Given the fact that she is not severely ill, is able to take oral fluids well, and has adequate follow-up, outpatient management after stabilization in the emergency department is appropriate. Patients who appear toxic, who have significant nausea and vomiting, who have significant comorbidity (e.g., diabetes mellitus), or in whom compliance is questionable should be admitted to the hospital. Follow-up in 48 to 72 hours is appropriate for outpatients to ensure improvement or resolution of symptoms and to review culture data. An important consideration in the selection of appropriate antibiotics for UTI is the emergence [illegible] studies have demonstrated a [illegible] resistance to ampicillin, first-generation cephalosporins, and trimethoprim-sulfamethoxazole in strains of** ***E. coli.*** **Thus, these agents are not recommended for use as monotherapy for acute pyelonephritis. In contrast, resistance to fluoroquinolones in strains causing UTI has been much less frequent, making these agents a reasonable choice.** *(Answer: C—Discharge the patient after giving her a prescription for oral ciprofloxacin and scheduling a follow-up visit in clinic within 2 days)*

43. A 60-year-old man with a history of type 2 diabetes mellitus and rheumatoid arthritis is admitted for knee arthroplasty. Four days postoperatively, you are consulted because he has developed fever and cough productive of blood-tinged sputum. Chest radiography reveals a left lower lobe infiltrate.

Which of the following is the most important pathogen to consider when choosing appropriate empirical antimicrobial therapy for this patient?

- ❑ **A. *Legionella* species**
- ❑ **B. *Klebsiella pneumoniae***
- ❑ **C. *Listeria monocytogenes***

❑ D. Nontyphoidal *Salmonella*

❑ E. *Staphylococcus epidermidis*

Key Concept/Objective: To understand that Klebsiella *and other enteric gram-negative rods are among the leading causes of nosocomial infections, including pneumonia*

This patient has developed hospital-acquired pneumonia. Although *Klebsiella* species only occasionally cause infection in otherwise healthy persons in the community, they are among the leading causative agents of nosocomial infections, including UTI, pneumonia, biliary infections, and bacteremia. Nosocomial pneumonias are often polymicrobial, with enteric gram-negative organisms (including *Klebsiella, E. coli,* and *Enterobacter*) playing a significant role. The other organisms most frequently implicated in causing nosocomial pneumonia are *Pseudomonas aeruginosa* and *Staphylococcus aureus. S. pneumoniae* and *Legionella* species are rarer causes of nosocomial pneumonia. Broad-spectrum agents should be used for empirical antimicrobial therapy in this setting. The agents chosen should have potent in vitro activity against enteric gram-negative rods; such agents include third-generation cephalosporins and combinations of β-lactam inhibitors and β-lactamase inhibitors. Nosocomial outbreaks of *Klebsiella* can be difficult to manage because these organisms may produce extended-spectrum β-lactamase and are often resistant to multiple drugs. *(Answer: B—*Klebsiella pneumoniae*)*

For more information, see Donnenberg MS: 7 Infectious Disease: VIII Infections Due to Escherichia coli and Other Enteric Gram-Negative Bacilli. ACP Medicine Online (www.acpmedicine.com). Dale DC, Federman DD, Eds. WebMD Inc., New York, February 2002

Campylobacter, Salmonella, Shigella, Yersinia, Vibrio, Helicobacter

44. A patient with a medical history of cirrhosis presents with fever, altered mental status, and bullous lesions on the legs and arms. His blood pressure is 60/30 mm Hg. An interview with family reveals that the patient was eating raw oysters in the Gulf Coast several days earlier.

Which of the following statements is true regarding this patient's illness?

❑ A. **Infection by *Vibrio* species is unlikely, because the patient did not have diarrhea**

❑ B. **The treatment of choice is azithromycin**

❑ C. **The organism causing this illness can also cause infection of a superficial wound that can lead to cellulitis or fasciitis**

❑ D. **When treated with appropriate antibiotics, mortality is approximately 10%**

❑ E. **Diagnosis is made clinically because the organism cannot be isolated from blood cultures**

Key Concept/Objective: To understand the presentation of Vibrio vulnificus *sepsis*

V. vulnificus can be isolated from waters of the eastern and western coasts of the United States. It can cause overwhelming sepsis in compromised individuals. Patients particularly at risk are those with chronic liver disease or iron-overload states. Hemorrhagic bullous skin lesions are characteristic. Patients need not have diarrhea that would be expected with *V. cholerae*. Another clinical syndrome associated with *V. vulnificus* is that of local wound infection that progresses to fasciitis. Although the diagnosis may be made clinically, the causative organism can be isolated from blood cultures. For treatment, the drug of choice is tetracycline, with or without cefotaxime. With bacteremia, the mortality is over 50% despite appropriate antibiotic therapy. *(Answer: C—The organism causing this illness can also cause infection of a superficial wound that can lead to cellulitis or fasciitis)*

45. A 40-year-old man presents with nausea, vomiting, low-grade fever, and midepigastric pain of 3 days' duration. A C-urea breath test is positive.

Which of the following is true regarding **Helicobacter pylori** ***infection?***

- ❑ **A. A positive C-urea breath test confirms a diagnosis of *H. pylori* gastroenteritis**
- ❑ **B. Hypochlorhydria and associated gastritis may be present for 2 to 8 months after initial infection with *H. pylori***
- ❑ **C. Treatment of *H. pylori* is warranted only if the patient has documented ulcer disease or gastritis**
- ❑ **D. The optimal method for checking for cure of patients undergoing treatment of *H. pylori* infection is the *H. pylori* serum antibody test**
- ❑ **E. *H. pylori* infection is the causative agent in the majority of cases of gastric adenocarcinomas**

Key Concept/Objective: To understand the clinical manifestations of acute H. pylori *infection and the treatment and complications of chronic* H. pylori *infection*

Acute infection with *H. pylori* causes gastroenteritis in up to 60% of patients. Although a positive result on the C-urea breath test confirms the presence of *H. pylori* , such a result does not necessarily mean that *H. pylori* is the cause of the infection. After acute infection, hypochlorhydria and associated gastritis may be present for several months. Because of the potential for long-term complications, any patient with *H. pylori* infection should undergo treatment. After a patient has completed treatment, the C-urea breath test or the stool antigen test can confirm that the patient is cured. Antibody levels cannot be used, because they will remain elevated for at least 9 months after disease resolution. Although *H. pylori* has been associated with gastric adenocarcinoma, it is not the cause of the majority of cases. *(Answer: B—Hypochlorhydria and associated gastritis may be present for 2 to 8 months after initial infection with* H. pylori*)*

46. A 32-year-old woman develops crampy periumbilical pain and fever over a period of several hours. The pain and fever are followed by profuse diarrhea.

Which of the following statements regarding the diagnosis of this patient is true?

- ❑ **A. The presence of fecal leukocytes is consistent with infection with *Shigella, Salmonella,* or *Vibrio cholerae***
- ❑ **B. Fever and abdominal pain are characteristically absent in patients with *V. cholerae* infections**
- ❑ **C. The presence of blood in the stool would make *Shigella* and [illegible]**
- ❑ **D. The most common cause of bacterial gastroenteritis in the United States is *Shigella***
- ❑ **E. For cases of acute infection, *Campylobacter, Shigella,* and *Salmonella* should grow on standard culture media**

Key Concept/Objective: To understand specific characteristics helpful in the diagnosis of bacterial gastroenteritis of various causes

The presence of fecal leukocytes is helpful in determining whether or not the cause of the diarrhea is an invasive infection or an inflammatory process such as inflammatory bowel disease. Other features associated with invasive infection are fever, abdominal pain, or even blood in the stool. Diarrhea caused by *Campylobacter, Shigella,* or *Salmonella* is characteristically associated with fecal leukocytes, fever, abdominal pain, and blood in the stool. (In patients with diarrhea caused by *Salmonella,* stools are less commonly heme-positive than in patients with diarrhea caused by the other pathogens.) This spectrum of clinical findings results from the fact that these pathogens invade intestinal epithelial cells. *V. cholerae,* on the other hand, colonizes the proximal

small intestine and secretes enterotoxins that cause the ensuing diarrhea. Thus, fecal leukocytes, fever, abdominal pain, and bloody stools are not expected. Many diagnostic features of diarrhea caused by *Campylobacter*, *Shigella*, and *Salmonella* overlap. The most common cause of bacterial gastroenteritis in the United States is *Campylobacter* (46%), followed by *Salmonella* (28%) and *Shigella* (17%). Stool culture can be helpful in identifying the specific etiologic agent if this is felt to be necessary. *Campylobacter* does not grow on standard media but will grow on specialized media. *Shigella* and *Salmonella* will grow on standard media. *(Answer: B—Fever and abdominal pain are characteristically absent in patients with* V. cholerae *infections)*

47. A 40-year-old man contracts a bacterial gastroenteritis associated with fever, severe abdominal pain, and profuse diarrhea. The etiologic agent is never determined.

Which of the following statements accurately characterizes the complications that may ensue in this patient?

- ❑ A. **As many as 40% of patients with Guillain-Barré syndrome had recent *Shigella* infection**
- ❑ B. **The arthritis associated with *Campylobacter* infection results from bacteremic spread of infection to joints**
- ❑ C. **Antibiotic treatment of infection caused by enterohemorrhagic *E. coli* (EHEC) may increase the risk of developing hemolytic-uremic syndrome (HUS)**
- ❑ D. **HUS most commonly results from infection with *Shigella***
- ❑ E. **The development of erythema nodosum suggests infection with *Salmonella***

Key Concept/Objective: To understand the various complications of infectious diarrhea

Infectious diarrhea can be associated with various complications. Postinfectious arthritis occurs in approximately 1% of patients with *Campylobacter* gastroenteritis. This is a sterile monoarticular or migratory polyarticular arthritis that particularly involves the knee. It begins 7 to 10 days after the onset of diarrhea and may persist for months. Up to 40% of patients with Guillain-Barré syndrome have evidence of recent *Campylobacter* infection. HUS is most commonly the result of infection with EHEC, but it can result from infection with *Shigella*. Antibiotic treatment of infection caused by EHEC may increase the risk of development of HUS. Thus, the clinician should not prescribe antibiotic therapy if EHEC is a real diagnostic possibility. Erythema nodosum complicates 1% to 5% of *Yersinia enterocolitica* infections in adults in the United States. It develops 2 to 20 days after the onset of gastrointestinal symptoms and typically resolves within a month. *(Answer: C—Antibiotic treatment of infection caused by enterohemorrhagic* E. coli *[EHEC] may increase the risk of developing hemolytic-uremic syndrome [HUS])*

48. A 60-year-old man presents with abdominal pain, fever, and profuse diarrhea. He has had diarrhea for 2 days; his symptoms started 2 days after eating at a cookout.

Which of the following statements regarding the treatment of this patient is true?

- ❑ A. **One positive blood culture with *Salmonella* suggests an endovascular nidus of infection**
- ❑ B. **No patient with *Salmonella* gastroenteritis should be treated with antibiotics because treatment merely prolongs the carrier state**
- ❑ C. **The decision to use antimotility agents such as Lomotil (diphenoxylate hydrochloride with atropine sulfate) should be based on the number of stools passed per day**
- ❑ D. **Erythromycin is the treatment of choice for gastroenteritis caused by *Campylobacter* if antibiotic therapy is deemed necessary**

❑ E. **Antibiotic treatment is indicated for *Shigella* gastroenteritis to shorten the period of fecal excretion**

Key Concept/Objective: To understand the basic concepts of the treatment of infectious diarrhea

Treatment of infectious diarrhea of most causes mostly involves supportive care. However, it is important to recognize specific indications and contraindications of certain treatments. *Campylobacter* enteritis is usually self-limited; therefore, specific therapy is often unnecessary. However, it may be prudent to administer antibiotics to those patients with moderately severe disease as well as to immunosuppressed patients, pregnant women, or patients with symptoms that worsen or persist for more than 7 days after diagnosis. For *Campylobacter* enteritis, erythromycin is the treatment of choice. For *Salmonella* gastroenteritis, treatment may prolong the carrier state. However, antibiotics should be administered to patients who are severely ill or who are at risk for extraintestinal spread of infection; these patients include infants, persons older than 50 years, patients with cardiac valvular or mural abnormalities, patients with prosthetic vascular grafts, and those receiving immunosuppression. Quinolones or third-generation cephalosporins are optimal. Nontyphoidal *Salmonella* has a propensity to colonize sites of vascular abnormality such as prosthetic vascular grafts, atherosclerotic grafts, and aneurysms. The presence of high-grade bacteremia (more than 50% of three or more blood cultures are positive) is suggestive of an endovascular infection. For *Shigella* gastroenteritis, antibiotics are not essential; however, for isolates that are known to be susceptible, ampicillin or tetracycline has been shown to shorten the clinical illness and the period of fecal excretion. Generally speaking, antimotility agents such as Lomotil should not be used in patients with infectious diarrhea. *(Answer: D—Erythromycin is the treatment of choice for gastroenteritis caused by* Campylobacter *if antibiotic therapy is deemed necessary)*

For more information, see Goldberg MB: 7 Infectious Disease: IX Infections Due to the Enteric Pathogens Campylobacter, Salmonella, Shigella, Yersinia, Vibrio, and Helicobacter. ACP Medicine Online (www.acpmedicine.com). Dale DC, Federman DD, Eds. WebMD Inc., New York, February 2002

Haemophilus, Moraxella, Legionella, Bordetella, Pseudomonas

49. A 68-year-old man presents to the emergency department with productive cough, shortness of breath, dizziness, and fever. His symptoms began 2 days ago and have been worsening. On presentation, the patient is febrile, hypoxic, tachycardic, and mildly confused. Chest x-ray shows an infiltrate in the left lower lobe. Gram stain of sputum is performed.

Which of the following statements is true regarding the cause of this patient's pneumonia?

❑ A. ***Pseudomonas aeruginosa*, *Legionella pneumophila*, *Haemophilus influenzae*, and *Moraxella* (*Branhamella*) *catarrhalis* generally are readily apparent on sputum Gram stain as gram-negative rods**

❑ B. **The apparent severity of the patient's illness suggests that *M. catarrhalis* is not the etiologic agent**

❑ C. **A third-generation cephalosporin would cover all important potential gram-negative pathogens**

❑ D. ***H. influenzae* pneumonia in adults is now rare because an effective vaccine is available**

❑ E. **The development of an empyema would be uncharacteristic of a gram-negative pathogen**

Key Concept/Objective: To understand various gram-negative pneumonias

***P. aeruginosa* is generally well visualized on Gram stain of sputum as a gram-negative rod. *Legionella* organisms are poorly seen on routine Gram stain, but visualization of these small, pleomorphic gram-negative bacilli is improved if basic fuchsin is used as**

the counterstain in place of safranin O. *H. influenzae* is often visible on Gram stain, but the morphology of the organism is often misleading: plump gram-negative rods, filamentous organisms, gram-negative diplococci, and under-decolorized gram-positive cocci have been described. *M. catarrhalis* is a gram-negative diplococcus that is morphologically indistinguishable from *Neisseria* species. This patient's signs and symptoms are not consistent with the usual presentation of pneumonia caused by *M. catarrhalis*. Pneumonia caused by *M. catarrhalis* occurs most often in the elderly, particularly those with underlying chronic obstructive pulmonary disease. The clinical features are those of a mild, acute pneumonia. A third-generation cephalosporin would cover *M. catarrhalis* and *H. influenzae* but would not cover Legionella. *H. influenzae* is the second or third most common cause of community-acquired pneumonia in adults. Most of the isolates in these cases are nontypeable strains not affected by the vaccine active against the type b capsular polysaccharide. Suppurative complications such as empyema can certainly be seen in pneumonia caused by *H. influenzae*, but empyema is rare in pneumonia caused by *L. pneumophila* and *M. catarrhalis*. *(Answer: B—The apparent severity of the patient's illness suggests that* M. catarrhalis *is not the etiologic agent)*

50. A 22-year-old man comes to your clinic with a cough that "won't go away"; he has had the cough for the past 2 to 3 weeks. He reports having episodes of severe coughing, and he has even experienced emesis with severe coughing spells. In your differential diagnosis, you consider *Bordetella pertussis* infection and atypical pneumonia.

Which of the following statements is true regarding B. pertussis infection?

- ❑ **A. If this illness is caused by *B. pertussis*, a marked lymphocytosis would be expected**
- ❑ **B. Adults infected with *B. pertussis* do not experience a catarrhal stage, as do children**
- ❑ **C. In adolescents and adults, *B. pertussis* infection generally occurs in those who were inadequately vaccinated**
- ❑ **D. Diagnosis can be reliably confirmed by use of acute and convalescent antibody titers**
- ❑ **E. Erythromycin is the treatment of choice for suspected *B. pertussis* infection in adults**

Key Concept/Objective: To understand the clinical features of B. pertussis *infection in children and adults*

In children, *B. pertussis* infection is generally associated with a marked lymphocytosis during the paroxysmal stage. However, in adolescents and adults, this lymphocytosis is usually absent. About half of adults do report a preceding catarrhal illness. *B. pertussis* infections in adolescents and adults probably occur as a result of the waning of immunity 5 to 10 years after vaccination; most *B. pertussis* infections that occur during early childhood now involve children who are either too young to have received vaccine or who were inadequately vaccinated. The interpretation of serologic results in vaccinated individuals can be difficult. A single elevated antibody titer should be interpreted in relation to age-matched, population-specific controls. Paired specimens have limited utility because a rapid amnestic response to infection usually precludes the detection of a significant rise in antibody concentrations between acute and convalescent sera. Cultures are usually negative in adults with persistent cough. Erythromycin is the treatment of choice. Erythromycin speeds elimination of *B. pertussis* from the nasopharynx, reduces transmission of infection, and may ameliorate the severity of disease, even if therapy is initiated during the paroxysmal phase. *(Answer: E—Erythromycin is the treatment of choice for suspected* B. pertussis *infection in adults)*

51. Several cases of pneumonia have developed in hospitalized patients at the hospital where you practice. The infection control team determines that the hospital water supply is contaminated with *L. pneumophila*.

Which of the following statements is true regarding infection caused by* L. pneumophila *in this setting?

- ❑ **A. Legionellosis is acquired mainly from upper airway colonization and aspiration of colonized secretions in hospitalized patients**
- ❑ **B. Legionellosis is more common in winter months because the causative organism does not proliferate in a hot environment**
- ❑ **C. Relative bradycardia can be a distinctive feature of *Legionella* pneumonia**
- ❑ **D. A patient exposed to *L. pneumophila* is more likely to contract *Legionella* pneumonia than Pontiac fever**
- ❑ **E. All forms of *Legionella* infection tend to attack a compromised host**

Key Concept/Objective: To understand the features of pneumonic and nonpneumonic legionellosis

Legionellosis is acquired mainly through the inhalation of aerosolized bacteria from an environmental source. The infection is more common during summer, when seasonal conditions promote the growth of legionellae in the environment and the use of air conditioners and other cooling devices facilitates the dissemination of airborne bacteria. Patients' temperatures may exceed 102.2° F (39° C), and relative bradycardia (a heart rate less than 100 beats/min despite a temperature of 104° F [40° C] or higher) may be present. During epidemics, the attack rate of *Legionella* pneumonia varies from 0.2% to 7%; nonpneumonic legionellosis afflicts over 65% of the people exposed. One or more risk factors, including immunosuppression, cancer, alcoholism, and diabetes mellitus, can be identified in most victims of *Legionella* pneumonia, but nonpneumonic legionellosis readily affects patients who are otherwise healthy. *(Answer: C—Relative bradycardia can be a distinctive feature of* Legionella *pneumonia)*

52. A patient who is currently neutropenic after induction of chemotherapy for acute myeloid leukemia becomes hypotensive and is transferred to the intensive care unit. He is given broad-spectrum antibiotics and shows initial improvement, but 36 hours later he becomes tachypneic and hypoxic and requires intubation and mechanical ventilation. By this time, blood cultures have grown *Pseudomonas aeruginosa*, and a chest x-ray shows multifocal infiltrates.

Which of the following statements correctly characterizes the complications of nosocomial* P. aeruginosa *infection?

- ❑ **A. Ecthyma gangrenosum, the characteristic skin lesion of *Pseudomonas* bacteremia, initially manifests as painful nodules and then undergoes central ulceration**
- ❑ **B. Sputum obtained from the endotracheal tube that grows [illegible] pneumonia**
- ❑ **C. Right lower quadrant abdominal pain in this patient would be characteristic of typhlitis**
- ❑ **D. Initial therapy of suspected pseudomonal bacteremia or pneumonia should be monotherapy with high doses of an antipseudomonal β-lactam**
- ❑ **E. Pseudomonal bacteremia commonly results in infective endocarditis**

Key Concept/Objective: To understand the clinical features and complications of nosocomial P. aeruginosa *infection*

***Pseudomonas* infection is associated with significant morbidity and high mortality in patients requiring intensive care. Ecthyma gangrenosum is a distinctive skin infection that occurs in the setting of bacteremia. The lesions may be discrete or multiple; they begin as painless macules or nodules and may become bullous. Lesions undergo central necrosis over a period of 12 to 24 hours; surrounding the lesion is a rim of tender erythema. *Pseudomonas* and other pathogens commonly colonize the trachea in intubat-**

ed patients without causing pneumonia. The diagnosis of *P. aeruginosa* pneumonia is most accurately made from quantitative cultures of bronchoscopic specimens. Whether bronchoscopy actually affects outcome is unclear. Typhlitis refers to localized gangrenous necrosis of the cecum that causes pain in the right lower quadrant. It is associated with neutropenia as well as *Pseudomonas* infection. Treatment of suspected *P. aeruginosa* infection should begin with high doses of an antipseudomonal β-lactam in combination with an aminoglycoside or fluoroquinolone. The use of two agents increases the likelihood of effective initial therapy. *P. aeruginosa* is a rare cause of infective endocarditis. Most reported cases have occurred in injection drug users; episodes have been known to complicate cardiac surgery. Hemodynamic decompensation in a bacteremic patient should always provoke consideration of infective endocarditis as the underlying cause. *(Answer: C—Right lower quadrant abdominal pain in this patient would be characteristic of typhlitis)*

53. A 23-year-old man who is status post splenectomy after a motor vehicle accident 1 year ago presents to the emergency department with fever, shortness of breath, and severe pain on swallowing. He is accompanied by his wife and their 6-month-old child. On physical examination, he has stridor and is sitting up with his neck extended and chin forward.

Which of the following statements is correct regarding the care of this patient and his family?

- ❑ **A. A lateral neck radiograph should be ordered, after which the patient should be reevaluated**
- ❑ **B. The patient's wife should receive chemoprophylaxis**
- ❑ **C. Chemoprophylaxis is not necessary for the patient's child**
- ❑ **D. This local infection rarely results in positive blood cultures**
- ❑ **E. Ampicillin is the drug of choice if the patient is not allergic to penicillin**

Key Concept/Objective: To understand the treatment of epiglottitis caused by H. influenzae *as well as basic fundamentals of chemoprophylaxis to prevent secondary cases*

This is a case of epiglottitis caused by *H. influenzae* in a patient predisposed because of having undergone splenectomy. Patients with epiglottitis can experience airway obstruction of rapid onset because of worsening inflammation. Therefore, a physician prepared to secure an airway should accompany this patient to the radiology suite. Rifampin prophylaxis should be administered to all adults and children in households with at least one member (other than the index case) who is younger than 4 years and who has not been immunized or whose immunization is incomplete. Thus, both wife and child should receive prophylaxis. This infection is most likely caused by *H. influenzae* type b, which does not colonize the airway as efficiently as unencapsulated strains but which has a much greater capacity to invade the bloodstream. Epiglottitis should be considered an invasive infection; blood cultures are positive in many cases. Patients can even die of septic shock. The antibiotic of choice is a third-generation cephalosporin. Ampicillin is highly effective against sensitive strains, but 35% to 40% of North American isolates of *H. influenzae* are resistant to ampicillin. *(Answer: B—The patient's wife should receive chemoprophylaxis)*

For more information, see Skerrett SJ: 7 Infectious Disease: X Infections Due to Haemophilus, Moraxella, Legionella, Bordetella, and Pseudomonas. ACP Medicine Online (www.acpmedicine.com). Dale DC, Federman DD, Eds. WebMD Inc., New York, April 2002

Brucella, Francisella, Yersinia Pestis, Bartonella

54. In Arkansas, a previously healthy 14-year-old boy presents to a clinic with fever, chills, headache, and malaise. Approximately 10 days earlier, he spent a day hunting rabbits with a relative. Examination reveals an ulcerated lesion with a black base on the left forearm as well as left axillary lymphadenopa-

thy. Laboratory tests are unremarkable except for a mildly elevated hepatic transaminase level. Tularemia is suspected.

Which of the following statements regarding the diagnosis of tularemia is false?

- ❑ A. **Serum agglutinins are usually detectable 2 to 3 weeks into the illness**
- ❑ B. **Pathology of infected lymph nodes is likely to reveal mononuclear cell infiltrate and granuloma formation**
- ❑ C. **Blood cultures are positive in a minority of patients**
- ❑ D. **Attempts to isolate and culture the organism should be made by routine hospital laboratories to define resistance patterns**
- ❑ E. **Definitive diagnosis is generally based on detection of antibodies to *Francisella tularensis***

Key Concept/Objective: To understand the diagnosis of tularemia

This patient displays symptoms typical of tularemia, which is a zoonotic illness caused by the gram-negative coccobacillus *F. tularensis*. Humans acquire tularemia through direct contact with infected wild mammals (including rabbits and muskrats) or from the bites of infected arthropods (typically, hard ticks). Hunters, trappers, veterinarians, and meat handlers are among those at increased risk for the disease. The ulceroglandular form of the disease is most common; in this form, affected patients develop an ulcer with surrounding erythema (and often a black base) at the site of inoculation. Spread of bacteria to regional lymph nodes results in lymphadenopathy, which histologically consists of monocytic infiltrates and granulomas. Definitive diagnosis of the disease is typically based on the detection of antibodies to *F. tularensis*, which are detectable 10 to 14 days after onset of illness and reach maximum titers at 2 to 6 weeks. Cultures of blood and lymph node tissue lead to the diagnosis in fewer than 10% of cases. However, routine attempts at isolation and culture of the organism should generally not be undertaken by most clinical hospital laboratories, given the highly infectious nature of the organism and the risk of airborne transmission to laboratory workers. As is the case with *Brucella* species and *Yersinia pestis*, these organisms can potentially be used as biologic weapons. *(Answer: D—Attempts to isolate and culture the organism should be made by routine hospital laboratories to define resistance patterns)*

55. A 50-year-old man is admitted to the hospital with a 3-week history of fever, chills, headache, malaise, and myalgias. One month before the onset of illness, he returned to the United States from an annual 2-week mission to Mexico, during which he stayed in a small village where he assisted farm workers. While there, he consumed foods produced locally on the farm, including vegetables, meat products, and goat's milk. On examination, he is febrile with nontender cervical lymphadenopathy and mild hepatomegaly. The results of initial laboratory workup are as follows: white cell count, 4,500/µl; hematocrit, 31%; platelet count, 138,000/µl; a slight elevation in hepatic transaminase level (less than twice the upper limit of normal). A biopsy of one of the lymph nodes reveals noncaseating granuloma formation.

Which of the following organisms is most likely the cause of this patient's illness?

- ❑ A. **Hepatitis A virus (HAV)**
- ❑ B. ***Mycobacterium avium* complex (MAC)**
- ❑ C. ***Mycobacterium tuberculosis***
- ❑ D. ***Plasmodium vivax***
- ❑ E. ***Brucella melitensis***

Key Concept/Objective: To know the epidemiologic associations and clinical findings of brucellosis

This patient has brucellosis, a zoonosis with protean manifestations. The animal reservoirs of brucellosis include goats (*B. melitensis*), cattle (*B. abortus*), pigs (*B. suis*), and dogs (*B. canis*). Brucellosis continues to be a major zoonosis worldwide. Infection in the United States is highest in people whose occupations bring them into direct contact

with animals or their bodily fluids; these persons include farmers, ranchers, veterinarians, and laboratory personnel. Another frequent source of infection is by ingestion of unpasteurized dairy products by travelers to countries such as Mexico, as is the case with this patient. After ingestion, incubation typically lasts 10 to 14 days, followed by the development of nonspecific symptoms such as those described. Once inoculated, bacteria travel to regional lymph nodes, where they multiply and enter the bloodstream, localizing in the cells of the reticuloendothelial system (including the liver, spleen, and bone marrow). Noncaseating granuloma formation typically occurs at sites of tissue infection. Metastatic spread to bone, joints, meninges, and cardiac valves is well described. Laboratory findings are often nonspecific and include normal or low white cell count, anemia, thrombocytopenia, and mild elevations of values in liver function tests. *Brucella* is a slow-growing organism that can be recovered from blood or bone marrow aspirates; the laboratory that performs the tests should be informed that *Brucella* is suspected, in order that the laboratory may keep blood cultures for 21 days. Agglutination titers can be helpful in making the diagnosis. *(Answer: E—*Brucella melitensis*)*

56. A 42-year-old woman with HIV presents to the office for evaluation of new skin lesions, malaise, and low-grade fever. She has advanced HIV disease (the results of her last $CD4^+$ T cell count was 75 cells/μl) and has had previous episodes of *Pneumocystis carinii* pneumonia and cryptococcal meningitis. She reports that she has had no recent contact with sick people and has not traveled recently. She has a dog and a cat at home but has suffered no bites or scratches. Examination of the skin reveals a few reddish-purple papules over the trunk and oral mucosa and a larger pedunculated mass with an angiomatous appearance on the right upper back. A biopsy is performed on one of the lesions; methenamine-silver staining of the specimen demonstrates lobular proliferation of new blood vessels and a neutrophilic inflammatory response that surrounds clumps of tiny bacilli.

Which of the following statements regarding this infection is false?

- ❑ **A. Dissemination with involvement of the lymph nodes, spleen, liver, and bone marrow may occur**
- ❑ **B. The causative organism is likely to be *Bartonella henselae***
- ❑ **C. A vigorous immune response to primary infection protects against subsequent relapse**
- ❑ **D. Treatment with erythromycin or doxycycline by mouth for at least 2 months is effective therapy**
- ❑ **E. Peliosis hepatis, which is characterized by the formation of venous lakes within the hepatic parenchyma, is a relatively common manifestation of the disease**

Key Concept/Objective: To understand the features of bacillary angiomatosis caused by Bartonella henselae

This patient has findings typical of bacillary angiomatosis, an infection with *B. henselae* that primarily involves the skin and lymph nodes; it is often seen in patients with AIDS whose $CD4^+$ T cell count is less than 100 cells/μl. Cutaneous lesions are produced by areas of neovascular proliferation associated with the inflammatory response to the bacteria. Lesions appear in crops and can have a papular, verrucous, or pedunculated appearance. They are typically red to purple and are difficult to distinguish from Kapsosi sarcoma. Regional lymphadenopathy is common. Systemic disease involving the liver, spleen, and bone also occurs. Peliosis hepatis is a characteristic finding in the liver and appears as hypodense lesions on abdominal CT. Treatment with erythromycin or doxycycline usually results in rapid improvement; this treatment should be continued for 2 months. Relapses are frequent after discontinuance of therapy, and some patients need lifelong treatment with tetracycline or a macrolide for disease control. *(Answer: C—A vigorous immune response to primary infection protects against subsequent relapse)*

57. A 15-year-old girl who works as a veterinary technician presents to clinic with complaints of painful swelling under her right arm that developed over the past 10 to 14 days. The swelling has been accompanied by low-grade fever, fatigue, and headache. She was previously healthy and is receiving no medications other than acetaminophen. On examination, you note a 3 by 3 cm tender lymph node in the right axilla, with overlying erythema and slight fluctuance. There is a small healing pustule on the dorsum of the right hand and several superficial linear abrasions over both forearms.

Which of the following statements regarding this infection is true?

- ❑ **A. Encephalitis, seizures, and coma are well-recognized sequelae of the illness**
- ❑ **B. Tissue aspirated from an affected lymph node is likely to reveal acid-fast bacilli**
- ❑ **C. Symptoms are unlikely to improve in the absence of sustained antimicrobial therapy**
- ❑ **D. Skin testing for a reaction to the causative organism is the diagnostic procedure of choice**
- ❑ **E. Person-to-person spread of the illness is a common mode of transmission**

Key Concept/Objective: To recognize cat-scratch disease (CSD) and its manifestations

CSD is one of several diseases caused by *Bartonella* species, which are small, fastidious gram-negative rods. The majority of cases of CSD are caused by *B. henselae*. After the scratch or bite of a cat (typically a kitten), a primary cutaneous papule or pustule typically develops at the site of inoculation. Regional lymphadenopathy and fever follow. Although in immunocompetent hosts the disease usually self-resolves within weeks to months, well-described neurologic complications occur in a minority of patients; these complications include encephalitis, seizures, and even coma. Another atypical presentation of the disease is Parinaud oculoglandular syndrome, which consists of granulomatous conjunctivitis and preauricular lymphadenitis. The differential diagnosis for CSD includes tularemia, mycobacterial infections, plague, brucellosis, sporotrichosis, and lymphogranuloma venereum. Diagnosis is often clinical but can be confirmed by demonstration of antibodies directed against *B. henselae*. Serologic studies have largely supplanted the use of CSD skin testing. Symptoms generally resolve without antimicrobial therapy. Only azithromycin has been demonstrated in a clinical trial to hasten resolution of lymphadenopathy in typical cases of CSD. *(Answer: A—Encephalitis, seizures, and coma are well-recognized sequelae of the illness)*

For more information, see Liles WC: 7 Infectious Disease: XI Infections Due to Brucella, Francisella, Yersinia Pestis, and Bartonella. ACP Medicine Online (www.acpmedicine.com). Dale DC, Federman DD, Eds. WebMD Inc., New York, March 2002

Diseases Due to Chlamydia

58. A 24-year-old man from sub-Saharan Africa comes to your office to establish primary care. He has been blind since 20 years of age because of a recurrent eye infection. He has no other significant medical history. You make a probable diagnosis of trachoma.

Which of the following statements about this patient's* Chlamydia *infection is false?

- ❑ **A. The infection is caused by *Chlamydia trachomatis*, which is an intracellular pathogen**
- ❑ **B. The organism causing blindness in this patient is identical to that causing sexually transmitted diseases such as urethritis and lymphogranuloma venereum (LGV)**
- ❑ **C. *Chlamydia pneumoniae* has been associated with an increased risk of cardiovascular disease**
- ❑ **D. *Chlamydia* organisms are widespread in nature and can cause infections in mammals and other animal species**

Key Concept/Objective: To understand the clinical presentations of infections caused by different species of Chlamydia

The chlamydiae are widespread obligate intracellular pathogens. These organisms produce a variety of infections in mammals and avian species. There are three species known to infect humans: *C. trachomatis*, *C. pneumoniae*, and *C. psittaci*. One of the best-known chlamydial reservoirs is parrots and parakeets; these birds can be infected (often asymptomatically) by *C. psittaci*. Human contact with these animals can cause psittacosis. This patient is likely to have trachoma, the most common cause of preventable blindness in the underdeveloped world. Recurrent episodes of infection cause progressive scarring of the cornea, leading ultimately to blindness. Trachoma is caused by *C. trachomatis*. There are 18 distinct serotypes of *C. trachomatis*. In different serotypes, tissue tropism and disease specificity differ. Serovars A, B, Ba, and C are associated with trachoma, whereas serovars D through K are associated with sexually transmitted and perinatally acquired infections. Serovars L1, L2, and L3 are more invasive than the other serovars and spread to lymphatic tissues. These serovars produce the clinical syndromes of LGV and hemorrhagic proctocolitis. In several epidemiologic studies, *C. pneumoniae* infection was linked to an increase in the risk of atherosclerotic disease. Randomized controlled trials are investigating the effect of therapy for subclinical *C. pneumoniae* infections on cardiovascular outcomes. *(Answer: B—The organism causing blindness in this patient is identical to that causing sexually transmitted diseases such as urethritis and lymphogranuloma venereum [LGV])*

59. A 35-year-old heterosexual man presents to your clinic with complaints of burning on urination, urethral discharge, and urethral itching. He denies having fever, chills, nausea, or vomiting. Physical examination is significant only for purulent discharge at the urethral meatus. Smear of the discharge shows the presence of polymorphonuclear leukocytes; however, the Gram stain is negative.

Which of the following statements regarding treatment of this patient is false?

- ❑ **A. Female partners of men with nongonococcal urethritis from *Chlamydia trachomatis* need to be treated with antibiotics**
- ❑ **B. Doxycycline, 100 mg p.o. twice a day for 7 days, is adequate therapy for this patient**
- ❑ **C. One dose of azithromycin, 1 g p.o., is adequate therapy for this patient**
- ❑ **D. If no bacteria are isolated on Gram stain, no further treatment is necessary**

Key Concept/Objective: To understand the treatment of nongonococcal urethritis

Nongonococcal urethritis (NGU) is the most common presentation of *C. trachomatis* infection in men. Presumptive diagnosis is made by demonstrating leukocyte predominance on urethral exudate smear in the absence of identifiable organisms on Gram stain. The specific presentation is variable; up to 50% of men with NGU are asymptomatic. Confirmatory diagnosis is made by either NAAT or culture. Treatment consists of either doxycycline taken twice daily for 1 week or azithromycin taken in a single dose of 1 g. Because these treatments are equally effective, cost and compliance often influence the specific choice of therapy. Female partners of patients with NGU should be presumptively treated as well. *(Answer: D—If no bacteria are isolated on Gram stain, no further treatment is necessary)*

60. A 27-year-old man presents to the emergency department with severe scrotal pain, nausea, vomiting, and fever. He denies having ever had a sexually transmitted disease, nor has he ever undergone surgery. He does report that for the past 2 weeks he has had a urethral discharge. On physical examination, the patient's temperature is 99.6° F (37.6° C), there is pain on palpation of the lateral aspect of the scrotum, and there is epididymal swelling.

Which of the following statements regarding the treatment of this patient is false?

❑ **A. Testicular torsion should be ruled out by ultrasound**

❑ **B. All patients with epididymitis should be admitted for intravenous antibiotics**

❑ **C. A presumptive diagnosis can be made on the basis of findings of pyuria on urinalysis or smear of urethral discharge**

❑ **D. The results of a nuclear acid amplification test (NAAT) of urine or a urethral discharge can confirm the diagnosis of epididymitis in this patient**

❑ **E. Ofloxacin, 300 mg b.i.d., should be started empirically until the causative agent is identified**

Key Concept/Objective: To understand the diagnosis and treatment of epididymitis

In a very small percentage of patients with urethritis, the infection may ascend to the genital tract and cause acute epididymitis. In heterosexual men younger than 35 years, *Chlamydia trachomatis* is the major cause of acute epididymitis. Most patients present with unilateral scrotal pain, fever, and epididymal tenderness; testicular torsion should therefore be ruled out in certain cases. The diagnosis of epididymitis is made in the same manner as urethritis. Empirical treatment should be started once cultures are obtained. In ill-appearing patients who are toxic and in severe pain, hospital admission is often warranted for administration of intravenous antibiotics and pain medication. However, if the patient is otherwise doing well, he may be treated as an outpatient and followed closely. *(Answer: B—All patients with epididymitis should be admitted for intravenous antibiotics)*

61. A 44-year-old woman presents to your clinic for evaluation of fever, chills, and malaise; she has had these symptoms for 4 days. In addition, she complains of a severe headache and a dry, nonproductive cough. Results of physical examination are as follows: temperature, 101.6° F (38.7° C); pulse, 62 beats/min, respiratory rate, 16 breaths/min; blood pressure, 136/82 mm Hg. HEENT, pulmonary, and cardiac examination results are within normal limits. Abdominal examination is significant for mild splenomegaly; but the abdomen is nontender and nondistended, and bowel sounds are normal. Upon further questioning, the patient reports that she visited her daughter 2 weeks earlier and that her daughter has a parrot. You suspect psittacosis.

Which of the following statements regarding diagnostic tests for psittacosis is false?

❑ **A. Abnormal results on liver function testing are commonly seen**

❑ **B. The white cell count is usually elevated**

❑ **C. The erythrocyte sedimentation rate (ESR) is usually not elevated**

❑ **D. Chest x-ray typically shows nonspecific, patchy infiltrates**

❑ **E. A fourfold increase in acute and convalescent antibody titers confirms the diagnosis**

Key Concept/Objective: To know the laboratory findings of psittacosis

***Chlamydia psittaci* has been isolated from the secretions, excretions, tissue, and feathers of both symptomatic and asymptomatic birds. In humans, the bacteria are inhaled and are then disseminated hematogenously; they primarily localize in the alveolar macrophages and the endothelial cells of the liver and spleen. The incubation period is from 7 to 14 days. At presentation, the disease can vary in severity from mild to life threatening. On rare occasions, psittacosis can be fatal. Common symptoms are fever, chills, malaise, headache, and nonproductive cough. Other features include an absence of consolidation and pleural effusion, relative bradycardia, splenomegaly, and a rash resembling the rose spots of typhoid fever. Diagnosis is made clinically. Treatment with tetracycline should be initiated while awaiting laboratory results. Abnormal results on liver function testing are commonly seen; the ESR is normal; and the chest x-ray shows a nonspecific pattern. The white cell count is usually normal or decreased. The diagno-**

sis is confirmed by a fourfold increase in acute and convalescent antibody titers. *(Answer: B—The white cell count is usually elevated)*

62. A 27-year-old man who recently returned from Southeast Asia presents to your clinic for evaluation of painful swelling of the left groin, fever, chills, headaches, and arthralgias. On physical examination, his temperature is 100.6° F (38.1° C), and matted, fluctuant, suppurative left inguinal lymphadenopathy is noted. The overlying skin is inflamed. LGV is diagnosed by complement fixation assay, and you treat the patient with doxycycline.

If the patient had gone untreated, which of the following complications could NOT develop?

- ❑ **A. Genital elephantiasis**
- ❑ **B. Encephalitis**
- ❑ **C. Penile fistulas**
- ❑ **D. Aseptic meningitis**
- ❑ **E. Chancroid**

Key Concept/Objective: To understand the complications of untreated LGV

LGV is a sexually transmitted disease caused by *C. trachomatis*. The disease begins with an isolated, transient genital, rectal, or oral lesion; suppurative regional lymphadenopathy then occurs. Although the disease is rare in the United States, it is endemic in many parts of the world, including Africa, Asia, South America, and the Caribbean. The primary lesion is often a painless genital papule or vesicle that usually heals without scarring. From this primary site, the infection spreads to regional lymph nodes; approximately 2 to 6 weeks after the primary infection, lymphadenopathy develops. Femoral and iliac lymph nodes enlarge progressively and become matted, fluctuant, and often suppurative, forming fistulas to the skin. In addition to lymphadenopathy developing, fever, chills, headache and meningismus can develop. The diagnosis is made serologically with complement fixation or microimmunofluorescence testing. Treatment consists of doxycycline, 100 mg b.i.d. for 21 days. If untreated, patients can develop genital elephantiasis as a late complication; aseptic meningitis; encephalitis; and penile fistulas. Chancroid is a sexually transmitted disease caused by *Haemophilus ducreyi* and is not a complication of LGV; however, chancroid must be included in the differential diagnosis of patients with genital ulcers and lymphadenopathy. *(Answer: E—Chancroid)*

63. A 22-year-old white woman presents to your clinic for routine yearly gynecologic examination. She is asymptomatic and has been doing well. Her medical history is unremarkable. In the social history, she states that she is sexually active and that she engages in unprotected sex. Upon further questioning, she states that she has had four sexual partners in the past year.

Which of the following measures is most appropriate for the prevention of pelvic inflammatory disease (PID) in this patient?

- ❑ **A. Empirical treatment of *N. gonorrhoeae* and *C. trachomatis* infections**
- ❑ **B. Counseling on the importance of minimizing high-risk behavior**
- ❑ **C. Screening for *Chlamydia* and *N. gonorrhoeae*; treatment should be initiated only if the patient starts having symptoms**
- ❑ **D. Screening for *Chlamydia* and *N. gonorrhoeae*; treatment should be initiated if cultures are positive**

Key Concept/Objective: To know the importance of screening for chlamydial cervical infections to prevent PID

Chlamydial mucopurulent cervicitis in women is a serious infection, especially if left untreated. Women often present with vaginal discharge, bleeding, and abdominal pain; however, a significant number of patients with cervical infection are asymptomatic. If untreated, ascending infection can develop into salpingitis and eventually PID. PID

caused by *C. trachomatis* has been linked with infertility as a result of fallopian tube scarring; ectopic pregnancy is another important sequela. A prospective cohort study showed that treatment of asymptomatic patients effectively prevented subsequent PID. Therefore, chlamydial screening of high-risk adolescents and women younger than 25 years who have new sexual partners is strongly recommended. *(Answer: D—Screening for* Chlamydia *and* N. gonorrhoeae*; treatment should be initiated if cultures are positive)*

For more information, see Stamm WE: 7 Infectious Disease: XIII Diseases Due to Chlamydia. ACP Medicine Online (www.acpmedicine.com). Dale DC, Federman DD, Eds. WebMD Inc., New York, May 2002

Antimicrobial Therapy

64. A 64-year-old man with long-standing diabetes mellitus presents to the emergency department for evaluation of shortness of breath. He was in his usual state of health until 2 days ago, when he developed cough with green sputum, dyspnea on exertion, and a fever of 102° F (38.9° C). He denies having been in contact with persons who were sick. He has no history of cigarette smoking or cardiac or pulmonary illnesses. The patient has never been vaccinated for pneumonia. On physical examination, the patient is tachycardic, is tachypneic, and has rales in the left midlung zone with associated egophony and increased fremitus. Laboratory studies reveal leukocytosis with a left shift. A chest x-ray reveals left-lower-lobe pneumonia.

For this patient, which of the following statements regarding penicillin and cephalosporin therapy is false?

- ❑ **A. Like the penicillins, the cephalosporins are bactericidal antibiotics**
- ❑ **B. Third-generation cephalosporins are active against most penicillin-nonsusceptible pneumococci**
- ❑ **C. In treating an infection with penicillin-resistant *Streptococcus pneumoniae*, adding a β-lactamase inhibitor to a regimen of penicillin will augment antibiotic killing**
- ❑ **D. Cefepime has activity against aerobic gram-positive bacteria, methicillin-susceptible *Staphylococcus aureus*, and gram-negative bacteria, including *Pseudomonas***

Key Concept/Objective: To understand the characteristics and spectrums of activity of penicillin and the cephalosporins

Like the penicillins, the cephalosporins are bactericidal antibiotics that inhibit bacterial cell wall synthesis and have a low intrinsic toxicity. Although third-generation agents are less active against many gram-positive cocci than the older cephalosporins, they are active against most penicillin-nonsusceptible pneumococci. Penicillin-resistant strains of *S. pneumoniae* have altered penicillin-binding proteins and are not affected by the addition of a β-lactamase inhibitor. Cefepime is a fourth-generation cephalosporin with broad antimicrobial activity against both aerobic gram-positive bacteria (e.g., penicillin-nonsusceptible *S. pneumoniae*) and methicillin-susceptible *S. aureus*; it is also effective against gram-negative bacteria, including *Haemophilus influenzae*, *Neisseria*, and Enterobacteriaceae. Its activity against *Pseudomonas* is similar to that of ceftazidime. *(Answer: C—In treating an infection with penicillin-resistant* Streptococcus pneumoniae*, adding a β-lactamase inhibitor to a regimen of penicillin will augment antibiotic killing)*

65. A 33-year-old man with AIDS was admitted to the hospital 3 days ago with cellulitis and an ulceration of his left lower extremity. He has suffered from several opportunistic infections over the past 2 years, including *Pneumocystis carinii* pneumonia, thrush, and disseminated *Mycobacterium avium-intracellulare*. He has had an uneventful hospital stay but remains febrile. His ulceration is deep, and the anterior surface of the tibia is visible on examination. The patient was started on empirical vancomycin therapy at the time of his admission. Bone biopsy cultures have grown methicillin-resistant *S. aureus*.

Which of the following statements regarding antibiotics with activity against methicillin-resistant* S. aureus *is false?

- ❑ **A. Vancomycin is the drug of choice in the treatment of infections caused by methicillin-resistant *S. aureus***
- ❑ **B. Because quinupristin-dalfopristin is associated with a high incidence of phlebitis, a central line should be used for intravenous delivery**
- ❑ **C. Daptomycin is a bactericidal agent currently approved only for complicated skin, skin structure, and pulmonary infections**
- ❑ **D. Linezolid, an agent that is bacteriostatic against *S. aureus*, is available in both intravenous and oral preparations**

Key Concept/Objective: To know the important features of antibiotics used in the treatment of infections caused by methicillin-resistant S. aureus

Vancomycin is the drug of choice in the treatment of infections caused by methicillin-resistant *S. aureus*. Because quinupristin-dalfopristin is associated with a high incidence of phlebitis, a central line should be used for intravenous delivery. Other adverse effects include arthralgias and myalgias, which may be severe, and elevations of the bilirubin level. Daptomycin is bactericidal, and synergy has been demonstrated with gentamicin against staphylococci and enterococci. Daptomycin is currently approved only for complicated skin and skin structure infections. Daptomycin achieves suboptimal levels in the lungs and should not be used for pulmonary infections. Linezolid is bacteriostatic against staphylococci and enterococci, but it is bactericidal against most streptococci. Intravenous and oral preparations of linezolid are available. *(Answer: C—Daptomycin is a bactericidal agent currently approved only for complicated skin, skin structure, and pulmonary infections)*

66. A 41-year-old woman is admitted to the hospital for evaluation of fever and abdominal pain. She was well until 2 days ago, when she developed dysuria and right flank pain. She denies having cough, dyspnea, nausea, emesis, or diarrhea. She has not traveled recently, and she is monogamous with her husband of 15 years. On physical examination, moderate tenderness to palpation is noted over the bladder, and costovertebral angle tenderness is noted on the right. The rest of the examination is unremarkable. Laboratory studies reveal leukocytosis and pyuria. A CT scan of her abdomen and pelvis is consistent with pyelonephritis without evidence of nephrolithiasis or obstructive uropathy. The patient is started on intravenous hydration and a fluoroquinolone antibiotic.

Which of the following statements regarding fluoroquinolones is false?

- ❑ **A. The fluoroquinolones are bactericidal compounds that inhibit DNA synthesis and introduce double-strand DNA breaks by targeting DNA gyrase and topoisomerase IV**
- ❑ **B. Ciprofloxacin is the drug of choice for *Bacillus anthracis***
- ❑ **C. The newer fluoroquinolones are preferred for the treatment of community-acquired pneumonia**
- ❑ **D. The bioavailability of the fluoroquinolones is greatly augmented when given intravenously**

Key Concept/Objective: To know the important clinical features of the fluoroquinolones

The fluoroquinolones are bactericidal compounds that inhibit DNA synthesis and introduce double-strand DNA breaks by targeting DNA gyrase and topoisomerase IV. Ciprofloxacin is the drug of choice for *B. anthracis*, though other fluoroquinolones are also active in vitro. Because the newer quinolones bind equally to DNA gyrase and topoisomerase IV and because they have enhanced pharmacokinetic and pharmacodynamic parameters for *S. pneumoniae*, it has been argued that they are the preferred quinolones for community-acquired pneumonia. The fluoroquinolones are rapidly absorbed from the gastrointestinal tract and have nearly 100% bioavailability. *(Answer: D—The bioavailability of the fluoroquinolones is greatly augmented when given intravenously)*

67. Antimicrobials play a fundamental role in the physician's ability to manage infections. To optimize therapy, clinicians must take into account several factors, including the causative microorganism, host comorbidities, and cost. The clinician must also be able to recognize and, if possible, prevent adverse reactions to commonly used antimicrobial agents.

Which of the following adverse reactions to antimicrobial agents is NOT a direct toxic effect of the drug?

- ❑ **A. In the intensive care unit, a patient with *Acinetobacter* pneumonia has a generalized seizure after being started on imipenem**
- ❑ **B. A patient receiving oral isoniazid for tuberculosis develops numbness and tingling in her hands after 5 weeks of therapy**
- ❑ **C. A 50-year-old man with an unknown medical history develops acute respiratory distress, hypotension, and urticaria 30 minutes after being given an intramuscular injection of penicillin G**
- ❑ **D. An elderly man with coronary disease who is hospitalized for pneumonia is being treated with erythromycin; the patient becomes pulseless, and the monitor shows ventricular fibrillation (torsades de pointes); review of rhythm strips before the arrest reveals a prolonged QT interval**
- ❑ **E. Four days after being started on gentamicin, a patient's creatinine level is noted to have doubled**

Key Concept/Objective: To know the direct toxic effects of antimicrobials and to understand the difference between direct toxic effects and hypersensitivity reactions

There are generally three different types of adverse reactions to antibiotics: direct drug toxicity, hypersensitivity (allergic) reactions, and microbial superinfection. Direct drug toxicity is generally dose related. Host susceptibility factors, such as renal or hepatic impairment, may greatly affect the likelihood of toxicity. For instance, patients with underlying renal insufficiency are at greater risk for developing azotemia and tubular damage when treated with aminoglycosides, vancomycin, or amphotericin B. Other examples of direct toxic effects of antibiotics include seizures induced by the carbapenem antibiotic imipenem; peripheral neuropathy caused by isoniazid; and conduction system abnormalities (prolongation of the QT interval) caused by macrolides, such as erythromycin. Hypersensitivity reactions, on the other hand, are generally not dose related but immune mediated. Allergies to penicillin have been most extensively studied. A careful history of allergic reactions should be obtained before prescribing any antibiotic. Microbial superinfection occurs when antimicrobial therapy reduces susceptible organisms from the normal flora of the skin, oral and genitourinary mucosae, and the gastrointestinal tract. *Clostridium difficile*–associated diarrhea is an example of a common adverse effect resulting from microbial superinfection. *(Answer: C—A 50-year-old man with an unknown medical history develops acute respiratory distress, hypotension, and urticaria 30 minutes after being given an intramuscular injection of penicillin G)*

68. Penicillin G was the first widely used antibiotic to treat systemic infections. The penicillin family of antibiotics remains an important weapon in the arsenal against invasive bacterial disease.

Which of the following statements regarding penicillin and its β-lactam derivatives is false?

- ❑ **A. The major mechanism by which bacteria develop resistance is through the production of enzymes that cleave the β-lactam ring (β-lactamases)**
- ❑ **B. Penicillins are bactericidal agents that bind to proteins known as penicillin-binding proteins; they inhibit bacterial cell wall synthesis**
- ❑ **C. High-level resistance of *Streptococcus pneumoniae* to penicillins can generally be overcome by the addition of a β-lactamase inhibitor, such as clavulanate or sulbactam**
- ❑ **D. Dicloxacillin, a penicillinase-resistant penicillin, has excellent gas-**

trointestinal absorption and is active against both streptococcal and staphylococcal organisms, making it an effective treatment for cellulitis in the outpatient setting

❑ **E. With increasing use of broad-spectrum penicillins such as ampicillin, resistance among *Escherichia coli* and nontyphoidal *Salmonella* strains has steadily increased**

Key Concept/Objective: To understand the mechanism of action of penicillin and its derivatives and the means by which resistance develops

The penicillins are bactericidal antibiotics that prevent synthesis of the bacterial cell wall peptidoglycan by attaching to various penicillin-binding proteins located on the inner surface of the cell membrane. In the treatment of infections caused by susceptible organisms, the penicillins remain a good choice for antimicrobial therapy because of their efficacy and safety profile and the fact that most practitioners are familiar with them. Alterations in the chemical structure of penicillin have resulted in the production of second-generation extended-spectrum penicillins (e.g., ampicillin), third- and fourth-generation extended-spectrum penicillins (e.g., ticarcillin and piperacillin), and penicillinase-resistant penicillins (e.g., nafcillin and dicloxacillin). These agents have greatly broadened the utility of this family of drugs. Resistance to penicillin and related β-lactams is well understood; such resistance occurs through a few major mechanisms. Several bacterial species (e.g., penicillin-resistant staphylococci, anaerobes, and *Haemophilus* species) produce enzymes that cleave the β-lactam ring (β-lactamases). Activity against these organisms can often be restored by combining the penicillin with a β-lactamase inhibitor, such as sulbactam or clavulanic acid. Although strains of *Escherichia coli* and *Salmonella* were previously almost uniformly susceptible to broad-spectrum aminopenicillins such as ampicillin, they have increasingly developed resistance by acquiring β-lactamase activity. Other species, such as resistant strains of *S. pneumoniae*, methicillin-resistant *Staphylococcus aureus*, and enterococci, have developed resistance as a result of alterations in the penicillin-binding proteins. The addition of a β-lactamase inhibitor will not overcome resistance in these organisms. *(Answer: C—High-level resistance of* Streptococcus pneumoniae *to penicillins can generally be overcome by the addition of a β-lactamase inhibitor, such as clavulanate or sulbactam)*

69. ***Which of the following antimicrobials does NOT require dose adjustment in a patient with significant renal impairment (creatinine clearance < 50 ml/min)?***

❑ **A. Levofloxacin**

❑ **B. Ceftazidime**

❑ **C. Gentamicin**

❑ **D. Vancomycin**

❑ **E. Nafcillin**

Key Concept/Objective: To know the importance of host factors such as renal or hepatic impairment in maintaining effective and safe levels of antimicrobials

Consideration of the mechanisms by which antibiotics are metabolized and cleared by the body is crucial in choosing the appropriate drug and dosage in an infected patient, especially one who is elderly or has comorbidities. Several commonly used antimicrobials (e.g., cephalosporins, aminoglycosides, fluoroquinolones, trimethoprim-sulfamethoxazole, and vancomycin) are excreted primarily by the kidney. Thus, in patients with diminished creatinine clearance or those undergoing dialysis, dose adjustments must be made to avoid dose-related toxic effects. Monitoring peak and trough levels of drugs such as the aminoglycosides and vancomycin can help guide therapy. Several other drugs are excreted primarily by the liver, including nafcillin, clindamycin, doxycycline, and the macrolides; adjustments of dosages of these compounds is generally not needed in patients with renal impairment, but care must be taken when using these agents in patients with cirrhosis or abnormal liver function. *(Answer: E—Nafcillin)*

70. The fluoroquinolones are among the most important of the newer antibiotics, largely because of their spectrum of activity, ease of administration, and favorable safety profile. With their increasing popularity and widespread use have come growing concerns about the emergence of bacterial resistance, and it is recommended that clinicians use such broad-spectrum antimicrobials judiciously.

Which of the following statements regarding fluoroquinolones is false?

❑ A. **In addition to having activity against enteric gram-negative organisms and intracellular organisms such as *Chlamydia*, ciprofloxacin and levofloxacin provide reasonable coverage against anaerobes**

❑ B. **The fluoroquinolones have been noted to cause arthropathy in young animals and are therefore generally not used in patients who are younger than 18 years or are pregnant**

❑ C. **Ciprofloxacin is the agent of choice for treating *Bacillus anthracis* (anthrax)**

❑ D. **The fluoroquinolones are absorbed rapidly through the GI tract; the bioavailability achieved through oral administration generally approaches that of parenteral administration**

❑ E. **The fluoroquinolones are bactericidal agents that work by inhibiting DNA gyrase**

Key Concept/Objective: To understand the advantages and limitations of the fluoroquinolones

The fluoroquinolones are among the most widely prescribed antimicrobials. These drugs have a broad spectrum of activity and rapidly kill bacteria by impairing DNA synthesis. High serum and tissue levels are achieved by intravenous and oral administration, and relatively long serum half-lives allow for once- and twice-daily dosing regimens. Given their good activity against both gram-positive organisms such as *S. pneumoniae* and aerobic gram-negative organisms, fluoroquinolones are among the first-line drugs used to treat community-acquired pneumonia and UTIs. The recent outbreaks of *B. anthracis* have demonstrated the efficacy of ciprofloxacin in the treatment and prevention of disease, and this agent is considered first-line therapy. Fluoroquinolones are generally not given to children or pregnant women because of studies in animals that suggest that these drugs induce arthropathy. In adults, the development of tendinitis (and even Achilles tendon rupture) is a well-described (but relatively rare) complication. Other than trovafloxacin, the use of which has been severely limited after reports of hepatotoxicity, the fluoroquinolones generally do not have sufficient activity against anaerobic organisms (e.g., *Bacteroides* species) to warrant their use when an anaerobic infection is suspected. *(Answer: A—In addition to having activity against enteric gram-negative organisms and intracellular organisms such as* Chlamydia, *ciprofloxacin and levofloxacin provide reasonable coverage against anaerobes)*

71. *For which of the following clinical situations would it be inappropriate to use vancomycin?*

❑ A. **In combination with imipenem as empirical therapy for a frequently hospitalized nursing home resident suspected of having septic shock**

❑ B. **As oral monotherapy in a hospitalized patient with pseudomembranous colitis caused by *C. difficile* who has not tolerated metronidazole**

❑ C. **In combination with gentamicin as intravenous therapy for the treatment of prosthetic valve endocarditis caused by coagulase-negative *Staphylococcus***

❑ D. **As intravenous monotherapy in a meningitis patient whose cerebrospinal fluid culture demonstrates pneumococcus that is sensitive to vancomycin and is intermediately resistant to ceftriaxone**

❑ E. **As intravenous monotherapy in a patient with methicillin-resistant *S. aureus* (MRSA) infection associated with the presence of a central venous catheter**

Key Concept/Objective: To understand the appropriate uses of vancomycin

Vancomycin is a glycopeptide that has very good activity against gram-positive organisms such as *S. aureus* (including MRSA), *S. epidermidis*, and *Enterococcus* species. It is frequently used empirically when methicillin-resistant staphylococcal infection may be a serious consideration (e.g., sepsis in a nursing home resident or hospitalized patient, hospital-acquired pneumonia, and *S. epidermidis* bacteremia related to line infection). In a patient with endocarditis, vancomycin is frequently used in combination with gentamicin to eradicate *Enterococcus* or *S. epidermidis*. (Patients with penicillin-susceptible strains of *Enterococcus* can be treated with penicillin and gentamicin.) In general, vancomycin is not appropriate as monotherapy for bacterial meningitis, because it has low and erratic penetration into the CSF. It is generally used in combination with a third-generation cephalosporin (which has excellent CSF penetration) when drug-resistant pneumococcal meningitis is a concern. Experience with vancomycin as monotherapy for meningitis is very limited. Vancomycin is not absorbed orally and is an effective treatment for *C. difficile* colitis. Increasing vancomycin resistance (most notably among *Enterococcus* strains) is a growing concern; judicious use of this antibiotic is crucial. *(Answer: D—As intravenous monotherapy in a meningitis patient whose cerebrospinal fluid culture demonstrates pneumococcus that is sensitive to vancomycin and is intermediately resistant to ceftriaxone)*

For more information, see Dellit TH, Simon HB, Hooton TM: 7 Infectious Disease: XIV Antimicrobial Therapy. ACP Medicine Online (www.acpmedicine.com). Dale DC, Federman DD, Eds. WebMD Inc., New York, August 2004

Septic Arthritis

72. A 53-year-old African-American woman presents to your clinic complaining of right knee pain of 12 hours' duration. She denies having any trauma and has never had any knee surgery, but she does report a history of osteoarthritis. However, this pain is nothing like the pain of her osteoarthritis. On examination, the patient's right knee has an effusion and is warm and red. You consider acute septic arthritis and crystal-induced arthritis as the diagnosis.

Which of the following statements regarding this patient's workup is false?

❑ A. **Synovial fluid analysis is the diagnostic test of choice to distinguish between crystal-induced arthritis and infection-induced arthritis**

❑ B. **On physical examination, the presence of fever is universal in patients with septic arthritis and is uncommon in patients with crystal-induced arthritis**

❑ C. **Important historical facts to elucidate include a history of trauma, immunosuppressive states, sexually transmitted diseases (STDs), and I.V. drug abuse or recent I.V. catheterization**

❑ D. **Radiographs are useful when there is clinical suspicion of chronic osteomyelitis, osteonecrosis, or pathologic or insufficiency fracture**

Key Concept/Objective: To understand the diagnostic workup of a patient with acute monoarthritis

Bacterial infections account for less than 20% of all cases of acute monoarticular and oligoarticular arthritis. Crystal-induced arthritis is approximately four times more common. Because septic arthritis represents a potential threat to life and limb, the possibility of infection dictates the sequence and pace of the diagnostic evaluation. A thorough history remains a key element in the diagnosis of septic arthritis. Pertinent features include acute onset of joint pain or a significant change in the pattern of chronic joint pain; a history of joint trauma; a history of prodromal extra-articular symptoms suggestive of bacteremia; any comorbid immunosuppression, including diabetes mellitus, intravenous drug use, or prior intravenous catheterization; the presence of STDs; and

geographic location (e.g., in the case of Lyme disease). Fever is not uniformly present in adults or children with septic arthritis. Fever may be present in fewer than 60% of patients with nongonococcal septic arthritis. Rigors may be present in fewer than 10% of patients. High spiking fevers (> 102.2° F [39° C]) and rigors can also occur in patients with crystal-induced arthritis. Thus, systemic features are neither sensitive enough nor specific enough to warrant making or excluding the diagnosis of septic arthritis without examination of the synovial fluid. Synovial fluid leukocyte count, polarized microscopy, Gram stain, and culture are the most important initial laboratory investigations in the evaluation of suspected septic arthritis. Acutely or painfully swollen joints should be aspirated and the synovial fluid analyzed. Synovial fluid analysis is the diagnostic test of choice to distinguish between crystal-induced arthritis and infection-induced arthritis. In the absence of trauma, radiographs are of limited utility in the diagnosis of acute synovitis. Radiographs are useful when there is clinical suspicion of chronic osteomyelitis, osteonecrosis, or pathologic or insufficiency fracture. Radionuclide scans and other imaging procedures are occasionally useful in localizing and defining the extent of infection. *(Answer: B—On physical examination, the presence of fever is universal in patients with septic arthritis and is uncommon in patients with crystal-induced arthritis)*

73. A 19-year-old white woman presents with a complaint of a painful and swollen left wrist; she has had these symptoms for 1 to 2 days. She has come to see you now because the pain is limiting her ability to pick up objects. She has no significant medical history. Her sexual history is significant for multiple sexual partners since the patient went to college, but she had no documented cases of STD. She reports that her menstrual period began 3 days ago.

Which of the following statements regarding gonococcal septic arthritis is true?

- ❑ A. The triad of disseminated gonococcal infection (DGI) includes tenosynovitis, dermatitis, and symptomatic vaginitis/cervicitis in women or urethritis in men
- ❑ B. Recurrent disseminated gonococcal infections have been associated with common variable immunodeficiency (CVID)
- ❑ C. Therapy for suspected gonococcal arthritis can be instituted with penicillin, because most gonococcal isolates remain sensitive to penicillin
- ❑ D. Rectal, cervical, pharyngeal, and urethral cultures for *Neisseria gonococcus* should be performed if gonococcal infection is suspected

Key Concept/Objective: To understand the clinical presentation and treatment of gonococcal arthritis and DGI

In some practice settings, DGI is a relatively common cause of septic arthritis and tenosynovitis in healthy, sexually active patients. In a review of 41 cases of gonococcal arthritis, 83% of patients were female, and the mean age was 23 years. Dermatitis (usually sparse peripheral necrotic pustules) and migratory polyarthralgias/polyarthritis were present in 39% and 66% of the patients, respectively. Along with tenosynovitis, these findings constitute the classic triad of DGI. Genitourinary involvement was noted in 63% of the patients, but women are often asymptomatic. If gonococcal infection is suspected, the workup should include rectal, cervical, urethral, and pharyngeal cultures—any of which may be positive, even in the absence of local symptoms. Data compiled by the Centers for Disease Control and Prevention indicate that up to 33% of gonococcal isolates obtained in STD clinics in the United States are resistant to penicillin or tetracycline. Resistant strains are capable of systemic dissemination. There have been only rare reports of resistance to ceftriaxone; therefore, initial therapy should include parenteral therapy with ceftriaxone or ciprofloxacin. Recognized infection should always prompt an evaluation for other STDs, including syphilis and HIV. Empirical treatment for *Chlamydia trachomatis* infection should also be given, because this infection is frequently asymptomatic and can result in infertility if untreated; both partners should be treated whenever possible. Disseminated *Neisseria* infections, which

may be recurrent, have been associated with the presence of terminal complement deficiencies. *(Answer: D—Rectal, cervical, pharyngeal, and urethral cultures for* Neisseria gonococcus *should be performed if gonococcal infection is suspected)*

74. A 59-year-old man presents to the emergency department with multiple painful joints; the pain began acutely 2 days ago. The patient has had fever and chills. On examination, you note synovitis of the left knee and right ankle. Aspiration of the knee synovial fluid reveals no crystals. A Gram stain shows gram-positive cocci.

Which of the following statements regarding gram-positive bacteria and septic arthritis is false?

- ❑ A. **Staphylococcal species are more common than streptococcal species as a cause of septic arthritis**
- ❑ B. **Group B streptococcal infection may be particularly virulent in diabetic patients and may involve the axial joints (i.e., the sacroiliac, sternoclavicular, and manubriosternal joints)**
- ❑ C. **Gram stain is a reliable tool to differentiate between *Staphylococcus* and *Streptococcus*, because *Staphylococcus* appears as clusters in biologic smears**
- ❑ D. **Initial therapy for suspected staphylococcal or streptococcal septic arthritis should be vancomycin**

Key Concept/Objective: To understand the presentation and treatment of septic arthritis caused by gram-positive bacteria

Gram-positive bacteria remain the most common cause of septic arthritis, accounting for 70% to 80% of cases. *S. aureus* accounts for more than half of the cases of culture-positive septic arthritis in studies at university hospitals and for even higher percentages of certain patient subgroups: 70% to 80% of patients with polyarticular septic arthritis; more than 80% of infected patients with RA; and 82% of infected hemodialysis patients. Staphylococcal arthritis was particularly frequent in a series of patients with endocarditis related to intravenous drug abuse. Gram stain cannot be relied on to differentiate between *Staphylococcus* and *Streptococcus*, because in biologic smears, *Staphylococcus* may not exhibit the clusters seen when grown in vitro. Suspected staphylococcal joint infection should be treated initially with vancomycin until methicillin resistance can be excluded. Non-group A, α-hemolytic streptococci are the second most common cause of septic arthritis, accounting for 10% to 21% of culture-positive cases. The number of reported group B (and to a lesser extent, groups C and G) streptococcal infections has been increasing. Group B streptococcal infection may be particularly virulent in diabetic patients and may involve axial joints (e.g., the sacroiliac, sternoclavicular, and manubriosternal joints) and may be associated with poor functional outcome. Other manifestations of group B streptococcal sepsis include myositis, fasciitis, and endophthalmitis. For initial therapy, vancomycin is a reasonable choice. Definitive therapy should be made on the basis of culture results. *(Answer: C—Gram stain is a reliable tool to differentiate between* Staphylococcus *and* Streptococcus, *because* Staphylococcus *appears as clusters in biologic smears)*

75. ***Which of the following statements about septic (bacterial) arthritis is true?***

- ❑ A. **Local inoculation of organisms into the joint space is the most common route of acquisition**
- ❑ B. **HIV-infected patients are at increased risk**
- ❑ C. **Patients with underlying joint disease (e.g., rheumatoid arthritis) are at increased risk**
- ❑ D. **The finger joints are the most commonly involved site**
- ❑ E. **Most cases are polyarticular**

Key Concept/Objective: To understand the epidemiology and pathogenesis of bacterial arthritis

Patients with underlying joint damage from any cause (e.g., rheumatoid arthritis, trauma) are at increased risk for developing septic arthritis. In the majority of cases, bacteria are presumed to reach the joint space via the bloodstream rather than by direct inoculation (as would occur with postarthroplasty infections or with infections associated with trauma). The knee and hip are the most commonly involved joints; bacterial arthritis of the small finger joints is uncommon. Only 10% to 15% of cases of septic arthritis are polyarticular. HIV infection has not been identified as a risk factor for septic arthritis. *(Answer: C—Patients with underlying joint disease [e.g., rheumatoid arthritis] are at increased risk)*

76. A 23-year-old sexually active woman presents with left knee and wrist pain. She initially experienced polyarthralgias and low-grade fevers for several days, after which she developed progressive left knee pain. On examination, she is febrile and has a significant effusion and pain with passive range of motion of the left knee. Tenosynovitis of the left wrist is also noted. A few scattered necrotic pustular lesions are present on the extremities. The rest of the examination (including pelvic examination) is negative. Appropriate cultures are obtained, and a diagnostic aspirate of the knee joint reveals a WBC count of 45,000/mm^3 (predominantly polymorphonuclear leukocytes), but the Gram stain is negative. Cultures of the joint fluid eventually yield *Neisseria gonorrhoeae.*

Which of the following statements about gonococcal arthritis is true?

- ❑ **A. Arthritis caused by this organism is more common in men than in women**
- ❑ **B. Progressive joint damage leading to permanent disability is likely**
- ❑ **C. Absence of clinical pelvic gonococcal infection rules out the diagnosis**
- ❑ **D. The synovial fluid usually tests positive on Gram staining**
- ❑ **E. The prognosis for patients with gonococcal arthritis is generally better than for patients with nongonococcal arthritis**

Key Concept/Objective: To be able to recognize the clinical features of gonococcal arthritis

Gonococcal arthritis is a relatively common cause of septic arthritis in young, otherwise healthy, sexually active patients. The majority of patients are women. Skin rash (scattered pustular skin lesions), migratory polyarthralgias/polyarthritis, and tenosynovitis constitute the classic triad of disseminated gonococcal infection. The distinction between gonococcal and nongonococcal arthritis is clinically useful, because gonococcal infections tend to have a better prognosis than nongonococcal arthritis. Progressive joint damage is uncommon in gonococcal arthritis. Diagnosis can be difficult, and the results of Gram staining of synovial fluid are usually negative. The frequency of positive cultures taken from various sites of infection is as follows: urogenital, 86%; synovial fluid, 44%; rectal, 86%; and pharyngeal, 7%. In order to maximize the diagnostic yield, it is important to obtain cultures from all sites of potential exposure (e.g., pharynx, rectum, vagina, cervix). Although genitourinary infection is present in the majority of patients, it may be asymptomatic in women. *(Answer: E—The prognosis for patients with gonococcal arthritis is generally better than for patients with nongonococcal arthritis)*

77. ***What is the best treatment for the patient described in Question 76?***

- ❑ **A. Penicillin and doxycycline**
- ❑ **B. Ceftriaxone and azithromycin**
- ❑ **C. Ceftriaxone alone**
- ❑ **D. Doxycycline and azithromycin**
- ❑ **E. Cefazolin alone**

Key Concept/Objective: To know the appropriate management of gonococcal arthritis

Up to one third of gonococcal isolates in the United States are resistant to penicillin or tetracycline; these agents are therefore not recommended for treatment of gonococcal

infection. Parenteral regimens of ceftriaxone, cefotaxime, or imipenem are recommended. It is important to treat any patient with documented gonococcal infection for concomitant *Chlamydia trachomatis* infection with either doxycycline (100 mg p.o., b.i.d. × 7 days) or azithromycin (1 g p.o. × 1 dose). Of the choices listed, only choice B includes therapy that is appropriate for both *N. gonorrhoeae* (ceftriaxone) and *C. trachomatis* (azithromycin). *(Answer: B—Ceftriaxone and azithromycin)*

78. A 68-year-old woman with gout and long-standing rheumatoid arthritis presents with progressive right hip pain of 3 days' duration. She was diagnosed with rheumatoid arthritis over 15 years ago and has been treated with methotrexate and low-dose prednisone (5 mg daily) for the past several years. Her rheumatoid arthritis has involved multiple joints, including the hands, shoulders, and knees. She had a single episode of gout of the right metatarsophalangeal joint 1 year ago. On examination, she is afebrile. Deformities consistent with rheumatoid arthritis are present. The right hip is slightly warm, and there is pain with passive range of motion of the joint. Laboratory results show a white blood cell count (WBC) of 7,600/mm^3 and an erythrocyte sedimentation rate of 54. Results of joint fluid analysis are as follows: very rare crystals; WBC, 84,000/mm^3 (95% polymorphonuclear leukocytes); Gram stain, negative; culture pending.

Which of the following findings reliably excludes bacterial arthritis in this patient?

- ❑ **A. Absence of fever**
- ❑ **B. Presence of crystals in synovial fluid**
- ❑ **C. Absence of peripheral blood leukocytosis**
- ❑ **D. Negative results on Gram staining of synovial fluid**
- ❑ **E. None of the above**

Key Concept/Objective: To understand the limitations of diagnostic tests in patients with suspected septic arthritis

Patients with underlying joint damage from any cause are at increased risk for developing septic arthritis. Unfortunately, no clinical signs or symptoms are pathognomonic for septic arthritis, nor are laboratory tests (other than culture) sufficiently sensitive or specific to confirm or exclude the diagnosis. Although crystal-induced arthritis is a possibility in this patient, a few crystals may be found in the synovial fluid of asymptomatic patients who have a history of gout. Also, crystal arthropathy and septic arthritis may coexist; thus, the presence of crystals does not rule out septic arthritis, and cultures should be obtained when there is a clinical suspicion of septic arthritis or when a regimen of intra-articular corticosteroid injections is planned. Fever is present in more than 60% of patients with nongonococcal arthritis. Similarly, the Gram stain of synovial fluid is positive in more than 50% of patients with culture-confirmed septic arthritis. *(Answer: E—None of the above)*

79. A diagnosis of possible crystal-induced arthropathy is made for the patient in Question 78. She is treated with colchicines, and the dosages of her systemic corticosteroids are increased. The next day, synovial fluid cultures are positive.

Which of the following is the most common cause of septic arthritis in patients with underlying rheumatoid arthritis, and what treatment should this patient receive?

- ❑ **A. *N. gonorrhoeae*; I.V. antibiotics and surgical drainage**
- ❑ **B. *Streptococcus pyogenes*; I.V. antibiotics**
- ❑ **C. *Staphylococcus aureus*; I.V. antibiotics and surgical drainage**
- ❑ **D. *Escherichia coli*; I.V. antibiotics and surgical drainage**
- ❑ **E. *Staphylococcus epidermidis*; I.V. antibiotics**

Key Concept/Objective: To understand the causative organisms and appropriate management of nongonococcal arthritis

Gram-positive organisms remain the most common cause of septic arthritis, accounting for 70% to 80% of cases. Among patients with rheumatoid arthritis, *S. aureus* accounts for more than 80% of cases. *N. gonorrhoeae, S. epidermidis, S. pyogenes,* and *E. coli* would be much less likely than *S. aureus* in this clinical setting. Management of septic arthritis consists of drainage (either repeated aspiration or surgical drainage), parenteral antibiotics, and temporary (not prolonged) joint immobilization for pain control. Surgical drainage is generally indicated in the following situations: septic arthritis of the hip or other joints that are difficult to aspirate or monitor for adequate drainage; extensive spread of infection to the soft tissues; and inadequate response to medical therapy. For this patient with *S. aureus* arthritis of the hip (a joint that is difficult to monitor for complete drainage), parenteral antibiotics (e.g., nafcillin or cefazolin if the strain of *S. aureus* is not methicillin resistant) and surgical drainage are the most appropriate therapy. *(Answer: C—*Staphylococcus aureus; *I.V. antibiotics and surgical drainage)*

For more information, see Mandell BF: 7 Infectious Disease: XV Septic Arthritis. ACP Medicine Online (www.acpmedicine.com). Dale DC, Federman DD, Eds. WebMD Inc., New York, July 2004

Osteomyelitis

80. A 32-year-old man presents to your clinic for the first time for evaluation of neck pain. He reports a 1-week history of worsening posterior neck pain. He denies having experienced any trauma; he also denies having any constitutional symptoms. His medical history is insignificant, but he admits to heavy alcohol use and the sporadic use of I.V. drugs; he last used I.V. drugs 2 weeks ago. On physical examination, the patient's temperature is 99.2° F (37.3° C). Severe tenderness to palpation is noted at C4-C5. The neurologic examination is normal.

Which of the following statements regarding vertebral osteomyelitis is true?

❑ A. **Neurologic deficits are present in the majority of patients with vertebral osteomyelitis**

❑ B. **Cervical spine involvement is often seen in patients who abuse I.V. drugs**

❑ C. **Most cases of vertebral osteomyelitis derive from a contiguous focus of infection**

❑ D. ***Salmonella* species are the most common organisms in cases of vertebral osteomyelitis associated with I.V. drug abuse**

Key Concept/Objective: To know the clinical features of vertebral osteomyelitis

In I.V. drug abusers, hematogenous osteomyelitis is associated with subtle clinical signs and symptoms. Patients may present with localized pain, but fever is usually absent. Although vertebral osteomyelitis is common, infection of the pubis and the clavicle is also seen. Culture of the infected site usually yields *Staphylococcus aureus* or *S. epidermidis*, although *Pseudomonas aeruginosa* is often seen. Neurologic signs are generally absent but, when present, may indicate an epidural abscess. Vertebral infection typically involves the vertebral body rather than the spinous or transverse processes; often, two adjacent vertebrae and the disk space between them are affected. The lumbar region is most frequently involved in pyogenic hematogenous osteomyelitis. Thoracic vertebrae are often infected in spinal tuberculosis (Pott disease). The cervical spine is often the site of infection in patients who abuse I.V. drugs. Vertebral osteomyelitis is almost always the result of hematogenous seeding. *(Answer: B—Cervical spine involvement is often seen in patients who abuse I.V. drugs)*

81. A 57-year-old man presents for evaluation of a left lower extremity ulcer. He has a history of hypertension and poorly controlled type 2 diabetes mellitus. The lesion began approximately 4 weeks ago in the absence of any known trauma. The patient reports experiencing subjective fevers, chills, and malaise over the past few days. On physical examination, the patient's temperature is 100.4° F (38° C). A nontender stage 3 ulceration of the plantar surface is noted on the patient's left first metatarsal, with surrounding erythema and mild discharge.

Which of the following statements regarding osteomyelitis in this patient is true?

- ❑ A. **The most likely reason for osteomyelitis in this patient is hematogenous seeding**
- ❑ B. **Prolonged antibiotic therapy alone cures the majority of these patients**
- ❑ C. **Infections are rarely polymicrobial**
- ❑ D. **Vascular insufficiency impairs wound healing and allows bacterial proliferation**

Key Concept/Objective: To know the clinical features of osteomyelitis in diabetic patients

Osteomyelitis secondary to vascular insufficiency occurs most frequently in older patients with diabetes mellitus or severe vascular impairment. In these patients, osteomyelitis usually develops by contiguous spread of infection from soft tissue to underlying bone; it often occurs in the small bones of the feet. Complex foot lesions in diabetic patients result from a combination of neuropathy, atherosclerotic peripheral vascular disease, and repetitive trauma to the area. Bone infections develop in about 25% of diabetic patients with superficial mild to moderate foot infections; however, of those patients with serious foot infections, over 50% will have osteomyelitis. Extensive debridement is necessary, and about two thirds of cases require bone resection or partial amputation. Limb ischemia, combined with poor collateral circulation, impairs wound healing in foot ulcers and allows for the contiguous spread of infection to bone. In addition, this anoxic environment contributes to the development of gangrenous changes and anaerobic infections. Furthermore, peripheral vascular disease may compromise the efficacy of antibiotic therapy by preventing the accumulation of adequate drug levels in the infected tissues. Although *S. aureus* is the most common pathogen isolated from patients with osteomyelitis associated with vascular insufficiency, multiple organisms, including both anaerobes and aerobes, may be present, especially in hospitalized patients. *(Answer: D—Vascular insufficiency impairs wound healing and allows bacterial proliferation)*

82. A 72-year-old woman returns to your clinic for hospital follow-up 8 days after undergoing replacement of the right hip. Her postoperative course was unremarkable until 2 days ago, when she experienced increasing right hip pain, fever, and purulent discharge from the surgical site. The patient is admitted to the hospital and is diagnosed with osteomyelitis of the right hip.

For this patient, which of the following statements regarding osteomyelitis is true?

- ❑ A. ***S. epidermidis*** **is the most likely organism, because of the abrupt onset of signs and symptoms**
- ❑ B. **The infection was likely introduced after discharge from the hospital**
- ❑ C. **Late-onset postoperative osteomyelitis is likely to be secondary to hematogenous seeding**
- ❑ D. **Osteomyelitis can be seen in the immediate postoperative period or as late as 2 years after joint replacement**

Key Concept/Objective: To know the clinical features of osteomyelitis that occurs after joint replacement surgery

Osteomyelitis may occur soon after surgery or later after replacement of the hip joint. Often evident within the first few days or weeks after surgery, acute contiguous infections result directly from infection of the skin, subcutaneous tissue, or muscle. Fever, pain, erythema, edema, and purulent drainage often occur when early infections are caused by pyogenic organisms such as *S. aureus*, streptococci, or enteric gram-negative bacilli. When early infections are caused by less pathogenic organisms, such as *S. epidermidis* or diphtheroids, the disease presents more insidiously. Chronic contiguous

infections are usually diagnosed 6 to 24 months after surgery. Most infections are probably introduced during surgery but remain quiescent for a long time. *(Answer: D—Osteomyelitis can be seen in the immediate postoperative period or as late as 2 years after joint replacement)*

83. A 13-year-old girl is brought to your office by her mother for evaluation of left leg pain. Two weeks ago, the patient began to experience anterior left leg pain, which caused a slight limp. Over the past 2 weeks, the pain has become more severe, and the patient has experienced temperatures of up to 101° F (38.3° C). The patient reports that approximately 4 weeks ago, she sustained an injury to her left leg during a soccer game. At that time, x-rays were negative for a fracture, and the swelling and bruising resolved with rest and the use of ice packs. Laboratory studies reveal leukocytosis with a left shift. X-rays at this time show deep soft tissue swelling and periosteal elevation.

Which of the following statements regarding osteomyelitis in children is true?

- ❑ **A. In over 50% of cases of osteomyelitis in children, blood cultures are positive**
- ❑ **B. In most cases of osteomyelitis in children, the infection has a single focus in the small bones of the feet and hands**
- ❑ **C. Most cases of osteomyelitis in children are polymicrobial**
- ❑ **D. Most cases of osteomyelitis in children are associated with marked drainage from the site of osteomyelitis**

Key Concept/Objective: To know the key features of osteomyelitis in children

Hematogenous osteomyelitis is usually seen in children between 1 and 15 years of age, in adults older than 50 years, or in persons who abuse I.V. drugs. In children, infection usually occurs as a single focus in the metaphyseal area of long bones (particularly the tibia and femur). Children may be predisposed to infection associated with minor trauma that causes a small hematoma, vessel obstruction, and bone necrosis. Drainage is not usually seen. Blood cultures are positive in more than half of patients. Although in most children, symptoms are present for 3 weeks or less, some children may present with vague symptoms of 1 to 3 months' duration. Most cases of hematogenous osteomyelitis are monomicrobial. Although *S. aureus* causes 60% to 90% of cases of hematogenous osteomyelitis, certain organisms tend to cause infections in certain age groups. In newborns, group B streptococci and gram-negative bacilli are common. In children, streptococci and *Haemophilus influenzae* are often seen. However, evidence from a retrospective study in Canada showed that vaccination of infants and children succeeded in eliminating *H. influenzae* type b as an infective agent in hematogenous osteomyelitis. Polymicrobial hematogenous osteomyelitis is usually caused by *S. aureus* and *Streptococcus*. *(Answer: A—In over 50% of cases of osteomyelitis in children, blood cultures are positive)*

For more information, see Gentry LO: 7 Infectious Disease: XVI Osteomyelitis. ACP Medicine Online (www.acpmedicine.com). Dale DC, Federman DD, Eds. WebMD Inc., New York, November 2004

Rickettsia, Ehrlichia, Coxiella

84. A 27-year-old man presents to the emergency department for evaluation of fever and rash. He was well until 4 days ago, when he developed fever, a rash on his left wrist and both ankles, and diffuse body aches. He states that he just returned from a trip to the mountains of northern Georgia, where he spent a week mountain biking. This is an annual trip that he and friends take in April. He denies having cough, shortness of breath, sore throat, or dysuria, but he has developed some moderate, constant abdominal pain. He denies having nausea or emesis. He states that his rash has now spread to involve most of his trunk. He is unaware of any tick exposure. He denies having any sexual contact other than with his wife of 4 years. He takes no prescription or over-the-counter medications.

Which of the following statements regarding Rocky Mountain spotted fever (RMSF) is false?

❑ A. Over 90% of all cases of RMSF occur from early spring to early autumn and are most often reported from the southeastern and south central United States

❑ B. The diagnosis of RMSF is made on the basis of the presence of the classic rash

❑ C. The diagnosis of RMSF is based on clinical features and an appropriate epidemiologic setting rather than on any single laboratory test

❑ D. Doxycycline is the preferred agent for the treatment of RMSF in all patients except pregnant women

Key Concept/Objective: To understand the diagnosis and management of RMSF

Over 90% of all cases of RMSF occur from early spring to early autumn. It is most often reported from the southeastern and south central United States. The rash typically develops on the third to the fifth day of illness. The appearance of the rash may be delayed, however, and in a small percentage of patients, the rash does not develop at all. Delay or absence of the rash greatly complicates clinical diagnosis. In one study, only 14% of RMSF patients had a rash on the first day of illness, and fewer than 50% developed a rash in the first 72 hours of illness. The absence of rash does not correspond to milder disease; a small percentage of patients with so-called spotless RMSF have fatal illness. The diagnosis of RMSF is notoriously difficult, even for experienced physicians in highly endemic areas. It is axiomatic that the diagnosis of RMSF must be based on the clinical features and an appropriate epidemiologic setting rather than on any single laboratory test. There is no completely reliable diagnostic test for RMSF in the early phases of illness; thus, therapy should always begin before laboratory confirmation is obtained. Doxycycline is the preferred agent in all patients except pregnant women, for whom chloramphenicol remains the agent of choice. *(Answer: B—The diagnosis of RMSF is made on the basis of the presence of the classic rash)*

85. A 55-year-old man with a history of hypertension and coronary artery disease presents to your office for evaluation. He was in his usual state of health until 2 days ago, when he developed fever, fatigue, and a persistent, dull headache. He denies having any cough, dysuria, urinary hesitancy, or rash, and he has not had any contact with sick persons. He generally feels very healthy, and he plays golf three times each week at his local golf course in Tennessee. He does state that the ticks have been especially bad this year at his golf course, and he notes that he has removed at least five ticks from his body this month alone. His chest x-ray is normal. His complete blood count reveals leukopenia and thrombocytopenia.

Which of the following statements regarding ehrlichiosis is true?

❑ A. Skin rash does not occur in patients with ehrlichiosis

❑ B. For this patient, human granulocytic ehrlichiosis (HGE) is more likely than human monocytic ehrlichiosis (HME)

❑ C. The common laboratory abnormalities associated with HME are leukopenia, thrombocytopenia, abnormal liver function tests, and elevation of lactate dehydrogenase (LDH) and alkaline phosphatase

❑ D. The principal animal reservoir for ***Ehrlichia chaffeensis*** is rabbits

Key Concept/Objective: To know the important clinical characteristics of Ehrlichia *infection*

Skin rash is uncommon in patients with HME, but when present, it may be macular, maculopapular, or petechial. Although skin rash was reported in 36% of cases in one case series of 211 patients with HME, skin rash has been less common in the experience of many clinicians working in HME-endemic regions. HME has been recognized as endemic throughout the southeastern and south central United States. First described in patients from the north central United States, HGE is now known to occur in Wisconsin, Minnesota, Connecticut, New York, Massachusetts, California, Florida, and western Europe. The most common laboratory abnormalities seen in patients with HME is leukopenia (often accompanied by a left shift), thrombocytopenia, and elevated plasma levels of aminotransferases (transaminases), lactate dehydrogenase, and alka-

line phosphatase. Anemia and an elevated plasma creatinine concentration also may be seen. Later in the course of illness or during recovery, a striking atypical lymphocytosis may occur. White-tailed deer are thought to be the principal animal reservoirs for *E. chaffeensis*. A study from Georgia found serologic evidence of *E. chaffeensis* infection in 27 of 35 deer and isolated *E. chaffeensis* from five of them, confirming that deer are naturally infected in endemic areas. *(Answer: C—The common laboratory abnormalities associated with HME are leukopenia, thrombocytopenia, abnormal liver function tests, and elevation of lactate dehydrogenase [LDH] and alkaline phosphatase)*

86. A 47-year-old man presents to your office for evaluation of fever. The patient was in his usual state of health until 10 days ago, when he developed a black "scab" with surrounding redness on his left leg. The lesion is still present. Four days after the development of the scab, the patient began to have persistent fever, and he is now experiencing headache, anorexia, and malaise. He also notes some "large glands" in his neck. His physical examination is significant for generalized lymphadenopathy and a 2 cm necrotic skin lesion on the anterior surface of his left lower extremity. He denies having a new sexual partner, as well as the use of illicit substances. He states that the scab originally appeared while he was in Bangkok on a business trip. He states that while in Bangkok, he toured the city and visited several parks and wooded areas.

Which of the following statements regarding scrub typhus is false?

- ❑ A. **The *Ixodes* tick is the common vector for scrub typhus, Lyme disease, babesiosis, and human granulocytic ehrlichiosis**
- ❑ B. ***Orientia tsutsugamushi* is distributed throughout the Pacific rim and is endemic in Korea, China, Taiwan, Japan, Pakistan, India, Thailand, Malaysia, and northern Australia**
- ❑ C. **Because of the ease of air travel and the long incubation period of scrub typhus (up to 2 weeks), tourists to endemic areas may fall ill after returning home**
- ❑ D. **A localized necrotic skin lesion or eschar is a hallmark of scrub typhus**

Key Concept/Objective: To know the important clinical features of scrub typhus

The reservoir and vector of scrub typhus are trombiculid mites of the genus *Leptotrombidium*. *O. tsutsugamushi* is distributed throughout the Pacific rim and is endemic in Korea, China, Taiwan, Japan, Pakistan, India, Thailand, Malaysia, and northern Australia. Most cases of scrub typhus occur in rural areas, but cases may also occur in suburban areas, such as those around Bangkok, where the seroprevalence in the general population may be as high as 20%. Because of the ease of air travel and the long incubation period of scrub typhus (up to 2 weeks), tourists to endemic areas may fall ill after returning home to regions where the illness is not familiar to physicians. Numerous cases of scrub typhus have been described in tourists returning to the United States, Europe, and Canada from endemic regions. A localized necrotic skin lesion or eschar is a hallmark of scrub typhus. Eschars typically occur at the site of the infected chigger bite and may appear before the onset of systemic symptoms. *(Answer: A—The* Ixodes *tick is the common vector for scrub typhus, Lyme disease, babesiosis, and human granulocytic ehrlichiosis)*

For more information, see Sexton DJ: 7 Infectious Disease: XVII Infections Due to Rickettsia, Ehrlichia, and Coxiella. ACP Medicine Online (www.acpmedicine.com). Dale DC, Federman DD, Eds. WebMD Inc., New York, August 2004

Infective Endocarditis

87. A 72-year-old man with a history of hypertension, diabetes mellitus, and aortic stenosis returns to your clinic 3 weeks after being diagnosed with a viral upper respiratory infection. Today he complains of continued fever, myalgias, malaise, and night sweats. At the time of initial presentation, the patient was

treated conservatively with acetaminophen and encouraged to maintain oral fluid intake. He denies having rigors, chest pain, dyspnea, cough, diarrhea, or dysuria. Results of physical examination are as follows: temperature, 100.5° F (38° C); blood pressure, 156/87 mm Hg; heart rate, 92 beats/min; respiratory rate, 14 breaths/min; and O_2 saturation, 99% on room air. The patient is in no acute distress. The lungs are clear to auscultation bilaterally. Heart examination reveals a regular heart rate with a 3/6 systolic ejection murmur that radiates to the carotid arteries bilaterally. There is no skin rash. The neurologic examination is nonfocal. You are concerned about the possibility of occult infection or malignancy and admit the patient for workup for fever of undetermined origin (FUO). A transthoracic echocardiogram demonstrates a 6 mm vegetation on the aortic valve. Blood cultures from three sites are obtained.

For this patient, which of the following statements about subacute bacterial endocarditis (SBE) is true?

- ❑ **A. Vegetations of more than 5 mm in size are associated with an increased risk of embolization**
- ❑ **B. In most patients with SBE, blood cultures will be positive in the absence of previous antibiotic use**
- ❑ **C. Over 50% of patients with SBE are afebrile**
- ❑ **D. Physical examination findings frequently include clubbing and splenomegaly**

Key Concept/Objective: To know the clinical features of SBE

The constitutional symptoms of SBE usually begin insidiously and often persist for weeks to months. Fevers, sweats, weakness, myalgias, arthralgias, malaise, anorexia, and easy fatigability are prominent. Fewer than 5% of patients are afebrile; such patients are often elderly, markedly malnourished, or azotemic. Fever and other nonspecific symptoms in the presence of a predisposing cardiac lesion may be the only clinical manifestations of SBE in some patients. In most patients with SBE, blood cultures drawn before initiation of antibiotic therapy are positive, reflecting the sustained bacteremia associated with an infected endothelial surface. Factors associated with an increased risk of embolization include vegetations of 10 mm or more in size as seen on echocardiography; vegetations on the mitral valve, particularly the anterior leaflet; vegetations that increase in size during therapy; and infection by *Staphylococcus aureus*. The incidence of arterial emboli decreases about 10-fold during the initial 2 weeks of antimicrobial therapy. *(Answer: B—In most patients with SBE, blood cultures will be positive in the absence of previous antibiotic use)*

88. A 35-year-old man presents in the urgent care clinic complaining of fever. He reports that for the past 2 days, he has been experiencing subjective fever, shaking chills, and pleuritic chest pain. Further history reveals a nonproductive cough. The patient denies having any underlying medical conditions. He admits to daily alcohol use and frequent I.V. drug use. Results of physical examination are as follows: temperature, 103.8° F (39.9° C); blood pressure, 109/62 mm Hg; heart rate, 110 beats/min; respiratory rate, 18 breaths/min; and O_2 saturation, 98% on room air. The lungs are clear bilaterally. The neck veins are flat, and the heart is tachycardic with a short systolic ejection murmur that is louder on inspiration. The skin is warm and diaphoretic without lesions.

For this patient, which of the following statements about infective endocarditis in intravenous drug users (IDUs) is true?

- ❑ **A. The mitral valve is the most commonly involved valve**
- ❑ **B. The majority of IDUs who develop endocarditis have preexisting valvular heart disease**
- ❑ **C. An empirical antibiotic regimen need not include vancomycin because the patient has not been exposed to the health care system recently**
- ❑ **D. The majority of IDUs with right-sided endocarditis have septic pulmonary emboli**

Key Concept/Objective: To know the common features of endocarditis in IDUs

The annual incidence of endocarditis in IDUs is 0.2% to 2.0%. At the time of their initial attack of endocarditis, 70% to 80% of IDUs have no history or findings of preexisting valvular heart disease. In IDUs, the tricuspid valve is infected more frequently (55%) than the aortic valve (35%) or mitral valve (30%). Septic pulmonary emboli occur in about 75% of cases—particularly in patients with *S. aureus* infection—and cause sputum production, hemoptysis, and initial radiologic findings suggestive of pneumonia. *S. aureus* accounts for almost 80% of right-sided endocarditis in IDUs. Vancomycin, although active against both methicillin-sensitive *S. aureus* (MSSA) and methicillin-resistant *S. aureus* (MRSA), is not the first choice, because it is somewhat less effective than the penicillinase-resistant penicillins. However, vancomycin should be added initially because of the increasing frequency of MRSA strains, not only in nosocomial infections but also in community-acquired infections. If the blood culture yields MSSA, vancomycin should be discontinued; if the blood culture yields MRSA, then vancomycin alone should be continued. *(Answer: D—The majority of IDUs with right-sided endocarditis have septic pulmonary emboli)*

89. A 62-year-old woman whom you have been following for hypertension and aortic stenosis returns to clinic 6 weeks after undergoing aortic valve replacement with a mechanical valve. Her immediate postoperative course was uneventful, but recently she has had difficulty regulating her international normalized ratio (INR), and she has noted subjective fevers over the past 3 days. Physical examination reveals a temperature of 101.5° F (38.6° C). The heart examination is consistent for a patient with a mechanical aortic valve. The patient's lungs are clear bilaterally. The neurologic examination is unremarkable. Examination of the skin reveals scattered petechiae. Laboratory data reveal a leukocytosis (WBC, 16,000/mm^3) with left shift; hematocrit, 38%; platelets, 210,000/mm^3; and INR, 2.6. You order three sets of blood cultures and admit the patient to the hospital with a presumptive diagnosis of infective endocarditis.

For this patient, which of the following statements concerning prosthetic valve endocarditis (PVE) is true?

- ❑ **A. The patient's risk of developing PVE is higher with a mechanical valve than it would be with a porcine valve**
- ❑ **B. Warfarin therapy should be withheld at this time because of the increased risk of embolic complications**
- ❑ **C. The most common organism causing PVE within the first year of valve replacement is *S. epidermidis***
- ❑ **D. Transthoracic echocardiography is superior to transesophageal echocardiography in the evaluation of PVE**

Key Concept/Objective: To understand the clinical features and diagnosis of PVE

The cumulative incidence of PVE is estimated to be 1% to 2% at 1 year and 4% to 5% at 4 years after valve implantation. Infection may be introduced at the time of valve placement or from transient bacteremia at any time thereafter. The overall risks of infection are similar for mechanical and porcine bioprosthetic valves and for aortic and mitral valve prostheses. The leading cause of PVE during the first year after surgery is methicillin-resistant coagulase-negative staphylococci, predominantly *S. epidermidis*. The dominant clinical feature of PVE that occurs during the first 60 days after surgery for early PVE is fever, whether or not there is a regurgitant murmur associated with the prosthetic valve. Transesophageal echocardiography is notably superior to transthoracic echocardiography in the evaluation of patients with suspected PVE. Transthoracic echocardiography has limited usefulness in the diagnosis of PVE because the prosthesis itself produces echoes that often obscure vegetations and abscesses. Anticoagulant therapy in a patient with endocarditis carries the potential risk of causing or worsening postembolization hemorrhage in the brain or other sites. However, the benefits of anticoagulation probably outweigh the risks if a strong indication exists, such as atrial fibrillation, cardiomyopathy, mural thrombus, or deep vein thrombophlebitis. Anticoagulation therapy may be carefully administered to patients with endocarditis when

it is so indicated. In patients with prosthetic valves who require long-term warfarin therapy, such therapy should be continued unless there are specific contraindications. *(Answer: C—The most common organism causing PVE within the first year of valve replacement is* S. epidermidis*)*

90. A 44-year-old woman presents to your clinic complaining of bloody bowel movements, which she has experienced intermittently over the past 2 weeks. She denies having any abdominal pain, constipation, diarrhea, or constitutional symptoms. She is worried because she has a family history of colon cancer. She was diagnosed in the past with mitral valve prolapse. She takes no medications. Digital rectal examination (DRE) reveals guaiac-positive brown stool without hemorrhoids or anal fissure. You decide to proceed with upper and lower endoscopy.

For this patient, which of the following statements is true?

- ❑ **A. An audible heart murmur is not an indication for antibiotic prophylaxis**
- ❑ **B. Echocardiographic evidence of mitral regurgitation is an indication for antibiotic prophylaxis**
- ❑ **C. Patients with mitral valve prolapse and echocardiographic evidence of thickened valves are not at increased risk for endocarditis**
- ❑ **D. Procedures involving manipulation of the lower GI tract are likely to produce streptococcal bacteremia**

Key Concept/Objective: To know the indications for antibiotic prophylaxis for patients with mitral valve prolapse

Patients who are at higher risk for endocarditis than the general population should be given prophylaxis when they undergo procedures likely to lead to bacteremia with organisms that commonly cause endocarditis. The need for prophylaxis in all patients with mitral valve prolapse is controversial. Nevertheless, prophylaxis is recommended when mitral valve prolapse is accompanied by an audible murmur, when there is echocardiographic evidence of mitral regurgitation, or when there are thickened valves. Prophylaxis is recommended for patients at high or moderate risk for endocarditis who undergo procedures that involve the oral cavity, the respiratory tract, or the esophagus and are likely to cause streptococcal bacteremia. Prophylaxis is indicated for patients at high or moderate risk for endocarditis who undergo procedures that involve the genitourinary tract, the GI tract distal to the stomach, or the biliary tract and that are likely to cause bacteremia with enterococci. *(Answer: B—Echocardiographic evidence of mitral regurgitation is an indication for antibiotic prophylaxis)*

For more information, see Durack DT, Karchmer AW: 7 Infectious Disease: XVIII Infective Endocarditis. ACP Medicine Online (www.acpmedicine.com). Dale DC, Federman DD, Eds. WebMD Inc., New York, December 2004

Bacterial Infections of the Upper Respiratory Tract

91. A 41-year-old woman presents to your office for the evaluation of fever. She was in her usual state of health until 7 days ago, when she developed fever and severe right facial pain. Her pain and fever have continued, and she has developed purulent nasal drainage and foul breath odor. She admits that she has suffered from similar symptoms in the past but never this severe. She denies having had any contact with sick persons. Her general state of health has been good, although she has a 30 pack-year smoking history. On physical examination, the patient's temperature is 100.5° F (38° C). Her pain is exacerbated when she leans forward, and there is tenderness to palpation over the right maxillary and right frontal sinuses. Each of these sinuses is opaque on transillumination. The rest of the examination is normal.

Which of the following statements regarding acute and chronic sinusitis is true?

- ❑ **A. Ethmoiditis is the most common form of sinusitis in adults**
- ❑ **B. The most useful criterion for the diagnosis of bacterial sinusitis is the presence of purulent nasal discharge**

❑ **C. Antihistamines are useful in the treatment of acute sinusitis**

❑ **D. Antibiotics should be used in patients who are moderately to seriously ill, in patients whose symptoms fail to respond to decongestants, and in those who have complications**

Key Concept/Objective: To understand the diagnosis and treatment of bacterial sinusitis

Antibiotics should be used in the following patients: those who are moderately to seriously ill; those whose symptoms fail to respond to decongestants; and those who have complications. Frontal sinusitis and maxillary sinusitis are most common in adults; ethmoiditis is most common in children. The diagnosis of acute sinusitis can usually be established on clinical grounds. Purulent nasal discharge is not specific for sinusitis and may occur in viral nasopharyngitis. Antihistamines are not indicated, because they thicken secretions and impair drainage. *(Answer: D—Antibiotics should be used in patients who are moderately to seriously ill, in patients whose symptoms fail to respond to decongestants, and in those who have complications)*

92. A 17-year-old male presents to your office for the evaluation of fever. He was in his usual state of health until 3 days ago, when he developed severe left ear pain and fever. He states that he is now having trouble hearing from his left ear. He denies having been in contact with sick persons, and he has been very healthy. On physical examination, the patient's temperature is 100.9° F (38.3° C). A bulging left tympanic membrane with obscuration of the bony landmarks is noted. The external ear and the postauricular area are without tenderness to palpation. On questioning, the patient reports that he had similar symptoms as a child on many occasions.

Which of the following statements regarding acute otitis media is true?

❑ **A. Purulent otitis media typically results from bacterial migration from the external auditory canal to the normally sterile middle ear**

❑ **B. The most common cause of purulent otitis media is group A streptococci**

❑ **C. The cornerstone of the clinical diagnosis is a bulging tympanic membrane, with impaired mobility and obscuration of the bony landmarks**

❑ **D. Drugs active against β-lactamase–producing bacteria have proved to be superior to amoxicillin in the treatment of acute otitis media**

Key Concept/Objective: To understand the diagnosis and treatment of acute otitis media

A bulging tympanic membrane with impaired mobility and obscuration of the bony landmarks is the cornerstone of the clinical diagnosis of acute otitis media. Tympanic membrane perforation and otorrhea may occur. The most common causes of purulent otitis media are the pneumococcus, nontypable strains of *H. influenzae*, and *M. cartarrhalis*; the previously important group A streptococci are now uncommon. Purulent otitis media results when bacteria ascend from the nasopharynx to the normally sterile middle ear. As in the case of sinusitis, drugs active against β-lactamase–producing bacteria have not proved to be superior to amoxicillin in the treatment of acute otitis media. *(Answer: C—The cornerstone of the clinical diagnosis is a bulging tympanic membrane, with impaired mobility and obscuration of the bony landmarks)*

93. A 21-year-old woman presents with a complaint of sore throat. She was in her usual state of health until 3 days ago, when she developed a nonproductive cough, nasal drainage, ear pain, and a sore throat. She denies having shortness of breath, sputum production, fever, rash, joint pains, or gastrointestinal symptoms. She also denies having been in contact with sick persons. For the past 2 years, she has been in a sexual relationship with a single sexual partner. On physical examination, the patient is found to have erythema of the posterior pharynx and nasal turbinates. Small, bilateral, serous, middle-ear fluid collections are noted. Lung examination is normal. The patient is afebrile. She requests antibiotics, stating that she always improves much more quickly with this therapy.

Which of the following statements regarding pharyngitis is true?

- ❑ A. **Group A streptococci are the most common cause of pharyngitis**
- ❑ B. **Four clinical criteria have been proposed as suggestive of group A streptococcal pharyngitis: tonsillar exudates, tender anterior adenopathy, absence of cough, and history of fever**
- ❑ C. **Office-based rapid diagnostic tests for group A streptococcal pharyngitis have a sensitivity of nearly 100%**
- ❑ D. **Pneumococci and staphylococci are emerging causes of pharyngitis**

Key Concept/Objective: To understand the diagnosis of group A streptococcal pharyngitis

The following four clinical criteria have been proposed as suggestive of group A streptococcal pharyngitis: tonsillar exudates, tender anterior adenopathy, absence of cough, and history of fever. Group A streptococci are the most therapeutically important cause of pharyngitis, although in terms of frequency, they cause as few as 5% of the cases of pharyngitis. Throat cultures remain the standard method for identifying group A streptococci in the pharynx. In addition, rapid diagnostic tests suitable for office use are available. These procedures entail the extraction of streptococcal antigens from throat swabs and the rapid identification of the antigens through immunologic tests such as latex agglutination or enzyme-linked immunosorbent assay. The sensitivity of these tests ranges from 77% to 95%; specificity ranges from 86% to 100%. Many other bacterial species can be cultured from the pharynges of both symptomatic and asymptomatic patients, but they almost never cause pharyngitis. *(Answer: B—Four clinical criteria have been proposed as suggestive of group A streptococcal pharyngitis: tonsillar exudates, tender anterior adenopathy, absence of cough, and history of fever)*

94. A 24-year-old man presents to the emergency department complaining of fever and sore throat. He is accompanied by his mother, who explains that the patient was well until 2 days ago, when he developed high fevers with severe throat pain. She says that his illness appears to have worsened and that he now has severe dysphagia and is actively drooling. On physical examination, the patient has a temperature of 102° F (38.9° C) and is stridorous. A stat lateral-view x-ray of the neck reveals marked epiglottal edema. The patient is emergently intubated and moved to the intensive care unit for further therapy.

Which of the following statements regarding epiglottitis is true?

- ❑ A. **The major cause of acute epiglottitis in children and adults is *Haemophilus influenzae* type b**
- ❑ B. **The incidence of epiglottitis is decreasing in both children and adults**
- ❑ C. **When epiglottitis is suspected, visual inspection with the assistance of a tongue blade should be the first action taken**
- ❑ D. **Steroids have been proved to be the best initial medical therapy**

Key Concept/Objective: To understand the diagnosis and treatment of epiglottitis

***H. influenzae* type b is the major cause of acute epiglottitis in children and adults. Other pathogens, including pneumococci, streptococci, staphylococci, and *Klebsiella pneumoniae*, can produce an identical syndrome. Acute epiglottitis occurs most commonly in children between 2 and 8 years of age and is more frequent in boys. The incidence of epiglottitis in childhood is declining rapidly in populations that have received *H. influenzae* type b vaccinations. Cases in adults appear to be increasing, however, perhaps because of improved diagnosis. Simple inspection of the pharynx is usually unrewarding. Furthermore, any instrumentation, even a tongue blade, can provoke spasm and total airway obstruction, although adults are at lower risk for this complication. Therefore, unless acute respiratory distress is present, a lateral-view x-ray of the neck should be taken immediately. If the film does not demonstrate epiglottal edema, indirect laryngoscopy can be undertaken; if edema is present, however, the diagnosis is confirmed, and instrumentation is unnecessary. Steroids are sometimes advocated to**

reduce the edema, but their effectiveness has not been tested in controlled clinical trials. *(Answer: A—The major cause of acute epiglottitis in children and adults is* Haemophilus influenzae *type b)*

95. A 4-year-old girl is brought to your office by her mother, whose chief complaint is that her daughter has an ear infection. The patient's immunizations are up to date. The patient is in the 60th percentile for height and weight. The mother states that her daughter has complained of right ear pain for 2 days but has not had any fever. Physical examination reveals a well-developed child in no acute distress. The oropharynx is clear. The right tympanic membrane appears to be bulging, with cloudy fluid behind and poor visualization of the ossicles. The mother asks if her daughter can be treated without use of antibiotics.

What might your response to the mother be, given the current guidelines for treatment for otitis media?

- ❑ **A. "Yes, antibiotics have no role in the treatment of otitis media."**
- ❑ **B. "If we do not give your daughter antibiotics soon, we risk systemic infection and possible death."**
- ❑ **C. "All middle ear infections require antibiotics; withholding treatment would be wrong."**
- ❑ **D. "If your daughter's symptoms do not improve within 3 days, we should start antibiotic therapy."**

Key Concept/Objective: To understand the role of antibiotics in uncomplicated otitis media

The utility of antibiotics in uncomplicated otitis media is being reappraised. Their benefits appear modest; a meta-analysis concluded that to prevent one child from experiencing pain by 2 to 7 days after infection, 17 children must be treated with antibiotics. Further studies are required to determine which patients are most likely to benefit from antibiotics, which drugs are best, and how long therapy should be continued. A new approach that merits study is a delayed-therapy strategy, in which an antibiotic is prescribed when otitis media is diagnosed, but the parents of the child are encouraged to fill the prescription only if the child's condition has not improved after 72 hours. Clearly, antibiotics do have a role in management of this common condition. To delay antibiotic therapy for longer than 3 days would jeopardize this patient's health. This parent's concern about the overuse of antibiotics in this common disease is warranted, and her interest in other treatment plans is reasonable. *(Answer: D—"If your daughter's symptoms do not improve within 3 days, we should start antibiotic therapy.")*

96. A 43-year-old man without any medical history comes to your office with complaints of sinusitis. He reports increased nasal drainage, facial tenderness, and a mild headache. Physical examination reveals a moderately ill man whose temperature, determined orally, is 100.8° F (38.2° C). His appearance is appropriate for his age. A strong odor of tobacco smoke emanates from his clothes. His oropharynx is erythematous. There is mild purulent drainage from his nares, and pain is elicited with maxillary percussion. Your diagnosis is acute sinusitis.

Which of the following treatments or medications should be avoided in this patient?

- ❑ **A. Smoking cessation**
- ❑ **B. Antibiotics**
- ❑ **C. Decongestants**
- ❑ **D. Antihistamines**

Key Concept/Objective: To understand the treatment of acute sinusitis

Acute sinusitis is treated with analgesics and topical heat for patient comfort. Decongestants are of paramount importance. Pseudoephedrine can be administered orally or by nasal spray. Antibiotics should be used in moderately to seriously ill patients, in patients whose symptoms fail to respond to decongestants, and in patients who have complications. Tobacco smoke is a known irritant of paranasal sinus respira-

tory epithelium. Antihistamines are not indicated, because they thicken secretions and impair sinus drainage. *(Answer: D—Antihistamines)*

97. A 39-year-old white man presents to your office with fever and ear pain of 2 days' duration. He has a 12-year history of diabetes mellitus. On physical examination, the patient appears acutely ill. His temperature is 99.8° F (37.7° C), his heart rate is 103 beats/min, and his blood pressure is 132/80 mm Hg. The left auditory canal shows erythema and purulent drainage.

How should this patient be managed?

- ❑ **A. Admission to hospital; initiation of I.V. antipseudomonal antibiotics; surgical consultation**
- ❑ **B. Polymyxin B eardrops**
- ❑ **C. An oral β-lactam**
- ❑ **D. Polymyxin B eardrops and an oral β-lactam**

Key Concept/Objective: To understand the diagnosis and treatment of malignant otitis externa

Malignant otitis externa, an infection with *Pseudomonas aeruginosa* that progressively invades the cartilage, soft tissue, and skull, is a rare condition that occurs in diabetic patients. Neurologic complications can be lethal. Prolonged, maximal parenteral therapy with combinations of antipseudomonal agents, such as tobramycin and piperacillin, is generally recommended. Monotherapy with intravenous ceftazidime and prolonged therapy with oral ciprofloxacin have been successful. Other antibiotics that may prove useful alone or in combination are aztreonam, cefepime, imipenem, and meropenem. Aggressive surgical debridement has been a mainstay of treatment but may be required less often in patients who are treated early and aggressively with antibiotics. CT scanning is superior to magnetic resonance imaging for early diagnosis, but either technique can be used to monitor patients for bone destruction and neurologic complications; should these sequelae occur, debridement is required. *(Answer: A—Admission to hospital; initiation of I.V. antipseudomonal antibiotics; surgical consultation)*

98. A 19-year-old white woman comes to your office with fever and a sore throat. The pain radiates to her right ear, and she has been having difficulty swallowing. During your interview with the patient, she has difficulty with oral secretions and appears to be drooling. On physical examination, the patient appears toxic. Her temperature is 100.7° F (38.2 ° C). The oropharynx shows an enlarged right tonsil, which is erythematous with whitish exudates; the affected tonsil appears to be displaced forward, downward, and toward the midline. The patient had some difficulty opening her mouth for full visualization.

On the basis of this clinical presentation, what is the correct diagnosis?

- ❑ **A. Viral pharyngitis**
- ❑ **B. Lemierre syndrome**
- ❑ **C. Peritonsillar abscess (Quinsy throat)**
- ❑ **D. Ludwig angina**

Key Concept/Objective: To know the clinical presentation of peritonsillar abcess

Peritonsillar abscess, also called Quinsy throat, is a complication of streptococcal tonsillitis most often seen in adolescents and young adults. Group A streptococci are the primary cause of the condition, although most peritonsillar abscesses also harbor mixed oral bacteria, with a predominance of anaerobes. Patients have fever and sore throat, often with pain referred to the ear. Dysphagia prevents the patient from swallowing saliva, commonly causing drooling; edema and pain produce a characteristic muffled, so-called hot-potato voice. The affected tonsil is visibly displaced forward, downward, and toward the midline; the soft palate may be edematous. Trismus occurs in some patients. Viral pharyngitis will not cause a patient to appear toxic. Both Lemierre syndrome (postanginal sepsis) and Ludwig angina are complications of pharyngeal infections, but the clinical presentations of those two entities are distinct and are not found

in this patient. Infection of the parapharyngeal space occasionally spreads to the jugular vein and causes Lemierre syndrome, characterized by septic phlebitis, septic pulmonary emboli, and anaerobic bacteremia. Pharyngitis and dental infections may also lead to Lemierre syndrome. Facial swelling is an early diagnostic clue. Ludwig angina is a cellulitis of the submandibular, sublingual, and submental regions. In 86% of patients, the infection originates from a dental focus. Clinical features include fever, marked toxicity, and a rapidly progressive, brawny edema in the floor of the mouth and the anterior neck. Elevation of the tongue impedes swallowing, and airway obstruction may be lethal. *(Answer: C—Peritonsillar abscess [Quinsy throat])*

99. A 45-year-old woman comes to your clinic complaining of fever, purulent nasal discharge, and left facial and upper molar pain of 3 days' duration. On physical examination, the patient appears well. Her temperature is 100.4° F (38.0° C), and she has tenderness to palpation and percussion over her left maxilla.

Which of the following statements is true regarding the treatment of this patient's sinusitis?

- ❑ **A. Antihistamines are helpful in promoting sinus drainage**
- ❑ **B. Antibiotics that are resistant to β-lactamases have greater efficacy than other antibiotics**
- ❑ **C. All cases of acute sinusitis require antibiotic therapy**
- ❑ **D. Nasal decongestants, such as pseudoephedrine, are a mainstay of therapy**
- ❑ **E. Surgical intervention is now indicated**

Key Concept/Objective: To know the treatment options for acute sinusitis

The treatment of acute sinusitis is aimed at promoting drainage of the sinuses. Nasal decongestants are of paramount importance, and physical measures such as sleeping at a 45° angle, sleeping with the unaffected side dependent, and inhalation of steam can also be helpful. Antihistamines may thicken nasal secretions and would not be helpful. Although it is traditional to prescribe antibiotics for 7 to 10 days for sinusitis, data suggest that in uncomplicated cases, antibiotics do not affect the clinical course of sinusitis, and antibiotics that are β-lactamase resistant have not been shown to have any greater efficacy than those that are not. Surgical intervention is reserved for patients who fail to respond to medical therapy or who have complications. *(Answer: D—Nasal decongestants, such as pseudoephedrine, are a mainstay of therapy)*

100. A 35-year-old man presents complaining of a sore throat of 2 days' duration. He has had low-grade fever, a temperature that rises to 100.4° F (38° C), and little coryza or cough. On physical examination, the patient appears well. He has a temperature of 99.5° F (37.5° C), with a markedly injected posterior pharynx and exudates over his tonsils. You suspect streptococcal pharyngitis.

Which of the following statements is true regarding streptococcal pharyngitis?

- ❑ **A. Immunologic tests based on throat swabs can distinguish the carrier state from infection**
- ❑ **B. Penicillin V, 250 mg q.i.d. or b.i.d. for 10 days, is effective in eradicating group A streptococci from the nasopharynx**
- ❑ **C. Treatment must be started within 5 days of the onset of symptoms to prevent rheumatic fever**
- ❑ **D. Group A streptococci are responsible for 10% to 15% of cases of pharyngitis in adults**
- ❑ **E. The need to culture asymptomatic family contacts of patients with streptococcal pharyngitis is well established**

Key Concept/Objective: To know the key aspects of diagnosis and treatment of streptococcal pharyngitis

Penicillin V is the drug of choice in treating streptococcal pharyngitis; b.i.d. dosing is as effective as q.i.d. dosing and may improve compliance. Throat swabs for immunologic testing for group A streptococci have adequate sensitivity and specificity for detecting the pathogen but cannot distinguish between active infection and the carrier state (the latter may approach 20% of the adult population). Treatment may be started within 9 days of the onset of symptoms to prevent rheumatic fever. Group A streptococci are responsible for only 5% of cases of pharyngitis in adults. Screening asymptomatic family contacts is controversial and probably unnecessary. *(Answer: B—Penicillin V, 250 mg q.i.d. or b.i.d. for 10 days, is effective in eradicating group A streptococci from the nasopharynx)*

101. A 67-year-old woman with poorly controlled diabetes comes to your clinic complaining of ear pain for the past day. She has noticed some purulent drainage. On physical examination, the patient's temperature is 38.9° C (102° F). The rest of her vital signs are stable. There is greenish drainage from the auditory canal, and the pinna is erythematous and swollen. The ear is exquisitely tender to manipulation; she cannot tolerate placement of the speculum in her ear.

Which of the following is appropriate management of this patient's condition?

- ❑ **A. Oral trimethoprim-sulfamethoxazole for 1 week**
- ❑ **B. A prolonged course of oral ciprofloxacin with close outpatient follow-up**
- ❑ **C. Hospital admission for intravenous antibiotics active against *Pseudomonas* and urgent consultation with an otolaryngologist**
- ❑ **D. Placement of a wick in the ear for easier administration of a 1-week course of eardrops of antibiotics, polymyxin B, and neomycin**

Key Concept/Objective: To be able to diagnose and treat pseudomonal (malignant) otitis externa

Otitis externa is a common infection that is often seen in patients with a history of exposure to water. Malignant otitis externa is a condition seen only in diabetic patients; it is characterized by invasion by *Pseudomonas aeruginosa* of the periauricular cartilage, soft tissue, and skull. It is usually treated with combination antipseudomonal antibiotics; hospital admission is highly recommended for patients who are febrile or who appear toxic. Oral ciprofloxacin has been effective in carefully selected patients who have milder disease than this patient. Surgical debridement may be necessary. Oral trimethoprim-sulfamethoxazole would not give antipseudomonal coverage. Placement of a wick in the ear and antibiotic eardrops are adequate therapy for ordinary otitis externa, but this patient's fever and her history of diabetes suggest a more serious infection. *(Answer: C—Hospital admission for intravenous antibiotics active against* Pseudomonas *and urgent consultation with an otolaryngologist)*

102. An 18-year-old woman presents at your clinic complaining of fevers, chills, tenderness along the left side of her neck, and pain when she turns her head to the right. Two weeks ago, she had a sore throat, cough, mild nausea, and vomiting, for which she did not seek care. On physical examination, the patient's temperature is 102.4° F (39.1° C). She is able to open her mouth easily. HEENT examination is remarkable for swelling of the face. The oropharynx is erythematous, and the side of the neck is tender but not swollen. On pulmonary examination, there are crackles and decreased fremitus at the left base.

Which of the following is appropriate for managing this patient's condition?

- ❑ **A. Contrast-enhanced CT scan of the neck and chest, two sets of blood cultures, and intravenous antibiotics effective against anaerobic bacteria**
- ❑ **B. Contrast-enhanced CT scan of the neck and chest, two sets of blood cultures, intravenous antibiotics effective against anaerobic bacteria, and heparin infusion**
- ❑ **C. Two sets of blood cultures, intravenous antibiotics effective against anaerobic bacteria, and heparin infusion**

❑ **D. Contrast-enhanced CT scan of the neck and chest, two sets of blood cultures, intravenous antibiotics effective against anaerobic bacteria, heparin infusion, and drainage/resection of the involved structure**

Key Concept/Objective: To be able to diagnose and treat septic thrombophlebitis of the internal jugular vein (Lemierre syndrome)

Lemierre syndrome occurs most commonly in children and young adults and is characterized by septic thrombophlebitis of the internal jugular vein, septic pulmonary emboli, and anaerobic bacteremia. It is typically caused by *Fusobacterium necrophorum*. Lemierre syndrome starts as pharyngitis with invasion into the deep pharyngeal tissue; this allows drainage into the lateral pharyngeal space and subsequent thrombosis of the internal jugular vein. CT scanning of the neck can lead to a diagnosis of thrombosis (ultrasound can also be used); blood cultures are important in identifying the pathogen. Penicillin G, metronidazole, and clindamycin have been the mainstays of therapy, although since the 1970s, *Fusobacterium* species have been found to be positive for β-lactamase, and some authors recommend using antibiotics that are β-lactamase-stable or antibiotic combinations that include β-lactamase inhibitors. Heparin therapy has not been conclusively shown to improve outcomes, and ligation and surgical resection of the internal jugular vein are rarely necessary with adequate antibiotic therapy. *(Answer: A—Contrast-enhanced CT scan of the neck and chest, two sets of blood cultures, and intravenous antibiotics effective against anaerobic bacteria)*

For more information, see Simon HB: 7 Infectious Disease: XIX Bacterial Infections of the Upper Respiratory Tract. ACP Medicine Online (www.acpmedicine.com). Dale DC, Federman DD, Eds. WebMD Inc., New York, October 2004

Pneumonia and Other Pulmonary Infections

103. A 53-year-old man with diabetes presents to the emergency department for the evaluation of fever. He was in his usual state of health until 36 hours ago, when he developed fever and fatigue; these symptoms were followed by a productive cough. Over the past few hours, he has developed worsening shortness of breath, cough, and dizziness. He has had diabetes mellitus for many years, and he states that he has not seen a physician in the past 12 months. On physical examination, the patient is tachycardic and tachypnic. His blood pressure is 94/46 mm Hg, he is orthostatic, and his temperature is 102.7° F (39.3° C). Hemoglobin O_2 saturation is 88% on room air. The patient has rales and dullness to percussion at the right pulmonary base. Chest x-ray reveals a right lower lobe infiltrate. Laboratory data reveal a leukocytosis with left shift, as well as mild renal insufficiency.

Which of the following statements regarding community-acquired pneumonia is true?

❑ **A. Bacterial pneumonia is principally spread person to person**

❑ **B. The inflammatory response to *Streptococcus pneumoniae* or *Haemophilus influenzae* often produces lobar consolidation and significant tissue necrosis**

❑ **C. For patients who do not require hospitalization, advanced macrolides, doxycycline, and respiratory fluoroquinolones are reasonable choices for therapy**

❑ **D. For patients with hospital-acquired pneumonia, advanced macrolides, vancomycin, or doxycycline will suffice as monotherapies**

Key Concept/Objective: To understand the diagnosis and treatment of community-acquired pneumonia

Erythromycin is cost-effective, but the so-called advanced macrolides clarithromycin and azithromycin may be preferable because of their better gastrointestinal tolerability and their activity against *Haemophilus* and *Moraxella* species. Doxycycline is an effective and inexpensive alternative. However, because of the increasing prevalence of drug-resistant pneumococci, use of one of the so-called respiratory fluoroquinolones

(i.e., levofloxacin, gatifloxacin, moxifloxacin, or gemifloxacin) is recommended. Pneumococci are spread from person to person by aerosolized droplets, but pneumococcal pneumonia is not highly contagious and is caused in many cases by aspiration of nasopharyngeal organisms, the second major mechanism of infection. The inflammatory response to *S. pneumoniae* or *H. influenzae* often produces lobar consolidation, but these infections rarely result in tissue necrosis. Initial treatment of hospital-acquired pneumonia includes ticarcillin-clavulanate or piperacillin-tazobactam; meropenem or imipenem-cilastatin; a third-generation cephalosporin plus nafcillin or vancomycin; a first-generation cephalosporin plus an aminoglycoside; or vancomycin plus an aminoglycoside. *(Answer: C—For patients who do not require hospitalization, advanced macrolides, doxycycline, and respiratory fluoroquinolones are reasonable choices for therapy)*

104. A 26-year-old woman presents to your office for the evaluation of fever. She was in her usual state of health until 24 hours ago, when she developed fatigue, myalgias, and severe headache. Her temperature rose to 102° F (38.9° C), and she developed a nonproductive cough and chest tightness. She reports worsening nausea and diarrhea over the same period. She denies having any sick contacts, and she was previously healthy. On physical examination, her temperature is 101.5° F (38.6° C). Bilateral rales with tachycardia are noted. She has no meningismus. Chest x-ray reveals bilateral, patchy air-space and interstitial infiltrates. She is admitted to the hospital for further evaluation and monitoring.

Which of the following statements regarding Legionnaires disease is true?

❑ A. **_Legionella pneumophila_ is typically acquired by person-to-person contact**

❑ B. **There are currently no available methods of rapidly diagnosing infection with _L. pneumophila_**

❑ C. **Current evidence indicates that azithromycin or levofloxacin is the treatment of choice**

❑ D. **In patients in whom monotherapy with azithromycin or levofloxacin fails, there are no other medical alternatives**

Key Concept/Objective: To understand the diagnosis and treatment of Legionnaires disease

On in vitro susceptibility testing, *L. pneumophila* has been shown to be susceptible to a variety of antimicrobial agents, including erythromycin, clarithromycin, azithromycin, tetracycline, rifampin, and the fluoroquinolones. According to current evidence, azithromycin or levofloxacin is the treatment of choice. Human disease is acquired primarily by inhalation of aerosols contaminated with organisms; person-to-person transmission has not been documented. A method of rapid diagnosis involves detection of *L. pneumophila* antigen in the urine; this radioimmunoassay test is highly specific and has a sensitivity of about 80% to 90%. However, the test is available only for *L. pneumophila* serogroup 1, which is the most common cause of Legionnaires disease. A combination of rifampin and either azithromycin or levofloxacin may be considered in patients who fail to respond to monotherapy and in immunologically impaired patients with overwhelming disease. *(Answer: C—Current evidence indicates that azithromycin or levofloxacin is the treatment of choice)*

105. A 61-year-old man with a history of alcoholism and seizure disorder arrives at the emergency department for evaluation. He was found lying on the sidewalk by passers-by, who notified the emergency medical system. The patient is partially arousable to pain and voice. His vital signs are stable. Hemoglobin O_2 saturation is 99% on 2 L/min O_2 by nasal cannula. Physical examination is remarkable for poor dentition, fetid breath, rales and egophony in the right midlung zone, and tachypnea. Chest x-ray reveals a dense infiltrate of the right lower lobe. He is treated for possible seizure, intubated for airway protection, and moved to the intensive care unit for further care.

Which of the following statements regarding the diagnosis and treatment of aspiration pneumonia is true?

❑ A. **Aspiration pneumonia always presents as an acute rather than indolent illness**

❑ B. ***Prevotella melaninogenica*, *Fusobacterium nucleatum*, and *Peptostreptococcus* are particularly important causes of aspiration pneumonia**

❑ C. **Radiographically, infiltrates are most common in the apices of the lungs**

❑ D. **Penicillin monotherapy is no longer considered appropriate therapy for aspiration pneumonia**

Key Concept/Objective: To understand the diagnosis and treatment of aspiration pneumonia

Because anaerobes are the dominant flora of the upper respiratory tract (outnumbering aerobic or facultative bacteria by 10 to 1), it is not surprising that anaerobes are the dominant organisms in aspiration pneumonia. Of particular importance are *P. melaninogenica* and other *Prevotella* species, *F. nucleatum*, and anaerobic or microaerophilic streptococci and *Peptostreptococcus*. As expected, multiple organisms are recovered from most patients. Patients with mixed aspiration pneumonia may present with an acute febrile illness, or the illness may follow a more indolent course, extending over many days or even weeks. Radiographically, infiltrates are most common in dependent areas of the lung, especially the apical segments of the lower lobes and the posterior segments of the upper lobes. With the exception of *Bacteroides fragilis*, which can be identified along with other anaerobic species in 17% of patients with classic aspiration pneumonia, all the anaerobes found are penicillin sensitive. Penicillin is effective when *B. fragilis* is present in addition to penicillin-sensitive organisms, suggesting that aspiration pneumonias are synergistic infections that can be treated successfully by elimination of most but not necessarily all of the organisms involved. *(Answer: B—*Prevotella melaninogenica, Fusobacterium nucleatum, *and* Peptostreptococcus *are particularly important causes of aspiration pneumonia)*

106. A 55-year-old alcoholic man presents with fever and shortness of breath. The patient was in his usual state of health until 10 days ago, when he developed intermittent fever; a productive, foul-smelling cough; and anorexia. He has been a heavy drinker for many years and admits to recent binges. He denies having urinary, abdominal, or gastrointestinal symptoms. On physical examination, the patient's temperature is 99.9° F (37.7° C). He has exceptionally poor dentition, and dullness to percussion is noted at the right pulmonary base. Chest x-ray reveals an air-space infiltrate in the right lower lobe, with an associated moderate pleural effusion. Thoracentesis reveals an exudative effusion of pH 6.95. Gram stain of the pleural fluid reveals gram-negative rods.

Which of the following statements regarding the diagnosis and treatment of empyema is true?

❑ A. ***Staphylococcus aureus*, various species of *Streptococcus*, and gram-negative bacilli are the most common causes of empyema**

❑ B. [illegible]

❑ C. **Gross purulence is diagnostic of empyema, and the absence of frank pus rules out infection**

❑ D. **Video-assisted thoracoscopic surgery (VATS) is the traditional method for draining empyemas**

Key Concept/Objective: To understand the diagnosis and treatment of empyema

The most common causes of empyema are *S. aureus*, various species of *Streptococcus*, and gram-negative bacilli. Among the gram-negative bacilli, *Klebsiella pneumoniae* has been linked with diabetes. Many infections are mixed. Anaerobes have been recognized in 25% to 76% of empyemas and may occur in pure culture or in combination with aerobic or facultative organisms. *Fusobacterium*, *Prevotella*, and anaerobic gram-positive cocci are the anaerobes most often seen. Bacteria can reach the pleural space by many routes. Most often, empyema results from the direct spread of bronchopulmonary infections, including pneumonias, lung abscesses, and bronchiectasis. Hematogenous seeding is an infrequent mechanism of empyema formation. Gross purulence is diagnostic of empyema, but the absence of frank pus does not rule out infection. Closed chest tube

drainage is the traditional method for draining empyemas, but image-guided catheter drainage is also effective, particularly when the fluid is loculated. If complete drainage cannot be achieved with chest tubes, VATS can often disrupt intrapleural adhesions and achieve excellent drainage of loculated effusions. *(Answer: A—*Staphylococcus aureus, *various species of* Streptococcus, *and gram-negative bacilli are the most common causes of empyema)*

107. A 68-year-old white woman presents to the hospital with fever, cough, sputum production, and dyspnea. The patient's medical history is significant for osteoarthritis and hypertension. The results of the physical examination are as follows: temperature, 102.4° F (39.1° C); heart rate, 114 beats/min; blood pressure, 106/72 mm Hg; respiratory rate, 24 breaths/min; O_2 saturation, 79% on room air. Pulmonary examination reveals crackles at the right base, with increased tactile fremitus. A chest radiograph reveals a right lower lobe infiltrate. The patient is admitted to the intensive care unit. Her husband asks about the likelihood of the patient's dying from her pneumonia.

Given recent mortality data, which of the following is the most appropriate response to the husband's question?

- ❑ **A. "It is very rare for anyone to die from pneumonia—less than 1%."**
- ❑ **B. "Although your wife is ill, I expect a full recovery; her chance of dying is nearly zero."**
- ❑ **C. "Your wife is very ill and is in the ICU; about 3 of 10 patients in her situation die."**
- ❑ **D. "Your wife's prognosis is guarded; I would estimate the mortality to be 90% for patients with this severity of illness."**

Key Concept/Objective: To understand mortality from pneumonia for patients admitted to the ICU

Community-acquired pneumonias are a major problem in the United States, with at least 924,000 cases reported annually. About 485,000 cases require hospitalization, and at least 50,000 result in death. The mortality of community-acquired pneumonia ranges from less than 1% in patients who are not ill enough to require hospitalization to 13.7% for hospitalized patients, 19.6% for bacteremic patients, and 36.5% for patients admitted to ICUs. Clinical and laboratory data can be used to determine which patients are at greatest risk for death and thus require hospitalization and aggressive therapy. *(Answer: C—"Your wife is very ill and is in the ICU; about 3 of 10 patients in her situation die.")*

108. A 75-year-old man was admitted to your service 48 hours ago because of pneumonia. At the time of admission, sputum and blood cultures were drawn. Despite receiving appropriate antibiotics for community-acquired pneumonia, his clinical picture continues to worsen. Respiratory failure ensues, requiring that the patient be mechanically ventilated. On hospital day 3, admission sputum and blood cultures reveal gram-negative rods.

Which of the following likely contributed to this patient's gram-negative pneumonia?

- ❑ **A. Age**
- ❑ **B. The patient's having been recently treated with antibiotics**
- ❑ **C. Sex**
- ❑ **D. Mechanical ventilation**

Key Concept/Objective: To understand the risk factors for gram-negative pneumonia

Staphylococci and gram-negative bacilli are much less common but more serious causes of community-acquired respiratory infections. Significant predisposing conditions are required for these organisms to produce pneumonia. In the community setting, staphylococcal pneumonia usually follows influenza. Gram-negative pneumonias in the community setting are most common in patients who have recently been hospitalized and treated with antibiotics, in smokers and others with chronic lung disease, and in immunosuppressed individuals. Because this patient was admitted with pneumonia

and because initial cultures were drawn on admission, mechanical ventilation cannot be a causal factor. Sex and age are not known risk factors for pneumonia caused by gram-negative rods. *(Answer: B—The patient's having been recently treated with antibiotics)*

109. A 34-year-old air-conditioning repairman is admitted to the hospital because of respiratory distress. He reports fever, chills, a mildly productive cough, myalgias, headache, and nausea. Physical examination shows a toxic-appearing man in moderate respiratory distress. His temperature is 102.2° F (39.0° C); his heart rate is 120 beats/min; his blood pressure is 124/78 mm Hg; and his respiratory rate is 24 breaths/min. Crackles at both lung bases with diffuse wheezes are noted. Laboratory data show profound leukocytosis with a left shift and a serum sodium level of 126 mEq/L. He is admitted to hospital for treatment of community-acquired pneumonia.

Which of the following is the best antibiotic regimen for this patient?

- ❑ A. **Penicillin**
- ❑ B. **Clindamycin**
- ❑ C. **Gentamicin**
- ❑ D. **Azithromycin or levofloxacin**

Key Concept/Objective: To understand the treatment of suspected Legionella *pneumonia*

Since it was first recognized in 1976, Legionnaires disease has become recognized as a common cause of both community-acquired and hospital-acquired pneumonia. In nature, *L. pneumophila* survives principally in water and, to a lesser extent, in soil. Contaminated water systems have been responsible for both community-acquired and hospital-acquired outbreaks. Legionnaires disease is characterized by a 1-day prodrome of myalgias, malaise, and slight headache after an incubation period of 2 to 10 days. Acute onset of high fever, shaking chills, nonproductive cough, tachypnea, and, often, pleuritic pain ensues. The cough may subsequently become slightly productive, but the sputum is not purulent. Hyponatremia, although common in many pathologic lung conditions, is suggestive of *Legionella* infection. On in vitro susceptibility testing, *L. pneumophila* is susceptible to a variety of antimicrobial agents, including erythromycin, clarithromycin, azithromycin, tetracycline, rifampin, and the fluoroquinolones. Current evidence indicates that azithromycin or levofloxacin is the treatment of choice. *(Answer: D—Azithromycin or levofloxacin)*

110. A 56-year-old patient who has smoked two packs of cigarettes a day for 40 years presents to your office for a second opinion. His previous physician recently diagnosed him as having chronic bronchitis. The patient reports that no work-up was done, "not even a chest x-ray." The patient asks, "How can my doctor know I have chronic bronchitis without doing any sort of examination or workup?"

Which of the following is the most appropriate response to this patient's question?

- ❑ A. **"You are right; at least a chest x-ray is needed to make this diagnosis."**
- ❑ B. **"You are right; you need some blood work, lung function tests, and a chest x-ray before this diagnosis can be made."**
- ❑ C. **"Given your history of smoking, you must have chronic bronchitis."**
- ❑ D. **"The diagnosis is made on the basis of history alone; given your smoking history, if you have a cough with sputum production for most days for at least 3 months each year for 2 or more years, chronic bronchitis is the correct diagnosis."**

Key Concept/Objective: To understand the diagnosis of chronic bronchitis

Patients with chronic bronchitis characteristically produce sputum on most days for at least 3 months each year for more than 2 years. The sputum is frequently colonized by *Haemophilus influenzae* (nontypable), *S. pneumoniae*, or *Mycoplasma catarrhalis*, either singly or in combination. Although it is uncertain whether the bacteria themselves produce additional airway damage, heavy bacterial loads correlate with increased

inflammation. Chronic bronchtitis is a clinical diagnosis. Workup, although beneficial to rule out other potential causes of lung dysfunction, is not necessary for diagnosis. *(Answer: D—"The diagnosis is made on the basis of history alone; given your smoking history, if you have a cough with sputum production for most days for at least 3 months each year for 2 or more years, chronic bronchitis is the correct diagnosis.")*

111. An 18-year-old college student comes to the student health clinic for evaluation of fever and cough. Headache, sore throat, runny nose, and fatigue began 5 days ago. Fever and cough began 2 days ago and steadily increased. The cough is hacking, occurs frequently, and produces small amounts of clear sputum with occasional flecks of purulent material and blood. The patient has a history of childhood asthma, occasional marijuana use, and acne. He takes no oral medications and has no known drug allergies. On physical examination, the patient appears ill but not toxic. He has a temperature of 100.9° F (38.3° C), mild pharyngeal erythema without thrush or oral hairy leukoplakia, and no adenopathy. Chest examination results are normal. Pulse oximetry, measured while the patient is breathing room air, is 98%. Chest x-ray reveals segmental opacities in the right and left lower lobes. Sputum Gram stain shows abundant polymorphonuclear cells without microorganisms. The white blood cell count is 12,000/mm^3, with 70% polymorphonuclear leukocytes and no left shift. A bedside test for cold agglutinins is positive.

Which of the following would be the most appropriate choice for antimicrobial treatment of this patient's condition?

- ❑ **A. No antimicrobial treatment**
- ❑ **B. Amoxicillin, 500 mg p.o., t.i.d., for 14 days**
- ❑ **C. Amoxicillin-clavulanate, 875 mg p.o., b.i.d., for 14 days**
- ❑ **D. Azithromycin, 500 mg p.o. once, then 250 mg p.o., q.d., for 4 days**
- ❑ **E. Ciprofloxacin, 500 mg p.o., b.i.d., for 10 days**

Key Concept/Objective: To understand the clinical presentation and treatment of mycoplasmal pneumonia

This previously healthy young man presents with bilateral pneumonia after an upper respiratory prodrome, hacking cough with minimal sputum production, absence of microorganisms on sputum Gram stain, and segmental pulmonary infiltrates. These features are consistent with either mycoplasmal or chlamydial pneumonia, with the presence of cold agglutinins favoring the former. Antimicrobial treatment can shorten the duration of symptoms (especially fever) in patients with mycoplasmal pneumonia. Of the choices given, only azithromycin would be expected to be effective against *Mycoplasma* and *Chlamydia*. *(Answer: D—Azithromycin, 500 mg p.o. once, then 250 mg p.o., q.d., for 4 days)*

112. A 34-year-old man seeks evaluation of a cough. His illness began with a sore throat and nasal congestion 5 days ago. He subsequently developed a cough productive of green sputum and a burning sensation in the retrosternal chest that occurs with coughing spells. He has felt cold at times but denies shaking chills, shortness of breath, and hemoptysis. There is a history of seasonal allergies, but he takes no medications and has no known drug allergies. He is a nonsmoker who typically jogs 3 miles, four times weekly. Pulse oximetry reveals a normal resting oxygen saturation; the patient's temperature is 100.2° F (37.9° C). The chest is clear to percussion, with audible expiratory wheezes. After taking a deep breath, the patient coughs, producing green sputum. A Gram stain of the specimen reveals polymorphonuclear and mononuclear cells without microorganisms. A chest x-ray is normal.

Which of the following would be the most appropriate choice for antimicrobial treatment of this patient's condition?

- ❑ **A. No antimicrobial treatment**
- ❑ **B. Amoxicillin-clavulanate, 875 mg p.o., b.i.d., for 10 days**
- ❑ **C. Trimethoprim-sulfamethoxazole, 1 double-strength tablet p.o., b.i.d., for 10 days**

❑ D. **Azithromycin, 500 mg p.o. once, then 250 mg p.o., q.d., for 4 days**

❑ E. **Levofloxacin, 250 mg p.o., q.d., for 10 days**

Key Concept/Objective: To understand that antimicrobial therapy is ineffective for acute bronchitis

This otherwise healthy man who is without underlying lung disease has acute bronchitis, an illness caused predominantly by respiratory viruses. Up to 85% of patients diagnosed with acute bronchitis in the United States receive antimicrobial therapy. This practice has likely contributed to the rapid emergence of drug-resistant strains of bacteria. *(Answer: A—No antimicrobial treatment)*

113. A 62-year woman with non-Hodgkin lymphoma is admitted after the abrupt onset of fever, chills, shortness of breath, and cough productive of brown sputum. She had been well until the morning of admission. In the emergency department, she complains of right-sided pleuritic chest pain. She denies having headache, stiff neck, and photophobia. The patient's lymphoma was treated with six cycles of chemotherapy that were completed 6 weeks before admission. On physical examination, the patient appears acutely ill, with a temperature of 103.1° F (39.5° C) and a respiratory rate of 32 breaths/min. Pulse oximetry reveals an oxygen saturation of 88% while the patient is breathing room air. Mental status is normal, and meningismus is not present. The right posterior chest is dull to percussion. Rhonchi and bronchial breath sounds are heard in the same area. Sputum Gram stain shows sheets of polymorphonuclear cells with abundant gram-positive diplococci. A chest x-ray demonstrates lobar opacification of the right lower lobe. The white blood cell count is 6,500, with 80% polymorphonuclear cells and increased band forms. Because you practice in a region in which up to 30% of invasive *Streptococcus pneumoniae* isolates show intermediate or high-grade resistance to penicillin, you are worried that this patient may be infected with a drug-resistant strain.

Which of the following would be the most appropriate initial choice for antimicrobial therapy in this patient?

❑ A. **Ampicillin-sulbactam, 1.5 g I.V., q. 6 hr**

❑ B. **Cefuroxime, 1.5 g I.V., q. 8 hr**

❑ C. **Erythromycin, 500 mg I.V., q. 6 hr**

❑ D. **Levofloxacin, 500 mg I.V., q. 24 hr**

❑ E. **Vancomycin, 1 g I.V., q. 12 hr**

Key Concept/Objective: To know how to treat pneumonia caused by drug-resistant Streptococcus pneumoniae

The prevalence of high-level antimicrobial drug resistance in *S. pneumoniae* isolates varies across geographic regions. When prescribing initial treatment for community-acquired pneumococcal pneumonia, a physician should be aware of both the regional prevalence of drug resistance and the typical patterns of antimicrobial cross-resistance. Of the choices given, only levofloxacin has a very low rate of cross-resistance. Because an alteration of penicillin-binding proteins is the usual mechanism of penicillin resistance in *S. pneumoniae*, the addition of a β-lactamase inhibitor does not result in greater effectiveness, and there is broad cross-resistance with first- and second-generation cephalosporins. In addition, drug-resistant *S. pneumoniae* isolates frequently carry plasmid-mediated cross-resistance against other classes of antimicrobial drugs, including macrolides, sulfas, and tetracyclines. Vancomycin resistance remains exceedingly rare among *S. pneumoniae* isolates; nevertheless, use of this agent in community-acquired pneumonia should be reserved for patients with suspected meningitis or neutropenia, those in whom therapy with first-line agents fail, or those whose infective organisms demonstrate resistance to other agents, to avoid promotion of vancomycin-resistant strains of bacteria, especially species of *Enterococcus* and *Staphylococcus*. *(Answer: D—Levofloxacin, 500 mg I.V., q. 24 hr)*

114. A homeless 56-year-old man is admitted with progressive fever and right-sided chest pain. He describes how for 3 weeks he has had anorexia, fatigue, and cough productive of profuse purulent sputum with occasional hemoptysis. Additional medical problems include a 60-pack-year history of cigarette smoking, chronic alcoholism, occasional injection drug use, and chronic hepatitis C infection. He takes no medications. On physical examination, the patient appears cachectic and acutely ill and has a temperature of 101.3° F (38.5° C). He has numerous injection track marks on his extremities but no cyanosis, clubbing, or peripheral edema. Severe periodontal disease is noted. The upper half of the right posterior chest is dull to percussion, and rhonchi are heard in the same region. A chest CT scan demonstrates opacification of the posterior segment of the right upper lobe, with a central fluid-filled and air-filled cavity. Sputum is foul smelling and brown in color. Gram stain demonstrates abundant polymorphonuclear leukocytes; gram-positive cocci of various sizes appear as single organisms and in pairs and chains, and occasional gram-positive rods, gram-negative cocci, and gram-negative rods are present. Sputum culture grows mixed oral flora.

Which of the following is the most likely diagnosis for this patient?

- ❑ **A. Tuberculosis**
- ❑ **B. Primary anaerobic lung abscess**
- ❑ **C. Squamous cell lung cancer with cavitation and postobstructive pneumonia**
- ❑ **D. Septic pulmonary embolism**
- ❑ **E. Wegener granulomatosis**

Key Concept/Objective: To know the clinical features of primary anaerobic lung abscess

Each of the conditions listed can produce cavitary lung lesions. Features of this patient's illness that favor the diagnosis of primary anaerobic lung abscess are the subacute course, weight loss, periodontal disease, use of substances that alter consciousness (alcohol, injection drugs), presence of profuse purulent sputum and hemoptysis, location in the posterior segment of the upper lobe, and Gram stain result. Tuberculosis would also be a key consideration, but the sputum Gram stain result precludes a diagnosis of tuberculosis. Nevertheless, it would be reasonable to place this patient in respiratory isolation, perform PPD skin testing (without controls), and send sputum for acid-fast bacilli staining and mycobacterial culture. This patient's presentation is also consistent with a diagnosis of lung cancer complicated by postobstructive pneumonia. Of the various histologic types of lung cancer, squamous cell tumors are the most likely to cavitate. Production of profuse sputum does not suggest obstruction, however. In injection drug users, septic pulmonary embolism is a common complication of tricuspid valve endocarditis. The slow progression of this patient's illness would be unusual for that condition, however, and septic embolization occurs most often in the lower lobes. Wegener granulomatosis is the least likely cause of this man's illness. *(Answer: B—Primary anaerobic lung abscess)*

115. A 68-year-old man with severe chronic obstructive pulmonary disease (COPD) (baseline FEV_1, 800 ml) is admitted to the intensive care unit with acute respiratory failure and fever. His wife reports that he was in his usual state of debilitated health until 4 days ago, when he developed myalgias, fever, chills, and a headache. Two days before admission, he experienced increasing shortness of breath and cough, and he passed several watery bowel movements. Symptoms did not improve with increased use of albuterol, which was administered at home with a nebulizer. On the day of admission, he appeared confused and severely short of breath. Paramedics were summoned and performed endotracheal intubation before transporting him to the hospital. In the intensive care unit, the patient is incapable of being aroused; he has a temperature of 104° F (40° C), a blood pressure of 130/90 mm Hg, and a pulse of 88 beats/min. Physical examination reveals normal extremities, no rashes, a supple neck, and a barrel-shaped chest with diffuse wheezes. The point of maximal impulse is felt in the epigastric region, and the heart sounds are muffled. The abdomen is soft without involuntary guarding. Laboratory results are notable for a white blood cell count of 14,250/mm^3, with normal differential; sodium, 128 mEq/L; alanine aminotransferase, 122 IU/L; and creatine phosphokinase, 450 IU/L (MB quotient, 3%). Chest x-ray demonstrates an endotracheal tube in good position, flattened hemidiaphragms, and a left lower lobe opacity that was not present on previous films.

While you await the results of further diagnostic studies, empirical antimicrobial therapy should be initiated against which of the following microorganisms?

- ❑ A. ***Streptococcus pneumoniae***
- ❑ B. ***Haemophilus influenzae***
- ❑ C. ***Chlamydia pneumoniae***
- ❑ D. ***Legionella pneumophila***
- ❑ E. **All of the above**

Key Concept/Objective: To know the most common causes of severe community-acquired pneumonia in patients with underlying lung disease

This patient is critically ill and should receive empirical treatment against each of the microorganisms listed. *S. pneumoniae, H. influenzae,* and *L. pneumophila* are widely recognized as important causes of pneumonia in this population. In addition, recent studies have demonstrated that *C. pneumoniae* also can cause illness ranging in severity from acute bronchitis to severe pneumonia in patients with COPD. *(Answer: E—All of the above)*

For more information, see Simon HB: 7 Infectious Disease: XX Pneumonia and Other Pulmonary Infections. ACP Medicine Online (www.acpmedicine.com). Dale DC, Federman DD, Eds. WebMD Inc., New York, October 2004

Peritonitis and Intra-abdominal Abscesses

116. A 47-year-old man with cirrhosis secondary to alcoholic liver disease is brought to the emergency department by his care provider because of mental status changes. He has a history of hepatic encephalopathy and ascites but no history of gastrointestinal bleeding. His medications are furosemide, spironolactone, and lactulose. He has had confusion and somnolence for the past 3 days. On physical examination, the patient is afebrile, with a temperature of 99° F (37.2° C); pulse, 90 beats/min; respirations, 20 breaths/min; and blood pressure, 100/60 mm Hg. He is somnolent and oriented only to person. Lungs are clear to auscultation. The abdomen is distended, with shifting dullness and bulging flanks; he has active bowel sounds and no tenderness on palpation. Stool is guaiac negative. Peripheral WBC is 9,400/mm^3; hematocrit, 33%; platelets, 93,000/mm^3. Peritoneal fluid reveals a WBC of 200/mm^3 with 80% polymorphonuclear leukocytes (PMNs). Gram stain of ascitic fluid reveals no organisms.

Which of the following makes the diagnosis of spontaneous bacterial peritonitis (SBP) unlikely?

- ❑ A. **Absence of fever**
- ❑ B. **Absence of elevated peripheral WBCs**
- ❑ C. **Absence of abdominal pain or tenderness on examination**
- ❑ D. **Gram stain of ascitic fluid revealing no organisms**
- ❑ E. **PMN count in the ascitic fluid < 250 cells/mm^3**

Key Concept/Objective: To understand the clinical presentation of SBP

The clinical presentation of SBP is often subtle. The diagnosis of SBP should be considered in any patient with known cirrhosis who has clinical deterioration, such as worsening of hepatic encephalopathy or hypotension. Paracentesis for evaluation of the ascitic fluid is necessary. Fever is a common symptom but is absent in 30% of patients with SBP. The peripheral WBC is not valuable in determining whether or not a patient has SBP. Abdominal pain is a common feature of SBP, but only half of patients will have tenderness on examination. The Gram stain of the ascitic fluid in SBP is typically negative, although visualization of a single bacterial type would be consistent with SBP (the presence of multiple bacterial forms would suggest secondary peritonitis). The diagnosis of SBP is made from the PMN count of the ascitic fluid. In typical SBP, the PMN count is > 250 cells/mm^3. *(Answer: E—PMN count in the ascitic fluid < 250 cells/mm^3)*

117. Cultures of the ascitic fluid from the patient in Question 116 grow *Escherichia coli.*

How would this patient's ascitic fluid be classified, and what is the recommended treatment?

❑ A. **Bacterascites; treat with antibiotics**

❑ B. **Bacterascites; do not treat with antibiotics**

❑ C. **Bacterascites; do not treat with antibiotics, and repeat paracentesis in 48 hours**

❑ D. **Spontaneous bacterial peritonitis; treat with antibiotics**

❑ E. **Culture-negative neutrophilic ascites (CNNA)**

Key Concept/Objective: To understand the variants of SBP and their appropriate treatment

Three variants of SBP are recognized on the basis of culture and neutrophil counts of the ascitic fluid. In a strict sense, SBP is defined by an ascitic fluid with a positive culture and a PMN count > 250 cells/mm^3. CNNA has a negative culture and a neutrocytic ascites (PMN count > 500 cells/mm^3). Bacterascites is characterized by a positive ascitic fluid culture in the absence of neutrocytic ascites (PMN count < 250 cells/mm^3). SBP and CNNA are indistinguishable clinically and are managed identically with antibiotics. Bacterascites in the absence of symptoms is usually self-limited and can be managed by observation and repeat paracentesis in 48 hours. In this case, however, the patient is symptomatic with mental status changes, and treatment with antibiotics is indicated. *(Answer: A—Bacterascites; treat with antibiotics)*

118. A 48-year-old woman with cirrhosis secondary to hepatitis C and a history of SBP presents with complaints of diffuse abdominal pain and fever. On physical examination, she is febrile, with a temperature of 102.6° F (39.2° C); pulse, 110 beats/min; respirations, 24 breaths/min; and blood pressure, 90/60 mm Hg. Her abdomen is distended and diffusely tender to palpation, without rebound or guarding; there is shifting dullness, and bowel sounds are present. Laboratory data show a peripheral WBC of 12,000; hematocrit, 30%; and platelets, 62,000. Ascitic fluid PMN count is 800 cells/mm^3. Gram stain reveals gram-negative rods.

Which of the following treatments is NOT appropriate in the management of this patient?

❑ A. **Cefotaxime I.V. for 5 days, provided the patient is clinically improved and repeat paracentesis is normal**

❑ B. **Cefotaxime I.V. for 10 to 14 days**

❑ C. **Ampicillin and gentamicin I.V. for 10 to 14 days**

❑ D. **Albumin infusion**

❑ E. **Norfloxacin, 400 mg/day, for an indefinite period after resolution of SBP**

Key Concept/Objective: To understand the treatment and prophylaxis of SBP

The initial antibiotic therapy for SBP is empirical. The most common pathogens are *E. coli*, pneumococcal and streptococcal species, *Klebsiella*, and anaerobes. Cefotaxime has emerged as the treatment of choice. Other third-generation cephalosporins—ampicillin-sulbactam, ticarcillin-clavulanic acid, meropenem, and imipenem—and combination therapy with aztreonam and clindamycin are also useful. Therapy with ampicillin and an aminoglycoside (e.g., gentamicin) was traditionally recommended as treatment for SBP. However, because of the potential for nephrotoxicity with aminoglycosides, this regimen should be avoided. The duration of treatment is typically 10 to 14 days, but short-duration therapy (5 days) is equally effective. Repeat paracentesis should have a PMN count < 250 cells/mm^3 and be culture-negative. Patients with SBP are at high risk for renal failure. The use of albumin infusion at the time of diagnosis and on day 3 was shown to reduce substantially the incidence of renal failure in a recent clinical trial. Patients who have a history of SBP are at high risk for recurrence (69% within 1 year). Prophylactic therapy with norfloxacin or trimethoprim-sulfamethoxazole has been shown to decrease the incidence of SBP, but no significant difference in survival has been noted. *(Answer: C—Ampicillin and gentamicin I.V. for 10 to 14 days)*

119. A 76-year-old woman presents with a 1-week history of spiking fevers with rigors, nausea, vomiting, and left lower quadrant pain. She has a history of steroid-dependent rheumatoid arthritis and diverticulosis. On physical examination, the patient is febrile, with a temperature of 103.1° F (39.5° C); pulse, 100 beats/min; respirations, 24 breaths/min; and blood pressure, 125/80 mm Hg. She appears to be in mild distress. Abdominal examination reveals moderate tenderness on deep palpation in the left lower quadrant, without rebound or guarding. Bowel sounds are present. Peripheral WBC is 22,000; hematocrit, 39%; and platelets, 390,000. Urine analysis of a catheterized specimen reveals 3+ WBCs and abundant gram-negative rods of different morphologies and gram-positive cocci.

Which of the following would be most useful to evaluate the possibility of intra-abdominal abscess in this patient?

- ❑ **A. Spiral CT scan**
- ❑ **B. MRI**
- ❑ **C. Ultrasound**
- ❑ **D. Paracentesis**
- ❑ **E. Gallium-67 scanning**

Key Concept/Objective: To understand the tests used in the diagnosis of intra-abdominal abscess

Intra-abdominal abscesses typically present with fever, abdominal pain, and leukocytosis. Patients who are elderly or on corticosteroids can present atypically. The presence of multiple bacterial species in the urine of this patient raises the possibility of vesicoenteric fistula and intra-abdominal abscess. The evaluation of suspected intra-abdominal abscess often begins with plain radiographs, which, given their speed and availability, are useful for revealing intra-abdominal free air, indicative of a perforated viscus. Ultrasound can be a very helpful imaging modality for the examination of the left and right upper quadrants and the true pelvis. It is limited by the inability to image through bowel gas. Spiral CT scanning is the most accurate study for the evaluation of intra-abdominal abscess, with specificity and sensitivity rates exceeding 90%. MRI and nuclear medicine studies are generally not useful in the diagnosis of intra-abdominal infections. In patients without ascites, the omentum is very much liable to contain intra-abdominal abscesses. For this reason, paracentesis is usually not helpful in making a diagnosis. Four-quadrant paracentesis is used in the setting of peritonitis secondary to diffuse bowel disease, trauma, or surgery. *(Answer: A—Spiral CT scan)*

120. The patient described in Question 119 is found to have a 5 cm × 5 cm × 8 cm abscess adjacent to the superior portion of the bladder.

Which of the following treatments would not be useful in the management of this patient?

- ❑ **A. Percutaneous drainage using ultrasound guidance**
- ❑ **B. Percutaneous drainage using CT guidance**
- ❑ **C. Delayed surgical exploration/repair**
- ❑ **D. Imipenem I.V.**
- ❑ **E. Peritoneal lavage with antibiotics**

Key Concept/Objective: To understand the treatment of intra-abdominal abscess

Intra-abdominal abscesses must be treated with drainage of the fluid collections. Ultrasound guidance can be used for superficial or large collections. CT-guided techniques can provide access to and drainage of smaller and deeper fluid collections. Intravenous antibiotics are essential in both preventing and treating bacteremia, but they will not eradicate infection and must be used in conjunction with drainage. Antibiotics should be chosen empirically to cover enteric flora (an example of such an antibiotic is imipenem). Surgical exploration, drainage, and repair may be used in patients who fail to respond to percutaneous drainage or have other conditions that mandate surgery. Often the approach is to treat the patient with antibiotics and percu-

taneous drainage initially to provide control of sepsis and create optimal conditions for surgery. Peritoneal lavage with antibiotics has no established role in the treatment of intra-abdominal abscess. *(Answer: E—Peritoneal lavage with antibiotics)*

For more information, see Liles WC, Dellinger EP: 7 Infectious Disease: XXI Peritonitis and Intra-abdominal Abscesses. ACP Medicine Online (www.acpmedicine.com). Dale DC, Federman DD, Eds. WebMD Inc., New York, March 2004

Vaginitis and Sexually Transmitted Diseases

121. A 25-year-old man presents for the evaluation of dysuria and urethral discharge. The patient is sexually active and reports having three female sexual partners over the past 6 months. When asked about condom use, he answers, "Occasionally." He denies having a history of sexually transmitted diseases (STDs). A urethral swab is performed; Gram stain reveals multiple polymorphonuclear leukocytes and gram-negative intracellular diplococci.

Which of the following antimicrobial regimens would be recommended in the treatment of this patient?

- ❑ **A. Ceftriaxone, 125 mg I.M.**
- ❑ **B. Doxycycline, 100 mg b.i.d. for 7 days**
- ❑ **C. Ceftriaxone, 125 mg I.M., and metronidazole, 2 g p.o.**
- ❑ **D. Ceftriaxone, 125 mg I.M., and azithromycin, 1 g p.o.**

Key Concept/Objective: To understand the need of treating patients with gonococcal urethritis for both Neisseia gonorrhea *and* Chlamydia trachomatis

Patients with evidence of gonococcal infection on urethral Gram stain should be treated for gonorrhea. Recommended regimens include single doses of the following agents: (1) cefixime, 400 mg p.o.; (2) ceftriaxone, 125 mg I.M.; (3) ciprofloxacin, 500 mg p.o.; (4) ofloxacin, 400 mg p.o.; and (5) levofloxacin, 250 mg p.o. Quinolone-resistant *N. gonorrhoeae* has recently emerged as a problem in Asia, the Pacific Islands, and, most recently, California. Consequently, quinolones are no longer recommended for the empirical treatment of gonorrhea in persons in these areas or in their contacts. Because of the high chlamydial coinfection rate, all patients with gonorrhea should also be treated for *Chlamydia*, unless that diagnosis has been microbiologically excluded. Treatment for presumptive chlamydial infection in men with nongonococcal urethritis is with azithromycin in a single 1 g oral dose or doxycycline, 100 mg orally twice a day for 7 days. *(Answer: D—Ceftriaxone, 125 mg I.M., and azithromycin, 1 g p.o.)*

122. A 28-year-old woman presents to clinic for the evaluation of vaginal discharge and pruritus. A pelvic examination is performed as part of this patient's evaluation.

Which of the following is NOT a component of the Amsel criteria for the diagnosis of bacterial vaginosis (BV)?

- ❑ **A. Presence of a homogeneous, thin vaginal discharge**
- ❑ **B. Vaginal pH less than 4.5**
- ❑ **C. Clue cells**
- ❑ **D. Presence of amine odor when vaginal fluid is mixed with 10% potassium hydroxide (KOH)**

Key Concept/Objective: To recognize the Amsel criteria for the diagnosis of BV

BV is the most common cause of vaginal discharge in women of reproductive age. Prevalence studies have found BV in 10% to 40% of women tested, with higher rates of infection in women tested in STD clinics and in African Americans. Douching and use of intrauterine devices (IUDs) have also been associated with BV. Physical examination

of women with BV typically reveals a homogeneous, white, uniformly adherent vaginal discharge. The Amsel criteria for the diagnosis of BV include the following: (1) presence of a homogeneous, thin vaginal discharge; (2) vaginal pH greater than 4.5; (3) clue cells (bacteria attached to vaginal epithelial cells on wet mount); and (4) presence of an amine (fishy) odor when vaginal fluid is mixed with 10% KOH. The presence of three of the four criteria establishes the diagnosis. *(Answer: B—Vaginal pH less than 4.5)*

123. A 24-year-old woman presents to the emergency department for evaluation of fever and dull lower-abdominal pain. The patient is sexually active; she reports the onset of her symptoms corresponded with the start of menses 10 days ago. Pelvic examination reveals cervical motion tenderness. Cervical swab specimens are sent for Gram stain and ligase chain reaction (LCR) for *Neisseria gonorrhoeae* and *Chlamydia.*

Which of the following is most appropriate in the management of this patient?

❑ **A. Empirical treatment for pelvic inflammatory disease (PID)**

❑ **B. Treatment for PID if Gram stain of cervical swab reveals gram-negative diplococci**

❑ **C. Treatment for PID if LCR for *N. gonorrhoeae* or *Chlamydia* is positive**

❑ **D. Discharge from the emergency department with clinic follow-up within 48 hours**

Key Concept/Objective: To know the Centers for Disease Control and Prevention's recommendation to initiate treatment of PID in all sexually active young women with cervical motion tenderness

PID is an inflammatory process involving a variable combination of endometritis, salpingitis, tubo-ovarian abscess, and pelvic peritonitis. PID can be bloodborne (e.g., tuberculosis) or result from extension of an intra-abdominal process. At present, however, PID most often develops when bacteria ascend from the vagina or cervix into the endometrium, fallopian tubes, and pelvic peritoneum. The diagnosis of PID is difficult. In clinically detected cases, the cardinal symptom of PID is pelvic or abdominal pain. The pain is typically dull or aching. Onset can be acute or subacute and frequently occurs at the beginning of menses. Typically, patients present after having symptoms for less than 2 weeks. Because the diagnosis of PID can be challenging, because the sequelae of PID can be severe, and because treatment is safe and inexpensive, all patients suspected of having PID should undergo treatment for PID. The CDC recommends initiating treatment of PID in all sexually active young women with adnexal tenderness or cervical motion tenderness. These criteria are likely to be sensitive, but they are also quite nonspecific. Treatment for PID is directed against *C. trachomatis, N. gonorrhoeae,* gram-negative facultative anaerobes, vaginal anaerobes, and streptococci. Numerous [illegible] *(Answer: A—Empirical treatment for pelvic inflammatory disease [PID])*

124. An 18-year-old man presents to clinic for the evaluation of genital ulcers. He is sexually active and reports having two female sexual partners over the past 12 months.

Which of the following is the most common cause of genital ulcer disease (GUD) in developed nations?

❑ **A. Syphilis (*Treponema pallidum*)**

❑ **B. Herpes (herpes simplex virus type 1 or type 2)**

❑ **C. Lymphogranuloma venereum (LGV) (L-serotypes of *Chlamydia trachomatis*)**

❑ **D. Chancroid (*Haemophilus ducreyi*)**

Key Concept/Objective: To understand that HSV is the most common cause of GUD in developed nations

Herpes, syphilis, and chancroid are the major causes of GUD. Less common causes include lymphogranuloma venereum (infection with L-serotypes of *C. trachomatis*); donovanosis (infection with *Calymmatobacterum granulomatis*); superinfection of ectoparasitic infections; trauma; neoplasm; Behçet syndrome; Reiter syndrome; and fixed drug eruptions (e.g., from doxycycline or sulfonamides). Herpes is the most common cause of GUD in developed nations. In the United States in 2000, over two million people sought care for genital herpes. In contrast, a total of 5,979 cases of primary and secondary syphilis and 82 cases of chancroid were reported to the CDC. A 1996 study of 516 STD clinic patients with genital ulcers found that 62% had HSV, 10% had syphilis, 3% had both syphilis and herpes, 3% had chancroid, and 22% had no identified pathogen. Traditionally, chancroid and syphilis have been the most common causes of genital ulcers in most developing nations. However, recent studies undertaken in sub-Saharan Africa have documented the increasing importance of herpes as a cause of GUD, particularly in areas where HIV is highly prevalent. *(Answer: B—Herpes [herpes simplex virus type 1 or type 2])*

For more information, see Golden MR: 7 Infectious Disease: XXII Vaginitis and Sexually Transmitted Diseases. ACP Medicine Online (www.acpmedicine.com). Dale DC, Federman DD, Eds. WebMD Inc., New York, April 2003

Urinary Tract Infections

125. A 35-year-old man presents to your clinic with complaints of dysuria. He reports no discharge, only burning and pain on urination. On physical examination, the patient is afebrile; all other vital signs are stable, and the examination is otherwise unremarkable. Results of urinalysis using the leukocyte esterase dipstick test were positive for leukocyte esterase, with 25 to 35 WBCs/µl, 0 to 5 RBCs/µl, and 3+ bacteria.

Which of the following statements is false regarding urinary tract infections (UTIs) in men?

- ❑ A. A 3- to 5-day antibiotic regimen is sufficient for treatment
- ❑ B. The incidence of UTI in men is low; such infections have been attributed to urologic abnormalities
- ❑ C. Uncomplicated UTIs can occur in men who have unprotected anal intercourse
- ❑ D. UTIs can occur in men with HIV whose $CD4^+$ T cell count is less than 200 cells/µl

Key Concept/Objective: To understand the risk factors for and treatment of UTI in men

In general, UTI occurs more commonly in females than males, except at the extremes of age. In men older than 50 years, the increasing incidence of prostatic hypertrophy accounts for the increased incidence of UTIs. The incidence of UTI is otherwise low except in young men with urologic abnormalities, in men who have unprotected anal intercourse, and in men with AIDS whose $CD4^+$ T cell count is less than 200 cells/µl. In these patients, treatment should not be limited to a short course of therapy but should be extended to a 7- to 14-day regimen of either trimethoprim-sulfamethoxazole or a fluoroquinolone. *(Answer: A—A 3- to 5-day antibiotic regimen is sufficient for treatment)*

126. A 26-year-old woman presents with complaints of dysuria. She denies having fever, chills, nausea, or vomiting; however, she states that she has had multiple UTIs in the past and that her present symptoms are similar to past UTI symptoms. She has no other medical history. The patient has a temperature of 100.6° F (38.1° C). The rest of the physical examination is unremarkable. Urinalysis with leukocyte esterase dipstick shows 1+ leukocyte esterase, 20 to 25 WBCs/µl, and bacteria that were too numerous to count.

Which of the following statements regarding recurrence of UTI is true?

- ❑ A. The majority of recurrent UTIs occur as a result of unsuccessful eradication of the primary infection

- ❑ B. **The use of spermicide is associated with a decreased rate of recurrence**
- ❑ C. **A maternal history of UTI is an independent risk factor for recurrent UTI**
- ❑ D. **A history of first UTI occurring before 18 years of age is associated with recurrent UTI**

Key Concept/Objective: To understand the risk factors and pathogenesis of recurrent UTI

Approximately one in three women with UTI will experience recurrence of infection. These recurrent infections are caused by either incomplete eradication (10%) or reinfection (90%). The average rate of recurrence is 2.6 infections a year; the likelihood of recurrence increases with decreased intervals between infections. Various risk factors have been associated with increased incidence of UTI, including increased frequency of sexual intercourse, use of spermicide, having a new sexual partner, a history of first UTI occurring before 15 years of age, and a maternal history of UTI. *(Answer: C—A maternal history of UTI is an independent risk factor for recurrent UTI)*

127. A 32-year-old woman presents to her obstetrics/gynecology clinic for routine follow-up. She is 18 weeks' pregnant and has been doing well. She states that she was experiencing nausea and vomiting until the 14th week, but since then she has had no complaints. She has no other significant medical history. Results of physical examination are normal. The results of laboratory studies are normal except for urinalysis, which shows 3+ bacteria.

Which of the following statements is true regarding asymptomatic bacteriuria in pregnant women?

- ❑ A. **Pregnant women with asymptomatic bacteriuria are not at increased risk for perinatal mortality or morbidity**
- ❑ B. **If not treated, 25% of pregnant women with asymptomatic bacteriuria will develop pyelonephritis later in pregnancy**
- ❑ C. **Pregnant women with asymptomatic bacteriuria have the same risk of UTI on long-term follow-up as women without bacteriuria**
- ❑ D. **Asymptomatic bacteriuria should be monitored closely but treated only after symptoms develop**

Key Concept/Objective: To understand the evaluation and treatment of pregnant women with asymptomatic bacteriuria

The approach to asymptomatic bacteriuria in pregnant women is significantly different from that in nonpregnant women. Because of the increased incidence of maternal mortality and premature births, asymptomatic bacteriuria in pregnant women is actively sought and is as aggressively treated and followed as symptomatic infection. Pregnant women with untreated bacteriuria are at increased risk for pyelonephritis later in the pregnancy, and there is an increased risk of recurrent UTI on long-term follow-up. Treatment of pregnant women with asymptomatic bacteriuria is also more aggressive (in nonpregnant women, bacteriuria is not treated unless symptoms develop). In addition, the duration of therapy is longer in pregnant women than in nonpregnant women. *(Answer: B—If not treated, 25% of pregnant women with asymptomatic bacteriuria will develop pyelonephritis later in pregnancy)*

128. A 23-year-old woman calls your office with a complaint of dysuria of 3 days' duration. She is in her 24th week of pregnancy. She denies having fever, chills, nausea, or vomiting. Previously, she had a UTI, and she wonders whether she can use some antibiotics left over from her previous regimen.

Which of the following antibiotics is NOT recommended for treatment of UTI during pregnancy?

- ❑ A. **Nitrofurantoin**
- ❑ B. **Ciprofloxacin**

❑ C. Ampicillin

❑ D. Ceftriaxone

Key Concept/Objective: To know which antibiotics are safe to use in pregnancy

For the pregnant patient with UTI, the antibiotic options are significantly decreased because of various fetal toxicities associated with some medications. Nitrofurantoin, ampicillin, ceftriaxone, and other cephalosporins have been considered safe for use in pregnancy. Fluoroquinolones are avoided because of fetal cartilage injury, and trimethoprim-sulfamethoxazole is avoided because of various other toxicities. Aminoglycosides are considered relatively safe and may be used in pregnant patients with pyelonephritis who require I.V. therapy. *(Answer: B—Ciprofloxacin)*

129. A 27-year-old woman with diabetes mellitus presents with fever, dysuria, nausea, vomiting, and flank tenderness. The patient's temperature is 101.4° F (38.6° C), her pulse is 110 beats/min, and her blood pressure is 90/50 mm Hg. Physical examination reveals a young woman in moderate distress. The chest is clear on examination, and the cardiac examination is normal except for tachycardia. The abdomen is benign except for marked costovertebral tenderness on the right. Laboratory results are as follows: WBC, 18,000 with a left shift; BUN and creatinine levels are within normal limits; urinalysis is positive for leukocyte esterase, with 30 to 40 WBC/high-power field; bacteria are too numerous to count. The patient is admitted to the hospital and is treated with I.V. fluids and levofloxacin. She improves only minimally overnight, and over the next 36 hours, she remains febrile. The WBC count remains elevated. Concerns for complications arise, and a CT scan of the abdomen is ordered.

Which of the following is NOT a likely diagnosis for this patient?

❑ A. Perinephric abscess

❑ B. Emphysematous pyelonephritis

❑ C. Uncomplicated cystitis

❑ D. Renal abscess

Key Concept/Objective: To understand and anticipate the complications of UTI

The degree of illness experienced by patients with UTI is broad: patients may be asymptomatic, or they may develop shock or disseminated intravascular coagulopathy. The majority of patients with uncomplicated UTI present with fever and dysuria; they can be treated with oral therapy. Patients with structural abnormalities or renal cyst or those who are immunosuppressed may develop complicated infections that require aggressive evaluation and therapy. Perinephric and renal abscesses are two forms of UTI that can present insidiously and can rapidly progress to more acute illness. Both diagnoses should be considered in patients who do not respond appropriately to antibiotic therapy. Definitive diagnosis depends on radiographic detection of a mass lesion; treatment with drainage may be indicated. Diabetic patients can experience a severe form of pyelonephritis that produces gas in the renal and perinephric tissues. This diagnosis should be considered in patients who have a delayed response to antibiotics; definitive diagnosis depends on radiographic detection. Uncomplicated cystitis is unlikely to cause the severity of symptoms seen in this patient, and uncomplicated cystitis should respond rapidly to antibiotic therapy. *(Answer: C—Uncomplicated cystitis)*

For more information, see Gupta K, Stamm WE: 7 Infectious Disease: XXIII Urinary Tract Infections. ACP Medicine Online (www.acpmedicine.com). Dale DC, Federman DD, Eds. WebMD Inc., New York, January 2005

Hyperthermia, Fever, and Fever of Undetermined Origin

130. A patient with a medical history significant for Graves disease develops a temperature of 106° F (41.1° C), tachycardia, and altered mental status 7 hours after undergoing elective cholecystectomy for symptomatic cholelithiasis. The differential diagnosis for this change of status includes infections, thyroid storm, and malignant hyperthermia of anesthesia.

Which of the following statements is true regarding this clinical scenario?

- ❑ A. **Employing external cooling methods (e.g., ice, cool I.V. fluids) is the appropriate first step to take in treating pyrexia, regardless of its etiology**
- ❑ B. **If the diagnosis is thyroid storm, antipyretics play a vital role in correcting the pyrexia**
- ❑ C. **If the diagnosis is malignant hyperthermia of anesthesia, treatment is purely supportive and involves use of external cooling techniques**
- ❑ D. **The development of rigors during external cooling after the patient's temperature had been lowered 2° would suggest that the source of his pyrexia is the hypothalamus**
- ❑ E. **Only the underlying etiology dictates the clinical consequences of this degree of pyrexia**

Key Concept/Objective: To understand the differences between hyperthermia and fever

In fever, the hypothalamic set point rises secondary to various inflammatory mediators. Intact thermal control mechanisms are brought into play to bring body temperature to the new set point. In hyperthermia, on the other hand, thermal control mechanisms fail, with the result that heat production exceeds dissipation. In the presence of infection, pyrexia results from an altered hypothalamic set point, producing fever. Pyrexia associated with thyroid storm or malignant hyperthermia of anesthesia results from excess heat generation in conjunction with ineffective thermal control mechanisms. External cooling methods are appropriate in the initial treatment of hyperthermia but not necessarily fever. In fever, antipyretics should be administered first if possible. If this is not done, the body will continually try to reach the abnormally high set point of the hypothalamus, potentially resulting in the development of rigors during the cooling process. Rigors could develop during treatment of hyperthermia if the patient's temperature is lowered below the normal level. However, one would not expect rigors after the temperature had been lowered just 2° unless the set point had been elevated. The onset of significant pyrexia shortly after surgery makes the diagnosis of malignant hyperthermia of anesthesia very likely. Malignant hyperthermia of anesthesia usually develops during the initial stages of surgery, but it can develop several hours later. Although external cooling plays a role, the cornerstone of therapy is I.V. dantrolene sodium. Dantrolene is a muscle relaxant; it decreases the heat generated by involuntary muscle contractions. In thyroid storm, the set point should be normal, so antipyretics would not play a role. *(Answer: D—The development of rigors during external cooling after the patient's temperature had been lowered 2° would suggest that the source of his pyrexia is the hypothalamus)*

131. A 42-year-old man presents with a 6-week history of symptomatic fever; during this period, his temperature has been between 101° and 102° F (38.3° to 38.9° C). He has also been experiencing drenching night sweats and generalized weakness. His medication profile has not been altered for the past 6 months. On review of symptoms, the patient has no shortness of breath or cough, and his bowel habits are normal. Results of physical examination are normal except for the finding of a soft systolic flow murmur. The chest x-ray is normal. CBC shows normocytic anemia, with an HCT of 34% (iron studies indicate chronic disease) and unremarkable electrolytes. Results of liver function tests are normal. Results of purified protein derivative (PPD) tuberculin skin testing are negative.

Which of the following statements regarding the workup and differential diagnosis of this fever of undetermined origin (FUO) is true?

- ❑ A. **On the assumption that the patient has not been receiving antibiotics, negative results on several blood cultures would effectively eliminate subacute infective endocarditis as a possibility**
- ❑ B. **The normal chest x-ray in conjunction with negative results on PPD testing effectively eliminates tuberculosis as a potential source**
- ❑ C. **Drug fever is not a consideration, because the patient has had the**

fever for only 6 weeks, yet his medications have not been changed for 6 months

❑ **D. An abdominal CT scan would be an important part of the workup if the diagnosis did not become rapidly apparent**

❑ **E. An erythrocyte sedimentation rate (ESR) that is elevated to greater than 100 mm/hr is virtually diagnostic of temporal arteritis or other vasculitis**

Key Concept/Objective: To understand the differential diagnosis of FUO

Negative blood cultures would not eliminate endocarditis as a possibility because of the possibility of infection with fastidious bacteria, chlamydial infection, or Q fever: these pathogens often do not grow on standard blood culture media. At presentation, patients with miliary tuberculosis often have negative results on PPD testing. In patients with miliary tuberculosis, the absence of miliary lesions on the chest x-ray is not uncommon. A bone marrow biopsy can be very helpful in making the diagnosis. The diagnosis of drug fever is considered within the first several weeks of the onset of FUO, and any recently administered drugs are discontinued early on. However, certain drugs, such as phenytoin, methyldopa, and isoniazid, may not produce fever until weeks or months after their initial use. For any person of this age with FUO, lymphoma is a diagnostic consideration. Thus, CT scanning may be useful in finding retroperitoneal adenopathy, especially in a patient who does not have peripheral adenopathy. Although an elevated ESR is suggestive of vasculitis, it is by no means specific. Patients with either malignancy or infection can present with an ESR elevated to this degree. *(Answer: D—An abdominal CT scan would be an important part of the workup if the diagnosis did not become rapidly apparent)*

132. A 37-year-old male marathon runner has a syncopal episode during the last mile of the 26.2-mile run. The outside temperature is 92° F, with almost 100% humidity. He is brought to the emergency department for presumed dehydration. The patient is awake and alert during the ambulance ride. Upon arrival at the emergency department, the patient says he is dizzy and that he has a severe headache and muscle cramps. His temperature, determined orally, is 104° F (40° C), his pulse is 115 beats/min, his respiratory rate is 24 breaths/min, and his blood pressure (taken both while sitting and standing) is 110/60 mm Hg.

Which of the following would be most helpful in determining whether this patient has heatstroke or heat exhaustion?

❑ **A. Normal mental status**

❑ **B. An HCT of 54%**

❑ **C. Arterial blood gas values as follows: arterial plasma pH, 7.35; arterial carbon dioxide tension (P_aco_2), 44 mm Hg; pulmonary arterial oxygen saturation, 86%; arterial carbon dioxide content, 24 mEq/L; arterial saturation, 98%**

❑ **D. A platelet count of 60,000**

❑ **E. Hemoglobinuria**

Key Concept/Objective: To understand the different clinical presentations of heat-related illnesses

Heat exhaustion is associated with temperatures of 99.5° to 102.2° F (37.5° to 39° C); heatstroke is associated with temperatures in excess of 105° F (40.5° C). This patient's temperature is not clearly within one range or the other; thus, the diagnosis is clouded, but there should be significant concern about heatstroke. Mental status is not a reliable indicator for differentiating between the two. Patients with heat exhaustion can have mild confusion, and patients with heatstroke do not have neurologic impairment. Dehydration with tachycardia, low blood pressure as determined orthostatically, and hemoconcentration can occur in either disorder. Two potential acid-base abnormalities in heatstroke are early respiratory alkalosis (associated with tachypnea) and late-occurring metabolic acidosis, resulting from an accumulation of lactic acid. Pure respiratory acidosis would not be expected, especially in a patient with normal mental status and

a normal state of alertness. Heatstroke is associated with several renal abnormalities, including hematuria, myoglobinuria, proteinuria, and casts. Hemoglobinuria, a manifestation of lysis of red cells, would not be expected as a result of heatstroke or heat exhaustion. However, it could result from the repetitive impact of this patient's feet on the road during the marathon: so-called march hemoglobinuria. Thrombocytopenia in this setting is ominous because it indicates the presence of disseminated intravascular coagulopathy (DIC), which is more common in exertional than in classic heatstroke. DIC would not be expected to be present with heat exhaustion. DIC is just one of many manifestations of organ dysfunction associated with heatstroke. The list includes acute respiratory distress syndrome, liver function abnormalities, renal failure with active sediment, and severe electrolyte derangements. *(Answer: D—A platelet count of 60,000)*

133. A patient with Parkinson disease runs out of her medication and does not obtain refills. After 2 days, she develops severe warmth, rigid arms and legs, and diaphoresis. She is brought to the emergency department. Her temperature is 106° F (41.1° C).

Which of the following statements regarding this patient is false?

- ❑ **A. Appropriate treatment includes fluid/electrolyte therapy and a trial of either dantrolene sodium or bromocriptine**
- ❑ **B. Hyponatremia would be a typical electrolyte abnormality**
- ❑ **C. External cooling plays a role in treatment**
- ❑ **D. Acute renal failure could occur secondary to the presence of an endogenous nephrotoxin**
- ❑ **E. A similar syndrome can be caused by certain antipsychotic medications**

Key Concept/Objective: To recognize the clinical manifestations of neuroleptic malignant syndrome

This patient has neuroleptic malignant syndrome, caused by rapid withdrawal of a dopaminergic drug used to treat Parkinson disease (e.g., amantadine or levodopa). Appropriate therapy includes fluid/electrolyte therapy and a trial of dantrolene sodium (a muscle relaxant) or bromocriptine (a dopamine agonist). External cooling is also important early on because the set point has not been altered. Potential complications include the development of rhabdomyolysis and resultant acute failure; there may be liver function abnormalities. Hypernatremia, not hyponatremia, is a typical electrolyte derangement. *(Answer: B—Hyponatremia would be a typical electrolyte abnormality)*

For more information, see Simon HB: 7 Infectious Disease: XXIV Hyperthermia, Fever, and Fever of Undetermined Origin. ACP Medicine Online (www.acpmedicine.com). Dale DC, Federman DD, Eds. WebMD Inc., New York, October 2003

Respiratory Viral Infections

134. A 19-year-old woman presents with complaints of sore throat; red, irritated eyes; and a progressively worsening nonproductive cough. She reports that she was well until she went swimming in a community pool 5 days ago. On examination, she is afebrile, the conjunctiva are injected bilaterally, the oropharnyx is erythematous, the lungs are clear, and there is no adenopathy.

Which of the following respiratory viruses is the most likely cause of this infection?

- ❑ **A. Adenovirus**
- ❑ **B. Parainfluenza virus**
- ❑ **C. Rhinovirus**
- ❑ **D. Respiratory syncytial virus**

Key Concept/Objective: To understand adenovirus infections

Adenoviruses cause a variety of respiratory tract syndromes, including pharyngoconjunctival fever, which is often contracted while swimming in contaminated water. In addition to transmission by direct contact with respiratory secretions or infectious aerosols, fecal-oral transmission can occur. Infection may be acquired by pharyngeal inoculation or conjunctival inoculation from contaminated water. The incubation period for adenovirus infection of the respiratory tract is usually 4 to 7 days. Adenovirus respiratory disease typically causes moderate to severe, sometimes exudative, pharyngitis and tracheobronchitis. Fever and systemic symptoms are often prominent, and rhinitis, cervical adenitis, and follicular conjunctivitis are common. Parainfluenza viruses are the most commonly recognized cause of croup, accounting for up to 75% of cases with a documented viral cause, and they are the second leading cause of lower respiratory tract disease resulting in hospitalization of infants. Respiratory syncytial virus is the major cause of lower respiratory tract disease in infants and young children, and it is also increasingly recognized as a cause of lower respiratory tract disease in older adults and immunocompromised persons. Febrile upper respiratory tract illness and otitis media are common. Rhinoviruses cause approximately one infection per person a year in adults, and rates are even higher in children. Rhinovirus causes about 50% of colds in adults each year and up to 90% during the fall months. *(Answer: A—Adenovirus)*

135. A 33-year-old man and his 29-year-old wife present to the emergency department in acute respiratory failure. They had gone camping in Arizona 2 weeks ago. Over the past 4 days, they both have had fever, myalgias, and gastrointestinal symptoms that included abdominal pain, nausea, and vomiting; they had no respiratory symptoms.

For these patients, which of the following statements is true?

- ❑ **A. The most likely etiologic agent is coronavirus**
- ❑ **B. Recovery will occur with antiviral and corticosteroid therapy**
- ❑ **C. A vaccine is available to prevent their type of infection**
- ❑ **D. The mortality is 50% for their type of infection**

Key Concept/Objective: To understand the hantavirus cardiopulmonary syndrome (HCPS)

The mortality from HCPS is about 50%; most deaths are caused by intractable hypotension and associated dysrhythmia. The causative agent is a hantavirus, for which the principal animal reservoir is the deer mouse. Human infections occur by inhalation of aerosols of infectious excreta. Most HCPS cases have occurred in young to middle-aged adults who have no underlying disease. The largest numbers of cases have occurred in New Mexico, Arizona, and California. The incubation period averages 12 to 16 days. A history of exposure to a rural setting, rodents or their dwellings, or agricultural work may suggest the diagnosis. The disease is primarily caused by increases in permeability of the pulmonary vascular endothelium that appears to be immune mediated. The pulmonary capillary leak and the development of noncardiogenic pulmonary edema lead to respiratory failure. Specific antiviral therapy has been attempted with intravenous ribavirin, but its value for patients with HCPS is uncertain; a controlled trial is in progress. Corticosteroids are also of uncertain value. There is currently no clinically available vaccine to prevent hantavirus infections. *(Answer: D—The mortality is 50% for their type of infection)*

136. A 66-year-old man presents in early January with fever, chills, headaches, malaise, and myalgias of 2 days' duration. His medical history is significant for type 2 diabetes, for which he takes glyburide. He was recently vaccinated for influenza. On examination, he has a temperature of 101.2° F (38.4° C), injected conjunctiva, clear nasal discharge, pharyngeal erythema with small tender cervical lymph nodes, and clear lung fields; his chest x-ray is normal.

For this patient, which of the following statements is true?

- ❑ **A. Antigenic drift is the major change that causes annual variation in this infectious agent**

❑ B. **Definitive diagnosis will have little impact on the treatment of this patient**

❑ C. **Vaccination in this patient rules out influenza as an etiologic agent**

❑ D. **Chemoprophylaxis is effective for one type of this infectious agent**

Key Concept/Objective: To know and understand influenza virus infections

Two major types of antigenic change can occur: drift and shift. Antigenic drift refers to relatively minor changes in hemagglutinin and less often with neuraminidase that occur frequently (usually every few years) and sequentially in the setting of selective immunologic pressure in the population. Drift results from point mutations of the corresponding RNA segment. The surface glycoproteins induce host humoral and cellular immune responses and are responsible for the changing antigenicity of influenza viruses. Antigenic shift occurs only in influenza A viruses and results from acquisition of a new gene segment for hemagglutinin with or without one for neuraminidase. Several rapid assays are commercially available in the United States to detect influenza A and B occurring together; one of these assays is able to rapidly differentiate between influenza A and influenza B. Making a definitive diagnosis can have a significant impact on medical management. The efficacy of the influenza vaccine is 70% to 90% in young adults, especially when the vaccine antigen and the circulating strain are closely matched. Although vaccination is less effective in elderly and immunocompromised patients, vaccination provides partial protection against pneumonia and death. Amantadine and rimantadine are active against influenza A only. A new class of compounds, the neuraminidase inhibitors, is active against influenza A and B viruses. The neuraminidase inhibitors are also effective for prophylaxis of influenza A and B infections. *(Answer: A—Antigenic drift is the major change that causes annual variation in this infectious agent)*

For more information, see Hayden FG, Ison MG: 7 Infectious Disease: XXV Respiratory Viral Infections. ACP Medicine Online (www.acpmedicine.com). Dale DC, Federman DD, Eds. WebMD Inc., New York, December 2004

Herpesvirus Infections

137. A 22-year-old female college student presents to your office as a new walk-in patient. She has no medical history and takes no medications. She comes today for evaluation of painful groin lesions of 3 days' duration. She states that she had unprotected sex with a new partner about 1 week ago. Four days ago, she developed fever and chills, severe fatigue, painful groin swellings, and "blisters" on her labia. She states that she has had a total of five sexual partners. On physical examination, the patient is afebrile, has tender superficial inguinal lymphadenopathy measuring 2 cm bilaterally, and has several clustered vesicular lesions on her labia majora

Which of the following statements regarding herpes simplex virus (HSV) infections is false?

❑ A. **Direct contact with infected secretions is the principal mode of transmission of HSV**

❑ B. **Herpes simplex virus type 2 (HSV-2) is transmitted more efficiently from males to females than from females to males**

❑ C. **HSV-2 is a local infection that is confined to the genitourinary system**

❑ D. **Among the general public, herpetic whitlow is typically caused by HSV-2**

Key Concept/Objective: To understand the important clinical features of HSV-2 infection

Direct contact with infected secretions is the principal mode of HSV transmission. HSV-1 is usually transmitted by an oral route and HSV-2 by a genital route. Transmission of HSV occurs frequently, even in the absence of lesions. HSV-2 is transmitted more efficiently from males to females than from females to males. Autoinoculation to other skin sites also occurs, more often with HSV-2 than with HSV-1. Extragenital lesions

develop during the course of primary infection in 10% to 18% of patients. Aseptic meningitis is not uncommon with primary genital herpes, particularly in women; in rare instances, herpetic sacral radiculomyelitis occurs. Primary finger infections, or whitlows, usually involve one digit and are characterized by intense itching or pain followed by the formation of deep vesicles that may coalesce. Among the general public, whitlows are most often caused by HSV-2, whereas among medical and dental personnel, HSV-1 is the principal culprit. *(Answer: C—HSV-2 is a local infection that is confined to the genitourinary system)*

138. A 70-year-old male patient who has diabetes and hypertension presents with a complaint of severe flank pain. He was in his usual state of health until 5 days ago, when he developed intermittent, severe, lancinating pain that radiated from his midchest to his right flank and then to his right middle back. He denies having undergone any trauma or having hematuria, dysuria, fever, chills, weight loss, or a history of renal stones. He also states that his shirt has been "sticking to his back" during this period. On physical examination, the patient is afebrile and has a diffuse vesicular eruption in a T4 distribution with severe pain to palpation. His physical examination is otherwise normal. The patient's diabetes has been under very poor control for many years because of the patient's failure to adhere to his medical regimen.

Which of the following statements regarding varicella-zoster virus (VZV) infection is true?

- ❑ **A. Primary varicella infection is communicable and can result in herpes zoster infection in a contact**
- ❑ **B. Hospitalized patients with varicella or herpes zoster infection should be isolated to prevent spread of the virus to other susceptible persons**
- ❑ **C. There is no available medical therapy for herpes zoster eruptions**
- ❑ **D. Ramsay Hunt syndrome is a herpes zoster eruption in the first branch of the trigeminal nerve**

Key Concept/Objective: To know the clinical concepts and features of VZV infection

Herpes zoster results from the reactivation of VZV infection. Varicella in one patient cannot produce herpes zoster in another; however, persons who are exposed to patients who have herpes zoster can contract varicella. Nosocomial transmission of VZV has been reported. Thus, hospitalized patients with varicella or herpes zoster should be isolated to prevent spread of the virus to other susceptible persons. High-dose oral acyclovir (800 mg five times daily for 7 days), when begun early, may shorten the course and reduce the severity of herpes zoster in otherwise healthy hosts. Oral valacyclovir (1 g three times daily) or famciclovir (500 mg three times daily) may also be used. Ramsay Hunt syndrome is an infection of the geniculate ganglion of the seventh cranial nerve that produces facial paralysis; vesicles on the eardrum and side of the tongue can also occur. *(Answer: B—Hospitalized patients with varicella or herpes zoster infection should be isolated to prevent spread of the virus to other susceptible persons)*

139. A 22-year-old man presents to your clinic with complaints of fever, sore throat, marked fatigue, and myalgias. He has had these symptoms for 7 days. He denies having had contact with anyone who was sick, and he denies ever having unprotected sexual intercourse. He does not drink and denies using illicit drugs. He has had only one sexual partner, with whom he has been having sexual relations for several months. His fever is low grade but constant. His sore throat has been improving, and he denies having cough or sputum production. His temperature is 100° F (37.8° C). On physical examination, moderate pharyngeal injection without exudates is noted, and the spleen tip is palpable and slightly tender. There are no other abnormal findings. Laboratory testing shows a normal WBC, mild elevations of aspartate aminotransferase (AST) and alanine aminotransferase (ALT) levels, a differential with 10% atypical lymphocytes, and a negative result on heterophil antibody screening.

Which of the following statements regarding cytomegalovirus (CMV) infection is true?

- ❑ **A. CMV pneumonitis is a common problem in patients during the first 4 months after organ transplantation**

- ❑ **B. Heterophil antibodies are formed in response to both CMV and Epstein-Barr virus (EBV) infections**
- ❑ **C. Despite profound immunosuppression, CMV is an uncommon cause of infection in patients with AIDS**
- ❑ **D. Detection of CMV in urine or saliva confirms active acute infection**

Key Concept/Objective: To know the clinical and diagnostic features of CMV infection

This otherwise healthy young man has a mononucleosis-like illness and tests negative for heterophil antibodies. CMV mononucleosis occurs in patients of any age but is most common in sexually active young adults. Heterophil antibodies are not formed in response to CMV infection. CMV is recognized as an important pathogen in patients with AIDS. The virus often contributes to the immunosuppression observed in such patients and may cause disseminated disease affecting the eyes, the gastrointestinal tract, or the central nervous system. At least 50% of patients with AIDS have CMV viremia, and 90% or more have evidence of CMV infection at autopsy. Demonstration of viremia is a better indicator of acute infection than the detection of virus in urine or saliva. CMV appears to be the most frequent and important viral pathogen in patients who have undergone organ transplantation. Most commonly, such patients with CMV syndromes present with fever and leukopenia, which may progress to pneumonitis or, in rare instances, to disseminated disease. The period of highest risk is 1 to 4 months after transplantation and appears to relate to the degree of host immunosuppression. *(Answer: A—CMV pneumonitis is a common problem in patients during the first 4 months after organ transplantation)*

140. A 28-year-old woman presents for her annual physical examination. She experiences painful genital herpes outbreaks three times a year and asks about treatment options.

Which of the following would you recommend for this patient?

- ❑ **A. Famciclovir, 250 mg b.i.d. for suppressive therapy**
- ❑ **B. Acyclovir, 800 mg t.i.d. for 10 days at onset of symptoms**
- ❑ **C. Denavir cream twice daily for outbreaks**
- ❑ **D. Acyclovir, 200 mg five times a day for 7 days at onset of symptoms**
- ❑ **E. Denavir cream daily for suppressive therapy**

Key Concept/Objective: To know the treatment options for genital herpes

Patients who have fewer than six episodes per year should be treated with an oral agent at the onset of symptoms. Oral acyclovir is one option; it is given at a lower dosage for herpes simplex virus type 2 than for herpes zoster (800 mg t.i.d.). Patients who experience frequent recurrences should be considered for daily suppressive therapy. In a recent randomized, double-blind, placebo-controlled trial, a regimen of daily famciclovir significantly reduced the median time between outbreaks in patients with six or more episodes a year. There is no role for topical agents, either for acute or suppressive therapy. In patients whose episodes are extremely severe or who do not respond to treatment, suppression should be considered even if they do not have more than six episodes a year. *(Answer: D—Acyclovir, 200 mg five times a day for 7 days at onset of symptoms)*

141. Three weeks ago, a 78-year-old man with coronary artery disease and diabetes developed herpes zoster of the right lateral chest wall. He was treated within 48 hours of symptom onset with oral acyclovir. He continues to have significant pain.

What would be appropriate therapy for this patient at this point?

- ❑ **A. Gabapentin**
- ❑ **B. Oxycodone**
- ❑ **C. Nortriptyline**

❑ D. Prednisone

❑ E. Repeat course of acyclovir

Key Concept/Objecetive: To be able to choose appropriate therapy in an elderly patient with postherpetic neuralgia

Treatment options for postherpetic neuralgia include topical anesthetics, oral analgesics, tricyclic antidepressants, and gabapentin. Neither oral steroids nor antiviral agents are effective in the long-term treatment of this syndrome. Although some patients need long-acting narcotics to control their pain, oxycodone would not be the initial drug of choice, especially in the elderly, who are at higher risk for CNS effects and falls. Tricyclic antidepressants are contraindicated in patients with active ischemic heart disease. *(Answer: A—Gabapentin)*

142. A 43-year-old man experienced a change in his vision and was diagnosed with cytomegalovirus (CMV) retinitis. He was subsequently diagnosed with AIDS, and his initial $CD4^+$ T cell count was 28 cells/µl. He was treated with I.V. ganciclovir and experienced improvement of vision; he was also started on antiretroviral therapy. His repeat $CD4^+$ T cell count was 315/µl. For the past 6 months, he has maintained a $CD4^+$ T cell count of greater than 300 cells/µl with a nondetectable RNA viral load.

What would be appropriate treatment of this patient's retinitis?

❑ A. Discontinue ganciclovir until he is found to have recurrent retinitis on serial retinal examinations

❑ B. Continue I.V. ganciclovir as maintenance therapy

❑ C. Switch to oral ganciclovir as maintenance therapy

❑ D. Discontinue ganciclovir until his $CD4^+$ T cell count count falls below 50 cells/µl

❑ E. Administer ganciclovir ocular implants

Key Concept/Objective: To understand the role of maintenance and prophylactic therapy for CMV retinitis in AIDS patients

CMV prophylaxis with oral ganciclovir is initiated in CMV-positive AIDS patients when their CD4 counts fall below 50. Intravenous ganciclovir is necessary for treatment of active CMV retinitis. Once initial treatment is complete, patients can be switched to oral ganciclovir for maintenance therapy. If a patient's CD4 count rises while on highly active antiretroviral therapy and is sustained above 100 in the absence of evidence of advancing HIV disease, then therapy for CMV retinitis can be stopped. Therapy should be restarted if the CD4 count drops below 50 or if retinitis recurs. *(Answer: D—Discontinue ganciclovir until his $CD4^+$ T cell count falls below 50 cells/µl)*

143. A 24-year-old woman presents to the clinic with fatigue, fever, sore throat, and puffy eyes. On examination, she is found to have lymphadenopathy and mild hepatosplenomegaly. She remembers having mononucleosis in college.

How would you interpret a positive heterophile antibody test result in this patient?

❑ A. Heterophile antibody testing would not be helpful for this patient, because the results may be positive owing to her previous episode of mononucleosis

❑ B. She has acute infectious mononucleosis from primary EBV

❑ C. She has a mononucleosis-like CMV infection

❑ D. A positive result indicates moderate to severe clinical disease

❑ E. She has acute rheumatoid arthritis

Key Concept/Objective: To understand the use of heterophile antibodies in the diagnosis of EBV mononucleosis

More than 90% of adolescents and adults with primary infectious mononucleosis test positive for heterophile antibodies. The monospot test is commonly used to test for heterophile antibodies. Patients test positive for 3 to 4 months after the onset of illness, and heterophile antibodies may persist for up to 9 months. Although CMV mononucleosis is often difficult to differentiate clinically from other forms of mononucleosis, patients with other forms of mononucleosis rarely test positive for heterophile antibodies. Heterophile antibodies can also be found in patients with rheumatoid arthritis, although this patient's current symptoms are not consistent with this diagnosis. The heterophile titer does not correlate with the severity of the illness. *(Answer: B—She has acute infectious mononucleosis from primary EBV)*

For more information, see Hirsch MS: 7 Infectious Disease: XXVI Herpesvirus Infections. ACP Medicine Online (www.acpmedicine.com). Dale DC, Federman DD, Eds. WebMD Inc., New York, June 2004

Enteric Viral Infections

144. A 24-year-old man presents to the emergency department complaining of headache, fever, nausea, and photophobia. On examination, the patient has a temperature of 101° F (38.3° C); nuchal rigidity is noted. A non–contrast-enhanced CT scan of the head shows no evidence of bleeding, trauma, or mass effect. You perform a lumbar puncture.

Which of the following cerebrospinal fluid profiles is most consistent with aseptic meningitis associated with enteroviral infection?

- ❑ **A. 10,000 WBC/mm^3 (predominantly neutrophils), low glucose level, high protein level**
- ❑ **B. 500 WBC/mm^3 (predominantly lymphocytes), low glucose level, high protein level**
- ❑ **C. 10,000 WBC/mm^3 (predominantly neutrophils), normal glucose level, normal to high protein level**
- ❑ **D. 500 WBC/mm^3 (predominantly lymphocytes), normal glucose level, normal to high protein level**

Key Concept/Objective: To know the typical cerebrospinal findings in a patient with enteroviral meningitis

Over 90% of cases of aseptic meningitis for which an etiology has been determined are enteroviral infections. In addition, aseptic meningitis is the most common central nervous system illness associated with enteroviruses. Typical CSF findings are a lymphocytic pleocytosis (usually < 1,000 WBC/mm^3) with a normal glucose level and normal to elevated protein level. It should be noted, however, that early in the course of the illness, polymorphonuclear cells may predominate. This is especially true in young children. Repeat lumbar punctures may be required to document a change in the typical lymphocytic predominance. It is important to differentiate aseptic meningitis from bacterial meningitis, for which a CSF profile similar to choice A would be expected. *(Answer: D—500 WBC/mm^3 [predominantly lymphocytes], normal glucose level, normal to high protein level)*

145. The 30-year-old mother of a healthy 4-year-old boy visits you for her annual physical examination and for health maintenance counseling. She is doing well, and after counseling her on various aspects of health maintenance, you ask if she has any questions for you. She states that she has no questions regarding herself but that she is concerned about her son. Several children at his day care facility have developed fever and respiratory symptoms, which were blamed on a virus. She wishes to know about factors that put one at risk for developing such an illness.

Which of the following is a risk factor for enteroviral illnesses, including minor febrile illness?

- ❑ **A. Female sex**
- ❑ **B. High socioeconomic status**

❑ C. Residence in urban areas

❑ D. Older age

Key Concept/Objective: To know the risk factors for enteroviral illnesses, including minor febrile illness

The children at your patient's day care facility might be suffering from minor febrile illness caused by an enterovirus. Enteroviruses are some of the most common viruses, and they have a wide geographic distribution. They are transmitted from person to person by fecal-oral and respiratory routes and may be transmitted by fomites. Young children are the most important transmitters of enteroviruses. Keeping these facts in mind, the risk factors for enteroviral illnesses include young age, low socioeconomic status, crowded living conditions, large households, living in an urban setting, poor hygiene and sanitation, and male sex. *(Answer: C—Residence in urban areas)*

146. A 45-year-old male patient notes that his sister's 2-year-old son has recently suffered a diarrheal illness. The illness was characterized by the abrupt onset of vomiting, followed by diarrhea and a fever to 101.5° F (38.6° C). You suspect the child had rotaviral gastroenteritis.

Which of the following statements regarding rotavirus is false?

❑ A. It is the most common cause of sporadic childhood viral gastroenteritis

❑ B. 50% of children are infected with rotavirus by 5 years of age

❑ C. The peak incidence of clinical illness occurs from 4 to 23 months of age

❑ D. Gastrointestinal symptoms resolve within 3 to 6 days

Key Concept/Objective: To understand the epidemiology and clinical presentation of rotavirus infection

Patients with viral gastroenteritis caused by rotavirus typically experience emesis of abrupt onset, followed by diarrhea. Many patients have fever. The illness usually resolves within 3 to 6 days. Rotavirus infects 95% of children by 3 to 5 years of age; the peak age range for the development of clinical illness is from 4 to 23 months. Rotaviruses are the most common cause of sporadic childhood gastroenteritis and severe childhood gastroenteritis. The major mode of transmission is thought to be through the fecal-oral route. *(Answer: B—50% of children are infected with rotavirus by 5 years of age)*

147. Several of your elderly patients from an assisted-living facility develop a diarrheal illness over a short period. Many complain of the sudden onset of nausea, abdominal cramping, and diarrhea associated with fever, chills, and myalgias. You worry about an epidemic of viral gastroenteritis.

What is the most common cause of epidemics of gastroenteritis?

❑ A. Rotavirus

❑ B. Enteric adenoviruses

❑ C. Norwalk-like viruses

❑ D. Astroviruses

Key Concept/Objective: To know the clinical presentation and the most common cause of epidemic viral gastroenteritis

Viral gastroenteritis occurs in two major epidemiologic forms: sporadic disease and epidemic disease. The latter affects both children and adults and is most commonly caused by Norwalk-like viruses. These viruses are very common; most children and virtually all adults demonstrate serum antibodies to Norwalk-like viruses. Unfortunately, these antibodies convey only transient immunity at best. Transmission is thought to be through the fecal-oral route; epidemics related to the consumption of water and foods contaminated by fecal material occur throughout the year. This patient's clinical presentation

is typical for adults. Serious consequences are rare and are related to dehydration. Treatment is supportive, with fluid administration as needed. The other viruses listed cause viral gastroenteritis but do not produce epidemics as frequently as the Norwalk-like viruses. *(Answer: C—Norwalk-like viruses)*

148. A 10-year-old boy presents with fever and unresponsiveness. His parents report that he was recently diagnosed with dermatomyositis and that he has a history of X-linked agammaglobulinemia. Examination reveals an ill-appearing, unresponsive child with fever, tachycardia, and nuchal rigidity. As you begin emergent evaluation and treatment for meningitis, he suffers a seizure. You worry that he has viral meningoencephalitis caused by an enterovirus.

Which of the following is NOT associated with severe, chronic enterovirus infections?

- ❑ **A. Severe combined immunodeficiency syndrome**
- ❑ **B. Bone marrow transplantation**
- ❑ **C. Long-term use of steroids**
- ❑ **D. X-linked agammaglobulinemia**

Key Concept/Objective: To know the clinical presentation of severe chronic enterovirus infection and to be able to identify the forms of immunosuppression that puts one at risk for this disease

The immune response to infections with enteroviruses is mediated by humoral mechanisms. These include an IgM response to primary infection and the subsequent production of IgA and IgG antibodies. Secondary infections promote an anamnestic response, resulting in high antibody titers. Circulating IgM and IgG antibodies neutralize enteroviruses; IgA antibodies are important in fighting mucosal invasion by the viruses. The importance of humoral immunity in defense against enterovirus infections is emphasized by the severe chronic enterovirus infection that can occur in patients with defective humoral immunity. Patients usually present with chronic, progressive meningoencephalitis. In addition, many patients have a syndrome resembling dermatomyositis. The prognosis is very poor. Conditions associated with defective humoral immunity include severe combined immunodeficiency syndrome, bone marrow transplantation, and X-linked agammaglobulinemia. Steroids are associated with impairment of cell-mediated immunity and do not put one at risk for this presentation of enterovirus infection. *(Answer: C—Long-term use of steroids)*

For more information, see Khetsuriani N, Parashar UD: 7 Infectious Disease: XXVIII Enteric Viral Infections. ACP Medicine Online (www.acpmedicine.com). Dale DC, Federman DD, Eds. WebMD Inc., New York, August 2002

Measles, Mumps, Rubella, Parvovirus, and Poxvirus

149. A 5-year-old Hispanic boy is brought by his mother to a same-day clinic with fever. The patient is originally from Central America and came to the United States the previous week. His symptoms are fever, coryza, dry cough, and red and swollen eyes; the patient has had these symptoms for 2 or 3 days. The fever and cough seem to be worsening, and the boy looks uncomfortable. On physical examination, the patient's temperature is 103° F (39.4° C); conjunctivitis and periorbital edema are present. The mouth examination shows several small white lesions on an erythematous base in the buccal mucosa close to the upper molars. The rest of the examination is unremarkable.

On the basis of history and physical examination, which of the following is the most likely diagnosis for this patient?

- ❑ **A. Kawasaki disease**
- ❑ **B. Measles**
- ❑ **C. Mumps**
- ❑ **D. Rubella**

Key Concept/Objective: To know the clinical picture of evolving measles

Measles is a highly infectious disease caused by a paramyxovirus of worldwide distribution. The portals of entry for measles are the respiratory tract and possibly the conjunctivae. Approximately 9 to 11 days after a person is exposed to the virus, malaise, fever, conjunctivitis, photophobia, periorbital edema, coryza, and cough develop. Cough may be severe, although it is generally nonproductive. Temperature may reach 105° F (40.6° C). Within 2 to 3 days, Koplik spots may appear on the buccal mucosa and occasionally on the conjunctivae. Koplik spots are lesions on the mucous membranes that appear as bluish-white specks on an erythematous base. The skin rash, which erupts 2 to 3 days later, usually appears at the hairline and spreads downward during the next 3 days as systemic symptoms subside. The rash lasts 4 to 6 days and then fades from the head downward. This patient's presentation, with high fever, coryza, conjunctivitis, periorbital edema, and Koplik spots, is typical of early measles. The rash should appear within the next couple of days. The diagnosis can be confirmed with demonstration of measles antigen by immunofluorescence on nasal secretion smears, by a measles-specific IgM enzyme immunoassay, or by rising titers of hemagglutination inhibition antibodies during a period of 2 to 3 weeks. Kawasaki syndrome is a multisystemic disorder that occurs mainly in children younger than 10 years. It is characterized by bilateral conjunctivitis, fever, strawberry tongue, edema of the extremities, polymorphous rash, and lymphadenopathy. Mumps is characterized by malaise, fever, and parotid swelling. Rubella patients present with a prodrome of fever, malaise, headache, and mild conjunctivitis. Postauricular, suboccipital, and posterior cervical lymphadenopathy often precede the rash. Within 1 to 5 days, the maculopapular rash appears and spreads from the face to the extremities. *(Answer: B—Measles)*

150. A 7-year-old girl is brought by her mother to your clinic with fever and facial swelling. She has had low-grade fever for 2 or 3 days, and the mother noticed the appearance of left facial swelling and tenderness 2 days ago. The patient's medical history is unremarkable except for the fact that she has not been vaccinated because of concerns about the development of autism. On physical examination, the patient's temperature is 101.1 F° (38.4° C), and there is parotid swelling and tenderness.

How would you proceed with the workup of this patient?

- ❑ **A. Parotid gland biopsy**
- ❑ **B. Cytomegalovirus (CMV) serology**
- ❑ **C. Bacterial culture of parotid gland secretion**
- ❑ **D. A clinical diagnosis can be made at this time; no further testing is indicated**

Key Concept/Objective: To know the characteristic clinical picture of mumps

Mumps virus has a worldwide distribution. A live mumps virus vaccine was approved for use in the United States in 1967; its use was facilitated by the subsequent incorporation with measles and rubella (MMR) vaccines. Approximately 11% of cases of mumps are observed in children from 1 to 4 years of age, 52% in children from 5 to 14 years of age, and 11% in persons older than 15 years. Two thirds of cases are symptomatic, with initial symptoms of malaise and fever predominating. Painful swelling of the parotid gland is the characteristic feature of infection. It may be unilateral, and other salivary glands may be involved. An unvaccinated child who presents with tender parotitis generally has mumps; further diagnostic testing is not required. In older age groups, other entities (sarcoidosis, tumors, alcohol abuse, drug side effects, and other viral or bacterial infections) should be considered. In persons without parotitis who have orchitis, aseptic meningitis, encephalitis, or other obscure syndromes (myocarditis or pancreatitis), mumps should be considered. Definitive diagnosis of mumps can be made by the isolation of virus from the oropharynx, cerebrospinal fluid, or urine or by virus serology. Rapid detection by polymerase chain reaction techniques is now possible in some laboratories. *(Answer: D—A clinical diagnosis can be made at this time; no further testing is indicated)*

151. A 22-year-old woman presents to clinic with fatigue of 1 week's duration. She had a febrile illness 2 or 3 weeks ago, during which she experienced a transient rash and joint pain. She works in a day care facility, where there has been an outbreak of a febrile illness with a rash during the past few weeks. The patient has a history of hereditary spherocytosis. She was prescribed a sulfa antibiotic for her febrile illness 2 weeks ago. Her physical examination is unremarkable except for the presence of pallor. Her laboratory tests show a hematocrit of 24%; the reticulocyte count is 0.5%.

Which of the following is the most likely diagnosis for this patient?

- ❑ **A. Hereditary spherocytosis in hemolytic crisis**
- ❑ **B. Aplastic crisis caused by parvovirus B19**
- ❑ **C. Glucose-6-phosphate dehydrogenase (G6PD) deficiency**
- ❑ **D. Systemic lupus erythematosus (SLE)**

Key Concept/Objective: To know the possible complications of parvovirus B19 infection

Parvovirus B19 causes erythema infectiosum (fifth disease) in otherwise healthy persons, aplastic crises in persons with hemolytic disorders, chronic anemia in immunocompromised hosts, and fetal loss in pregnant women. The rash of erythema infectiosum usually appears without prodromal symptoms after an incubation period of 4 to 14 days. The rash starts as a fiery-red rash on both cheeks; it then extends as an erythematous maculopapular eruption on the proximal extremities and trunk in a reticular pattern. The rash may wax and wane for weeks. Arthralgia and arthritis are seen in up to 80% of infected adults. Transient aplastic crises associated with parvovirus B19 occur in patients who have sickle cell anemia, hereditary spherocytosis, thalassemia, and various other hemolytic anemias. These aplastic crises are abrupt in onset and are associated with giant pronormoblasts in the bone marrow. They generally resolve spontaneously after 1 or 2 weeks. In immunocompromised patients, acute infection may lead to viral persistence and chronic bone marrow suppression. Pneumonia, hepatitis, and myocarditis have also been associated with parvovirus B19 infection. In this patient, the anemia with a low reticulocyte count suggests a transient aplastic process and not a hemolytic crisis. G6PD deficiency is an X-linked recessive disorder commonly seen in African-American men who present with episodes of hemolytic anemia in association with the use of oxidant drugs or with infections. The absence of reticulocytes and the patient's sex make this diagnosis unlikely. SLE can present with fever, rash, joint pain, and a hemolytic anemia. Parvovirus B19 is the most likely diagnosis.
(Answer: B—Aplastic crisis caused by parvovirus B19)

152. A 46-year-old man is seen in the dermatology clinic for a skin nodule. He developed a small nodule on his hand 2 weeks ago. He lives and works on a farm, where they keep dogs, chickens, and cows. The patient has no significant medical history. His physical examination is unremarkable except for the presence of a 5 × 5 mm tender pustular vesicle with surrounding erythema on his right middle finger at the level of the proximal interphalangeal (PIP) joint.

Which of the following is the most likely diagnosis and what is the appropriate management for this patient?

- ❑ **A. Paronychia; start fluconazole**
- ❑ **B. Orf virus infection; proceed with surgical removal**
- ❑ **C. Paravaccinia; observe**
- ❑ **D. Paravaccinia; start cidofovir**

Key Concept/Objective: To understand paravaccinia infections

Human paravaccinia, orf, and monkeypox infections result from direct contact with natural animal reservoirs of these agents; humans are only incidental hosts. Paravaccinia is an infection that produces lesions on the teats and oral mucosa of calves and milk cows. When humans are infected by direct contact, so-called milker's nodules develop on the fingers or hands; these nodules are occasionally associated with lymphadenitis. Lesions develop over a period of 1 to 2 weeks and resolve in 3 to 8 weeks.

Orf causes pustular dermatitis on the mucous membranes and corneas of sheep and goats. Lesions in humans resemble those caused by paravaccinia. Most cases are benign; immunocompromised patients have been successfully treated with cidofovir. This patient's presentation is clinically and epidemiologically consistent with paravaccinia (milker's nodule); the lesion should resolve in the next few weeks. Paronychia is an infection of the soft tissue around the nail, not the PIP joint. *(Answer: C—Paravaccinia; observe)*

For more information, see Hirsch MS: 7 Infectious Disease: XXIX Measles, Mumps, Rubella, Parvovirus, and Poxvirus. ACP Medicine Online (www.acpmedicine.com). Dale DC, Federman DD, Eds. WebMD Inc., New York, June 2003

Viral Zoonoses

153. A 47-year-old man who recently returned from a vacation to Arizona presents to your clinic with complaints of fever, myalgias, malaise, headache, nausea, and vomiting. Through clinical history and laboratory tests, you make a diagnosis of hantavirus pulmonary syndrome. You admit the patient to the intensive care unit for supportive care and correction of electrolyte, pulmonary, and hemodynamic abnormalities. The patient and his family ask what they can expect regarding the course of the disease. You reply that there are four phases of the disease and that mortality is, on average, 40% but that mortality can vary.

Which of the following is NOT one of the four phases of hantavirus pulmonary syndrome?

- ❑ **A. Febrile phase**
- ❑ **B. Diuretic phase**
- ❑ **C. Convalescent phase**
- ❑ **D. Renal phase**

Key Concept/Objective: To understand the four phases of hantavirus pulmonary syndrome

Hantavirus pulmonary syndrome is one of two common rodent-borne hantavirus syndromes in humans. The other is known as hemorrhagic fever with renal syndrome (HFRS). HFRS is more common in Europe and Asia; hantavirus pulmonary syndrome occurs in the Americas. Hantaviruses are maintained in nature by chronic infection of rodent hosts. Humans are infected after exposure to infectious excreta or by bites. Clinical disease can be divided into four phases: febrile, cardiopulmonary, diuretic, and convalescent. The febrile phase, typically lasting 3 to 5 days, is characterized by fever, myalgia, and malaise. Headache, dizziness, anorexia, nausea, vomiting, and diarrhea may occur. The cardiopulmonary phase is marked by pulmonary edema and shock. Once pulmonary edema develops, rapid onset of circulatory compromise and hypoxia often leads to death. During the diuretic phase, pulmonary edema clears and fever and shock resolve. The convalescent phase may last several months. *(Answer: D—Renal phase)*

154. A 36-year-old woman who recently returned from Africa after spending 6 months there on a medical mission presents to your clinic with complaints of fever, diarrhea, nausea, vomiting, abdominal pain, and rash. You are concerned about her symptoms and travel history, and you admit her to the hospital for observation. She remains ill and develops worsening symptoms of odynophagia, sore throat, and conjunctivitis. Finally, she develops disseminated intravascular coagulation, mucosal bleeding, altered mental status, and anuria, and she dies 9 days later.

Which of the following is the most likely diagnosis for this patient?

- ❑ **A. Lassa fever**
- ❑ **B. Ebola virus**
- ❑ **C. Yellow fever**
- ❑ **D. Sabia virus**

Key Concept/Objective: To know the symptoms and clinical course of Ebola virus infection and to be able to differentiate this disease from other African diseases

Marburg and Ebola viruses are two of the most severe filoviruses to emerge as recent pathogens. Ebola virus was first discovered in Sudan in 1976; since then, over 1,000 deaths have resulted from infection with the virus. Of the four known genetic subtypes of Ebola virus, only Zaire, Côte d'Ivoire, and Sudan have been associated with human disease in West and Central Africa. Ebola-Reston was the fourth subtype discovered in macaques imported from the Philippines for medical research. There are two clinical phases of Ebola virus infection. Early symptoms include fever, asthenia, diarrhea, nausea, vomiting, anorexia, abdominal pain, headaches, arthralgia, back pain, bilateral conjunctivitis, nonpruritic rash, sore throat, and odynophagia. The second phase, characterized by hemorrhagic manifestations, neuropsychiatric abnormalities, and oliguria/anuria, portends a worse outcome. Diagnosis can be made with enzyme-linked immunosorbent assay, polymerase chain reaction, and virus isolation. Treatment is supportive; efforts are focused on control of outbreaks through early diagnosis, case isolation, and other infection-control practices.

Lassa fever should be considered in this case. Patients with Lassa fever may present with symptoms similar to those of Ebola: fever, malaise, gastrointestinal symptoms, and hemorrhage. However, this patient's course was very specific to Ebola, with early symptoms of conjunctivitis, odynophagia, and rash and late symptoms of hemorrhage, altered mental status, and oliguria. Yellow fever is also a deadly disease in Africa that should be considered; however, hemorrhage is not likely with yellow fever, and this patient's symptoms are much more specific to Ebola. Finally, Sabia virus is a hemorrhagic fever found more commonly in Brazil. *(Answer: B—Ebola virus)*

155. A 26-year-old man presents to your clinic after being bitten on the arm by a bat. He has no symptoms and has never been vaccinated for rabies. He is treated with prompt postexposure prophylaxis, consisting of thorough washing of the bite wound and irrigation of the site with povidine-iodine solution. He is given human rabies immunoglobulin and rabies vaccine and is monitored closely.

Which of the following statements regarding the infectivity of rabies virus is false?

- ❑ **A. A bite on the face is associated with a 60% chance of disease**
- ❑ **B. A bite on the arm is associated with a 75% chance of disease**
- ❑ **C. A bite on the leg is associated with a 3% to 10% chance of disease**
- ❑ **D. A bite on the hand is associated with a 15% to 40% chance of disease**

Key Concept/Objective: To understand the relationship between site of infection and risk of disease

Rabies virus is of the family Rhabdoviridae, genus *Lyssavirus*. It occurs worldwide. Dogs remain the major source of human rabies. However, in the United States, canine rabies has been sharply limited, and therefore, wildlife rabies has increased in importance; 90% of all reported cases of animal rabies now occur in wildlife, particularly wild carnivores and bats. The infectivity of rabies virus varies with the site and mode of transmission. A bite on the face presents a 60% chance of disease; a bite on the hand or arm reduces the chance of disease to between 15% and 40%, and a bite on the leg presents only a 3% to 10% chance of disease. The risk of disease from a bite is almost 50 times greater than the risk from scratches by a rabid animal. The virus can be inhaled; inhalation of virus can cause rabies in laboratory workers exposed to viral aerosols and in explorers of bat-infested caves. *(Answer: B—A bite on the arm is associated with a 75% chance of disease)*

156. ***Which of the following causes of mosquito-transmitted meningoencephalitis has a rodent vertebrate host?***

- ❑ **A. La Crosse virus**
- ❑ **B. Murray Valley encephalitis virus**

❑ C. St. Louis encephalitis virus

❑ D. West Nile virus

Key Concept/Objective: To know the vertebrate host of various viruses that cause meningoencephalitis

Viral encephalitis is caused by a number of arboviruses belonging to the families Flaviviridae, Togaviridae, Bunyaviridae, and Reoviridae; other zoonotic viruses can also cause viral encephalitis. Almost all viruses that cause encephalitis are transmitted by either mosquitoes or ticks. Of those transmitted by mosquitoes, the majority have a bird vertebrate host. The exceptions are the encephalitides caused by Bunyaviridae, which include La Crosse encephalitis; California encephalitis; some viruses of the Togaviridae family, including Venezuelan equine encephalitis; and some cases of Western equine encephalitis. St. Louis encephalitis, West Nile encephalitis, and Murray Valley encephalitis are all transmitted by mosquitoes that have birds as their vertebrate host. *(Answer: A—La Crosse virus)*

157. A 42-year-old man presents to your clinic with complaints of fever, rigors, headache, and backache. The onset of symptoms was sudden and began 5 days ago. He reports that he recently traveled to Brazil for a 2-month vacation on the Amazon and that symptoms began 1 week after he returned. He reports that the symptoms subsided somewhat approximately 2 days ago but that he again feels ill. In addition to fever, rigors, headache, and backache, his symptoms now include nausea, vomiting, and decreased urine output. He has no other significant medical history or family history, and he takes no medications. On physical examination, the patient appears ill, restless, and flushed. Vital signs are as follows: temperature, 104 F° (40° C); blood pressure, 97/74 mm Hg; respiratory rate, 19 breaths/min; heart rate, 69 beats/min. HEENT examination is significant for flushing, swollen lips, and red tongue. The chest is clear on auscultation. The cardiovascular examination is normal, and no gallop or murmurs are heard. The abdomen and extremities are normal on examination. You admit the patient to the hospital and treat with supportive care. The patient improves; however, he develops significant jaundice while convalescing.

What is the vector responsible for this patient's disease?

❑ A. ***Aedes aegypti*** **mosquito**

❑ B. ***Haemaphysalis spinigera*** **tick**

❑ C. ***Hyalomma*** **tick**

❑ D. ***Dermacentor pictus*** **tick**

Key Concept/Objective: To understand yellow fever and its vector of infection

This patient has yellow fever, caused by the yellow fever virus, which is believed to have originated in Africa. The virus is now present in tropical America and Africa but does not occur in Asia. Yellow fever virus has two transmission cycles: jungle yellow fever and urban yellow fever. The forest or jungle transmission cycle involves canopy-dwelling mosquitoes and monkeys. In the urban cycle, humans are the vertebrate host and the *Aedes aegypti* mosquito is the principal vector. In dry areas and urban centers where water storage practices promote the breeding of *Aedes aegypti*, this mosquito is responsible for epidemic transmission. Several hundred thousand people are infected yearly, and outbreaks are frequent. Cases among unvaccinated travelers are rare. Yellow fever causes a full spectrum of disease, from subclinical infection to fatal, fulminant disease. Three common stages of the disease are noted (all of which were experienced by this patient): infection, remission, and intoxication. Bradycardia relative to fever is a nonspecific sign associated with yellow fever. *Aedes aegypti* is also the primary vector for Dengue fever; however, this patient did not exhibit the characteristic symptoms of myalgias, arthralgias, retroorbital pain, and rash. *Haemaphysalis spinigera* tick is the vector for Kyasanur Forest disease virus, which is found primarily in Mysore, India. The *Hyalomma* tick is the vector for Crimean-Congo hemorrhagic fever, which is found in sub-Saharan Africa, Eastern Europe, Russia, the Middle East, and western China. Finally, the *Dermacentor pictus* tick is the vector for Omsk hemorrhagic fever virus, which is found primarily in western Siberia. *(Answer: A—*Aedes aegypti *mosquito)*

For more information, see Gubler DJ, Petersen LR: 7 Infectious Disease: XXXI Viral Zoonoses. ACP Medicine Online (www.acpmedicine.com). Dale DC, Federman DD, Eds. WebMD Inc., New York, August 2002

Human Retroviral Infections

158. A young woman presents to your office with concerns about HIV infection because of previous I.V. drug abuse. Results of enzyme-linked immunosorbent assay (ELISA) and Western blot assay are positive for HIV.

Which of the following statements is true regarding the classification of this patient's infection?

- ❑ A. **If she is not treated for her HIV infection and gradually develops a low CD4⁺ T cell count with clinical manifestations of HIV, she has chronic infection**
- ❑ B. **If she is not treated for her HIV infection and gradually develops a low CD4⁺ T cell count without clinical manifestations of HIV, she has latent infection**
- ❑ C. **If she receives antiretroviral therapy and maintains an elevated CD4⁺ T cell count but maintains low but detectable plasma levels of HIV-1 RNA, she has persistent infection**
- ❑ D. **If she receives antiretroviral therapy and achieves an undetectable level of HIV-1 RNA, she has latent infection**
- ❑ E. **If she is also coinfected with HTLV-I and develops manifestations 40 years later, she can be said to have had chronic infection**

Key Concept/Objective: To understand the difference between latent, chronic, and persistent infection in the context of retroviral infection

Three patterns of restricted viral expression are known; all three patterns are important for retroviral infections. Latent infection is characterized by intermittent episodes of acute or subclinical disease with no virus detected between episodes. For example, when HIV-1 RNA levels are suppressed below detectable levels with antiretroviral therapy, the infection is described as latent infection. This should be distinguished from clinical latency, in which manifestations of disease disappear in the setting of ongoing viral replication. Chronic infection implies that the virus is demonstrable but disease is absent. Persistent infection is associated with a long incubation period, slowly increasing amounts of virus, and, eventually, symptomatic disease. Thus, the asymptomatic patient who is receiving therapy but in whom viral RNA is still detectable has chronic infection, whereas the untreated patient who has slowly increasing amounts of virus and in whom clinical signs and symptoms will eventually manifest has persistent infection. *(Answer: D—If she receives antiretroviral therapy and achieves an undetectable level of HIV-1 RNA, she has latent infection)*

159. An I.V. drug abuser becomes infected with HTLV-I.

Which of the following statements regarding various clinical manifestations of HTLV-I infection is true?

- ❑ A. **HTLV-I has a high disease penetrance, meaning that most infected patients will eventually show clinical manifestations of infection**
- ❑ B. **Patients with adult T cell leukemia (ATL) most commonly present with lymphadenopathy in the absence of circulating morphologically abnormal lymphocytes**
- ❑ C. **Patients with HTLV-I–associated myelopathy (HAM) characteristically have hyperreflexia, ankle clonus, extensor plantar responses, and spastic paraparesis**
- ❑ D. **Hypocalcemia is a classic manifestation of acute and lymphomatous ATL**
- ❑ E. **HAM characteristically leads to a deterioration of cognitive function**

Key Concept/Objective: To understand the various clinical manifestations of HTLV-I infection

HTLV-I only infrequently becomes established as a latent infection with expression of viral gene products. The virus thus has a very low level of disease penetrance. For example, the transformation of an infected cell is a rare event, and the cumulative lifetime risk of infected patients' developing ATL is 1% to 5%. One manifestation of HTLV-I infection is adult T cell leukemia (ATL). Four clinical types have been described: acute, lymphomatous, chronic, and smoldering. The most common by far is acute ATL. Acute ATL is characterized by a short clinical prodrome with an average of 2 weeks between the onset of symptoms and diagnosis. The clinical picture is characterized by rapidly progressive skin lesions, pulmonary infiltrates, and diarrhea. Patients with acute ATL have abnormal circulating lymphocytes with little lymphadenopathy. Lymphomatous ATL, the second most common type, accounting for 20% of cases, presents as lymphadenopathy in the absence of abnormal circulating cells. Both acute ATL and lymphomatous ATL are associated with hypercalcemia, not hypocalcemia. The other major manifestation of HTLV-I infection is HAM. This is a slowly progressive thoracic myelopathy. At onset, symptoms include weakness or stiffness in one or both legs, back pain, and urinary incontinence. On examination, patients characteristically have hyperreflexia, ankle clonus, extensor plantar responses, and spastic paraparesis. Cognitive function is generally not impaired. *(Answer: C—Patients with HTLV-I–associated myelopathy [HAM] characteristically have hyperreflexia, ankle clonus, extensor plantar responses, and spastic paraparesis)*

160. A patient presents to you in clinic and states that he recently donated blood for the first time. He was informed by the blood bank that he may have HIV infection and was advised to seek medical care. After a thorough interview, you decide that he does not have risk factors for HIV. You conduct your own serologic tests.

Which of the following is true regarding the serologic tests for diagnosing HIV infection?

- ❑ A. **The blood supply in the United States is screened only for HIV-1 infection, because HIV-2 infection has not been reported in the United States**
- ❑ B. **The positive predictive value of a positive enzyme immunoassay (EIA) for HIV infection is the same in all patients tested**
- ❑ C. **The current generation EIAs will miss acute infection of less than 6 months' duration**
- ❑ D. **Patients with positive EIA results and indeterminate results on Western blot assay can be retested in a year for definitive results**
- ❑ E. **Viral RNA detection is a more sensitive test for acute HIV infection than is detection of p24 antigenemia**

Key Concept/Objective: To understand various features of the tests used to diagnose acute and chronic HIV infection

HIV-1 infection is far more common in the United States than is HIV-2 infection. However, cases of HIV-2 have been reported in the United States, generally in patients who were born in, had traveled to, or had a sex partner from western Africa. Thus, both HIV-1 and HIV-2 pose a danger to blood recipients. The positive predictive value of a positive result on EIA depends on the seroprevalence of HIV-1 antibody in the population from which the individual is being tested. Thus, in a patient with no risk factors, the positive predictive value is lower, necessitating a confirmatory test: the Western blot assay. The current generation of EIAs have shortened the estimated antibody-negative window period of primary infection to approximately 1 month or less. The results of Western blot assay are indeterminate in 4% to 20% of patients whose serum samples are repeatedly reactive on HIV-1 EIA. Many of these patients have recently undergone seroconversion and should be followed very closely with repeat serologic testing to confirm or eliminate the diagnosis of HIV infection. Viral RNA detection is a more sensitive and specific way to diagnose acute HIV infection than is p24 antigenemia testing. Both tests

are used in practice. *(Answer: E—Viral RNA detection is a more sensitive test for acute HIV infection than is detection of p24 antigenemia)*

161. A patient with HIV infection who is receiving retroviral therapy presents to you for the first time after being relocated by his employer. He has had HIV infection for 12 years; his first viral load was 100,000 copies/ml of plasma. He currently has a $CD4^+$ T cell count of 400 cells/µl and a viral load of 10,000 copies/ml. He states that he has not missed a single dose of his medication.

Which of the following statements is true regarding this patient's $CD4^+$ T cell count, viral load, and prognosis?

- ❑ **A. In patients with long-standing HIV, the $CD4^+$ T cell count will become more predictive of disease progression than will viral load**
- ❑ **B. The risk of disease progression in a patient on antiretroviral therapy depends solely on the degree of reduction of the viral load and not on the initial viral load**
- ❑ **C. The goal of antiretroviral therapy is to decrease the viral load to below 5,000 copies/ml of plasma**
- ❑ **D. The regimen can be declared a therapeutic failure because the $CD4^+$ T cell count is below 500 cells/µl**

Key Concept/Objective: To understand the methods of monitoring HIV infection and their implications on prognosis

The magnitude of HIV-1 replication in infected persons is directly associated with the rate of disease progression. This quasi–steady-state has been referred to as the viral set point. Importantly, the predictive value of high plasma viral RNA levels decreases over time, while the predictive values of low $CD4^+$ T cell counts and $CD4^+$ T cell function increase over time. In late stages of disease, immune deficiency is most predictive of disease progression. The relative clinical benefit of any given decline in viral RNA does not depend on the baseline viral RNA level, but the absolute risk of progression to clinical disease remains higher in the patient with higher pretherapy plasma viral RNA levels. The goal of therapy is a durable reduction in the plasma viral RNA level by at least threefold or more from pretherapy levels, to below 1,000 copies/ml, and, preferably, to an undetectable level, which is now 50 RNA copies/ml of plasma. A suboptimal response or therapeutic failure can be defined as a failure of the plasma viral RNA level to decline by at least 30-fold or more from baseline after 4 to 8 weeks. Many clinicians also consider the inability to achieve undetectable plasma viral RNA levels by 12 to 24 weeks as evidence of therapeutic failure. In as many as 15% of patients who receive antiretroviral therapy, the plasma viral RNA level increases while the $CD4^+$ T cell count remains stable or continues to rise in response to therapy. At this time, if the increase in plasma viral RNA level is less than 0.5 log_{10} or 5,000 copies/ml, whichever is less, in a patient with an improved $CD4^+$ T cell count, serious consideration should be given to continuing the same treatment regimen and monitoring the patient's $CD4^+$ T cell count closely for deterioration. *(Answer: A—In patients with long-standing HIV, the $CD4^+$ T cell count will become more predictive of disease progression than will viral load)*

For more information, see Coombs RW: 7 Infectious Disease: XXXII Human Retroviral Infections. ACP Medicine Online (www.acpmedicine.com). Dale DC, Federman DD, Eds. WebMD Inc., New York, January 2002

HIV and AIDS

162. A 27-year-old man presents to your office with what he describes as a cold. During the interview, the patient notes that he has had unprotected heterosexual intercourse, and he is worried about contracting HIV. He asks you how the virus is transmitted.

Which of the following is NOT a mode of transmission of HIV?

❑ A. **Heterosexual intercourse; anal or oral-genital sexual intercourse**

❑ B. **Transmission from mother to child during gestation or delivery or during breast-feeding**

❑ C. **Sharing of needles when injecting drugs**

❑ D. **Needle-stick injuries**

❑ E. **Exposure of intact skin to contaminated blood products**

Key Concept/Objective: To understand how HIV is transmitted

Person-to-person transmission of HIV may occur through numerous routes, including heterosexual intercourse. This form of transmission is extremely common in underdeveloped nations and is not infrequently seen in large urban areas in the United States. Transmission of HIV via contaminated blood products, such as fresh frozen plasma and factor VIII, is extremely rare in the United States. Needle-stick injuries, especially with large-bore, hollow needles, are a well-recognized risk factor for transmission. There have been no reported cases of transmission of HIV from exposures to intact skin. Globally, sexual contact is the most common route of HIV transmission. The form of sexual contact associated with the highest risk is receptive anal intercourse. *(Answer: E—Exposure of intact skin to contaminated blood products)*

163. A 35-year-old male intravenous drug user comes to see you. He tested negative for HIV 6 months ago. He is worried because he has not been feeling well lately. He describes the recent onset of a cold, characterized by subjective fever, fatigue, and aching joints. On examination, you note generalized lymphadenopathy and a morbilliform rash. You are concerned that the patient may have acute infection with HIV.

What test or tests should be ordered in diagnosing this patient?

❑ A. **Enzyme-linked immunosorbent assay (ELISA) for HIV antibody**

❑ B. **$CD4^+$ T cell count**

❑ C. **Complete blood count for lymphopenia and thrombocytopenia**

❑ D. **p24 antigen test of HIV RNA**

❑ E. **HIV antibody test and a test for p24 antigen of HIV RNA**

Key Concept/Objective: To know the laboratory tests used to diagnose acute HIV infection

After acquiring HIV, infected persons may develop a nonspecific illness. This typically begins 7 to 14 days after acquiring HIV and is usually similar to influenza or mononucleosis in character. A high level of suspicion is required to make the diagnosis. Laboratory testing often reveals lymphopenia and thrombocytopenia, but these findings are not diagnostic. Results of HIV antibody testing are usually negative because it typically takes 22 to 27 days for the HIV antibody to manifest, and the $CD4^+$ T cell count may be normal. The plasma p24 antigen test is highly specific for HIV infection but is not as sensitive as the HIV RNA assay (the latter turns positive 3 to 5 days earlier than the p24 antigen test but is slightly less specific than that test). Patients typically have a high level of viremia, usually characterized by a plasma HIV RNA level of several million HIV RNA copies per milliliter of plasma. The combination of a strongly positive HIV RNA test result and a negative HIV antibody test result confirms the diagnosis of acute HIV infection. *(Answer: E—HIV antibody test and a test for p24 antigen of HIV RNA)*

164. A 45-year-old female patient of yours was diagnosed with AIDS over 10 years ago. Despite receiving highly active antiretroviral therapy (HAART) that you prescribed in consultation with a specialist in infectious diseases, her most recent $CD4^+$ T cell count was 180 cells/µl. You are worried about the patient's risk of acquiring an opportunistic infection and wish to begin prophylactic therapy.

For which of the following opportunistic infections is this patient at risk?

❑ A. ***Pneumocystis carinii*** **pneumonia**

❑ B. **CNS toxoplasmosis**

❑ C. **Cryptococcal meningitis**

❑ D. **Disseminated *Mycobacterium avium* complex infection**

❑ E. **Cytomegalovirus retinitis**

Key Concept/Objective: To know the $CD4^+$ T cell levels at which a patient with HIV is at risk for opportunistic infections

The risk of various opportunistic infections can be categorized on the basis of the patient's $CD4^+$ T cell count. A $CD4^+$ T cell count of less than 350 cells/µl places the patient at risk for *Mycobacterium tuberculosis* infection. When the $CD4^+$ T cell count is less than 200 cells/µl, there is a dramatic increase in risk of *P. carinii* pneumonia; Kaposi sarcoma is also seen in patients with this level of immunosuppression. For patients whose $CD4^+$ T cell counts are less than 100 cells/µl, CNS toxoplasmosis and cryptococcal meningitis are considerations. With very severe immunosuppression (i.e., $CD4^+$ T cell counts of less than 50 cells/µl), other infections and malignancies should be considered; these include disseminated *M. avium* infection, cytomegalovirus retinitis, CNS lymphoma, and progressive multifocal leukoencephalopathy. This patient should receive prophylaxis for *P. carinii* pneumonia with trimethoprim-sulfamethoxazole. *(Answer: A—*Pneumocystis carinii *pneumonia)*

165. A 37-year-old female patient who is known to be HIV positive presents to the emergency department complaining of shortness of breath and cough of several days' duration. On further questioning, she reports that her $CD4^+$ T cell count is less than 200 cells/µl. She has not been taking the trimethoprim-sulfamethoxazole that her physician prescribed for her. Her illness was gradual in onset, but it has progessed with associated subjective fever and fatigue. On examination, her temperature is 101° F (38.3° C), her respiratory rate is 26 breaths/min, and rhonchi are noted in both lung fields. An arterial blood gas measurement shows her oxygen tension (Po_2) to be 65 mm Hg, and a chest radiograph shows bilateral reticulonodular infiltrates. You make the presumptive diagnosis of *P. carinii* pneumonia.

With regard to this patient, which of the following statements is false?

❑ A. **This patient should be treated with trimethoprim-sulfamethoxazole**

❑ B. **To establish the diagnosis with certainty, the presence of the infecting organism needs to be confirmed; this is done by inducing sputum or taking samples during bronchoscopy**

❑ C. **The patient should receive corticosteroids**

❑ D. **A patient with *P. carinii* pneumonia may have a normal chest radiograph**

❑ E. **Patients with HIV who have been diagnosed with *P. carinii* pneumonia in the past must continue to receive prophylactic therapy indefinitely, regardless of their $CD4^+$ T cell counts**

Key Concept/Objective: To understand the clinical setting, presentation, and management of P. carinii *pneumonia in patients with HIV*

Patients with HIV who have *P. carinii* pneumonia typically have $CD4^+$ T cell counts of less than 200 cells/µl and present with shortness of breath of gradual onset, a nonproductive cough, and fever. The illness can be very serious and can cause hypoxemia, characterized by a large alveolar-arterial difference in oxygen (A-aDo_2). Chest radiographs typically show the pattern seen in this patient, but up to 30% of patients have a normal chest x-ray early in the course of their disease. The first-line therapy is trimethoprim-sulfamethoxazole. Corticosteroids should also be given if the PO_2 is less than 70 mm Hg or the A-aDo_2 gradient is greater than 35. If a patient who previously suffered *P. carinii* pneumonia can achieve sustained $CD4^+$ T cell counts of more than 200 cells/µl, they may discontinue secondary prophylaxis. *(Answer: E—Patients with HIV who have been diagnosed with* P. carinii *pneumonia in the past must continue to receive prophylactic therapy indefinitely, regardless of their $CD4^+$ T cell counts)*

166. A 37-year-old man with B3 HIV disease presents with fatigue. He is found to be anemic, with a hematocrit of 23. Workup reveals hemolytic anemia caused by the dapsone he is taking for *Pneumocystis carinii* pneumonia prophylaxis. He previously had a severe allergic reaction (Stevens-Johnson syndrome) to trimethoprim-sulfamethoxazole. He has been on highly active antiretroviral therapy for 2 years. When he started therapy, his $CD4^+$ T cell count was 125 cells/µl, and he had a viral load of 75,000 copies/ml. He now has a $CD4^+$ T cell count of 313 cells/µl, and the viral load is nondetectable (< 50 copies/ml).

What would you recommend for this patient?

❑ **A. Rechallenge with trimethoprim-sulfamethoxazole for *P. carinii* pneumonia prophylaxis**

❑ **B. Begin aerosolized pentamidine for *P. carinii* pneumonia prophylaxis**

❑ **C. Begin azithromycin for *P. carinii* pneumonia prophylaxis**

❑ **D. Begin desensitization protocol for trimethoprim-sulfamethoxazole**

❑ **E. Stop *P. carinii* pneumonia prophylaxis**

Key Concept/Objective: To understand that for some patients who have an excellent response to HAART (highly active antiretroviral therapy), P. carinii *pneumonia prophylaxis can be stopped*

This patient has had a severe reaction to trimethoprim-sulfamethoxazole in the past (Stevens-Johnson syndrome) and now cannot tolerate dapsone because of severe hemolytic anemia. He should not be rechallenged with trimethoprim-sulfamethoxazole, and desensitization should not be attempted. Both are reasonable options for patients without life-threatening reactions, but this patient's previous history of Stevens-Johnson syndrome contraindicates these options. Aerosolized pentamidine is expensive and not very effective. Azithromycin is not of proven efficacy. The best approach would be to discontinue *P. carinii* pneumonia prophylaxis altogether. Occurrence of *P. carinii* pneumonia in patients with $CD4^+$ T cell counts greater than 200 cells/µl and viral loads that are nondetectable on HAART are extremely uncommon. If patients have a $CD4^+$ T cell count greater than 200 cells/µl and a nondetectable viral load for 6 months on HAART, it is appropriate to consider stopping *P. carinii* pneumonia prophylaxis. *(Answer: E—Stop* P. carinii *pneumonia prophylaxis)*

167. A 33-year-old man with C3 HIV disease presents with fever, nausea, vomiting, and hypotension. The patient was on zidovudine, lamivudine (3TC), abacavir, and indinavir. He developed some nausea, malaise, and a mild rash 4 weeks ago, so he stopped the medications. He became alarmed at his most recent viral load (100,000 copies/ml) and restarted his antiretroviral medications. On examination, the patient is ill with a blood pressure of 70/40 mm Hg; pulse, 140 beats/min; and temperature, 102.5° F (39.2° C). He has a faint rash. His laboratory findings are as follows: $CD4^+$ T cell count, 6; viral load, 100,000; Hb, 10; HCT, 31; WBC, 2.2; AST, 30; ALT, 38; ALK phos, 120; bilirubin, 2.0 (indirect, 1.4; direct, 6).

What is the most likely cause of this patient's symptoms?

❑ **A. Side effect of abacavir**

❑ **B. Side effect of 3TC**

❑ **C. Side effect of zidovudine (AZT)**

❑ **D. Disseminated *Mycobacterium avium* complex**

❑ **E. Cholecystitis caused by indinavir**

Key Concept/Objective: To be able to recognize severe hypersensitivity reaction associated with abacavir rechallenge

This patient is manifesting symptoms of a hypersensitivity reaction to abacavir. About 3% of patients treated with abacavir have an allergic reaction to it. These reactions usually include rash and nausea and sometimes include fever. If a patient with a previous reaction to abacavir is rechallenged with the medicine, he or she can develop a much more severe life-threatening reaction with marked hypotension. 3TC has minimal side effects. The major side effects of zidovudine are myositis and anemia. Rarely, zidovu-

dine can cause severe liver disease. The sudden onset of symptoms is not typical for *Mycobacterium avium* complex. Indinavir can cause nephrolithiasis but does not cause cholelithiasis. Indinavir can cause an unconjugated hyperbilirubinemia (as this patient has), but it is always asymptomatic. *(Answer: A—Side effect of abacavir)*

168. A 27-year-old pregnant woman is found to be HIV positive on prenatal blood testing. Her CD4$^+$ T cell count is 410 cells/µl, and she has a viral load of 35,000 copies/ml of plasma. She does not wish to take any antiretroviral medications.

What should you advise her to do to best decrease the risk of transmission of HIV virus to her child?

- ❑ **A. Do nothing, because she already has a very low risk, because her CD4$^+$ T cell count is > 200 cells/µl**
- ❑ **B. Breast-feed the child until the age of 6 months**
- ❑ **C. Have a cesarean section**
- ❑ **D. Receive prophylaxis for HSV II**

Key Concept/Objective: To understand the factors that can decrease the risk of HIV transmission to the fetus

The best option to decrease the risk of transmission of HIV to the child would be maternal antiretroviral therapy. Single-drug treatment with zidovudine in the mother can reduce risk from about 25% to 8%. Treatment with neverapine at the time of delivery can lead to similar decreases in transmission. Combination antiretroviral therapy is even more successful at decreasing the risk. Unfortunately, this patient does not want to take medication, so the next best option would be cesarean section. In a recent prospective study, transmission rate was reduced from 10.5% in the vaginal delivery group to 1.8% in the cesarean group. Breast-feeding increases the risk of transmission. The risk of transmission is related to both the CD4$^+$ T cell count and the viral load. This patient's risk would not be low because of her high viral load. *(Answer: C—Have a cesarean section)*

169. A 37-year-old man with C3 HIV disease presents for follow-up. He is concerned because his face is becoming thinner, especially in regard to temporal wasting. He has also noticed development of increased fat in his central abdominal region and a buffalo hump. He is being treated with ritonavir, saquinavir, 3TC, and neverapine.

What laboratory abnormality would likely be seen in this patient?

- ❑ **A. Increased uric acid level**
- ❑ **B. Increased triglyceride level**
- ❑ **C. Increased creatine phosphokinase level**
- ❑ **D. Low platelet count**
- ❑ **E. High calcium level**

Key Concept/Objective: To be able to recognize hyperlipidemia associated with lipodystrophy syndrome

This patient presents with lipodystrophy. It is more common in patients on protease inhibitors. Patients with lipodystrophy are also likely to have hyperlipidemia (especially high triglycerides and low HDL cholesterol) and insulin resistance. Lipodystrophy develops most rapidly in the setting of combination protease inhibitor therapy with ritonavir and saquinavir. The most common lab abnormality seen in patients with lipodystrophy is hyperlipidemia. *(Answer: B—Increased triglyceride level)*

For more information, see Harrington H, Spach DH: 7 Infectious Disease: XXXIII HIV and AIDS. ACP Medicine Online (www.acpmedicine.com). Dale DC, Federman DD, Eds. WebMD Inc., New York, January 2005

Protozoan Infections

170. A 58-year-old man presents to your office complaining of fever, chills, muscle aches, and diarrhea of 3 days' duration. He returned from an East African safari about 3 weeks ago. The patient's symptoms began 3 days ago. During his trip, he took doxycycline for prophylaxis against malaria; he took his last pill 2 weeks after arriving back in the United States. The patient thinks he probably has a viral illness, but he asks you if it is possible that he has malaria.

For this patient, which of the following statements is true?

- ❑ **A. It is unlikely that the patient has malaria because his symptoms are too nonspecific**
- ❑ **B. It is unlikely that the patient has malaria because he was taking prophylactic antimalarial medication**
- ❑ **C. It is very likely that the patient has malaria because he was taking a medicine that is inappropriate for prophylaxis against malaria**
- ❑ **D. It is possible that the patient has malaria because he took his prophylactic medication for an inadequate duration**

Key Concept/Objective: To understand malaria prophylaxis for persons traveling to areas endemic for malaria

Persons infected with malaria remain asymptomatic during the time between the infecting mosquito bite and the erythrocytic stage of infection, a period that may range from about 1 to 4 weeks for *Plasmodium falciparum* infection. Because malaria chemoprophylaxis does not actually prevent malaria but rather treats erythrocytic-stage infection, chemoprophylactic medication must be continued for a full 4 weeks after a person returns from a malarious area. Failure to do so permits the development of malarial infection. An exception to this is with so-called causal prophylactic medications, such as atovaquone-proguanil, which also kills liver-stage parasites. This form of prophylaxis can be discontinued a week after leaving a malarious area. The appropriate choice of prophylactic medication depends on the travel destination and includes chloroquine, mefloquine, doxycycline, atovaquone-proguanil, and primaquine. It is important to note that in someone at risk for malaria, the constellations of symptoms are nonspecific and may suggest diagnoses other than malaria; however, in a patient with fever who has recently returned from a trip to a known malarious area, this diagnosis should be considered carefully in spite of the nonspecific nature of the symptoms. *(Answer: D—It is possible that the patient has malaria because he took his prophylactic medication for an inadequate duration)*

171. A 46-year-old white man with AIDS ($CD4^+$ T cell count, 42 cells/µl) presents to the emergency department after having a seizure. He reports that for the past 3 weeks, he has been experiencing worsening tremor, visual disturbances, and headaches. CT scan of the brain with contrast reveals a single rounded lesion with ring enhancement. You suspect infection with *Toxoplasma gondii.*

Which of the following statements regarding cerebral toxoplasmosis in AIDS patients is true?

- ❑ **A. Reactivation of latent *Toxoplasma* infection is unlikely to occur until the $CD4^+$ T cell count falls below 50 cells/µl**
- ❑ **B. Antibodies against *Toxoplasma* are rarely present in the cerebrospinal fluid of AIDS patients, because of their level of immunosuppression**
- ❑ **C. During treatment for cerebral toxoplasmosis, clinical and radiologic improvement is often observed within 2 weeks after initiating therapy**
- ❑ **D. After acute treatment of cerebral toxoplasmosis, patients must remain on lifelong suppressive therapy, independent of $CD4^+$ T cell count**

Key Concept/Objective: To understand the diagnosis and treatment of cerebral toxoplasmosis in AIDS patients

Most cases of toxoplasmosis in patients with AIDS result from reactivation of latent *Toxoplasma* cysts acquired before infection with HIV; reactivation is particularly likely when the CD4⁺ T cell count falls below 100 cells/µl. Serum antibody tests cannot be relied on in the diagnosis of primary toxoplasmosis in patients with AIDS; antibody titers do not reach the high levels typical of immunocompetent patients with toxoplasmosis, nor are IgM antibodies present in patients with AIDS. However, antibodies against *Toxoplasma* are present in the CSF in nearly two thirds of AIDS patients with cerebral toxoplasmosis, and their detection may assist in the diagnosis. With appropriate therapy, clinical and radiologic improvement is often observed within 1 to 2 weeks. If patients respond poorly to treatment and are seronegative or belong to population groups at high risk for tuberculosis, biopsy should be strongly considered. Patients with AIDS who have been treated for toxoplasmosis require prolonged suppressive therapy. If the CD4⁺ T cell count rises above 200 cells/µl for 3 months, secondary prophylaxis for toxoplasmosis can be stopped. *(Answer: C—During treatment for cerebral toxoplasmosis, clinical and radiologic improvement is often observed within 2 weeks after initiating therapy)*

172. A 37-year-old woman presents with complaints of foul-smelling, greasy diarrhea; nausea; and excessive flatulence. She has had these symptoms for 8 days. She states that she returned from a camping trip about 2 weeks ago. Immunologic assay detects giardial antigen in the stool.

Which of the following statements about treatment and prevention of giardiasis is true?

- ❑ **A. The most effective treatment is metronidazole, 250 mg three times a day for 5 days**
- ❑ **B. When drinking water comes from a potentially contaminated source, it is essential that it be heated or, preferably, boiled for at least 10 minutes**
- ❑ **C. On a camping trip, iodine-based water treatments can provide rapid decontamination in a few minutes**
- ❑ **D. Metronidazole is generally considered to be safe in pregnant patients**

Key Concept/Objective: To understand prophylaxis against and treatment of giardiasis

Boiling water or heating water to at least 158° F for 10 minutes renders water noninfectious. For hikers and campers, iodine-based water treatments are more effective than chlorine-based treatments; iodine disinfection must be carried out for at least 8 hours to be 99.9% effective. Metronidazole is the principal drug used to treat giardiasis; however, the usual dosage of 250 mg orally three times a day for 5 days may lead to recurrences in up to 40% of patients. Between 500 and 750 mg given orally three times a day for 10 days is 60% to 95% effective. Administration of 2 g of metronidazole once daily for 3 consecutive days is associated with the highest cure rates, yielding 93% to 100% efficacy. Treatment of giardiasis in pregnancy can be difficult. Metronidazole is often avoided, although studies have not documented teratogenic risks of metronidazole during pregnancy. *(Answer: B—When drinking water comes from a potentially contaminated source, it is essential that it be heated or, preferably, boiled for at least 10 minutes)*

173. A 39-year-old man with AIDS (CD4⁺ T cell count, 100 cells/µl) presents with a complaint of profuse, watery diarrhea. He has had these symptoms for 2 weeks. Conservative treatment measures have been unsuccessful. Evaluation of the stool reveals oocysts consistent with infection with *Cryptosporidium*.

Which of the following statements about cryptosporidiosis is true?

- ❑ **A. Cryptosporidiosis is usually self-limited in AIDS patients unless CD4⁺ T cell counts are below 100 cells/µl**

❑ **B. AIDS patients infected with *Cryptosporidium* are at risk for bacterial invasion of the biliary tract, which can cause complications that include cholecystitis and cholangitis**

❑ **C. Paromomycin has been proved to be highly effective in treating cryptosporidiosis in patients with HIV**

❑ **D. Antiretroviral therapy should be withheld during acute infection with *Cryptosporidium***

Key Concept/Objective: To understand the characteristics of cryptosporidiosis in immunocompromised patients

In immunocompromised patients, cryptosporidiosis can be persistent and severe. In HIV-infected patients with CD4⁺ T cell levels greater than 180 cells/µl, cryptosporidiosis can be self-limited. With more profound immunocompromise, however, the secretory diarrhea, which is chronic and profuse, is usually unremitting. In these persons, *Cryptosporidium* organisms may cause hepatobiliary disease, including cholecystitis, cholangitis, and papillary stenosis. Chemotherapy would be valuable in immunocompromised patients, but an effective regimen for cryptosporidiosis has not been established. For some HIV-infected patients, paromomycin may be at least partially beneficial in treating cryptosporidiosis, though in small controlled trials, no benefit was seen with this approach, as compared with placebo. Improvement of CD4⁺ T cell counts in HIV-infected patients through highly active antiretroviral therapy has put an end to life-threatening cryptosporidial diarrhea. *(Answer: B—AIDS patients infected with* Cryptosporidium *are at risk for bacterial invasion of the biliary tract, which can cause complications that include cholecystitis and cholangitis)*

For more information, see Van Voorhis WC, Weller PF: 7 Infectious Disease: XXXIV Protozoan Infections. ACP Medicine Online (www.acpmedicine.com). Dale DC, Federman DD, Eds. WebMD Inc., New York, November 2004

Bacterial Infections of the Central Nervous System

174. A 68-year-old man with underlying diabetes mellitus and alcoholic cirrhosis is brought to the emergency department for evaluation of fever of acute onset and deteriorated mental status. He has no known allergies and is not taking any medications. On examination, he is febrile and confused, and meningismus is present. Acute bacterial meningitis is suspected, and a lumbar puncture shows the following: total protein, 100 mg/dl; glucose, 60 mg/dl (blood, 240 mg/dl); and WBC, 460 cells/mm^3 (74% PMN). Results of CSF Gram stain and culture are pending.

Which of the following would be the best choice for empirical antibiotic therapy for acute bacterial meningitis in this patient?

❑ A. Ceftriaxone and vancomycin

❑ B. Vancomycin

❑ C. Ampicillin and ceftriaxone

❑ D. Vancomycin, ceftriaxone, and ampicillin

❑ E. Meropenem

Key Concept/Objective: To be able to select appropriate empirical antibiotics for a patient with acute bacterial meningitis

Among adults with acute community-acquired bacterial meningitis, *Streptococcus pneumoniae, Neisseria meningitidis, Haemophilus influenzae*, and *Listeria monocytogenes* are the most common pathogens. Prompt initiation of appropriate I.V. antibiotics is critical; antibiotic therapy should be started before definitive microbiologic results are available. The possibilities of highly penicillin-resistant *S. pneumoniae* and *L. monocytogenes* should be considered (especially given this patient's underlying diabetes and liver disease). Although ceftriaxone is appropriate for susceptible *S. pneumoniae*, it

would not be adequate for highly penicillin-resistant strains; thus, vancomycin should be given until definitive microbiologic results are available. The patient's advanced age and underlying medical conditions (i.e., diabetes, liver disease) predispose him to *L. monocytogenes* infection. Ampicillin is the antibiotic of choice for *Listeria* infections and should also be given empirically in this patient (cephalosporins, vancomycin, and meropenem are not sufficiently active against Listeria). Of the choices listed, only choice D provides coverage against highly penicillin-resistant *S. pneumoniae, L. monocytogenes, H. influenzae,* and *N. meningitidis.* *(Answer: D—Vancomycin, ceftriaxone, and ampicillin)*

175. For the patient in Question 174, I.V. antibiotics are begun, and the patient is admitted to the intensive care unit. The CSF Gram stain is reported as negative, but the culture eventually grows *Listeria monocytogenes.*

Which of the following statements about listerial meningitis in adults is true?

- ❑ **A. It typically occurs in elderly or immunocompromised persons**
- ❑ **B. It is usually associated with a positive CSF Gram stain**
- ❑ **C. Ceftriaxone is the antibiotic of choice**
- ❑ **D. It can usually be distinguished from meningitis of other causes by clinical findings**
- ❑ **E. Vancomycin is the treatment of choice**

Key Concept/Objective: To know the risk factors and clinical features of L. monocytogenes *meningitis*

L. monocytogenes* accounts for approximately 10% to 15% of cases of bacterial meningitis in adults. Listerial meningitis typically occurs in elderly patients, immunocompromised persons, or patients with serious underlying medical conditions (e.g., liver disease or diabetes). No clinical findings are helpful for reliably distinguishing *L. monocytogenes* from other pathogens that commonly cause acute bacterial meningitis. The CSF Gram stain is positive in only approximately 30% of patients with listerial meningitis (as compared to 60% to 90% of patients with meningitis caused by other bacteria). In addition, approximately 25% of patients with listerial meningitis have a lymphocytic predominance in the CSF (an uncommon finding in meningitis caused by other types of bacteria). The antibiotic of choice for listerial meningitis is ampicillin (or trimethoprim-sulfamethoxazole for the penicillin-allergic patient). Vancomycin, the cephalosporins (e.g., ceftriaxone), and the carbapenems (e.g., imipenem or meropenem) do not adequately cover *Listeria. *(Answer: A—It typically occurs in elderly or immunocompromised persons)*

176. ***Which of the following CSF profiles is most compatible with acute Streptococcus pneumoniae meningitis?***

- ❑ **A. Normal glucose level, normal total protein level, normal cell count**
- ❑ **B. Decreased glucose level; increased total protein level; increased cell count with a neutrophilic predominance**
- ❑ **C. Normal glucose level; increased total protein; increased cell count with a lymphocytic predominance**
- ❑ **D. Decreased glucose level; increased total protein level; increased cell count with a lymphocytic predominance**
- ❑ **E. Normal glucose level; increased total protein level; increased cell count with a red cell predominance**

Key Concept/Objective: To know the typical CSF profile in acute bacterial meningitis

The glucose and total protein levels and the WBC count and differential in the CSF are helpful in differentiating bacterial meningitis from viral and fungal meningitis. It is important to note that there may be overlap in the CSF abnormalities seen with meningitis from different causes. Typically, in acute bacterial meningitis (e.g., meningitis

caused by *S. pneumoniae*), the CSF glucose level is decreased, the total protein level is elevated, and the WBC count is elevated and has a neutrophilic predominance. The profile shown in choice C (normal glucose level, increased total protein level, increased number of lymphocytes) is typical of viral meningitis. The CSF profile shown in choice D (decreased glucose level, elevated protein level, increased number of lymphocytes) can be seen in meningitis caused by syphilis, Lyme disease, or *Mycobacterium tuberculosis.* The CSF profile shown in choice E (normal glucose level, elevated protein level, increased number of RBCs) may be seen after trauma or subarachnoid hemorrhage. *(Answer: B—Decreased glucose level; increased total protein level; increased cell count with a neutrophilic predominance)*

177. A 22-year-old man, who is an active injecting drug user, presents for evaluation of worsening localized back pain and intermittent fever of 3 days' duration. On examination, he is febrile, and focal tenderness is present over the L4-5 region. A detailed neurologic examination and the rest of the physical examination are normal. Laboratory data show a WBC count of 9.6 and an ESR of 64. X-rays of the lumbar spine are unremarkable.

Which of the following would be the most appropriate step to take next in treating this patient?

- ❑ A. Prescribe back exercises and ibuprofen for musculoskeletal back pain
- ❑ B. Prescribe oral cephalexin for possible myositis
- ❑ C. Obtain a spinal MRI
- ❑ D. Obtain a bone scan
- ❑ E. Obtain additional spinal x-rays in 48 hours

Key Concept/Objective: To know the clinical presentation and best diagnostic method for suspected spinal epidural abscess

Spinal epidural abscess must be considered early in any patient with fever and localized back pain, because delay in diagnosis and treatment can lead to serious neurologic sequelae. Injection drug users are at increased risk. Laboratory findings are nonspecific, although the ESR is elevated in most patients. When spinal epidural abscess is suspected, early imaging is warranted. MRI (if available) is the best choice for delineating an epidural abscess. If MRI is unavailable, CT should be performed. Although many patients with spinal epidural abscess have concomitant vertebral osteomyelitis, spinal x-rays are not sensitive enough to exclude the diagnosis. In this patient with fever, focal back pain, and an elevated ESR, spinal epidural abscess must be strongly considered and evaluated even if initial spinal x-rays are negative. Given this patient's clinical presentation and laboratory findings, a diagnosis of musculoskeletal back pain should be made only after thorough evaluation for epidural abscess. A bone scan would not adequately differentiate vertebral osteomyelitis from epidural abscess. *(Answer: C—Obtain a spinal MRI)*

178. The patient described in Question 177 is ultimately diagnosed with spinal epidural abscess at the L4-5 level.

Which of the following organisms is the most likely cause of this patient's spinal epidural abscess?

- ❑ A. *Haemophilus influenzae*
- ❑ B. *Staphylococcus aureus*
- ❑ C. *S. epidermidis*
- ❑ D. *Pseudomonas aeruginosa*
- ❑ E. *Enterococcus faecalis*

Key Concept/Objective: To know the most common pathogen(s) implicated in spinal epidural abscess

Most cases of spinal epidural abscess are caused by a single organism, although polymicrobial infections occur in approximately 5% to 10% of cases. *S. aureus* is the most common isolate. Other organisms include *M. tuberculosis*, streptococci, and gram-negative bacilli. *(Answer: B—Staphylococcus aureus)*

179. ***Which of the following is the most appropriate treatment for spinal epidural abscess?***

- ❑ **A. I.V. antibiotics**
- ❑ **B. Observation alone**
- ❑ **C. Oral antibiotics**
- ❑ **D. I.V. antibiotics and surgical drainage**

Key Concept/Objective: To know the optimal management of spinal epidural abscess

In addition to I.V. antibiotics, the most important element of therapy for spinal epidural abscess is urgent surgery for drainage of pus and removal of granulation tissue. Although some patients respond to antibiotics alone, rapid neurologic deterioration can occur without warning. Thus, unless there is an absolute contraindication for surgery, most patients with epidural abscess should undergo routine surgical intervention. *(Answer: D—I.V. antibiotics and surgical drainage)*

For more information, see Hirschmann JV: 7 Infectious Disease: XXXVI Bacterial Infections of the Central Nervous System. ACP Medicine Online (www.acpmedicine.com). Dale DC, Federman DD, Eds. WebMD Inc., New York, May 2001

Mycotic Infections

180. A 32-year-old woman with acute lymphoblastic leukemia is treated with induction chemotherapy. One week after the initiation of therapy, the patient develops a fever and is started on intravenous antibiotics. The patient remains febrile, neutropenic, and thrombocytopenic and is noted to be short of breath. Chest x-rays show a consolidated pulmonary infiltrate in the right lung zone. A sputum culture demonstrates several colonies of *Aspergillus*.

Which of the following statements regarding the diagnosis of this patient is false?

- ❑ **A. The patient most likely has invasive pulmonary aspergillosis**
- ❑ **B. Standard therapy involves intravenous amphotericin**
- ❑ **C. Biopsy is required for a definitive diagnosis**
- ❑ **D. The patient most likely has viral pneumonitis**
- ❑ **E. CT scans of the chest would show air crescents and halos**

Key Concept/Objective: To understand the clinical characteristics of invasive aspergillosis

***Aspergillus* species are commonly found in the environment, but invasive infection is rare except in immunosuppressed patients. The most common pathogen is *Aspergillus fumigatus*. Invasive *Aspergillus* in an immunocompromised host usually presents as a pulmonary infiltrate that is rapidly progressive. The organism spreads by vascular invasion that commonly progresses to tissue necrosis. A definitive diagnosis is difficult to make and requires biopsy; however, the isolation of a single colony of *Aspergillus* from the sputum of a neutropenic patient with pneumonia suggests the diagnosis of invasive *Aspergillus*. Although some patients may be treated with resection, most patients require prolonged therapy with amphotericin B.** *(Answer: D—The patient most likely has viral pneumonitis)*

181. A 46-year-old woman who is known to be HIV positive presents with fever and shortness of breath of 1 week's duration. Chest x-ray reveals bilateral alveolar infiltrates. The arterial oxygen tension (P_aO_2) is 48

mm Hg on room air. Results of methenamine-silver staining of material from bronchoalveolar lavage (BAL) are positive.

Which of the following statements regarding the treatment of this patient is true?

- ❑ A. **Transbronchial biopsy should be carried out to confirm the diagnosis**
- ❑ B. **Corticosteroids are contraindicated, given the risk of other opportunistic infections**
- ❑ C. **Aerosolized pentamidine would be appropriate if the patient is allergic to sulfa drugs**
- ❑ D. **After this patient is treated, secondary prophylaxis is unnecessary**
- ❑ E. **Intravenous trimethoprim-sulfamethoxazole alone should be administered**

Key Concept/Objective: To understand the risk factors, diagnosis, treatment, and prophylaxis of Pneumocystis carinii *infections*

Patients with AIDS and patients receiving immunosuppressive therapy are at risk for developing *Pneumocystis carinii* pneumonia. In this patient, bronchoalveolar lavage alone provides the diagnosis. Further diagnostic studies are not required in this setting, and treatment should be undertaken. For patients with severe hypoxemia who have a P_aO_2 of less than 70 mm Hg or an alveolar-to-arterial (A-a) gradient greater than 30, corticosteroids may be effective in treating lung damage. Steroids should be administered with appropriate antimicrobial therapy, which includes intravenous trimethoprim-sulfamethoxazole. Intravenous pentamidine should be reserved for patients who are allergic to sulfa drugs; aerosolized pentamidine is effective and is indicated as a second-line agent for prophylaxis, but it is not indicated in primary infections. Primary and secondary prophylaxis is indicated for patients with HIV whose $CD4^+$ T cell counts are below 200 cells/µl and for those with severe immunosuppression (i.e., transplant recipients). The preferred agent for prophylaxis is trimethoprim-sulfamethoxazole. *(Answer: E—Intravenous trimethoprim-sulfamethoxazole alone should be administered)*

182. A 60-year-old man with type 1 diabetes mellitus has been experiencing purulent drainage from his nose for 1 week. Suddenly, he develops fever, sinus pain, and headache, and a black eschar appears on the nasal mucosa.

What is the most likely causative agent of this patient's infection?

- ❑ A. ***Aspergillus***
- ❑ B. ***Mucor***
- ❑ C. ***Pseudomonas***
- ❑ D. ***Staphylococcus aureus***
- ❑ E. ***Haemophilus influenzae***

Key Concept/Objective: To understand the risk factors, clinical presentation, and therapy of zygomycosis

Zygomycosis is an opportunistic fungal infection that affects predominantly skin and soft tissues. Different species are classified under the phylum of Zygomycota, including *Rhizopus*, *Mucor*, and *Rhizomucor*. Predisposing conditions include diabetes in association with poor glycemic control; in addition, patients receiving long-term steroid therapy and patients with iron overload—especially those receiving multiple blood transfusions and those receiving the iron chelating agent desferoxamine—are at risk. Mucormycosis can develop into a rapidly invasive infection of the sinuses that results in extensive necrosis. Aggressive surgical debridement and parenteral administration of antibiotics are required. Mucormycosis must be considered in any seriously ill diabetic patient with sinus or ocular involvement, especially those experiencing ketoacidosis. Infection usually spreads from the nasal cavity and can rapidly involve the brain and meninges. Treatment involves accurate, early diagnosis, use of amphotericin at the

maximal systemic dosage, and aggressive debridement until the tissue cultures are negative. Prognosis is poor despite aggressive antifungal therapy and surgical debridement. *(Answer: B—*Mucor*)*

183. A 35-year-old woman who is known to be HIV positive presents to the emergency department with nausea, dizziness, confusion, and a stiff neck of 1 week's duration. On physical examination, her temperature is 101.6° F (38.7° C), and mild neck stiffness is present; other examination results are normal. Except for mild leukopenia, complete blood count and routine chemistries are normal. Head CT is performed, and no masses or bleeding is found. Lumbar puncture is performed, with the following results: an opening pressure of 32 cm H_2O; a low glucose level; an elevated protein level; and an elevated white cell count, with neutrophil predominance. Cryptococcal meningitis is suspected.

Which of the following will provide a definitive diagnosis?

- ❑ **A. Latex agglutination antigen in cerebrospinal fluid (CSF), followed by culture**
- ❑ **B. Latex agglutination antigen in CSF alone**
- ❑ **C. India ink smear alone for definitive diagnosis**
- ❑ **D. MRI of the head**
- ❑ **E. Latex agglutination titers in CSF**

Key Concept/Objective: To understand how to definitively diagnose cryptococcal meningitis

***Cryptococcus* is yeast that is widely disseminated in nature. In many immunocompetent patients, the organism is inhaled, and asymptomatic pulmonary infection develops. In patients with cell-mediated immunity, pulmonary infection may progress to central nervous system infection because CSF lacks several soluble anticryptococcal factors that are present in serum, such as complement components. Patients with cryptococcal meningitis often present with nonspecific complaints, such as headache, nausea, dizziness, and irritability. They may or may not have the usual signs of neck stiffness and fever. Diagnosis is made on the basis of CSF evaluation: an elevated opening pressure, an elevated white cell count with neutrophil predominance, an elevated protein level, and a decrease in the glucose level. Latex agglutination alone detects antigen in 90% of patients with cryptococcal meningitis and can provide a definitive diagnosis when confirmed by culture. India ink smear detects cryptococci in only 25% to 60% of patients, and antigen titers are only used to follow the course of disease. CT or MRI may be normal or result in findings that are nonspecific for meningitis.** *(Answer: A—Latex agglutination antigen in cerebrospinal fluid [CSF], followed by culture)*

For more information, see Kauffman CA: 7 Infectious Disease: XXXVII Mycotic Infections. ACP Medicine Online (www.acpmedicine.com). Dale DC, Federman DD, Eds. WebMD Inc., New York, February 2003

SECTION 8

INTERDISCIPLINARY MEDICINE

Management of Poisoning and Drug Overdose

1. A 48-year-old white man arrives at the emergency department obtunded. He is accompanied by his wife, who states, "He took a lot of pills, trying to hurt himself." She also reports that he drinks a pint of whiskey every day and more on the weekends and that he has prescription pain pills for chronic back pain. The patient is taken to an examination room; a brief clinical assessment reveals a patent and protected airway. The patient has pinpoint pupils.

Which of the following medications is NOT appropriate for this patient?

❑ **A. 25 g of 50% dextrose**

❑ **B. 100 mg of vitamin B_1 (thiamine)**

❑ **C. Nalaxone, 0.2 to 0.4 mg**

❑ **D. Flumazenil**

Key Concept/Objective: To know the appropriate pharmacotherapy for an overdose patient with decreased sensorioum

Poisoning or drug overdose depresses the sensorium; symptoms may range from stupor or obtundation to unresponsive coma. All patients with a depressed sensorium should be evaluated for hypoglycemia because many drugs and poisons can directly reduce or contribute to the reduction of blood glucose levels. A fingerstick blood glucose test and bedside assessment should be performed immediately; if such testing and assessment are impractical, an intravenous bolus of 25 g of 50% dextrose in water should be administered empirically before the laboratory report arrives. For alcoholic or malnourished persons, who may have vitamin deficiencies, 50 to 100 mg of vitamin B_1 (thiamine) should be administered I.V. or I.M. to prevent the development of Wernicke syndrome. If signs of recent opioid use (e.g., suspicious-looking pill bottles or I.V. drug paraphernalia) are in evidence or if the patient has clinical manifestations of excessive opioid effect (e.g., miosis or respiratory depression), the administration of naloxone may have both therapeutic and diagnostic value. Flumazenil, a short-acting, specific benzodiazepine antagonist with no intrinsic agonist effects, can rapidly reverse coma caused by diazepam and other benzodiazepines. However, it has not found a place in the routine management of unconscious patients with drug overdose, because it has the potential to cause seizures in patients who are chronically consuming large quantities of benzodiazepines or who have ingested an acute overdose of benzodiazepines and a tricyclic antidepressant or other potentially convulsant drug. *(Answer: D—Flumazenil)*

2. A 26-year-old African-American man is brought to the emergency department by his roommate. The roommate discovered the patient 1 hour ago taking a handful of pills. When he asked the patient what he was doing, the patient replied, "I am going to sleep for a very long time and I am not going to wake up." The patient confirms the roommate's story. Physical examination reveals a healthy, well-nourished, well-developed man in no acute distress. Vital signs are stable; his affect is mildly depressed, but he is neurologically alert.

Which of the following decontamination methods is NOT appropriate in this patient?

❑ **A. Gastric lavage**

❑ B. Activated charcoal administration

❑ C. Ipecac-induced emesis

❑ D. Whole bowel irrigation (Colyte or GoLYTELY)

Key Concept/Objective: To know the appropriate decontamination methods for a patient after acute ingestion

Gastric lavage is still an accepted method for gut decontamination in hospitalized patients who are obtunded or comatose, but several prospective, randomized, controlled trials have failed to show that emesis or lavage and charcoal provide better clinical results than administration of activated charcoal alone. Activated charcoal, a finely divided product of the distillation of various organic materials, has a large surface area that is capable of adsorbing many drugs and poisons. In the awake patient who has taken a moderate overdose of a drug or poison, most clinicians now employ oral activated charcoal without first emptying the gut; some clinicians still recommend lavage after a massive ingestion of a highly toxic drug. Whole bowel irrigation is a technique that involves the use of a large volume of an osmotically balanced electrolyte solution, such as Colyte or GoLYTELY, that contains nonabsorbable polyethylene glycol and that cleans the gut by mechanical action without net gain or loss of fluids or electrolytes. Although no controlled clinical trials to date have demonstrated improved outcome, it is recommended for those who have ingested large doses of poisons that are not well adsorbed by charcoal (e.g., iron or lithium), for those who have ingested sustained-release or enteric-coated products, and for those who have ingested drug packets or other potentially toxic foreign bodies. *(Answer: C—Ipecac-induced emesis)*

3. A 75-year-old woman comes to the emergency department after experiencing a presyncope event approximately 1 hour ago. Her daughter informs you that the patient saw her primary care physician yesterday and that she is now taking a new medication for high blood pressure. The patient reports she occasionally takes an extra dose of her blood pressure medicine when she has a headache, but on this day, she took two extra pills because she also forgot to take her medicine the day before. The patient brought the new medicine with her; it is atenolol, 100 mg tablets. Physical examination reveals an elderly woman in no distress. Her pulse is 32 beats/min, her blood pressure is 78/43 mm Hg, and her respiratory rate is 14 breaths/min. She is afebrile.

After I.V. access is established, what is the preferred antidote for this patient's hypotension and bradycardia?

❑ A. Atropine, 1 mg I.V.

❑ B. Dopamine drip, titrate to desired effect

❑ C. Glucagon, 5 to 10 mg I.V.

❑ D. Isoproterenol drip, titrate to desired effect

Key Concept/Objective: To understand the treatment of a patient with beta-blocker toxicity

Treatment of overdose with a beta blocker includes aggressive gut decontamination. In cases involving a large or recent ingestion, gastric lavage and the administration of activated charcoal and a cathartic agent should be initiated. Hypotension and bradycardia are unlikely to respond to beta-adrenergic–mediated agents such as dopamine and isoproterenol; instead, the patient should receive high dosages of glucagon (5 to 10 mg I.V., followed by 5 to 10 mg/hr). Glucagon is a potent inotropic agent that does not require beta-adrenergic receptors to activate cells. When glucagon fails, an epinephrine drip may be more beneficial in increasing heart rate and contractility than isoproterenol or dopamine. If pharmacologic therapy is unsuccessful, transvenous or external pacing should be used to maintain heart rate. Use of hemodialysis in atenolol poisoning has been reported. *(Answer: C—Glucagon, 5 to 10 mg I.V.)*

4. A 75-year-old man is admitted to the intensive care unit for confusion, repeated emesis, and tachycardia. His medical history is significant only for chronic obstructive pulmonary disease, for which he uses ipratropium bromide, albuterol inhalers, and theophylline. After 2 hours in the ICU, his theophylline

level is found to be 55 mg/L (10 to 20 mg/L is therapeutic). The electrocardiogram was significant only for sinus tachycardia of 132 beats/min. Activated charcoal is given. Over the next hour, despite two 500 ml boluses of normal saline, the patient's hypotension worsens.

What is the preferred method of treating this patient's hypotension?

- ❑ **A. External overdrive pacing to slow the heart rate**
- ❑ **B. Dopamine drip, titrated to the desired mean arterial pressure**
- ❑ **C. Hemodialysis**
- ❑ **D. Esmolol drip, titrated to the desired mean arterial pressure**

Key Concept/Objective: To understand the treatment of theophylline-induced hypotension

This patient's hypotension is caused by toxic levels of theophylline; because the hypotension is probably caused by beta$_2$-adrenergic–mediated vasodilatation, it should be treated with esmolol, 25 to 100 mg/kg/min, rather than a beta-adrenergic agonist such as dopamine. External pacing plays no role in the management of hypotension in a patient with sinus tachycardia. Hemodialysis has a role in the management of theophylline toxicity, especially if seizures develop or levels are greater than 100 mg/L; however, hemodialysis would likely worsen the existing hypotension acutely, and the hypotension would have to be improved before dialysis could be implemented. *(Answer: D—Esmolol drip, titrated to the desired mean arterial pressure)*

5. A 70-year-old woman with chronic atrial fibrillation who is on warfarin therapy was prescribed erythromycin 10 days ago for a community-acquired pneumonia. Today, she is found comatose. A CT scan of the head reveals a large intracranial hemorrhage, and her prothrombin time (international normalized ratio [INR]) is 20.

Overanticoagulation may have been avoided if, instead of erythromycin, this patient had been prescribed which of the following?

- ❑ **A. Cefoxitin**
- ❑ **B. Clarithromycin**
- ❑ **C. Ofloxacin**
- ❑ **D. Trimethoprim-sulfamethoxazole**
- ❑ **E. None of the above**

Key Concept/Objective: To know that warfarin interacts with a vast number of commonly prescribed drugs

Drugs that interact with warfarin include many antibiotics that are frequently used to treat community-acquired pneumonia (cephalosporins, quinolones, macrolides, tetracyclines, and long-acting sulfonamides). Use of these antibiotics in patients on warfarin requires vigilant monitoring of their anticoagulation status. Among the available newer-generation quinolone antibiotics, trovafloxacin and sparfloxacin do not seem to interact with warfarin. *(Answer: E—None of the above)*

6. A 33-year-old man who suffers from depression and chronic pain attempts suicide by overdosing on the collection of pain killers he has accumulated from multiple physicians. He is in the emergency department with stupor, pinpoint pupils, and hypotension.

Which of the following tests should you order for this patient?

- ❑ **A. Electrocardiogram**
- ❑ **B. Benzodiazepine level**
- ❑ **C. Acetaminophen level**
- ❑ **D. Aspirin level**
- ❑ **E. Electrocardiogram, acetaminophen level, and aspirin level**

Key Concept/Objective: To understand that intentional overdose may involve multiple substances

Prescription narcotic pain killers are often compounded with either aspirin or acetaminophen. Early recognition and treatment of toxic levels of either of these are critical to preventing subsequent metabolic acidosis (aspirin) or hepatic injury (acetaminophen). This patient, who has had multiple physicians and has been diagnosed with depression, may also have ingested tricyclic antidepressants. Electrocardiographic abnormalities, including widening of the QRS interval, prolongation of the QT interval, and right axis deviation of the terminal 40 msec of the QRS complex, may provide early clues to this potentially lethal ingestion. Although this patient is at risk for having a coexistent benzodiazepine ingestion, management is limited to supportive measures, so there is no clinical utility to checking a serum level. If he has or is suspected of having also ingested tricyclic antidepressants, use of flumazenil is contraindicated because of the risk of seizures. *(Answer: E—Electrocardiogram, acetaminophen level, and aspirin level)*

7. Having misunderstood your instructions on how she should adjust the dosages of her 12 different medications, a 68-year-old woman is now in the intensive care unit after taking an excess of propranolol. Her pulse is 35 beats/min, her blood pressure is 65/35 mm Hg, she is unresponsive, and her skin is mottled.

Therapeutic options for this patient include which of the following?

- ❑ **A. Dopamine drip**
- ❑ **B. Intravenous glucagon**
- ❑ **C. Isoproterenol drip**
- ❑ **D. Epinephrine drip**
- ❑ **E. Intravenous glucagon and epinephrine drip**

Key Concept/Objective: To understand that dopamine and isoproterenol exert their effects primarily through beta-adrenergic pathways

In the setting of profound beta blockade, dopamine and isoproterenol are likely to be ineffective. Glucagon does not require beta-adrenergic receptors to exert its positive inotropic effect. Epinephrine works through alpha-adrenergic receptors. *(Answer: E—Intravenous glucagon and epinephrine drip)*

8. A 58-year-old farmer is brought in from the fields to the emergency department sweating, vomiting, and confused. On examination, his blood pressure is 100/60 mm Hg, his pulse is 80 beats/min, and his respiratory rate is 24 breaths/min. He appears to be in moderate respiratory distress and has generalized muscle weakness. His pupils are pinpoint. He is salivating profusely and has gurgling upper respiratory sounds.

This patient most likely is suffering from which of the following conditions?

- ❑ **A. Heatstroke and dehydration**
- ❑ **B. Illicit opiate use/overdose**
- ❑ **C. Organophosphate poisoning**
- ❑ **D. Myocardial infarction**
- ❑ **E. Mushroom poisoning**

Key Concept: To know the constellation of cholinergic symptoms created by organophosphate poisoning

Agricultural workers are at risk for exposure to organophosphates, which are widely used in pesticides. Organophosphates are absorbed from the skin, lungs, gut, and conjunctiva. They inhibit acetylcholinesterase; therefore, presenting signs and symptoms are those of cholinergic excess. Prompt diagnosis and treatment are essential because some organophosphates undergo aging, whereby they become permanently bound to

acetylcholinesterase. After this occurs, treatment with pralidoxime becomes much less effective. *(Answer: C—Organophosphate poisoning)*

9. A 44-year-old chronic alcoholic man is once again in the emergency department, intoxicated. He is stuporous and has slurred speech. His blood pressure is 130/85 mm Hg, his pulse is 89 beats/min, and his respiratory rate is 26 breaths/min. His skin is warm, dry, and pink. Besides his altered mental status, his neurologic examination is nonfocal, and he has no external evidence of trauma. Laboratory results are as follows: WBC, 7,400; HCT, 45; platelets, 200,000; Na, 130; K, 3.5; Cl, 90; HCO_3, 15; Glu, 110.

You should order a serum level of which of the following for this patient?

❑ **A. Methanol**

❑ **B. Ethylene glycol**

❑ **C. Aspirin**

❑ **D. Methanol and ethylene glycol**

❑ **E. Methanol, ethylene glycol, and aspirin**

Key Concept/Objective: To be able to recognize anion-gap metabolic acidosis and to know the differential diagnosis

The differential diagnosis for anion-gap metabolic acidosis includes methanol overdose, uremia, diabetic ketoacidosis, paraldehyde overdose, aspirin overdose, lactic acidosis, and ethylene glycol overdose (MUDPALE). *(Answer: E—Methanol, ethylene glycol, and aspirin)*

For more information, see Olson KR, Patel MM: 8 Interdisciplinary Medicine: I Management of Poisoning and Drug Overdose. ACP Medicine Online (www.acpmedicine.com). Dale DC, Federman DD, Eds. WebMD Inc., New York, January 2003

Bites and Stings

10. A mother brings her 2-year-old son to the acute care clinic. She explains that when she picked him up from day care, she was told he had suffered some sort of bite in the playground. It is unclear who or what bit him, but there are puncture wounds in his right hand, which is red and swollen. The mother is worried about infection.

The bite of which of the following mammals is LEAST likely to result in infection?

❑ **A. Human**

❑ **B. Cat**

❑ **C. Dog**

❑ **D. Rat**

Key Concept/Objective: To recognize the risk of infection associated with various mammalian bites

Infection is the most common complication of bite wounds. The microbes responsible for infection originate either from the mouth of the mammal inflicting the wound or the victim's skin flora. Most infections resulting from the bites of mammals are polymicrobial. The incidence of infection depends on the location of the bite and the type of mammal inflicting the wound. The infection rate for dog bites is 2% to 20%; the infection rate for human bites is 10% to 50%; the rate for cat bites is 30% to 50%. Infections from rat bites are very infrequent. Prophylactic use of antibiotics for bites from mammals is debatable. The decision should be based on the location and appearance of the wound and the type of animal involved. For most mammalian bites, amoxicillin-clavulanic acid is the drug of choice. *(Answer: D—Rat)*

11. A 30-year-old man presents to the emergency department with a bite wound. He had been camping at a local wildlife preserve. While he was looking for firewood, his hand was bitten by what he thought was a squirrel. He was not able to capture the animal, but he did not think the animal was acting strangely. He believes he just "scared the critter." You are worried about the risk of rabies.

Which of the following animals should be regarded as rabid if it bites someone (assuming the animal cannot be tested for rabies in the laboratory)?

- ❑ **A. Squirrel**
- ❑ **B. Skunk**
- ❑ **C. Rabbit**
- ❑ **D. Rat**

Key Concept/Objective: To know common animals that have a very low probability of causing rabies

The clinician should always consider the possibility of rabies exposure in patients suffering bite wounds. The use of soap and a virucidal agent to clean the wound has been shown to help prevent rabies. With domestic-animal bites, postexposure rabies prophylaxis is warranted if (1) the animal is observed to be abnormal; (2) the animal is not available for observation and the rate of rabies in domestic animals in the region is high; or (3) the animal exhibited abnormal behavior, such as an unprovoked attack. With bites from wild animals, recommendations for rabies prophylaxis depend on the species. Skunks, bats, raccoons, foxes, and most other carnivores should be regarded as rabid unless immediate brain testing can be performed on the animal. The bites of squirrels, rats, rabbits, mice, hamsters, guinea pigs, gerbils, chipmunks, and other small rodents virtually never require postexposure prophylaxis for rabies. *(Answer: B—Skunk)*

12. A 42-year-old park ranger presents after being bitten by a snake on his right forearm. He informs you that the snake was a copperhead. He complains of pain and swelling at the site of the bite. Examination shows two puncture wounds on his right forearm. An area of tenderness, erythema, and swelling, which measures approximately 2 in. in diameter, surrounds the wounds. The patient is otherwise asymptomatic.

For which of the following patients is antivenin therapy most appropriate?

- ❑ **A. A 42-year-old man presenting 2 hours after a copperhead bite who is experiencing a grade 1 envenomation**
- ❑ **B. A 42-year-old man presenting 2 hours after a rattlesnake bite who is experiencing a grade 3 envenomation**
- ❑ **C. A 42-year-old man presenting 24 hours after a copperhead bite who is experiencing a grade 1 envenomation**
- ❑ **D. A 42-year-old man presenting 24 hours after a rattlesnake bite who is experiencing a grade 3 envenomation**

Key Concept/Objective: To be able to identify those patients most likely to benefit from therapy with antivenin and to be familiar with the classification system for envenomation

This patient has a grade 1 envenomation, characterized by pain and throbbing at the site of the bite, with 1 to 5 in. of surrounding erythema and edema and with no evidence of systemic involvement. Grade 0 envenomation is characterized by minimal local findings; grade 2 envenomation is characterized by severe pain over a larger area, with possible systemic involvement; envenomations of grades 3 and 4 are severe and are characterized by systemic manifestations such as fever, nausea, emesis, tachycardia, hypotension, diaphoresis, or mental status changes. Antivenins are available for North American pit vipers and eastern coral snakes, but they are indicated only for severe envenomations. Water moccasin and copperhead bites are usually managed without antivenin. Most antivenins are horse-serum based and can therefore cause serum sickness. Antivenin is most effective when given within 4 hours of the snakebite. It is of little value if administered more than 12 hours after the patient was bitten. Before using antivenin, the clinician should consider potential adverse effects and the situations in

which antivenin is most effective. This patient does not need antivenin at this time. *(Answer: B—A 42-year-old man presenting 2 hours after a rattlesnake bite who is experiencing a grade 3 envenomation)*

13. A 25-year-old woman presents to your office in Missouri with a spider bite. She states that she was getting firewood from the woodpile outside of her house the evening before and felt a sharp pain on the back of her right hand. She was unable to bring the spider to your office. On examination, you note an area of pallor with surrounding erythema over the dorsum of the patient's right hand. You suspect that she was bitten by a brown recluse spider.

Which of the following therapies is LEAST likely to benefit the victim of a brown recluse spider bite?

- ❑ **A. Administraton of steroids within 24 hours of the bite**
- ❑ **B. Administration of dapsone in patients who do not have glucose-6-phosphate dehydrogenase deficiency**
- ❑ **C. Use of antibiotics if there are signs of infection at the bite site**
- ❑ **D. Use of hyperbaric oxygen**

Key Concept/Objective: To know the therapies that have proven roles in the treatment of brown recluse spider bites

This patient's history is typical for someone who has suffered a brown recluse spider bite. These spiders are found under rocks and woodpiles in the south central United States. Brown recluses are more active at night. Their bite can cause pain within the first few hours of envenomation. Physical findings are a ring of pallor surrounded by erythema. These may eventually evolve to form a bleb, which can become necrotic. The necrosis can spread and may eventually form an eschar. There is some evidence of benefit from treatment with systemic steroids within 24 hours of envenomation. Dapsone has been shown to be helpful in treating the local damage caused by the venom. However, dapsone can cause a serious hemolytic reaction in those with glucose-6-phosphate dehydrogenase deficiency. Antibiotics are useful if there is evidence of infection. Hyperbaric oxygen has not been conclusively proven to be effective for brown recluse spider envenomations. *(Answer: D—Use of hyperbaric oxygen)*

For more information, see Lewis LM, Levine MD, Dribben WH: 8 Interdisciplinary Medicine: II Bites and Stings. ACP Medicine Online (www.acpmedicine.com). Dale DC, Federman DD, Eds. WebMD Inc., New York, September 2002

Cardiac Resuscitation

14. You find a 72-year-old man lying unresponsive in a restroom of a local airport. He is alone, and you don't know how long he has been unconscious. You speak loudly, trying to wake him up, and you shake him; he continues to be unresponsive.

On the basis of the chain of survival, what should be your sequential response in this situation?

- ❑ **A. Start cardiopulmonary response (CPR); call for help by activating the emergency medical system (EMS); and call for a defibrillator**
- ❑ **B. Look in his pocket or wallet for information about his medical history; start CPR; call for help by activating EMS; and call for a defibrillator**
- ❑ **C. Immediately call for help by activating EMS; call for a defibrillator; and start CPR**
- ❑ **D. Immediately call for help by activating EMS; call for a defibrillator; wait for EMS to come and to start an I.V.; and start CPR**

Key Concept/Objective: To understand the chain of survival

The resuscitation of an adult victim of sudden cardiac arrest should follow an orderly sequence, no matter where the patient collapse occurs. This sequence is called the chain

of survival. It comprises four elements: activation of EMS, CPR, defibrillation, and provision of advanced care. When a person is found to be unresponsive, the first thing to do is to confirm the unresponsiveness by speaking loudly and shaking the patient. If the patient remains unresponsive, the next step should be to call for help by activating EMS. If an automated external defibrillator is available, also call for it. After this is done, the next step is to assess the patient's airway, breathing, and circulation. CPR should then be initiated, and advanced care should begin once EMS arrives. *(Answer: C—Immediately call for help by activating EMS; call for a defibrillator; and start CPR)*

15. A 56-year-old woman is found pulseless in her room at a local hospital. The nurse calls "code blue," and you are the first doctor responding. The nurse has started CPR, and the patient has a patent I.V. line. After 2 minutes, the patient is still pulseless. A defibrillator has now been brought to the room.

What is the best intervention to take next in the care of this patient?

- ❑ **A. Continue CPR; look for a pulse again; establish an airway; give 1 mg of epinephrine I.V.; and repeat these measures until circulation has been restored**
- ❑ **B. Attach the defibrillator; analyze the rhythm; attempt to defibrillate if the rhythm is ventricular tachycardia (VT) or ventricular fibrillation (VF); continue CPR if unsuccessful; establish an airway; and proceed with I.V. medications**
- ❑ **C. Establish an airway; give 1 mg of epinephrine I.V.; continue CPR; attach the defibrillator and analyze the rhythm; and defibrillate if the rhythm is VF or VT**
- ❑ **D. Immediately give 1 mg of atropine; attach the defibrillator and analyze the rhythm; defibrillate if the rhythm is VF or VT; continue with CPR if unsuccessful; and establish an airway**

Key Concept/Objective: To understand the importance of analyzing the rhythm and providing immediate defibrillation if needed

In the chain of survival, the importance of rapid access to defibrillation cannot be overemphasized. In a patient who is dying from a shockable rhythm, the chance of survival declines by 7% to 10% for every minute that defibrillation is delayed. When provided immediately after the onset of VT, the success of defibrillation is extremely high. Early defibrillation is so critical that if a defibrillator is immediately available, its use takes precedence over CPR in patients with pulseless VT or VF. If CPR is already in progress, it should be halted while defibrillation takes place. *(Answer: B—Attach the defibrillator; analyze the rhythm; attempt to defibrillate if the rhythm is ventricular tachycardia [VT] or ventricular fibrillation [VF]; continue CPR [illegible]*

16. A 66-year-old male patient in the intensive care unit (ICU) is found in pulseless VT. He is intubated, and the nurse has started CPR. You try to defibrillate him three times without success, using shocks of 200 joules, 300 joules, and 360 joules.

What is the best step to take next in the treatment of this patient?

- ❑ **A. Continue CPR and try to defibrillate again with repeated shocks of 360 joules every 1 min**
- ❑ **B. Give 1 mg of epinephrine I.V., continue CPR, and give another shock of 360 joules in 30 to 60 sec**
- ❑ **C. Give 1 mg of atropine, continue CPR, and give another shock of 360 joules in 30 to 60 sec**
- ❑ **D. Give 300 mg of amiodarone I.V., continue CPR, and give another shock of 360 joules after 1 min**

Key Concept/Objective: To understand the appropriate management of pulseless VT and VF

When a monitor-defibrillator is available, the patient's rhythm is immediately analyzed. There are four rhythm possibilities: pulseless VT, pulseless VF, pulseless electrical activity, and asystole. Pulseless VT and pulseless VF are managed identically. The first step is to try to defibrillate with 200 joules; if the VT or VF persists, subsequent attempts should use 200 to 300 joules and 360 joules. After these attempts, the next action is to administer drug therapy. The first medication to be given is a vasoconstrictor (either epinephrine or vasopressin). If there is no I.V. access, these drugs can be given endotracheally. The rescuer should continue with CPR for 30 to 60 sec to allow the drug to reach the heart, then defibrillation should be attempted again. If pulseless VT or VF persists, antiarrhythmic drug therapy (i.e., amiodarone or lidocaine) should be added. *(Answer: B—Give 1 mg of epinephrine I.V., continue CPR, and give another shock of 360 joules in 30 to 60 sec)*

17. A 60-year-old homeless man is found unresponsive in a park. There are no witnesses. EMS is called and finds him in asystole. The appropriate protocol for asystole, including epinephrine, is started. The patient is intubated, and he is brought to a local emergency department after 12 minutes. On physical examination, there is no pulse; temperature is 80° F (26.7° C).

What is the best step to take next in the treatment of this patient?

- ❑ **A. Attach a monitor; confirm asystole; defibrillate; and proceed with CPR**
- ❑ **B. Consider stopping measures after 10 min if resuscitation has been unsuccessful and the patient remains in asystole**
- ❑ **C. Treat the hypothermia aggressively; continue with resuscitation and asystole protocol**
- ❑ **D. Attach a monitor; confirm asystole; administer 40 mg of vasopressin I.V., followed by CPR for 1 min, and then defibrillate; continue CPR**

Key Concept/Objective: To understand the appropriate management of asystole

The prognosis for asystole is generally regarded as dismal unless the patient is hypothermic or there are other extenuating but treatable circumstances. The sequence of resuscitation steps in the management of asystole is as follows: activation of EMS; CPR, rhythm evaluation, and asystole confirmation; intubation; I.V. access with epinephrine and atropine administration; and immediate transcutaneous pacing, if available. If asystole persists for more than 10 min despite optimal CPR, oxygenation, ventilation, and epinephrine or atropine administration, efforts should stop unless there is hypothermia or drug overdose. *(Answer: C—Treat the hypothermia aggressively; continue with resuscitation and asystole protocol)*

For more information, see Mengert TJ: 8 Interdisciplinary Medicine: III Cardiac Resucitation. ACP Medicine Online (www.acpmedicine.com). Dale DC, Federman DD, Eds. WebMD Inc., New York, April 2003

Preoperative Assessment

18. A 66-year-old female patient is admitted to the orthopedic surgery service with a left hip fracture. She has a history of hypertension and osteoporosis but is otherwise in good health. She has no history of chest pain, but she says she gets short of breath when she walks about a half mile. She smoked one pack of cigarettes a day for 30 years, but she quit 5 years ago. She is taking an ACE inhibitor for her hypertension. Review of systems is otherwise negative.

Which of the following statements regarding preoperative cardiovascular risk assessment is true?

- ❑ **A. The most important risk factor for cardiac death or complication perioperatively is a recent myocardial infarction**
- ❑ **B. The most important preoperative use of echocardiography is to assess the degree of systolic dysfunction**

- ❑ C. Most patients who do not have an independent clinical need for coronary revascularization can proceed to surgery without further cardiac investigation
- ❑ D. There is good evidence that diastolic dysfunction increases perioperative risk significantly

Key Concept/Objective: To understand the basic principles of preoperative cardiovascular risk assessment

Uncontrolled heart failure is the most important risk factor for cardiac death or complications. A history of functional limitation appears to be the most helpful of all the historical points in this assessment. Patients who can perform activities that require four metabolic equivalents have a good chance of survival for most surgical procedures; such patients require no further testing. The use of echocardiography as a predictive tool is controversial. Although many experts advocate echocardiography as a good tool for assessing heart failure control, the procedure may provide little prognostic information beyond that available from a careful history and physical examination. The most important preoperative use of echocardiography is in the differentiation of systolic dysfunction from diastolic dysfunction in patients with new-onset heart failure. The distinction is important, because data clearly show that systolic dysfunction, in a patient with substantial clinical manifestations (i.e., overt congestive failure), adds significantly to the risk of surgery. On the other hand, there are no data showing that echocardiographic evidence of systolic dysfunction in a patient without symptoms or signs of heart failure has any prognostic implications. There are also no good data indicating that diastolic dysfunction increases risk significantly. The preoperative evaluation of the patient with established or probable coronary artery disease (CAD) is of great importance. Recent myocardial infarction is second only to decompensated heart failure as a risk factor for perioperative complications. Decisions regarding the evaluation of chest pain in patients without a history of CAD can be difficult under any circumstance. The American College of Physicians clinical guidelines on the perioperative assessment and management of risk from CAD state that most patients who do not have an independent clinical need for coronary revascularization can proceed to surgery without further cardiac investigation. In other words, if there is no prior reason to perform coronary artery bypass surgery, further cardiac investigation usually does not need to be carried out for the anticipated surgery, unless there is some other overriding consideration. *(Answer: C—Most patients who do not have an independent clinical need for coronary revascularization can proceed to surgery without further cardiac investigation)*

19. A 63-year-old white man has severe osteoarthritis and wants to have knee replacement surgery. His orthopedic surgeon has referred him to you for preoperative evaluation. The patient has smoked 1.5 packs of cigarettes a day for 50 years and states that he has a chronic productive cough, dyspnea, and wheezing. The patient uses an albuterol and ipratropium bromide combination inhaler.

Which of the following statements regarding assessment of preoperative pulmonary risk is false?

- ❑ A. Performance on pulmonary function tests (PFTs) correlates well with mortality
- ❑ B. Acute reversible pulmonary disease, such as asthma or a respiratory tract infection, must be identified and treated before surgery
- ❑ C. Any patient with cardiovascular or pulmonary disease should receive a chest x-ray before surgery
- ❑ D. Patients who can exercise without significant symptoms are at low risk

Key Concept/Objective: To understand the basic principles of preoperative pulmonary risk assessment

The pulmonary evaluation process is unfortunately much more subjective than the cardiac evaluation. Acute reversible disease, such as asthma or a respiratory tract infection,

must be identified so that it can be treated and reversed before the procedure, if possible. Patients who can exercise without significant symptoms are at low risk. Shortness of breath on exercise, in the absence of heart disease, identifies patients at higher risk. Preoperative use of PFTs is controversial. PFTs do not readily identify individual patients who are at prohibitive risk of mortality; there is poor correlation between PFT results and mortality, despite some statistical correlation. If the history and physical examination do not suggest significant pulmonary disease, there is no advantage in performing PFTs. Most experts believe that any patient older than 60 years should have a baseline chest x-ray. Clearly, any patient with cardiovascular or pulmonary disease needs a chest x-ray. *(Answer: A—Performance on pulmonary function tests [PFTs] correlates well with mortality)*

20. A 59-year-old African-American man is admitted to the trauma surgery service after sustaining fractures of the tibia and fibula in a motor vehicle accident. You are consulted for perioperative management. The patient's medical history is significant for hypertension, which is uncontrolled; CAD status post myocardial infarction 5 years ago; and benign prostatic hypertrophy. The patient lost his job, as well as health insurance coverage, 6 months ago and is currently on no medications.

Which of the following statements regarding medical management of the surgical patient is false?

❑ A. **In patients with CAD, use of perioperative beta blockers can prevent complications after surgery, both short term and long term**

❑ B. **Patients with diastolic blood pressure below 100 mm Hg can proceed with surgical procedures**

❑ C. **Asymptomatic patients with hypothyroidism are at significant risk for myxedema coma**

❑ D. **Patients who are receiving long-term corticosteroid therapy need replacement therapy perioperatively**

Key Concept/Objective: To understand the management of surgical risk factors

It is now clear that the use of perioperative beta blockers can prevent complications after surgery, both short term and long term. Patients with known CAD who can tolerate beta blockers should already be taking these drugs. If they are not, a beta blocker should be started. Many experts recommend starting beta blockade before surgery in patients at high risk for CAD. Patients with a diastolic blood pressure below 110 mm Hg are not at significantly greater risk and do not require specific blood pressure management. However, it is clear that in patients with poorly controlled blood pressure who undergo surgery, blood pressure may swing widely, both in hypertensive and hypotensive directions. Both high and low blood pressures can cause problems perioperatively. Unless surgery is urgent or emergent, hurried attempts at blood pressure control are not advised. Patients with hypothyroidism, provided they are functional, do not have significant problems with surgery and do not require special treatment. Patients who are clinically hyperthyroid are at risk for thyroid storm perioperatively, so hyperthyroidism should be well controlled before surgery is undertaken. Patients who are taking corticosteroids (e.g., for rheumatic disease or asthma) usually need replacement therapy perioperatively. In normal persons, the daily output of cortisone is approximately 30 mg; peak stress levels are approximately 300 mg a day. Unfortunately, no good studies have been done to determine which patients definitely need supplementation and how long the increase in dose should be maintained. Current practice is to give additional medication to patients who are taking the equivalent of 30 mg or more of hydrocortisone a day. For patients at lower dosage ranges, supplemental doses (e.g., 50 mg) given twice daily are adequate; for those taking more than 150 mg a day, three doses a day of 50 to 100 mg are usually recommended. *(Answer: C—Asymptomatic patients with hypothyroidism are at significant risk for myxedema coma)*

For more information, see Lubin MF: 8 Interdisciplinary Medicine: IV Preoperative Assessment. ACP Medicine Online (www.acpmedicine.com). Dale DC, Federman DD, Eds. WebMD Inc., New York, July 2004

Bioterrorism

21. A 24-year-old man presents to the emergency department for evaluation. He is accompanied by his wife. The patient was in his usual state of health until 7 days ago, when he developed fever and malaise with headache, backache, nausea, vomiting, and abdominal pain. Five days ago, he developed a rash on his face and arms, which has spread over most of his body. He takes no medications. Physical examination is remarkable for a prominent rash consisting of diffuse, small macules and papules and occasional pustules. Your first consideration is that the patient may have a viral syndrome, such as varicella infection. The possibility occurs to you that a patient with smallpox could present in this way.

Which of the following statements regarding smallpox infection is true?

- ❑ **A. In infections of smallpox or varicella, skin lesions typically appear in different stages of development on any given part of the body**
- ❑ **B. Infectious mononucleosis is the disease most likely to be confused with smallpox**
- ❑ **C. Patients suspected of having smallpox require significant contact precautions, but airborne precautions are not required**
- ❑ **D. Only personnel who have been successfully vaccinated within 3 years and who are wearing appropriate barrier protection should be involved in specimen collection for suspected cases of smallpox**

Key Concept/Objective: To know the clinical manifestations of and appropriate containment methods for smallpox virus

Severe varicella is the disease most likely to be confused with smallpox. However, familiarity with the clinical features of the two diseases, particularly the rash, should help differentiate them. In smallpox infection, lesions are in the same stage of development on any given part of the body, whereas lesions in varicella are polymorphic. In the event of a limited outbreak, patients should be admitted to the hospital and confined to rooms that are under negative atmospheric pressure and equipped with high-efficiency particulate air (HEPA) filtration. Standard, contact, and airborne precautions, including use of gloves, gowns, and masks, should be strictly observed. Unvaccinated personnel caring for patients suspected of having smallpox should wear fit-tested N95 or higher-quality respirators. Only personnel who have undergone successful smallpox vaccination within 3 years and who are wearing appropriate barrier protection (i.e., gloves, gown, and shoe covers) should be involved in specimen collection for suspected cases of smallpox. *(Answer: D—Only personnel who have been successfully vaccinated within 3 years and who are wearing appropriate barrier protection should be involved in specimen collection for suspected cases of smallpox)*

22. A 22-year-old man who is in the military visits your clinic complaining of diffuse body aches, fatigue, shortness of breath, and midsternal chest pain. He has had these symptoms for 3 days. He notes that his chest pain worsens with deep inspiration. He has no significant medical history and takes no medications. He has a patch on his arm, which he explains was placed there by medical personnel to cover his smallpox vaccination site. He states that he received his vaccination 2 weeks ago. On physical examination, the patient's temperature is 99.9° F (37.7° C). His heart rate is 110 beats/min, and he has a pericardial rub on auscultation. His physical examination is otherwise normal. An electrocardiogram reveals sinus tachycardia, diffuse ST segment elevation, and PR interval depression.

Which of the following statements regarding smallpox vaccination is true?

- ❑ **A. The most common complication of smallpox vaccination is eczema vaccinatum**
- ❑ **B. The occurrence of myopericarditis after smallpox vaccination has been reported**
- ❑ **C. Complications of smallpox vaccination are more common after revaccination**
- ❑ **D. The most common serious complication of smallpox vaccination is myopericarditis**

Key Concept/Objective: To know the complications of smallpox vaccination

Moderate and severe complications of vaccinia vaccination include eczema vaccinatum, generalized vaccinia, progressive vaccinia, and postvaccinial encephalitis. These complications are rare but are at least 10 times more common after primary vaccination than after revaccination. The most common complication of smallpox vaccination, occurring in 529.2 cases per million doses, is localized vaccinia infection resulting from inadvertent transfer (autoinoculation) of vaccinia from the vaccination site to other parts of the body. Eczema vaccinatum (38.5/million doses) is a localized or systemic dissemination of vaccinia virus that occurs in persons who have eczema or a history of eczema or other chronic or exfoliative skin conditions (e.g., atopic dermatitis). The most common serious complication is postvaccinial encephalitis (12.3/million doses). It occurs mostly in infants younger than 1 year and, less often, in adolescents and adults receiving a primary vaccination. Among 450,293 United States military service members vaccinated from December 2002 to May 2003, 37 cases of suspected, probable, or confirmed myopericarditis were observed. Symptoms of myopericarditis after smallpox vaccination began 7 to 19 days after vaccination (range, 1 to 42 days). *(Answer: B—The occurrence of myopericarditis after smallpox vaccination has been reported)*

23. You are called urgently to the emergency department to evaluate a 35-year-old man who is suspected of having undergone a cerebrovascular accident. The patient's wife is at his bedside. On questioning, she states that the patient has no medical history and was in his usual state of health until 24 hours ago, when he developed double vision and had difficulty speaking and swallowing. His illness has been rapidly progressive. He is now almost mute and has developed severe shortness of breath. He has had no contact with persons who are ill. The emergency department physician informs you that two other patients with similar presentations were seen earlier today and that one more patient with the same complaints is in triage. Further discussions with these patients reveal that they were all at the same music concert 2 days ago.

Which of the following statements regarding botulism is true?

- ❑ A. **The classic clinical triad in patients with botulism is lack of fever, symmetrical descending flaccid paralysis with prominent bulbar palsies, and a clear sensorium**
- ❑ B. **Contamination of food supplies is the most likely way that botulinum toxin would be used in bioterrorism**
- ❑ C. **Botulism is easily confused with Guillain-Barré syndrome, because both illnesses are typified by descending flaccid paralysis**
- ❑ D. **Initiation of treatment with botulinum antitoxin should be withheld until botulism is confirmed by laboratory testing**

Key Concept/Objective: To know the clinical presentation of and appropriate therapy for botulism

The so-called classic triad of botulism summarizes the clinical presentation: an afebrile patient, symmetrical descending flaccid paralysis with prominent bulbar palsies, and a clear sensorium. Symptoms of cranial nerve abnormalities nearly always begin in the bulbar musculature; patients typically present with difficulty seeing, speaking, or swallowing. Clinical hallmarks include ptosis, blurred vision, and the so-called four Ds: diplopia, dysarthria, dysphonia, and dysphagia. Cranial nerve abnormalities and bulbar weakness are followed by symmetrical descending weakness and paralysis with progression from the head to the arms, thorax, and legs. Guillain-Barré syndrome typically results in ascending paralysis and sensory abnormalities. An aerosol attack is considered the most likely use of botulinum toxin for bioterrorism, although intentional contamination of food supplies is possible. Initiation of treatment with botulinum antitoxin should be based on the clinical diagnosis and should not await laboratory confirmation. A clinician who suspects botulism should immediately contact the local or state health department to facilitate procurement of antitoxin for treatment. *(Answer: A—The classic clinical triad in patients with botulism is lack of fever, symmetrical descending flaccid paralysis with prominent bulbar palsies, and a clear sensorium)*

24. A 35-year-old white man presents with fever, malaise, muscle aches, and cough. He reports no significant medical history. He works for the state government, and a letter with an unknown powder was sent to his office 3 days ago. He is concerned that he has anthrax. Four other people in his office have developed similar symptoms. Results of physical examination are as follows: heart rate, 106 beats/min; respiratory rate, 24 breaths/min; temperature, 101.8° F (38.8° C); and blood pressure, 124/78 mm Hg. The patient is in mild distress, and he is profusely diaphoretic. Pulmonary examination shows decreased breath sounds at the right base, with scattered crackles. The heart examination is significant only for tachycardia.

Given the likelihood of anthrax exposure in this patient, which of the following test would NOT be indicated to confirm the diagnosis of inhalational anthrax?

- ❑ **A. Blood cultures**
- ❑ **B. Chest x-ray**
- ❑ **C. Chest CT scan**
- ❑ **D. Sputum culture and Gram stain**

Key Concept/Objective: To understand the diagnosis of anthrax

There is no rapid screening test to diagnose inhalational anthrax in its early stages. In persons with a compatible clinical illness for whom there is a heightened suspicion of anthrax based on clinical and epidemiologic data, the appropriate initial diagnostic tests are (1) a chest x-ray, chest CT scan, or both and (2) culture and smear of peripheral blood. Mediastinal widening or hyperdense mediastinal lymphadenopathy (secondary to hemorrhagic lymph nodes) on a nonenhanced CT scan should raise the suspicion of pulmonary anthrax. Most persons with flulike illnesses do not have radiologic findings of pneumonia; those findings occur most often in the very young, the elderly, and persons with chronic lung disease. Pleural fluid and cerebrospinal fluid, as well as biopsy specimens taken from the pleura and lung, are also potentially useful for culture and other testing when disease is present in these sites, whereas sputum culture and Gram stain are unlikely to be useful. *(Answer: D—Sputum culture and Gram stain)*

25. A 56-year-old African-American woman comes to the clinic with complaints of blurred vision, difficulty speaking, and difficulty swallowing solids and liquids. She has recently returned from North Africa, where she serves in a United States government post. Upon further questioning, she remembers that some other people in her office had similar symptoms. Review of systems reveals xerostomia, nausea, and constipation. Physical examination reveals a middle-aged woman who is alert and oriented. There is prominent bilateral ptosis, and the patient has 4+/5 strength in deltoids and triceps bilaterally. Sensory examination is unremarkable.

What is the most likely diagnosis for this patient, given her constellation of symptoms?

- ❑ **A. Guillain-Barré syndrome**
- ❑ **B. Myasthenia gravis**
- ❑ **C. Botulism**
- ❑ **D. Cerebral vascular accident**

Key Concept/Objective: To understand the symptoms and signs of botulism

The incubation period for foodborne botulism is 2 hours to 8 days; the typical incubation period is 12 to 72 hours. The so-called classic triad of botulism summarizes the clinical presentation: an afebrile patient, symmetrical descending flaccid paralysis with prominent bulbar palsies, and a clear sensorium. Clinical hallmarks include ptosis, blurred vision, and the so-called four Ds: diplopia, dysarthria, dysphonia, and dysphagia. Cranial nerve abnormalities and bulbar weakness are followed by symmetrical descending weakness and paralysis with progression from the head to the arms, thorax, and legs. Anticholinergic symptoms are common; such symptoms include dry mouth, ileus, constipation, nausea and vomiting, urinary retention, and mydriasis. The differential diagnosis of botulism includes stroke, myasthenia gravis, Guillain-Barré syndrome, tick paralysis; poliomyelitis; Eaton-Lambert syndrome; paralytic shellfish poisoning; pufferfish ingestion; and anticholinesterase intoxication with organophos-

phates, atropine, carbon monoxide, or aminoglycosides. Because other people in the office where this patient worked had similar symptoms and because it is likely they shared a common source of food, botulism poisoning should be highly suspected. *(Answer: C—Botulism)*

26. A 45-year-old Asian man who is currently serving in the United States Marine Corps comes to the emergency department because of fever, which has persisted for 8 days. He reports returning from the Middle East 2 days ago. He states that, before his departure, several other marines had become ill and that some of them were so ill that they had to be transported to a hospital off the base. His symptoms also include headache, muscle aches, diarrhea with blood, and a rash on his extremities. On physical examination, the patient's temperature is 103.4° F (39.7° C); his heart rate is 73 beats/min; his respiratory rate is 23 breaths/min; and his blood pressure is 103/67 mm Hg. The patient is in moderate distress. Petechiae are noted on the oral pharynx. The lungs show crackles throughout. A digital rectal examination is positive for heme. The skin shows diffuse purpura.

On the basis of World Health Organization (WHO) data, which of the following findings would NOT support the diagnosis of acute hemorrhagic fever?

- ❑ **A. Temperature of 101° F (38.3° C) persisting for more than 1 month**
- ❑ **B. Blood in stools**
- ❑ **C. Severe illness and no predisposing factors for hemorrhagic manifestations**
- ❑ **D. Hemorrhagic rash**

Key Concept/Objective: To understand the diagnosis and presentation of hemorrhagic fever viruses

Initial symptoms of the acute hemorrhagic fever virus syndrome may include fever, headache, myalgia, rash, nausea, vomiting, diarrhea, abdominal pain, arthralgias, myalgias, and malaise. Illness caused by Ebola virus, Marburg virus, Rift Valley fever virus, yellow fever virus, Omsk hemorrhagic fever virus, and Kyasanur Forest disease virus has an abrupt onset, whereas Lassa fever and the diseases caused by Machupo, Junin, Guarinito, and Sabia viruses have a more insidious onset. Initial signs may include fever, tachypnea, relative bradycardia, hypotension (which may progress to circulatory shock), conjunctival injection, pharyngitis, and lymphadenopathy. Hemorrhagic symptoms, when they occur, develop later in the course of illness and include petechiae, purpura, bleeding into mucous membranes and conjunctiva, hematuria, hematemesis, and melena. Hepatic involvement is common, and renal involvement is proportional to cardiovascular compromise. Clinical diagnostic criteria based on WHO surveillance standards for acute hemorrhagic fever syndrome include temperature greater than 101° F (38.3° C) of less than 3 weeks' duration; severe illness and no predisposing factors for hemorrhagic manifestations; and at least two of the following hemorrhagic symptoms: hemorrhagic or purple rash, epistaxis, hematemesis, hematuria, hemoptysis, blood in stools, or other hemorrhagic symptom with no established alternative diagnosis. *(Answer: A—Temperature of 101° F [38.3° C] persisting for more than 1 month)*

For more information, see Duchin JS: 8 Interdisciplinary Medicine: V Bioterrorism. ACP Medicine Online (www.acpmedicine.com). Dale DC, Federman DD, Eds. WebMD Inc., New York, June 2004

Assessment of the Geriatric Patient

27. A 90-year-old man presents to his primary care physician with his 87-year-old wife, who is his primary caregiver. The patient has fallen once at home, and his appetite has diminished recently. The physician adjusts the patient's antihypertensive regimen, and the patient is scheduled to undergo a follow-up examination in 3 months. He returns in 3 months after having fallen two more times. He is generally failing to thrive.

Which of the following interventions is NOT consistent with the general principles of geriatric assessment?

- ❑ A Arranging for the patient to see a social worker, physical therapist, and home nurse in addition to his primary care physician
- ❑ B. Addressing the falls to prevent injury from subsequent falls
- ❑ C. Monitoring results of dietary recommendations to assess improvement in intake
- ❑ D. Always placing the physician in charge of the geriatric assessment team because he is most qualified to direct patient care
- ❑ E. Questioning the patient about issues related to sexuality

Key Concept/Objective: To understand the fundamental principles of geriatric assessment

General features of geriatric assessment include the following: (1) an interdisciplinary team approach to patient care; (2) a focus on prevention, including the prevention of decline (maintaining functional status); and (3) a feedback loop to promote adherence to recommendations by other health care providers, patients, and caregivers, as well as to promote patient self-efficacy or confidence in the ability to perform specific activities. This patient will benefit from seeing members of an interdisciplinary team, with team leadership rotating, depending on the major concern for the patient at any particular time. The prevention of falls will promote well-being. Addressing sexuality in this age group represents another form of preventive care that may require special intervention. Any intervention, such as a dietary modification, needs to be monitored for success or failure so that further adjustments can be made. *(Answer: D—Always placing the physician in charge of the geriatric assessment team because he is most qualified to direct patient care)*

28. An 85-year-old man is admitted to a geriatric acute care unit from home for treatment of nausea and vomiting related to a urinary tract infection.

Which of the following statements does NOT accurately characterize the benefits of a geriatric acute care unit over a general inpatient ward?

- ❑ A. The geriatric acute care unit provides a specially prepared environment
- ❑ B. Patients who receive care in a geriatric acute care unit have improved functional status 3 months after discharge, compared with those in a general inpatient ward
- ❑ C. The geriatric acute care unit provides patient-centered care that emphasizes independence
- ❑ D. There is an increased likelihood that patients receiving care in a geriatric acute care unit will be able to return home upon discharge
- ❑ E. The geriatric acute care unit provides intensive review of medical care to minimize the adverse effects of medications

Key Concept/Objective: To understand the benefits of specialized geriatric inpatient care

Geriatric acute care units were designed to improve functional outcomes for older patients. The programs comprise four key elements: (1) a specially prepared environment (e.g., uncluttered hallways, large clocks and calendars, and handrails); (2) patient-centered care emphasizing independence, including specific protocols for prevention of disability and for rehabilitation; (3) discharge planning, with the goal of returning the patient home; and (4) intensive review of medical care to minimize the adverse effects of procedures and medications. A randomized, controlled trial of 651 acutely ill patients 70 years of age or older demonstrated that at the time of hospital discharge, patients admitted to the geriatric acute care unit were better able to perform basic activities of daily living and were more likely to return home. However, by 90 days after discharge, the functional status of patients receiving care in the acute care unit was similar to those receiving usual care. *(Answer: B—Patients who receive care in a geriatric acute care unit have improved functional status 3 months after discharge, compared with those in a general inpatient ward)*

29. A 90-year-old man is brought by his daughter to see a geriatrician for the first time. He had formerly been cared for by a general internist. The geriatrician employs a trained receptionist, a nurse practitioner, and a social worker to help perform geriatric assessment on her patients.

Which of the following statements regarding outpatient geriatric assessment for this patient is false?

- ❑ **A. The patient completes a questionnaire in the waiting room to screen for common conditions in older persons**
- ❑ **B. The patient completes easily observed tasks, and his performance is assessed**
- ❑ **C. The daughter may be less likely to report increased burden of care during the ensuing year**
- ❑ **D. The cost of the assessment is covered by Medicare**

Key Concept/Objective: To understand methods of geriatric assessment in the outpatient setting

Outpatient geriatric assessment programs may be used as an adjunct to or a substitute for routine primary care. These programs utilize self-administered questionnaires to screen for common conditions in older persons. Patients can complete these questionnaires themselves or with the assistance of a trained receptionist. The questionnaire can be used to evaluate malnutrition, visual impairment, hearing loss, cognitive impairment, urinary incontinence, depression, physical limitations, and reduced leg mobility. The patient may be asked to perform easily observed tasks that relate to daily life, such as instrumental and basic activities of daily living. Outpatient geriatric assessment can benefit caregivers as well as patients. At present, Medicare does not cover hospital or physician geriatric assessment services. *(Answer: D—The cost of the assessment is covered by Medicare)*

30. A 76-year-old woman who is recovering from a hip fracture is hospitalized at a regional hospital, where she is to undergo geriatric assessment.

Which of the following statements regarding geriatric assessment units is true?

- ❑ **A. Although geriatric assessment units improve quality of life, they do not affect the risk of nursing home placement**
- ❑ **B. The costs associated with geriatric assessment units are universally offset by decreased institutional charges the following year**
- ❑ **C. A shortage of trained geriatricians nationwide may prevent formation of a formal geriatric assessment unit**
- ❑ **D. Geriatric assessment units are more likely to be found in the private setting because of their ability to generate revenue**

Key Concept/Objective: To understand the role of formal geriatric assessment programs

Treatment in a geriatric assessment unit results in improved function and decreased risk of nursing home placement. The availability of formal geriatric assessment programs is limited because of the nationwide shortage of trained geriatricians. Assessment programs are more likely to be found in large regional or academic medical centers. *(Answer: C—A shortage of trained geriatricians nationwide may prevent formation of a formal geriatric assessment unit)*

For more information, see Edelberg HK: 8 Interdisciplinary Medicine: VIII Assessment of the Geriatric Patient. ACP Medicine Online (www.acpmedicine.com). Dale DC, Federman DD, Eds. WebMD Inc., New York, September 2002

Disorders in Geriatric Patients

31. A 79-year-old woman is admitted to the hospital with productive cough, fever, and dyspnea. She has a fever of 101.9° F (38.8° C) and rales in the right base of her posterior lung fields. A chest x-ray reveals a

right-lower-lobe infiltrate. The patient is treated with a third-generation cephalosporin and a macrolide for community-acquired pneumonia. On her second day of hospitalization, the patient becomes becomes acutely confused, is throwing food in the room, and is attempting to get out of bed.

Which of the following statements regarding delirium in the elderly patient is false?

- ❑ **A. In medically ill patients, delirium is most commonly associated with acute infections, hypoxemia, hypotension, and the use of psychoactive medications**
- ❑ **B. By definition, delirium can be an acute or chronic disorder**
- ❑ **C. Medications frequently associated with delirium include antiarrhythmic agents, tricyclic antidepressants, neuroleptics, gastrointestinal medications, and antihistamines**
- ❑ **D. Patients with delirium can have perceptual disturbances such as hallucinations and can have a fluctuating level of alertness**

Key Concept/Objective: To understand the definition, etiology, and clinical features of delirium

Common causes of cognitive dysfunction in elderly patients are delirium, dementia, and depression. Delirium, an acute disorder of attention and global cognitive function, is a common and potentially preventable cause of adverse health outcomes. The criteria for delirium caused by a general medical condition include the following: disturbance of consciousness (i.e., reduced awareness of the environment), with reduced ability to focus, sustain, or shift attention; change in cognition (e.g., memory deficit, disorientation, language disturbance) or perceptual disturbance that is not better accounted for by a preexisting, established, or evolving dementia; increased or reduced psychomotor activity; disorganized sleep-wake cycle; acute onset of disturbance (usually hours to days), with fluctuation over the course of the day; and evidence from the history, physical examination, or laboratory findings that the disturbance is caused by an etiologically related general medical condition. Independent risk factors for delirium in elderly medical patients during hospitalization include the use of psychoactive medications, severe illness, cognitive impairment (dementia), vision impairment, and a high ratio of BUN to creatinine, implying dehydration. Precipitating factors for delirium in hospitalized elderly persons include the use of physical restraints, more than three medications added to the patient's drug regimen, bladder catheterization, and any iatrogenic event (e.g., unintentional injury). In medically ill patients, delirium is most commonly associated with acute infections, such as pneumonia and urosepsis; hypoxemia; hypotension; and the use of psychoactive medications. Psychoactive medications include many antiarrhythmic agents, tricyclic antidepressants, neuroleptics, gastrointestinal medications, and antihistamines. When used in large doses or in combination at therapeutic doses, these agents may induce delirium. The patient with delirium presents with an acute change in mental status and clinical features of disturbed consciousness, impaired cognition, and a fluctuating course. Perceptual disturbances, such as misperceptions, illusions or frank delusions, and hallucinations, are often accompanied by increased psychomotor activity. Most patients with delirium vacillate between hypoalertness and hyperalertness. *(Answer: B—By definition, delirium can be an acute or chronic disorder)*

32. A 76-year-old white woman presents to your clinic with a complaint of incontinence. She says that she has had this problem for "years" and has never undergone evaluation for it. She denies having dysuria or hematuria. The patient has five grown children.

Which of the following statements regarding urinary incontinence in the geriatric population is true?

- ❑ **A. The most common predisposing factors are overactive bladder resulting from changes in the bladder smooth muscle; prostatic hypertrophy; bladder wall relaxation or prolapse; medication side effects; and cognitive impairment**
- ❑ **B. The preferred management strategy includes thorough diagnostic workup before implementation of therapy, because empirical management is largely unsuccessful**

❑ C. In female patients with stress incontinence, first-line therapy includes medications

❑ D. To be considered abnormal, the postvoiding residual volume (PVR) of urine must be greater than 500 ml

Key Concept/Objective: To understand the causes, diagnostic workup, and management of urinary incontinence in the geriatric population

Urinary incontinence—the involuntary loss of urine of sufficient severity to be a social or health problem—is a common, costly, and potentially disabling condition that is never a consequence of normal aging. It is always treatable and often curable. An overactive bladder associated with changes in the smooth muscle of the bladder, prostatic hyperplasia in men, bladder wall relaxation or prolapse in women, medication side effects, and cognitive impairment are the most common factors predisposing older patients to urinary incontinence. Acute incontinence typically has a sudden onset and is associated with an acute illness (e.g., infection or delirium) or iatrogenic event (e.g., polypharmacy or restricted mobility). There are four basic types of established incontinence: stress, urge, overflow, and functional incontinence. In patients with established incontinence, blood tests should measure renal function, electrolytes, blood glucose, and serum calcium; these measurements help to exclude polyuric conditions that may cause incontinence. The most useful bedside test of lower urinary tract function is measurement of the PVR urine. Accurate measurement of the PVR is most often accomplished by straight catheterization of the urinary bladder after the patient attempts complete voiding. Pelvic ultrasonography and portable bladder scanning are safe and accurate alternative methods of estimating PVR. A PVR of less than 50 ml of urine is considered normal. A PVR of greater than 150 ml is abnormal even in elderly patients and indicates the need for further urologic evaluation or repeat measurement of PVR. Strategies for the management of urinary incontinence include behavioral modification techniques, medications, patient and caregiver education, surgical procedures, catheter placement, and incontinence supplies. The acute onset of incontinence should be evaluated and treated promptly. Urinary tract infection, acute urinary retention, stool impaction, and adverse effects of medications (e.g., diuretics) should be excluded. After the initial diagnostic evaluation, most patients should be treated on the basis of the most likely type of incontinence. This empirical approach will lead to successful management of a large percentage of incontinent patients. In female outpatients, behavioral interventions (e.g., biofeedback), bladder training, and pelvic muscle exercises are effective first-line therapies for established stress incontinence. Medications play a modest role in the treatment of stress incontinence. *(Answer: A—The most common predisposing factors are overactive bladder resulting from changes in the bladder smooth muscle; prostatic hypertrophy; bladder wall relaxation or prolapse; medication side effects; and cognitive impairment)*

33. An 80-year-old man comes to your clinic accompanied by his daughter. She is concerned because her father recently lost his balance while walking through the house. The daughter explains that if she hadn't been walking with her father, he would have fallen and injured himself. He has hypertension, benign prostatic hypertrophy, and coronary artery disease but is able to perform activities of daily living.

Which of the following statements regarding the primary care assessment of gait and falls in elderly patients is false?

❑ A. Older patients should be assessed yearly for risk of falls

❑ B. Risk factors for falls include weakness, gait and balance deficits, visual impairment, depression, poor lighting, and loose carpet in the home

❑ C. Exercise programs such as Tai Chi have not been shown to reduce the fall rate, although they do improve balance

❑ D. Medications associated with falls include loop diuretics, vasodilators, adrenergic antagonists, antidepressants, and sedative-hypnotic agents

Key Concept/Objective: To understand the risk factors for falls in the geriatric population, as well as the prevention and management of falls in this population

Accidental falls are common and potentially preventable causes of morbidity and mortality in elderly adults. The risk factors for falls and the effectiveness of multifactorial interventions to prevent recurrent falls in carefully targeted patients are well established. Intrinsic risk factors include lower extremity weakness, poor grip strength, gait and balance deficits, impaired performance of daily activities, visual impairment, cognitive impairment, and depression. Extrinsic risk factors include use of four or more prescription drugs and environmental impediments such as poor lighting, loose carpets, and the absence of bathroom safety equipment. The maintenance of normal balance and gait requires the successful integration of sensory (afferent), central nervous (brain and spinal cord), and musculoskeletal systems. A disturbance in sensory input (e.g., peripheral neuropathy), central nervous system functioning (e.g., dementia), or motor function (e.g., arthritis or muscle weakness) will predispose elderly patients to falls. The aging process may also predispose patients to falls by increasing postural sway and reducing adaptive reflexes. Patients at risk for falls can be identified through a medical history, physical examination, and a few laboratory studies. Older persons should be asked at least once a year whether they experience falls. Among those reporting a fall, a review of the circumstances surrounding the fall, including symptoms before and after the event, provides clues to the likely causes. Medications associated with falls most notably include those that cause postural hypotension, such as loop diuretics, vasodilators, or adrenergic antagonists, and those with psychotropic properties, such as antidepressants and sedative-hypnotic agents. Successful components of interventions used in clinical trials include review and alterations in medications, balance and gait training, muscle-strengthening exercises, improvement of postural hypotension, home-hazard modifications, and specific medical and cardiovascular treatments. Tai Chi exercises to enhance balance and body awareness, when combined with balance training, may also reduce the rate of falls. A randomized trial of Tai Chi exercise for 15 weeks in 200 persons 70 years of age and older resulted in a 47% decrease in falls after a 4-month follow-up period. *(Answer: C—Exercise programs such as Tai Chi have not been shown to reduce the fall rate, although they do improve balance)*

34. A 77-year-old man presented to your clinic for evaluation 2 weeks ago and was noted to be hypertensive (this was the second time his blood pressure was determined to be elevated). The patient was started on a diuretic and an ACE inhibitor for his hypertension. He was also started on a regimen of daily low-dose aspirin. Today the patient is brought in by family members for evaluation of confusion. They state that his change in mental status is new and began after he started taking his new medications.

Which of the following statements regarding iatrogenic illness in the geriatric population is false?

- ❑ A. **The most common documented cause of iatrogenic illness is adverse drug reactions, usually associated with polypharmacy**
- ❑ B. **Because most drugs are eliminated via the hepatic system, lower maintenance doses of medications are needed to avoid iatrogenic side effects of prescribed medications**
- ❑ C. **Ways to prevent nosocomial infections include hand washing, elevating the patient's head to prevent aspiration, and using narrow-spectrum antibiotic agents when indicated**
- ❑ D. **Drug distribution is altered by aging, primarily because of body-composition changes, with a decrease in total body water and lean body mass and a relative increase in body fat**

Key Concept/Objective: To understand the most common causes of iatrogenic illnesses in geriatric patients and how to prevent them

Iatrogenic, or physician-induced, illness results from a diagnostic procedure or therapeutic intervention that is not a natural consequence of the patient's disease. Iatrogenic illnesses include complications of drug therapy and of diagnostic or therapeutic procedures, nosocomial infections, fluid and electrolyte disorders, and trauma. The most

common documented cause of iatrogenic illness is adverse drug reactions, usually associated with polypharmacy. Adverse drug events are more likely to occur in elderly patients because of the age-related changes in drug metabolism, the occurrence of multiple comorbidities, and the use of polypharmacy. The incidence of adverse drug reactions increases with advancing age and the number of chronic diseases requiring drug therapy. The concomitant use of several medications increases the risk of drug interactions, unwanted effects, and adverse reactions. Many medications should be used with special caution in elderly patients because of age-related changes in drug pharmacokinetics (drug disposition) and pharmacodynamics (target tissue effects). Although drug absorption is not reduced in healthy elderly persons, absorption of medications can be reduced by disease states (e.g., malabsorption) or concomitant administration of drugs that decrease absorption of medications (e.g., antacids). Drug distribution is altered by aging, primarily because of body-composition changes, with a decrease in total body water and lean body mass and a relative increase in body fat. Consequently, water-soluble drugs achieve a higher serum concentration, whereas lipid-soluble drugs have a prolonged elimination half-life. Drug elimination is mainly influenced by renal function. The age-associated decrease in renal function, which results in decreased creatinine clearance, necessitates lower maintenance doses of renally excreted drugs in elderly patients. The prevention of iatrogenic illness resulting from the inappropriate prescribing of drugs begins with an understanding of the rational use of medications in elderly patients. In general, prescribing the fewest medications at the lowest needed dosages is a rational approach to the prevention of iatrogenic illness. Nosocomial pathogens are primarily transmitted through contact with hospital or nursing home personnel. Nosocomial infection can be prevented by washing hands and cleaning medical equipment (e.g., stethoscopes) between patient contacts, by wearing gloves during invasive procedures or during contact with wounds or mucous membranes, by using aseptic techniques when inserting or changing urinary catheters, by isolating infected patients (e.g., in nursing homes), by elevating the patient's head (to lessen the risk of aspiration), by replacing broad-spectrum antibiotics with narrow-spectrum antibiotics on the basis of bacterial sensitivity reports, and by limiting the use of urinary catheters. Prophylactic antimicrobial therapies and routine catheter replacement are not recommended. *(Answer: B—Because most drugs are eliminated via the hepatic system, lower maintenance doses of medications are needed to avoid iatrogenic side effects of prescribed medications)*

35. An 80-year-old male nursing home resident with a history of Alzheimer disease, atrial fibrillation, and congestive heart failure is admitted to the hospital with pneumonia and poor oral intake. His medications include lisinopril, warfarin, donepezil, and digoxin. The initial examination reveals a cognitively impaired man who is alert and oriented to person and place. The patient's score on the Mini-Mental State examination is 24/30. After 48 hours, you are called to see him because of altered mental status. Nurses report that over the past shift, the patient has become increasingly disoriented and agitated. On examination, he has a temperature of 100.4° F (38° C), he is lethargic, and he cannot sustain attention or follow commands.

Which of the following statements regarding the development of delirium is false?

- ❑ **A. The most important risk factor for delirium in this patient is his underlying dementia**
- ❑ **B. The therapeutic dosage of digoxin excludes this medication as a contributing cause of this patient's delirium**
- ❑ **C. Delirium develops in up to 15% of older hospitalized patients**
- ❑ **D. This patient's risk of mortality or of further decline in activities of daily living and cognitive function is significantly higher than would be the case in a similar patient who has not experienced delirium**
- ❑ **E. The use of physical restraints has been associated with the precipitation of delirium in elderly hospitalized patients**

Key Concept/Objective: To understand the significant risks of delirium in elderly hospitalized patients

Elderly patients are at increased risk for developing delirium during hospitalization. Delirium is an important condition to recognize, as the majority of cases are reversible with treatment of the underlying illness. Dementia or cognitive impairment is the single most important risk factor for the development of delirium. Other factors include acute infections, hypoxemia, and medications with psychoactive or anticholinergic effects. Cardiac medications such as digoxin and other antiarrhythmics can also cause delirium; elderly patients may be susceptible even when taking the drug at therapeutic doses. In addition, studies have linked the use of physical restraints and the addition of more than three medications to a patient's regimen during hospitalization to the development of delirium. In a multicenter cohort study, delirium in the hospital setting was associated with higher rates of mortality and future nursing home admissions. *(Answer: B—The therapeutic dosage of digoxin excludes this medication as a contributing cause of this patient's delirium)*

36. A 71-year-old woman presents to your clinic complaining of urinary incontinence of several months' duration. She has hypertension that is well controlled on hydrochlorothiazide. She states that intermittently, she experiences a sudden overwhelming need to void, which often results in loss of urine before she is able to reach the toilet. She denies having dysuria or abdominal pain. She is otherwise active and highly functional but has lately been limiting her social activities because of embarrassment. She has no loss of urine with coughing or ambulation. Her physical examination is unremarkable, and the results of urinalysis are within normal limits. Postvoid residual urine volume obtained in the office is 45 ml.

What is the appropriate classification and the best initial approach to the management of this patient's urinary incontinence?

- ❑ A. **Stress incontinence; prescribe an intravaginal estrogen preparation and consider surgical referral**
- ❑ B. **Overflow incontinence; discontinue the diuretic and teach the patient intermittent self-catheterization**
- ❑ C. **Urge incontinence; recommend behavioral therapies, including scheduled voiding and bladder retraining**
- ❑ D. **Functional incontinence; reassure the patient that the changes are age-related, and recommend diapers during excursions out of the house**
- ❑ E. **Detrusor hyperactivity secondary to chronic urinary tract infection; check urine culture and prescribe appropriate antibiotics**

Key Concept/Objective: To recognize and treat urinary incontinence in the elderly

Urinary incontinence is an important condition in elderly patients; it is not a normal consequence of aging and is often curable. This patient describes symptoms of urge incontinence caused by involuntary detrusor muscle contractions at relatively low bladder volumes. Urge incontinence can be improved with bladder retraining and scheduled voiding. Additionally, bladder relaxant medications such as oxybutinin or tolterodine are frequently helpful. This patient's history is not suggestive of stress incontinence, which would be characterized by loss of variable amounts of urine with coughing or straining and is caused by failure of sphincter mechanisms to remain closed during bladder filling. This patient's normal postvoid residual urine volume (less than 50 ml) helps rule out overflow incontinence, which is caused by detrusor inactivity or bladder outlet obstruction. Functional incontinence describes an inability or refusal to toilet, usually as a result of cognitive impairment or physical limitations. There is no evidence on urinalysis that this patient has a urinary tract infection, and culture in this setting would not be helpful. *(Answer: C—Urge incontinence; recommend behavioral therapies, including scheduled voiding and bladder retraining)*

37. An 86-year-old resident of a long-term care facility who has suffered multiple strokes in the past is noted to have an ulcer measuring 2 × 2 cm over the sacrum. On examination, the wound appears to extend partially through the dermis but not to the fascial plane (i.e., the patient has a stage II ulcer). There is minimal surrounding erythema and no apparent eschar formation or undermining.

Which of the following interventions is most likely to prevent progression and promote healing of the ulcer?

- ❑ **A. Daily topical antibiotic therapy with silver sulfadiazene**
- ❑ **B. Dressings with povidone-iodine–soaked gauze applied daily**
- ❑ **C. Sharp debridement followed by wet-to-dry dressings**
- ❑ **D. Frequent turning and use of a low-air-loss mattress to reduce pressure under bony prominences**
- ❑ **E. Initiation of tube feeding to improve nutrition**

Key Concept/Objective: To understand the treatment of pressure ulcers in the elderly

Pressure is the most important factor in the development and progression of pressure ulcers. Other etiologic factors include shearing forces, moisture, and injury from friction. The first step in managing ulcers of all stages is pressure reduction. This patient does not have evidence of full-thickness ulcer or eschar that would require surgical debridement. Topical antibiotics are appropriate for use in clean ulcers that are not healing with pressure relief and dressings, but their use alone is unlikely to result in healing. It is also important to optimize nutrition to promote wound healing, but it would be inappropriate to initiate tube feeding without first attempting local measures, such as pressure relief and use of wet-to-dry dressings with saline-soaked gauze. Povidone-iodine should not be applied to open wounds because of its toxic cellular effects. *(Answer: D—Frequent turning and use of a low-air-loss mattress to reduce pressure under bony prominences)*

38. A 78-year-old man is brought to clinic from a nursing home for evaluation after a fall. He has a history of hypertension, benign prostatic hypertrophy, and Parkinson disease, which was diagnosed 5 years ago. The fall was unwitnessed and occurred shortly after the patient had breakfast. He was awake and oriented to person and place after the fall. His medications include terazosin, hydrochlorothiazide, aspirin, carbidopa-levodopa, and temazepam. On physical examination, the patient appears frail; he has an unsteady, shuffling gait, and he uses a cane for support. No significant change in heart rate or blood pressure is found on orthostatic testing. There is a contusion over the left trochanter. Radiography is negative for fracture.

Which of the following statements regarding falls in nursing home residents receiving long-term care is false?

- ❑ **A. There is a consistent association between falling and the use of psychotropic medications such as neuroleptics and antidepressants**
- ❑ **B. Widespread use of physical restraints has been shown to reduce the rates of falls in long-term care facilities**
- ❑ **C. The incidence of falls among nursing home residents is close to three times that of the community-dwelling elderly**
- ❑ **D. A timed "get up and go" test performed in clinic (consisting of observing the patient stand up, walk 10 ft, turn, walk back, and sit down unassisted) is a valid tool that can predict gait impairment and falls**
- ❑ **E. A significant proportion of patients who fall develop a fear of falling that is itself associated with an increased risk of gait problems**

Key Concept/Objective: To know the risk factors for falls in elderly patients

Accidental falls are a common and serious problem in elderly patients. Multiple studies have identified risk factors for falling; these risk factors are either intrinsic (e.g., muscular weakness, poor balance) or extrinsic (e.g., poor lighting, polypharmacy). Among the most important are muscle weakness, a history of falls, gait and balance deficits, visual deficits, cognitive impairment, and age greater than 80 years. In studies both of patients receiving care in the home and of those receiving care in long-term care facilities, an association between psychotropic medications and falls has been demonstrated. The

American Geriatrics Society recommends that all older persons be asked at least once a year about falls, and any patient who reports a single fall should be observed performing "get up and go" maneuvers (described in choice D).[1] Patients demonstrating difficulty with this test should undergo further assessment, including review of the circumstances associated with the fall, medications, and directed assessment of vision and neurologic and cardiac function, as indicated. There is no evidence to support the routine use of restraints for the prevention of falls, given their significant drawbacks, which include deconditioning, depression, and development of pressure sores. *(Answer: B—Widespread use of physical restraints has been shown to reduce the rates of falls in long-term care facilities)*

1. Guideline for the prevention of falls in older persons. American Geriatrics Society, British Geriatrics Society, and American Academy of Orthopaedic Surgeons Panel on Falls Prevention. J Am Geriatr Soc 49:664, 2001

For more information, see Palmer RM: 8 Interdisciplinary Medicine: IX Management of Common Clinical Disorders in Geriatric Patients. ACP Medicine Online (www.acpmedicine.com). Dale DC, Federman DD, Eds. WebMD Inc., New York, August 2004

Rehabilitation of Geriatric Patients

39. A 75-year-old male patient is considered to be medically stable for discharge after suffering a stroke 5 days ago. His neurologic deficits include hemiplegia of his right arm and mild cognitive disturbances; he scored 2.0 on the Orpington Prognostic Scale. His medical history is significant for diabetes and hypertension, which is well controlled. Before his stroke, he was living by himself.

Which of the following is true regarding rehabilitation for this patient?

- ❑ A. **Rehabilitation should be deferred until the patient is discharged from the hospital, and the patient should receive therapy in an outpatient setting**
- ❑ B. **His initial Orpington Prognostic Scale score indicates only a 20% chance of independence in personal care and homemaking activities at 6 months**
- ❑ C. **Rehabilitation efforts need not be extended beyond the first 3 months, because functional recovery will not occur after this period**
- ❑ D. **The patient should be screened and treated for depression during rehabilitation**
- ❑ E. **During the rehabilitation of his right hemiplegia, aggressive therapy can be undertaken without concern for pain or shoulder dislocation, owing to muscle flaccidity**

Key Concept/Objective: To understand the rehabilitation for geriatric stroke patients

Major depression occurs in at least one third of patients after stroke. Poststroke rehabilitation should include screening for and treatment of this commonly overlooked complication. Increased socialization, counseling, and medication are appropriate. Cognitive impairment caused by depression may improve with treatment of depression and use of medications that cause less sedation and fewer anticholinergic side effects. In the first weeks after stroke, the patient's motor function, sensory function, balance, and cognition can be assessed through use of the Orpington Prognostic Scale. The patient's score is a strong predictor of functional status at 3 and 6 months; a score of 2.4 or less is associated with an 80% chance of the patient's being independent with regard to personal care and homemaking activities at 6 months. The potential for neuroplastic change is revolutionizing approaches to neurologic rehabilitation. The potential for neural reorganization is also changing the timing of rehabilitation; recent studies have demonstrated significant gains in function in chronic stroke patients who undergo treatments that focus on repetitive and forced practice. Shoulder pain and dislocation are especially likely in patients with a flaccid upper extremity, and reflex sympathetic dystrophy occurs in as many as 25% of patients with hemiplegia. *(Answer: D—The patient should be screened and treated for depression during rehabilitation)*

40. A 76-year-old female patient with diabetes and severe peripheral vascular disease undergoes a left below-the-knee amputation. Before the surgery, she was ambulatory and had no difficulty in weight bearing with the contralateral leg. Her diabetes is moderately well stabilized with insulin, and she has no other medical history. She smokes approximately 1 pack of cigarettes a day and has been doing so for 50 years.

Which of the following is NOT a key aspect in rehabilitation for this patient?

- ❑ **A. The patient should be counseled to stop smoking to promote wound healing and decrease the risk of future amputations**
- ❑ **B. The patient should be instructed as to the proper care of the contralateral leg**
- ❑ **C. The physician should be actively involved in the choice of the prosthetic limb and in the training of the patient**
- ❑ **D. Weight bearing and mobilization should be delayed until full healing of the residual limb has taken place**
- ❑ **E. Early angioplasty of the contralateral leg should be performed to prevent the need for its amputation**

Key Concept/Objective: To understand the rehabilitation of geriatric amputation patients

Early mobilization using a rigid, removable dressing and sometimes a temporary artificial leg can simultaneously protect the fragile healing tissues and prevent complications caused by prolonged immobility. About 25% of patients who undergo unilateral amputation because of peripheral vascular disease and 50% of patients who undergo the procedure because of diabetes will need to have the other leg amputated within 5 years. Care of the contralateral extremity is essential, and each amputee should have a program of regular foot care that includes checking for foot lesions; in addition, each amputee should practice peripheral vascular control measures, including smoking cessation and control of diabetes. Smoking delays wound healing. The role of angioplasty in reducing the need for amputation is unclear. Successful prosthetic ambulation depends on selection of an appropriate device, progressive ambulation, and management of concurrent problems. The physician should form a relationship with a reputable prosthetist who can integrate the technical issues involved in designing a prosthetic with the medical and functional status of the amputee. The prosthetic limb should be adapted to existing comorbidity, and the patient should be examined for signs of skin breakdown, edema, and infection occurring in association with use of the prosthesis. *(Answer: D—Weight bearing and mobilization should be delayed until full healing of the residual limb has taken place)*

41. An 87-year-old woman with severe dementia and advanced renal disease sustains a nondisplacement fracture across the trochanter of the left hip. She is a nursing home resident but was able to ambulate with assistance before sustaining the hip fracture.

When considering rehabilitation for this patient, which of the following considerations is most pertinent?

- ❑ **A. An inpatient multidisciplinary approach to rehabilitation can significantly improve the prognosis after surgery**
- ❑ **B. Rehabilitation without surgical intervention would be beneficial**
- ❑ **C. To prevent complications, early mobilization should be avoided in this patient**
- ❑ **D. This type of hip fracture is associated with avascular necrosis and nonunion**
- ❑ **E. This type of hip fracture usually requires a complete hip arthroplasty**

Key Concept/Objective: To understand the importance of rehabilitation for geriatric patients with hip fractures

Rehabilitation should be offered to all patients in the absence of near-terminal conditions and possibly to bedridden patients with end-stage dementia. Such patients may

be treated nonsurgically with early mobilization from bed to chair, control of pain, and treatment of complications. Patients with even mild to moderate dementia can benefit from rehabilitation after fracture. Hip fractures in elderly patients result in increased mortality. For such patients, 1-year mortality is 20%. After hip fracture, the care setting may not influence outcome much, and coordinated multidisciplinary approaches to inpatient rehabilitation of older patients have been found to have borderline effectiveness in reducing outcomes such as death and institutionalization. Early mobilization reduces all the complications of immobility, including bedsores, constipation, loss of strength, and risk of thromboembolism. Two thirds of hip fractures occur across the trochanter. Intertrochanteric fractures are often associated with significant bleeding into the surrounding soft tissue. Femoral neck fractures occur in the remaining one third of hip fractures; such fractures are likely to disrupt blood supply to the femoral head and may lead to avascular necrosis and nonunion. Surgical treatment of trochanteric fractures usually consists of open reduction and internal fixation, but femoral neck fractures may require complete hip arthroplasty. *(Answer: B—Rehabilitation without surgical intervention would be beneficial)*

42. An 82-year-old male patient with severe osteoarthritis of his left knee has been advised to have a total left knee replacement by an orthopedist. Until now, he has needed narcotic pain medications. He has diabetes and hypertension, both of which are moderately well controlled. He inquires about rehabilitation after the surgery.

Which of the following is true regarding rehabilitation after total knee replacement?

- ❑ A. **Total knee replacement in patients older than 80 years is associated with an increased rate of complications and increased length of hospital stay**
- ❑ B. **Strength training is an important component of rehabilitation and should be instituted within the first week after surgery**
- ❑ C. **After surgery, long-term benefits of rehabilitation include significant pain relief, improved function, and an increase in strength and mobility to a degree that is similar to that of other persons of the same age**
- ❑ D. **Aggressive physical therapy alone is adequate in the rehabilitation process after surgery**
- ❑ E. **Use of a machine that provides continuous passive motion helps with recovery and may shorten the length of stay in the hospital**

Key Concept/Objective: To understand the rehabilitation of geriatric arthroplasty patients

Improved range of motion is a critical step in recovery after below-the-knee amputations and is often aided by the use of a continuous passive motion (CPM) machine. Early postoperative CPM has been shown to be more effective than physical therapy alone in reducing flexion contracture and shortening length of stay. Home CPM produced satisfactory range of motion at about half the cost of home physical therapy in a recent clinical trial. Joint replacement in selected patients older than 80 years does not increase complication rates or length of stay. Strength training is often deferred for several weeks to promote stable healing of tissues, and isometric and resistive exercise with gradually increasing loads can be introduced safely by 8 weeks after surgery. Long-term outcomes include significant pain relief and improved function, although many patients do not achieve levels of strength or mobility comparable to those of age-matched control subjects. *(Answer: E—Use of a machine that provides continuous passive motion helps with recovery and may shorten the length of stay in the hospital)*

For more information, see Studenski S, Brown CJ: 8 Interdisciplinary Medicine: X Rehabilitation of Geriatric Patients. ACP Medicine Online (www.acpmedicine.com). Dale DC, Federman DD, Eds. WebMD Inc., New York, March 2004

SECTION 9

METABOLISM

Diagnosis and Treatment of Dyslipidemia

1. A 46-year-old woman visits your office as a new patient. She has recently moved to town and wishes to establish new primary care. She has no complaint today. She is moderately obese, with central adiposity. She has moderate hypertension, for which she has been undergoing treatment with a thiazide diuretic. The rest of her medical history is unremarkable. Her laboratory data reveal that her renal function is normal. Her blood glucose level is in the normal range, but her triglyceride level is elevated, and her high-density lipoprotein (HDL) cholesterol level is low. The rest of the physical examination is normal.

   Which of the following statements regarding the metabolic syndrome is true?

   - ❑ **A. An accumulation of visceral rather than subcutaneous fat has been observed in individuals with the metabolic syndrome**
   - ❑ **B. First-line therapy for treatment of the metabolic syndrome is high-dose statin therapy**
   - ❑ **C. The lipid abnormalities associated with the metabolic syndrome are a very high total low-density lipoprotein (LDL) cholesterol level and normal HDL cholesterol and triglyceride levels**
   - ❑ **D. This patient should not be diagnosed as having metabolic syndrome because she meets only four of the five diagnostic criteria for that disorder**

   Key Concept/Objective: To know the characteristics of the metabolic syndrome

   An accumulation of visceral rather than subcutaneous fat has been observed in individuals with the central body fat distribution characteristic of the metabolic syndrome. The lipid abnormalities associated with the metabolic syndrome are increased levels of triglyceride; increased numbers of small, dense LDL and apolipoprotein B particles; and decreased levels of HDL_2 cholesterol. The National Cholesterol Education Program Adult Treatment Panel III has suggested five clinical variables as diagnostic criteria for the metabolic syndrome: (1) increased waist circumference, (2) increased triglyceride level, (3) decreased HDL cholesterol level, (4) increased blood pressure, and (5) elevated level of fasting plasma glucose. A diagnosis of the metabolic syndrome is made when three or more of these clinical variables are present. Aerobic exercise and a diet low in saturated fat are indicated as therapy for most people with the metabolic syndrome. More aggressive therapy is indicated if the metabolic syndrome is severe or if the patient has familial combined hyperlipidemia or type 2 diabetes mellitus. *(Answer: A—An accumulation of visceral rather than subcutaneous fat has been observed in individuals with the metabolic syndrome)*

2. A 28-year-old white man visits your office for a routine physical examination. He has had no medical problems, he exercises regularly, and his weight is very near his ideal body weight. His family history is significant in that his father and two uncles each had heart attacks and underwent revascularization procedures between the ages of 49 and 55 years. On physical examination, tendon xanthomas are noted on the Achilles tendons and the extensor tendons of the patient's hands, and bilateral xanthelasma is present. The rest of the physical examination is normal.

Which of the following statements regarding familial hypercholesterolemia (FH) is true?

- ❑ A. It is inherited in an autosomal recessive fashion
- ❑ B. It is atypical for this patient with heterozygous FH to have developed xanthomas at only 28 years of age
- ❑ C. In patients with heterozygous FH, coronary artery disease develops early, with symptoms often manifesting in men in their fourth or fifth decade
- ❑ D. Although tendon xanthomas do occur with this illness, the xanthelasmas are a highly specific finding, indicating FH in this patient

Key Concept/Objective: To understand the physical examination findings and medical implications of FH

FH is an autosomal dominant disorder caused by a mutation in the gene encoding the LDL receptor protein. Tendon xanthomas begin to appear by 20 years of age and may be present in up to 70% of older individuals. Xanthelasma (cutaneous xanthomas on the palpebra) and corneal arcus are common after 30 years of age. Tendon xanthomas are a highly specific sign of FH, but xanthelasma and corneal arcus may occur in normocholesterolemic persons. Coronary artery disease develops early, with symptoms often manifesting in men in the fourth or fifth decade. By 60 years of age, at least 50% of men with FH experience myocardial infarction; in women, symptoms tend to develop about 10 years later. *(Answer: C—In patients with heterozygous FH, coronary artery disease develops early, with symptoms often manifesting in men in their fourth or fifth decade)*

3. A 35-year-old male patient visits your office asking for information about his medical condition. He states that several years ago, his physician told him that on the basis of his cholesterol profile and the presence of characteristic skin lesions on his ankles and hands, he likely had FH. The patient chose to ignore his previous doctor's advice regarding therapy, but he has now decided that he should seek medical attention. He asks you for general information regarding the treatment of his condition.

Which of the following statements regarding the treatment of heterozygous FH is true?

- ❑ A. Because it is an acquired illness, the screening of first-degree relatives is not necessary
- ❑ B. Aggressive diet therapy alone is adequate therapy for most patients with this illness
- ❑ C. Despite appropriate therapy for this illness, tendon xanthomas will not regress
- ❑ D. Effective treatment for this illness is possible with statins, intestinally active drugs, and nicotinic acid

Key Concept/Objective: To understand the appropriate therapy for patients with FH

FH is a primary cause of isolated, severely elevated cholesterol levels. The ability to diagnose FH is valuable because affected individuals will require drug therapy from a relatively young age. Careful attention to family members is mandatory; 50% of them will be affected and will require aggressive lipid-lowering therapy. In patients with heterozygous FH, it is possible to stimulate the one normal gene; in such patients, effective treatment is possible with statins, intestinally active drugs, and nicotinic acid. Because LDL cholesterol levels tend to be very high, combination therapy with two drugs is often required, and three drugs may be necessary. Although diet therapy alone is not sufficient for patients with heterozygous FH, reducing saturated fatty acid and cholesterol intake will lower LDL levels and reduce the amount of medication required. Tendon xanthomas have been shown to regress when LDL levels are maintained in a desirable range. *(Answer: D—Effective treatment for this illness is possible with statins, intestinally active drugs, and nicotinic acid)*

For more information, see Brunzell JD: 9 Metabolism: II Diagnosis and Treatment of Dyslipidemia. ACP Medicine Online (www.acpmedicine.com). Dale DC, Federman DD, Eds. WebMD Inc., New York, January 2004

The Porphyrias

4. A concerned young mother brings her 10-month-old son to your clinic for treatment of severe sunburn. She recently took her son to the beach and noticed the rapid appearance of large blisters and erosions after only a short period in the sun. The mother reports that two uncles sunburned easily and had "blood problems." You suspect congenital erythropoietic porphyria. Urinary, fecal, and erythrocyte porphyrin levels confirm the diagnosis.

Which of the following measures has NOT been shown to be helpful for patients with erythropoietic porphyria?

- ❑ **A. Bone marrow transplantation**
- ❑ **B. Avoidance of sunlight**
- ❑ **C. Vitamin B_{12} supplementation**
- ❑ **D. Oral β-carotene**

Key Concept/Objective: To understand the treatment of congenital erythropoietic porphyria

Congenital erythropoietic porphyria is an autosomal recessive disorder that results from a deficiency of the uroporphyrinogen cosynthase enzyme. It typically presents in infancy; patients have photosensitivity, hypertrichosis, hemolytic anemia, and erythrodontia. Treatment is aimed at protection from sun damage, decreasing hemolysis, increasing red blood cell production, or curing the disorder. Avoidance of sunlight and administration of β-carotene can help prevent photosensitivity reactions. Red blood cell transfusion has been helpful transiently in decreasing hemolysis and erythropoiesis, and bone marrow transplantation is curative. Vitamin B_{12} supplementation has not been successful in the treatment of congenital erythropoietic porphyria. *(Answer: C—Vitamin B_{12} supplementation)*

5. A 24-year-old woman with a history of acute intermittent porphyria (AIP) presents to the emergency department with diffuse abdominal pain, nausea, and vomiting of 24 hours' duration. She states that her symptoms are identical to those she experiences during acute attacks of AIP.

Which of the following, if found, is NOT consistent with an acute attack of AIP?

- ❑ **A. Photosensitive rash**
- ❑ **B. Hypertension**
- ❑ **C. Peripheral neuropathy**
- ❑ **D. Seizure**

Key Concept/Objective: To know the symptoms of attacks of AIP

AIP is an autosomal dominant disorder caused by a deficiency in porphobilinogen deaminase. Its course tends to be marked by asymptomatic periods that are interrupted by acute attacks. These attacks are marked by severe abdominal complaints, including pain, which may be localized or generalized; nausea; vomiting, and bowel disturbances. Urinary complaints, tachycardia, hypertension, fever, and tremor are also common. Neurologic symptoms can include weakness, peripheral neuropathy, and seizure, particularly in patients with coexisting hyponatremia. In severe cases, the urine may be the color of port wine because of the accumulation of porphobilin. Unlike most other porphyrias, no cutaneous manifestations are associated with this enzyme deficiency. *(Answer: A—Photosensitive rash)*

6. A 26-year-old woman with known AIP is brought to the hospital with abdominal pain after using narcotic analgesics after a tooth extraction. On examination, she is found to have fever, tachycardia, hypertension, and tremor. Urinalysis shows the urine to be deep red in color; there is no evidence of red blood cells. Soon after admission to the hospital for treatment, the patient suffers a generalized tonic-clonic seizure.

Which of the following would NOT be expected to help in the treatment of this patient's exacerbation of AIP?

❑ **A. Intravenous phenobarbital**

❑ **B. Intravenous fluids with sodium chloride**

❑ **C. Intravenous fluids with dextrose**

❑ **D. Intravenous hematin**

Key Concept/Objective: To understand the treatment of an attack of AIP

This patient appears to be suffering a severe attack of AIP. Treatment of her attack is aimed at eliminating or avoiding any inciting factors; achieving appropriate volume resuscitation with attention to sodium disorders; maintaining adequate nutrition, particularly carbohydrates; and temporarily blocking porphyrin synthesis. Thus, intravenous administration of fluid with both sodium chloride and dextrose is appropriate, as is identification and treatment of infection. Hematin, an inhibitor of porphyrin synthesis, is also effective in stopping acute attacks. However, phenobarbital is a potent inducer of the hepatic cytochrome P-450 system, which stimulates heme synthesis; this is a precipitating factor. *(Answer: A—Intravenous phenobarbital)*

7. A 45-year-old man with a long history of heavy alcohol ingestion presents with vesicles on sun-exposed areas of his body, particularly the dorsum of his hands. Some areas have become atrophic and hyperpigmented.

Which of the following laboratory findings would be consistent with a diagnosis of porphyria cutanea tarda (PCT) for this patient?

❑ **A. Normal serum ferritin level**

❑ **B. Isocoproporphyrin in the stool**

❑ **C. Normal plasma porphyrin level**

❑ **D. Urinary fluorescence under infrared light**

Key Concept/Objective: To understand the laboratory tests used to diagnose PCT

PCT is probably the most common of the porphyrias. It manifests as vesicle formation in sun-exposed areas, particularly the dorsum of the hands, followed by scarring and hyperpigmentation. It is frequently associated with liver abnormalities. PCT results from an inherited or acquired deficiency in uroporphyrinogen decarboxylase; the acquired form is frequently associated with excessive alcohol ingestion and iron overload. Therefore, the serum ferritin level is typically elevated. Plasma porphyrin levels are also elevated, as are urinary porphyrin levels, leading to urinary fluorescence under ultraviolet light. A finding that is virtually diagnostic of PCT is the presence of isocoproporphyrin in stool. *(Answer: B—Isocoproporphyrin in the stool)*

For more information, see Sassa S, Kappas A: 9 Metabolism: V The Porphyrias. ACP Medicine Online (www.acpmedicine.com). Dale DC, Federman DD, Eds. WebMD Inc., New York, December 2003

Diabetes Mellitus

8. A 38-year-old woman presents with symptoms of recurrent so-called yeast infection. Over the past 2 years, she has had repeated episodes of similar infections that have been only partially responsive to over-the-counter treatments. She has not seen a physician in the 10 years since her last pregnancy and denies knowledge of major medical illness. She has been moderately obese for most of her adult life; her maximal weight was 234 lb, although she recently lost 9 lb. She reports that she has had nocturia for the past several months. Physical examination is remarkable for a blood pressure of 145/92 mm Hg, obesity, and findings consistent with vaginal candidiasis.

Which of the following would be the most useful test for diagnosing diabetes in this patient?

- ❑ **A. Immediate measurement of blood glucose concentration**
- ❑ **B. Determination of hemoglobin A_{1c} (HbA_{1c}) level**
- ❑ **C. A 50 g oral glucose tolerance test**
- ❑ **D. Measurement of blood glucose after an overnight fast**
- ❑ **E. A 100 g oral glucose tolerance test**

Key Concept/Objective: To understand that measurement of fasting blood glucose (FBG) is the preferred diagnostic test for patients suspected of having type 2 diabetes

The standard means of diagnosing diabetes is measurement of FBG; the measurement should be repeated if the value is greater than 110 mg/dl. The current criteria considered diagnostic of diabetes is the finding of an FBG level of 126 mg/dl on more than one occasion. It must be realized that this value is somewhat arbitrary, and FBG values are distributed along a continuum from normal to diabetic. An FBG of 110 to 126 mg/dl is indicative of abnormal glucose metabolism, with higher values indicating an increased likelihood of progression to diabetes. A determination of random blood glucose level is diagnostic if that level is greater than 200 mg/dl in a symptomatic patient. This woman's nocturia and her recurrent vaginal candidiasis, which is a common correlate of hyperglycemia in women, are symptoms of diabetes. Random blood glucose values vary considerably more than do FBG values and so are not as reliable for establishing a diagnosis. The HbA_{1c} level reflects glycosylation of red cell proteins and is proportional to the glucose concentration over the preceding 2 to 3 months. Although FBG measurements are very useful for monitoring the course of patients with an established diagnosis, standards have not been established to enable clinicians to effectively distinguish diabetes from less serious causes of abnormalities in glucose metabolism. Glucose tolerance tests are quite sensitive in the detection of diabetes, and the 50 g and 100 g tests have a clear place in the diagnosis of gestational diabetes. However, these tests are more expensive and inconvenient for patients than measurement of FBG, and their results are less reproducible. Because abnormalities in fasting and postprandial glycemia tend to progress in tandem, FBG measurement has supplanted the oral glucose tolerance test for the diagnosis of diabetes except during pregnancy. *(Answer: D—Measurement of blood glucose after an overnight fast)*

9. A 25-year-old woman with a 12-year history of type 1 diabetes presents with complaints of recurrent nocturnal hypoglycemia. She reports that she has had repeated episodes of early morning awakening, during which she has experienced confusion and profound diaphoresis. She also experiences midday hypoglycemia when she eats lunch later than usual. These symptoms developed coincidently with her joining a health club, at which she engages in an aerobic training program five afternoons a week. She has been on a regimen of twice-daily injections of 45 units of a fixed mixture of 70% neutral protamine Hagedorn (NPH) insulin and 30% regular insulin (she has followed this regimen since she was a teenager). Despite the more frequent hypoglycemia, her HbA_{1c} level is 8.9%; evaluation of her home glucose monitoring results reveals morning fasting glucose levels that frequently exceed 250 mg/dl and afternoon values that average 185 mg/dl.

Which of the following steps is most appropriate for this patient?

❑ A. **Decreasing her evening insulin level by discontinuing the 70/30 insulin therapy and starting her on 12 U of regular insulin before dinner and 20 U of NPH insulin at bedtime**

❑ B. **A thorough diagnostic evaluation of pituitary and adrenal function**

❑ C. **Decreasing her evening insulin level by discontinuing the 70/30 insulin therapy and starting 12 U of lispro and 25 U of NPH insulin at dinner**

❑ D. **Measurement of plasma glucagon and epinephrine after induction of hypoglycemia**

❑ E. **Asking the patient to decrease the overall intensity of her physical training and to increase the amount of resistance training**

Key Concept/Objective: To understand that twice-daily insulin regimens are often ineffective in the treatment of type 1 diabetes

This patient's hypoglycemia has increased because of an increase in physical activity. It is not unusual for diabetic patients who require insulin to have delayed hypoglycemia in response to exercise. Her current regimen of NPH administered before dinner results in insulin action peaking in the early morning; because of her recent increase in daily glucose use with exercise, having insulin action peak at this time makes her susceptible to hypoglycemia. In addition, the poor overall glycemic control and the presence of fasting hyperglycemia indicate that she does not have effective overnight insulin action. Changing the time of administration of NPH from the evening to bedtime will shift the time of peak effect from between midnight and 3:00 A.M. to between 4:00 A.M. and 7:00 A.M.; this should result in a lower fasting glucose level as well as a decrease in the incidence of hypoglycemia. Increasing the number of insulin doses often results in better glycemic control, even when the total amount of insulin is decreased, because the timing of peak effects that results from increasing the number of doses is often more appropriate to the patient's needs. The use of lispro insulin can provide increased flexibility for patients who require insulin because the period of action of lispro is much shorter than that of regular insulin. In this case, substituting lispro for regular insulin might decrease the early morning insulin action that is causing the hypoglycemia, but continuing to administer NPH before dinner would still likely cause problems. The new onset of unexplained hypoglycemia in persons with type 1 diabetes should always raise concern that adrenal or thyroid insufficiency or some other autoimmune disease has developed. However, in this patient, these relatively rare conditions can be dismissed unless the patient continues to have hypoglycemia after adjustments are made to her insulin regimen. There are no standardized values for plasma glucagon and epinephrine levels that reliably indicate alpha cell, or autonomic nervous system, dysfunction. Aerobic exercise is as beneficial for persons with type 1 diabetes as it is for nondiabetic individuals, and although it frequently requires vigilant glucose monitoring and insulin adjustment, it should be encouraged in most cases. *(Answer: A—Decreasing her evening insulin level by discontinuing the 70/30 insulin therapy and starting her on 12 U of regular insulin before dinner and 20 U of NPH insulin at bedtime)*

10. A 42-year-old man with long-standing type 1 diabetes presents with gastroenteritis that has been worsening for 5 days. His serum biochemistry values are consistent with diabetic ketoacidosis (DKA); his blood pressure is 90/55 mm Hg, and his heart rate is 135 beats/min. Other laboratory findings are as follows: blood glucose, 656 mg/dl; sodium, 127 mEq/L; potassium, 4.2 mEq/L; HCO_3, 14 mEq/L; anion gap, 25; and pH, 7.05.

Which of the following would not be an appropriate step in the immediate treatment of this patient?

❑ A. **I.V. administration of 0.9% saline**

❑ B. **Admission to the intensive care unit**

❑ C. **I.V. administration of potassium chloride**

❑ **D. I.V. administration of insulin**

❑ **E. I.V. administration of sodium bicarbonate**

Key Concept/Objective: To understand that in most cases, successful treatment of DKA does not require bicarbonate administration

This patient's vital signs suggest moderate to severe dehydration, and volume replacement with normal saline is critical in the early management of his DKA. The severity of his metabolic derangements indicates that he should be treated in the intensive care unit. Insulin should be started immediately; the intravenous route is preferred because the rate of absorption of subcutaneous and intramuscular injections can vary in dehydrated individuals. The combination of volume expansion, diuresis, and insulin-dependent glucose disposal will lower the blood glucose level at a modest rate. More important, insulin will inhibit lipolysis and ketogenesis, reducing the acidosis. This patient is likely to have a large deficit in total body potassium, and with hydration and insulin treatment, his serum potassium level will decrease. Failure to adequately replace potassium can have severe consequences in patients with DKA, and potassium should be started immediately unless urine output is compromised or hyperkalemia exists. Administration of bicarbonate is not generally required in most cases of DKA and is generally reserved for treatment of severe acidosis (pH < 7.0 or HCO_3 < 10) or hemodynamic instability. Studies have indicated that the use of bicarbonate does not affect the course of most cases of DKA, and there is some theoretical rationale for not using bicarbonate unless clearly necessary. *(Answer: E—I.V. administration of sodium bicarbonate)*

11. A 49-year-old man was referred from a walk-in clinic when he was discovered to have a blood glucose level of 246 mg/dl during evaluation of an acute GI syndrome. Subsequently, a diagnosis of diabetes was confirmed by a finding of fasting blood glucose values of 190 mg/dl and 176 mg/dl, measured when the patient was not ill. Overall, this patient's clinical picture is consistent with type 2 diabetes. He has not received medical treatment or been evaluated for many years but reports being in generally good health.

Which of the following is the most reasonable approach for evaluating this patient's renal status?

❑ **A. Perform 24-hour urine collection, obtain an estimate of his creatinine clearance, and measure total protein excretion**

❑ **B. Measure the albumin-creatinine ratio on a spot urine sample**

❑ **C. Defer specific assessment because he has just been diagnosed, and diabetic nephropathy is unlikely to have developed**

❑ **D. Measure serum BUN and creatinine concentrations**

❑ **E. Perform renal ultrasound**

Key Concept/Objective: To know that urinary albumin excretion is the most sensitive means of detecting early diabetic nephropathy

An abnormally high rate of albumin excretion is the earliest manifestation of diabetic nephropathy, and microalbuminuria can be detected well before changes in creatinine clearance and pathologic proteinuria occur. Microalbuminuria is predictive of the progression of renal disease in most cases, and its occurrence marks the point in the course of nephropathy at which treatment is most efficacious. Therefore, all patients who are diagnosed with diabetes should undergo screening for renal albumin excretion. For patients with type 1 diabetes, formal evaluation can be deferred for several years because the time of disease onset is generally clear, and abnormalities in renal function do not occur during the first 5 years after onset. Patients with type 2 diabetes should be screened at the time of diagnosis because the time of onset of type 2 diabetes is often hard to discern, and asymptomatic hyperglycemia may have been present for several years. Screening for microalbuminuria can be done with a 24-hour urine collection, an overnight collection, a 4-hour timed collection, or a spot collection with determination

of albumin-creatinine ratio. All these measures require a specific assay for albumin because standard clinical laboratory measurements of urinary protein are not sensitive enough to detect microalbuminuria. Diabetic nephropathy is usually quite advanced before changes in the BUN and serum creatinine levels occur. Although one of the earliest renal manifestations of diabetes is transient kidney enlargement, renal ultrasound is not useful for screening for diabetic nephropathy. *(Answer: B—Measure the albumin-creatinine ratio on a spot urine sample)*

For more information, see Genuth S: 9 Metabolism: VI Diabetes Mellitus. ACP Medicine Online (www.acpmedicine.com). Dale DC, Federman DD, Eds. WebMD Inc., New York, May 2004

SECTION 10

NEPHROLOGY

Renal Function and Disorders of Water and Sodium Balance

1. A 52-year-old woman presents to the emergency department after experiencing 4 days of worsening mental status. She has not seen a doctor in over 20 years. Her medical history is unremarkable. She takes no medications. Physical examination shows a somnolent, obese woman with dry mucous membranes. The neurologic examination is nonfocal. Results of laboratory studies are as follows: sodium concentration, 128 mEq/L; potassium concentration, 4.5 mEq/L; chloride concentration, 94 mEq/L; serum glucose level, 810 mg/dl; renal function, normal.

Which of the following would be the most appropriate intervention in the care of this patient?

❑ **A. Fluid restriction and loop diuretics**

❑ **B. Administration of hypertonic saline**

❑ **C. Administration of normal saline and insulin**

❑ **D. Demeclocycline**

Key Concept/Objective: To be able to recognize hyperglycemic hyponatremia

Hyperglycemia lowers the plasma sodium concentration; in the absence of insulin, glucose is an effective osmole that attracts water from cells and thereby dilutes extracellular sodium. Therefore, the blood glucose level should always be examined when a low plasma sodium concentration is being evaluated. The plasma sodium concentration falls by approximately 3 mEq for every 200 mg/dl (10 mmol) increase in blood glucose and will increase by this amount when hyperglycemia is corrected with insulin. To evaluate hyponatremia in the presence of hyperglycemia, the serum sodium concentration must be "corrected" for the osmotic effect of glucose. In this patient, the corrected sodium concentration is within normal limits, and the sodium value will normalize once the high glucose level is treated. Hypertonic fluid, fluid restriction, loop diuretics, and demeclocycline can all be used in the management of hyponatremia, depending on the etiology of the problem. *(Answer: C—Administration of normal saline and insulin)*

2. A 60-year-old man comes to your clinic for follow-up. He has no new complaints. He has a history of hypothyroidism and mild asthma. His medications include levothyroxine and albuterol. The patient has been smoking two packs of cigarettes a day for 30 years. His physical examination is unremarkable. Results of laboratory studies are as follows: sodium concentration, 126 mEq/L; potassium concentration, 3.8 mEq/L; chloride concentration, 96 mEq/L; bicarbonate level, 24 mEq/L; blood urea nitrogen (BUN), 6 mg/dl; glucose and creatinine levels, normal; serum osmolality, 258 mOsm/L; urinary sodium, 56 mEq/L; urinary osmolality, 360 mOsm/kg. Thyroid function tests are within normal limits.

Which of the following interventions is most likely to normalize this patient's sodium level?

❑ **A. Increasing the dose of levothyroxine**

❑ **B. Restricting fluid intake**

❑ **C. Administering intravenous normal saline**

❑ **D. Starting a thiazide**

Key Concept/Objective: To understand the diagnosis and treatment of the syndrome of inappropriate antidiuretic hormone secretion (SIADH)

SIADH is a nonosmotic release of vasopressin in the absence of a hemodynamic stimulus to account for it. In SIADH, urinary sodium matches intake; as the urine is usually concentrated, the urinary sodium concentration exceeds 40 mEq/L unless dietary sodium intake is very low. The urinary osmolality also is inappropriately increased. BUN and serum uric acid are usually low in patients with SIADH. A number of disorders can be associated with SIADH. Tumors (most commonly small cell carcinoma of the lung) can ectopically synthesize and secrete vasopressin. Unexplained, persistent hyponatremia should be considered a marker for an underlying malignancy. SIADH is a mechanism for developing hyponatremia, not a diagnosis. In all patients with SIADH, a specific etiology for inappropriate vasopressin secretion should be sought. In a patient with clinical features of SIADH that has no obvious cause, a more extensive evaluation is indicated. The workup should include a careful search for malignancy and central nervous system pathology and an endocrine evaluation to exclude hypothyroidism and hypocortisolism. In patients with asymptomatic hyponatremia secondary to SIADH, the treatment of choice is fluid restriction. In this patient, there is no laboratory evidence of hypothyroidism, so increasing the dose of levothyroxine will not be helpful. Administration of normal saline in patients with SIADH can worsen the hyponatremia. Thiazides block the reabsorption of sodium and chloride in the distal tubule and can lead to severe hyponatremia. *(Answer: B—Restricting fluid intake)*

3. A 34-year-old woman presents to your clinic complaining of polyuria and polydipsia of 4 months' duration. She says she is urinating between 20 to 30 times every day. Her medical history is unremarkable. She takes oral contraceptives and a multivitamin. Her family history is significant for diabetes and coronary artery disease. Physical examination is unremarkable. Her sodium concentration is 143 mEq/L; her potassium, creatinine, and glucose levels are normal. Urine osmolality is 160 mOsm/kg.

Which of the following is the most likely diagnosis for this patient?

- ❑ **A. Diabetes insipidus**
- ❑ **B. Psychogenic polydipsia**
- ❑ **C. Beer potomania**
- ❑ **D. Salt poisoning**

Key Concept/Objective: To be able to recognize diabetes insipidus

This patient has polyuria with diluted urine and a serum sodium level in the high normal range. A diagnosis of diabetes insipidus can be made if the urine osmolality is less than 250 mOsm/kg despite hypernatremia (a serum sodium level greater than 143 mEq/L). When the disease is suspected in a polyuric patient whose serum sodium concentration is normal, the urine osmolality can be monitored while the patient is deprived of water, allowing the serum sodium level to increase to 143 mEq/L. Exogenous vasopressin increases urine osmolality by more than 150 mOsm/kg in patients with neurogenic (but not nephrogenic) diabetes insipidus. It is possible to misdiagnose diabetes insipidus in patients who actually have a primary thirst disorder. Excessive water intake suppresses vasopressin secretion and causes polyuria with dilute urine. Because patients with primary polydipsia secrete vasopressin normally, they do not become hypernatremic during diagnostic water deprivation. Correlation with plasma vasopressin levels is often necessary in borderline cases. Diabetes insipidus can be classified as neurogenic or nephrogenic. Neurogenic diabetes insipidus is caused by deficient secretion of vasopressin; nephrogenic diabetes insipidus results from the kidney's unresponsiveness to normally secreted hormone. With either disorder, patients present with polyuria and polydipsia. Most patients with polyuria do not become hypernatremic, because thirst maintains electrolyte-free water balance. Beer potomania will typically cause dilutional hyponatremia. Salt poisoning can cause hypernatremia with a high urinary osmolality. *(Answer: A—Diabetes insipidus)*

For more information, see Sterns RH: 10 Nephrology: I Renal Function and Disorders of Water and Sodium Balance. ACP Medicine Online (www.acpmedicine.com). Dale DC, Federman DD, Eds. WebMD Inc., New York, September 2003

Disorders of Acid-Base and Potassium Balance

4. A 22-year-old woman presents to the emergency department with nausea, vomiting, and abdominal pain of 4 days' duration. Her fluid balance profile is as follows: Na^+, 145; K^+, 5.0; Cl^-, 105; HCO_3^-, 15; BUN, 37; Cr, 1.6; glucose, 780; UA, 4+ ketones.

What is the best initial treatment of this patient's acid-base disorder?

- ❑ **A. Free water**
- ❑ **B. Normal saline**
- ❑ **C. Normal saline, sodium bicarbonate, and insulin**
- ❑ **D. Half-normal saline and insulin**
- ❑ **E. Normal saline and insulin**

Key Concept/Objective: To understand the diagnosis and treatment of diabetic ketoacidosis

Metabolic acidosis can be classified into two types: that associated with an elevation in the anion gap, and that in which the anion gap is normal. A calculation of the anion gap in this patient reveals a gap of 25. Among the causes of acidosis associated with an elevated anion gap are alcoholic ketoacidosis, lactic acidosis, starvation, ingestion of alcohols, ingestion of salicylates, and diabetic ketoacidosis. In patients with diabetic ketoacidosis (such as this patient), optimal initial treatment includes fluid replacement with normal saline to promote ketonuria and insulin to facilitate glucose transport. Bicarbonate therapy is not usually indicated unless the acidosis is severe or severe hyperkalemia is present. *(Answer: E—Normal saline and insulin)*

5. A 42-year-old woman presents with nausea, vomiting, and left flank pain with radiation to the groin; these symptoms have persisted for 3 days. A helical CT scan reveals a stone in the left ureter. On the basis of urinalysis and serum chemistries, a diagnosis of type 1 renal tubular acidosis (RTA) is made.

Which of the following is NOT consistent with type 1 RTA?

- ❑ **A. Normal-anion-gap metabolic acidosis**
- ❑ **B. Urine pH < 5.3**
- ❑ **C. Hypokalemia**
- ❑ **D. Urinary calcium phosphate crystals**
- ❑ **E. Sjögren syndrome**

Key Concept/Objective: To understand the diagnosis of type 1 RTA

Renal tubular acidosis is one of the causes of normal-anion-gap metabolic acidosis. Other causes are administration of HCl and losses of bicarbonate from the gastrointestinal tract. Type 1 RTA may be congenital, or it may occur in association with various immune disorders, such as Sjögren syndrome. The underlying defect involves the inability of the intercalated cells of the collecting tubule to pump out hydrogen ions. As a result, the urine pH is always greater that 5.3. Hypokalemia occurs secondary to enhanced Na^+-K^+ exchange in the distal tubule, because hydrogen ions are not secreted in response to sodium reabsorption. A major complication of type 1 RTA is nephrocalcinosis. Nephrocalcinosis is caused by calcium phosphate crystals, which occur secondary to an increase in the resorption of proximal tubular citrate through metabolic acidosis. The decrease in urinary citrate facilitates the precipitation of calcium phosphate crystals in the collecting tubule. *(Answer: B—Urine pH < 5.3)*

6. A 68-year-old man with chronic renal insufficiency presents with weakness, paresthesias, and progressively worsening shortness of breath. He has been experiencing these symptoms for 4 days. Laboratory findings show a potassium level of 7.2; an electrocardiogram reveals peaked T waves and widening of the QRS complex.

Which of the following is NOT indicated in the initial treatment of this patient?

- ❑ **A. Intravenous calcium**

❑ B. **Intravenous glucose and insulin**

❑ C. **Dialysis**

❑ D. **Sodium polystyrene sulfonate (Kayexalate, Kionex)**

❑ E. **Beta blockers**

Key Concept/Objective: To understand the diagnosis and treatment of hyperkalemia

The initial manifestations of hyperkalemia are usually neuromuscular in origin and are nonspecific. Diagnosis is based on serum potassium level; emergent treatment is based on whether cardiac arrhythmias are present or electrocardiographic changes are occurring. Treatment involves the use of intravenous calcium to reduce the excitability of cardiac cell membrane and use of intravenous glucose and insulin to facilitate transport of potassium into the intracellular space. Sodium polystyrene sulfonate is used to increase the excretion of potassium in the colon. In refractory cases, dialysis may be initiated to rapidly remove serum potassium. In addition, intranasal beta agonists may be used to transiently reduce serum potassium levels in the acute setting. Beta blockers can increase potassium levels. *(Answer: E—Beta blockers)*

7. A 35-year-old woman presents to your clinic with a history of headaches, weakness, fatigue, and polyuria. Her blood pressure is 210/94 mm Hg. Laboratory tests reveal the following abnormalities: arterial pH, 7.48; sodium, 148; potassium, 2.7; HCO_3^-, 37; plasma renin level is low; urine chloride, 28 mEq/L.

Which of the following is the most likely diagnosis?

❑ A. **Secondary hyperaldosteronism**

❑ B. **Diuretic abuse**

❑ C. **Milk-alkali syndrome**

❑ D. **Primary hyperaldosteronism**

❑ E. **Type 4 RTA**

Key Concept/Objective: To be able to differentiate between the various causes of metabolic alkalosis

Metabolic alkalosis is characterized by an elevation in serum bicarbonate level and a concomitant elevation of arterial pH. The causes of metabolic alkalosis include GI and renal losses of hydrogen ions; hypercalcemia; hypokalemia; excess alkali administration; and receiving thiazide or a loop diuretic. Primary hyperaldosteronism is characterized by hypertension, hypokalemia, hypernatremia, a low plasma renin level, and an elevated urine chloride level (as are seen in this patient). Secondary hyperaldosteronism is not usually associated with hypokalemia or metabolic alkalosis; it is usually associated with a high plasma renin level. Patients who have been abusing diuretics or who have milk-alkali syndrome often present with the serum values seen in this patient. However, in such patients, the urine chloride level is usually low (< 10), and these patients often present with volume depletion, whereas mild volume expansion is characteristic of primary hyperaldosteronism. Type IV RTA causes a metabolic acidosis. *(Answer: D—Primary hyperaldosteronism)*

For more information, see Black RM: 10 Nephrology: II Disorders of Acid-Base and Potassium Balance. ACP Medicine Online (www.acpmedicine.com). Dale DC, Federman DD, Eds. WebMD Inc., New York, December 2001

Approach to the Patient with Renal Disease

8. A 77-year-old man presents to the emergency department complaining that for the past 24 hours, he has been unable to void. The patient reports that he has had this problem intermittently and that he has been diagnosed with benign prostatic hyperplasia. He has an upper respiratory infection and has been taking over-the-counter pseudoephedrine. The patient also reports that a year ago, he was admitted to the hospital for unstable angina. At that time, his creatinine level was 1.1 mg/dl. In the emergency department, the patient's serum creatinine level is determined to be 4.2 mg/dl.

Regarding this patient's renal failure, which of the following statements is false?

- ❑ A. **Renal ultrasound should show bilateral hydronephrosis, suggesting obstructive uropathy as the cause of acute renal failure**
- ❑ B. **The use of pseudoephedrine has contributed to the development of urinary obstruction**
- ❑ C. **Urinalysis is commonly abnormal in obstructive uropathy; an abnormal result supports the diagnosis of obstruction**
- ❑ D. **Obstruction impairs the ability of the kidneys to concentrate the urine and thus contributes to a polyuric state**
- ❑ E. **Common causes of obstruction include nephrolithiasis and neurogenic bladder (and, in women, an enlarging cervical cancer)**

Key Concept/Objective: To be able to recognize urinary obstruction as a cause of acute renal failure

Obstruction of urine flow can occur anywhere along the urinary tract, from the renal pelvis to the urethra. Anuria suggests complete urinary obstruction, although anuria can also be a feature of bilateral renal artery thrombosis, acute cortical necrosis, or severe acute tubular necrosis. In the absence of complete obstruction, urine flow may not necessarily be decreased and in fact is often increased. Chronic partial obstruction of the ureters leads to ureteral dilatation, which overcomes the blockage of urine flow. In addition, obstruction impairs the urinary concentrating ability and thus contributes to a polyuric state. Common causes of urinary obstruction include nephrolithiasis, prostate enlargement in men, neurogenic bladder in diabetic patients, and an enlarging cervical cancer in women. The urinalysis result is typically unremarkable in obstructive uropathy. The diagnosis is most often made by demonstrating ureteral dilatation on renal sonography. *(Answer: C—Urinalysis is commonly abnormal in obstructive uropathy; an abnormal result supports the diagnosis of obstruction)*

9. A 75-year-old woman with diabetes and hypertension is admitted to the hospital with nausea, vomiting, and abdominal pain. At admission, laboratory values include a blood urea nitrogen (BUN) measurement of 18 and a plasma creatinine measurement of 0.5 mg/dl. As part of her workup, she undergoes a contrast-enhanced CT scan of the abdomen. During the first 48 hours of the hospital stay, repeat laboratory studies reveal a plasma creatinine level of 1.1 mg/dl.

Which of the following statements is false regarding estimates of this patient's glomerular filtration rate (GFR)?

- ❑ A. **A low baseline plasma creatinine value may lead to an overestimation of GFR because of decreased muscle mass in this elderly patient**
- ❑ B. **The change in plasma creatinine level of 0.6 mg/dl represents an approximately 50% decrease in the patient's GFR**
- ❑ C. **The use of drugs such as cimetidine and trimethoprim increase plasma creatinine levels without affecting true GFR because of inhibition of tubular secretion of creatinine**
- ❑ D. **The patient's ideal body weight correlates inversely with GFR**

Key Concept/Objective: To understand the use of creatinine clearance to estimate GFR and common factors that affect creatinine clearance

GFR is generally thought to be the best measure of renal function because filtration capacity correlates directly with the function of the nephron. Creatinine is produced at a relatively constant rate by hepatic conversion of skeletal muscle creatine, and the clearance of creatinine is used as an estimate of filtration. Creatinine clearance (C_{Cr}) can be measured by 24-hour collection of urine, or it can be estimated through use of a formula that involves the patient's age, ideal body weight (IBW), and plasma creatinine (Cr): $C_{Cr} = (140 - \text{age}) \times (\text{IBW in kg})/(72 \times \text{Cr})$. In females, the results are multiplied by a correction factor of 0.85. Because the production of creatinine is dependent on muscle mass, plasma levels are typically lower in elderly patients and in patients with conditions that result in profound muscle wasting. From the equation for estimating creatinine, it can be seen that creatinine clearance and GFR correlate directly with patient's

ideal body weight. Additionally, because creatinine clearance correlates inversely with plasma creatinine levels, a doubling of the plasma creatinine value (as seen in this patient) reflects a reduction in creatinine clearance by about half. It is important to note that creatinine clearance is not a perfect reflection of GFR because creatinine, in addition to being filtered, is also secreted in the tubules. Certain drugs, such as cimetidine, trimethoprim, and probenecid, inhibit this tubular secretion; this results in a decrease in creatinine clearance, but this decrease has no bearing on GFR. *(Answer: D—The patient's ideal body weight correlates inversely with GFR)*

10. A 60-year-old man who presented with fatigue and bone pain is found to be anemic and thrombocytopenic. Examination reveals pale conjunctivae and thigh tenderness but no peripheral edema. Radiographs demonstrate osteolytic lesions in several thoracic vertebrae and the left femur. Serum chemistries reveal a creatinine level of 1.2 mg/dl, a calcium level of 9.5 mg/dl, a total protein level of 11 mg/dl, and an albumin level of 3.2 mg/dl. On bone marrow biopsy, there is replacement of normal marrow with sheets of plasma cells. Urinalysis is unremarkable, but a 24-hour urine study reveals proteinuria of 2.0 g/day.

Which of the following statements regarding this patient's proteinuria is true?

- ❑ **A. The likely underlying pathology involves a structural abnormality of the filtration barrier that results in loss of negatively charged proteins**
- ❑ **B. It is likely that the results of the 24-hour urine study are falsely elevated because the urine dipstick test is sensitive for most protein species, including albumin and paraproteins**
- ❑ **C. The proteinuria reflects an overproduction of normally filtered proteins, which overwhelms the reabsorptive capacity of the tubules**
- ❑ **D. The patient's degree of proteinuria and spectrum of clinical findings is consistent with the nephrotic syndrome**

Key Concept/Objective: To understand the mechanisms of proteinuria and the means of detecting it

This patient has multiple myeloma, which is associated with an elevation in total protein level consistent with the production of immunoglobulin light chain paraproteins (Bence-Jones proteins). These positively charged proteins are filtered in large quantities and overwhelm the reabsorptive capacity of the tubules, resulting in significant proteinuria (overflow proteinuria). This finding is in contrast to those seen in conditions such as membranous nephropathy, diabetes mellitus, or minimal change disease; in these disorders, there is an alteration in the filtration barrier of the glomerulus, which allows negatively charged proteins such as albumin to be filtered excessively (glomerular proteinuria). These conditions can lead to the nephrotic syndrome, which is characterized by heavy proteinuria (> 3.5g/day) and concomitant hypoalbuminemia, edema, and hyperlipidemia. Results of standard dipstick testing will be positive only with negatively charged proteins such as albumin: thus, dipstick testing is insensitive with regard to the detection of Bence-Jones proteins, which are often positively charged. *(Answer: C—The proteinuria reflects an overproduction of normally filtered proteins, which overwhelms the reabsorptive capacity of the tubules)*

11. A 28-year-old man presents to clinic with a complaint of hematuria of 1 day's duration. He was well until 3 days ago, when he developed a sore throat, low-grade fever, and malaise, which lasted for approximately 48 hours. He had a similar episode approximately 1 year ago. He denies having rash, joint pains, or dysuria. On examination, he appears well, and he is afebrile. His blood pressure is 118/62 mm Hg. Urine dipstick assay is significant for 2+ blood and trace protein. Microscopic examination of the urine reveals 10 to 15 red cells per high-powered field; dysmorphic red cells and occasional red cell casts are noted as well. Further testing reveals a normal antistreptolysin-O (ASO) titer and serum complement level.

Which of the following statements regarding this patient's condition is false?

- ❑ **A. Findings on urinalysis identify the source of bleeding as glomerular in origin**
- ❑ **B. Renal biopsy is likely to reveal mesangial deposition of immunoglobulin A (IgA) on immunofluorescence microscopy**
- ❑ **C. Results of analysis of the urine sediment are consistent with a finding of hypercalciuria as a cause of the hematuria**

❑ D. **The time course of the illness and the serum complement level help to differentiate this patient's condition from acute postinfectious glomerulonephritis**

Key Concept/Objective: To recognize Berger disease and the urinary findings associated with glomerulonephritis

Microscopic evaluation of urinary sediment is an important component of the workup of hematuria because it may help localize the bleeding to either the upper urinary tract (i.e., glomeruli) or the lower urinary tract (i.e., renal pelvis, ureters, bladder, urethra). The presence of red cell casts (formed from erythrocytes passing through the renal tubules) is virtually pathognomonic for acute glomerulonephritis. Dysmorphic red cells and red cell casts would not typically be seen in patients with hematuria caused by abnormalities of the lower urinary tract, such as nephrolithiasis, malignancy, or prostatitis. This patient presented with recurrent episodes of macroscopic hematuria following an upper respiratory infection, which is a common finding in patients with IgA nephropathy (Berger disease). This condition constitutes 10% to 40% of all cases of primary glomerulonephritis and is associated with increased serum IgA levels and mesangial deposition of IgA. Onset is typically in the second and third decades of life; although the disease typically progresses slowly, approximately one half of patients with IgA nephropathy will develop end-stage renal disease within 25 years of onset. Hypertension and proteinuria are predictive of more rapid disease progression. Serum complement levels are typically normal: a finding that helps to differentiate Berger disease from other causes of acute glomerulonephritis, such as acute postinfectious glomerulonephritis and lupus, in which complement levels are typically low. *(Answer: C—Results of analysis of the urine sediment are consistent with a finding of hypercalciuria as a cause of the hematuria)*

12. A 45-year-old man with a history of alcohol abuse is brought to the emergency department after being found lying on the floor of his apartment by a neighbor. On examination, he is unresponsive and appears dehydrated. Initial blood work reveals a hematocrit of 41%, a BUN of 60 mg/dl, and a creatinine level of 3.2 mg/dl. Creatine kinase and lactose dehydrogenase (LDH) levels are elevated at 12,000 U/L and 475 U/L, respectively. Urinalysis shows reddish urine with a specific gravity of 1.020; dipstick assay shows 3+ blood and 1+ protein. Microscopic examination of urine sediment demonstrates 0 to 2 red cells and 0 to 5 white cells per high-powered field; hyaline casts are also observed.

The urinary findings are suggestive of which of the following conditions?

❑ A. **Acute glomerulonephritis**

❑ B. **Hemoglobinuria**

❑ C. **Allergic interstitial nephritis**

❑ D. **Myoglobinuria**

Key Concept/Objective: To recognize the findings associated with myoglobinuria

This patient presents with rhabdomyolysis related to alcohol intoxication and prolonged immobilization. Myoglobin released from the breakdown of skeletal muscle is an endogenous nephrotoxin that can induce acute renal failure (ARF) by direct injury to tubular epithelial cells. ARF is a complication in up to one third of patients with rhabdomyolysis; factors that predispose to ARF in this setting include hypovolemia and acidosis. The prompt recognition of myoglobinuria is thus of paramount importance in this clinical setting and can be aided greatly by careful examination of the urine. Both myoglobin and hemoglobin (released from the breakdown of red cells in hemolytic processes) will react with the urine dipstick test for blood. The presence of pigments in the urine should be suspected when the results of dipstick testing are strongly positive for blood in the absence of red cells on microscopic examination. Acute glomerulonephritis is characterized by the finding of red cells and red cell casts on urinalysis. Acute (allergic) interstitial nephritis is suggested by the presence of white cell casts and nonpigmented granular casts. Eosinophiluria is an additional finding that suggests interstitial nephritis, though a finding of eosinophiluria is not highly sensitive. *(Answer: D—Myoglobinuria)*

For more information, see Palmer BF: 10 Nephrology: III Approach to the Patient with Renal Disease. ACP Medicine Online (www.acpmedicine.com). Dale DC, Federman DD, Eds. WebMD Inc., New York, April 2004

Management of Chronic Kidney Disease

13. A 57-year-old woman with hypertension, mitral valve prolapse with regurgitation, asthma, and a history of alcoholism presents to your office to establish primary care. Because the patient has hypertension, you order a basic metabolic profile and urinalysis as a part of your initial evaluation. The laboratory calls to notify you that the patient's serum creatinine level is 2.3 mg/dl.

Which of the following statements regarding chronic kidney disease (CKD) is true?

- ❑ **A. CKD is defined as a glomerular filtration rate (GFR) of less than 30 ml/min/1.73 m^2 for longer than 3 months**
- ❑ **B. Persistently increased proteinuria in the setting of a normal or increased GFR signifies the presence of stage 1 CKD**
- ❑ **C. Measurement of 24-hour creatinine clearance to assess GFR is more accurate than estimating GFR from the Modification of Diet in Renal Disease (MDRD) equation**
- ❑ **D. Treatment of comorbid conditions, interventions to slow progression of kidney disease, and measures to reduce cardiovascular disease should begin during CKD stage 3**

Key Concept/Objective: To understand the basic principles of the diagnosis and treatment of CKD

CKD is defined as either kidney damage or a GFR of less than 60 ml/min/1.73 m^2 for longer than 3 months. The MDRD and Cockcroft-Gault equations provide useful estimates of GFR in adults. Clinical practice guidelines point out that clinicians should not use serum creatinine concentration as the sole means of assessing the level of kidney function. In addition, measurement of 24-hour creatinine clearance to assess GFR is not more accurate than estimating GFR from the MDRD equation. Evaluation of all patients with CKD should include testing for proteinuria. Persistently increased proteinuria is usually a marker of kidney damage; in the setting of a normal or increased GFR, it signifies the presence of stage 1 CKD. Treatment of comorbid conditions, interventions to slow progression of kidney disease, and measures to reduce cardiovascular disease should begin during stages 1 and 2. *(Answer: B—Persistently increased proteinuria in the setting of a normal or increased GFR signifies the presence of stage 1 CKD)*

14. A 46-year-old male patient with long-standing CKD, diabetes, and hypertension presents for routine follow-up. The patient is taking an ACE inhibitor and insulin. The patient's GFR is 42 ml/min/1.73 m^2, as calculated using the MDRD equation.

Which of the following statements regarding the management of complications associated with CKD is false?

- ❑ **A. Potassium balance is generally maintained within normal limits until the GFR falls to less than 10 ml/min**
- ❑ **B. When a patient is normotensive and maintains a constant weight with only trace edema, the patient has achieved the goal for salt intake**
- ❑ **C. Initially, patients with CKD have an anion gap metabolic acidosis, but over time, they develop a non–anion gap metabolic acidosis**
- ❑ **D. Initially in CKD, the parathyroid hormone level rises, resulting in fairly normal serum calcium and phosphate levels**

Key Concept/Objective: To understand the basic principles of the management of the complications associated with CKD

The goal of salt intake should be a quantity that results in the patient's being normotensive and maintaining a constant weight, with only trace edema present. Potassium balance is generally maintained within normal limits until the GFR falls to less than 10 ml/min. This balance is achieved by an increased potassium excretion rate per remaining nephron, as well as an increase in extrarenal potassium excretion, primarily effected via the colon. The development of hyperkalemia at higher levels of renal function suggests the presence of tubulointerstitial disease or disturbances in the renin-angiotensin-aldosterone axis. As renal insufficiency progresses, patients typically become

acidotic. Initially, the acidosis is of the non–anion gap type, but as renal insufficiency becomes far advanced, an anion gap acidosis supervenes. As GFR declines, the serum phosphate level begins to increase, causing a reciprocal decrease in the serum calcium concentration. In response, parathyroid hormone (PTH) is released, resulting in increased phosphate excretion in each of the remaining nephrons; thus, calcium and phosphorus levels return to normal. As renal function continues to decline, calcium and phosphorus levels remain within the normal range but at the expense of an ever-increasing level of PTH. *(Answer: C—Initially, patients with CKD have an anion gap metabolic acidosis, but over time, they develop a non–anion gap metabolic acidosis)*

15. A 53-year-old man with type 2 diabetes presents to your office to establish primary care. You measure his serum creatinine level.

Which of the following statements is true regarding assessment of renal function?

- ❑ A. **A serum creatinine value that is within the normal range indicates that the patient's GFR has declined by less than 25%**
- ❑ B. **If the patient has renal insufficiency, use of creatinine clearance, as determined by 24-hour urine collection, to assess GFR can lead to an underestimation of the GFR**
- ❑ C. **The Cockcroft-Gault formula estimates GFR while taking into account the increase in creatinine production with increasing weight and age**
- ❑ D. **Averaging the urea and creatinine clearance values will provide a more accurate estimation of GFR than use of the creatinine clearance value alone**
- ❑ E. **Creatinine clearance should provide an equally accurate estimation of GFR, regardless of the patient's current creatinine level**

Key Concept/Objective: To understand the various methods of estimating GFR

Various tools are available to assess renal function. The major limitation of the use of the serum creatinine level to assess GFR is that it cannot detect loss of renal function until the GFR has declined by more than 50%. Thus, a normal creatinine level does not rule out the possibility that the GFR has declined by more than 25%. The Cockcroft-Gault formula takes into account the increase in creatinine production that occurs with increasing weight and the decrease in production that occurs with advancing age. The most accurate way of following renal function is to directly measure the GFR by measuring the clearance of a compound that is freely filtered by the glomerulus but that is neither secreted nor absorbed. Use of creatinine clearance provides a fairly accurate measure of GFR because at normal levels of renal function, only a small percentage of creatinine appears in the urine through tubular secretion. The bulk of creatinine is filtered by the glomerulus. With advancing renal insufficiency, however, the percentage of creatinine that reaches the final urine through tubular secretion increases. As a result, use of creatinine clearance tends to lead to progressively larger overestimations of GFR with advancing renal insufficiency. Urea is filtered by the glomerulus and is reabsorbed by the tubule; thus, use of urea clearance leads to underestimations of GFR. However, the extent to which urea clearance leads to underestimations of GFR is similar to the extent to which creatinine clearance leads to overestimations of GFR. Thus, taking the average of urea and creatinine clearance values will give a very accurate estimation of GFR. *(Answer: D—Averaging the urea and creatinine clearance values will provide a more accurate estimation of GFR than use of the creatinine clearance value alone)*

16. You are managing a man with long-standing hypertension, diabetes, and chronic renal insufficiency. He has gradually developed anemia and edema and has recently developed hyperkalemia and acidosis as the time approaches when he will require hemodialysis.

Which of the following statements is true regarding the etiology and management of these typical abnormalities associated with chronic renal insufficiency?

- ❑ A. **Alkali therapy can help treat the acidosis but is unlikely to improve the hyperkalemia**

❑ B. Constipation should be avoided because it can cause the hyperkalemia to worsen

❑ C. The target hematocrit value for erythropoietin therapy is 30%

❑ D. Alkali should not be administered as sodium bicarbonate to patients receiving aluminum-containing phosphate binders

❑ E. Failure to respond to erythropoietin therapy is most commonly the result of underlying anemia of chronic renal disease

Key Concept/Objective: To understand the principles of management of metabolic and hematologic abnormalities in chronic renal failure

In chronic renal failure, hyperkalemia and acidosis are interrelated. Alkali therapy will certainly help to improve the acidosis and may improve the hyperkalemia through several mechanisms. First, alkalinization causes a shift of potassium into cells. Also, sodium bicarbonate enhances distal sodium delivery and therefore augments potassium secretion from the distal tubule. One should not administer citrate-containing alkali to patients receiving aluminum-containing phosphate binders, because citrate is known to enhance the gastrointestinal absorption of aluminum. In this setting, sodium bicarbonate diminishes the risk of aluminum toxicity. Constipation can cause hyperkalemia to worsen because potassium secretion by the colon is substantial in patients with advanced renal failure.

Severe anemia contributes to the development of left ventricular hypertrophy, which in turn is an important predictor of subsequent cardiac morbidity and mortality in patients receiving dialysis. Thus, early institution of erythropoietin therapy can improve dialysis outcomes. This is an important reason for timely referral of the patient with renal insufficiency to a nephrologist. A target hematocrit value of 30% in young patients who have no evidence of cardiovascular disease should provide relief of symptoms attributable to anemia. By contrast, older patients with comorbidities may benefit by targeting the hematocrit value closer to normal. Failure to respond to erythropoietin therapy is most commonly the result of iron deficiency. *(Answer: B—Constipation should be avoided because it can cause the hyperkalemia to worsen)*

17. A 34-year-old man with diabetes and hypertension comes for a check-up. His creatinine level is normal at 1.0 mg/dl, and he has microalbuminuria of 120 mg/24 hr.

Which of the following statements is true regarding the appropriate measures to slow progression of renal disease?

❑ A. Aggressive control of hyperglycemia may be more likely to slow progression of renal disease in patients with type 1 diabetes mellitus than in patients with type 2 diabetes mellitus

❑ B. The targeted blood pressure should be below 140/90 mm Hg

❑ C. Because this patient has diabetes, microalbuminuria is predictive of progression of renal disease

❑ D. Smoking is a risk factor for microalbuminuria because of its association with hypertension

❑ E. Although not clearly of benefit, a low-protein diet can be prescribed with little concern about deleterious effects

Key Concept/Objective: To understand the risk factors for renal disease progression

Evidence clearly shows that aggressive control of hyperglycemia in patients with type 1 diabetes mellitus will reduce the occurrence of microalbuminuria and macroalbuminuria and will slow the progression of nephropathy. Control of hyperglycemia in patients with type 2 diabetes mellitus is more controversial, as there are conflicting results of this approach in the literature. This may be related to the fact that renal lesions resulting from type 2 diabetes are more heterogeneous than the typical lesion from type 1 diabetes. Because uncontrolled hypertension can contribute to the progression of renal disease, target blood pressure values have been established. These values vary slightly, depending on the source of the recommendation, but in general, a blood pressure of 130/80 mm Hg or less should be sought. Microalbuminuria is a risk factor for progression to end-stage renal disease in diabetic and nondiabetic patients

with renal disease. Smoking is an independent risk factor for microalbuminuria in both hypertensive and normotensive patients. Finally, a low-protein diet can easily lead to malnutrition and calorie deficiency and therefore must be closely monitored. *(Answer: A—Aggressive control of hyperglycemia may be more likely to slow progression of renal disease in patients with type 1 diabetes mellitus than in patients with type 2 diabetes mellitus)*

For more information, see Palmer BF: 10 Nephrology: IV Management of Chronic Kidney Disease. ACP Medicine Online (www.acpmedicine.com). Dale DC, Federman DD, Eds. WebMD Inc., New York, September 2004

Glomerular Diseases

18. A previously healthy 54-year-old woman presents with a 3-week history of arthralgias and edema. Her examination is remarkable for a blood pressure of 170/106 mm Hg, bibasilar pulmonary crackles, and lower extremity edema. A freshly voided urine reveals red blood cells and red cell casts. A diagnosis of glomerulonephritis is made. Her serology is positive for antineutrophil cytoplasmic antibody (ANCA).

For this patient, a renal biopsy with immunofluorescent staining would be expected to show which of the following?

- ❑ **A. Positive staining for immune complexes**
- ❑ **B. Positive staining for immune deposits IgG and C3**
- ❑ **C. Positive staining for IgA and C3**
- ❑ **D. Positive staining for linear deposition of IgG and C3**
- ❑ **E. Negative staining for antibody or C3**

Key Concept/Objective: To understand that ANCA–associated glomerulonephritis is not associated with staining for immunoglobulin, complement, or immune deposits

ANCA-associated glomerulonephritis involves a vasculitic process of the small- and medium-sized blood vessels that usually presents as a focal segmental necrotizing glomerulonephritis. Renal involvement is usually acute, severe, and progressive, and glomeruli contain crescents. ANCA-associated glomerulonephritis is one of the causes of rapidly progressive glomerulonephritis, which many authors consider a medical emergency. ANCA-associated glomerulonephritis can be limited to the kidney or coexist with systemic illness such as Wegener granulomatosis. In contrast to many other kinds of glomerulonephritis, immunofluorescent staining fails to reveal the presence of antibody, complement, or immune complexes. This type of glomerulonephritis is also referred to as pauci-immune glomerulonephritis. If the disease is left untreated, the prognosis is poor. Initial treatment consists of corticosteroids and immunosuppressive therapy. *(Answer: E—Negative staining for antibody or C3)*

19. A 45-year-old man presents for a routine examination. His history is remarkable for a bleeding peptic ulcer at age 30 that required transfusion of several units of packed red blood cells. He has been without peptic symptoms since then. He consumes no alcohol. His physical examination reveals a blood pressure of 154/98 mm Hg, confirmed on several occasions, but is otherwise not remarkable. His laboratory evaluation was remarkable for ALT and AST levels that were 2.5 times normal and a dipstick that was positive for blood and protein.

What should be the next step in this patient's management?

- ❑ **A. Referral for a liver biopsy**
- ❑ **B. Renal arteriogram**
- ❑ **C. *Helicobacter pylori* antibody testing**
- ❑ **D. Serum renin measurement**
- ❑ **E. Serum antibody testing for hepatitis C**

Key Concept/Objective: To understand the pathogenic link between chronic hepatitis C infection and glomerulonephritis

Membranoproliferative glomerulonephritis can present with either the nephrotic syndrome or the nephritic syndrome. Type 1 membranoproliferative glomerulonephritis is caused by immune complex deposition in the subendothelium, most commonly immune deposits from hepatitis C virus (HCV) antigens and cryoglobulins. Approximately one third of patients present with microscopic hematuria and nonnephrotic proteinuria, and another third presents with nephrotic-range proteinuria with a mild decrease in renal function. Hypertension is a very common finding on initial presentation. HCV-associated membranoproliferative glomerulonephritis is usually treated with antiviral therapy when remission is common and relapse is frequent. *(Answer: E—Serum antibody testing for hepatitis C)*

20. A 21-year-old woman of Peruvian descent presents with hypertension, fatigue, and microscopic hematuria. A renal biopsy demonstrates glomerulonephritis secondary to focal segmental glomerulosclerosis (FSGS).

Which of the following would be the most appropriate step to take next in the treatment of this patient's disease?

- ❑ **A. Renal dialysis**
- ❑ **B. Cyclosporine**
- ❑ **C. Prednisone**
- ❑ **D. Cyclophosphamide**
- ❑ **E. Captopril**

Key Concept/Objective: To understand that glucocorticoids represent the key initial medical therapy for patients diagnosed with FSGS

FSGS is one of the most common causes of nephrotic syndrome in adults. In addition to the signs and symptoms of nephrotic syndrome, hypertension and hematuria occur in 50% of adults with FSGS. As in all glomerular diseases, if a secondary cause can be found (e.g., HIV, heroin, analgesics), correcting the underlying cause is the first priority. However, many causes are idiopathic. The first line of therapy in adults with FSGS is prednisone. It should be emphasized that the duration of therapy is critical in preventing relapses. Shortening the duration of prednisone treatment from the recommended 6 to 8 months is a risk factor for relapse. Of patients treated initially with prednisone, 55% respond to this treatment. For the 45% who do not respond, cytotoxic agents (e.g., cyclophosphamide) should be tried. Interestingly, if a patient undergoes a renal transplantation, there is a 20% to 30% chance that native disease will recur in the transplanted kidney within 3 years. *(Answer: C—Prednisone)*

21. A 45-year-old man presents with acute onset of flank pain and hematuria. He gives a history of several months of increasing peripheral edema in his lower extremities. His urinary protein-to-creatinine ratio is 3.9.

What would be the best step to take next in this patient's management?

- ❑ **A. Renal ultrasound and duplex scan**
- ❑ **B. Gram-negative antimicrobial therapy**
- ❑ **C. Intravenous furosemide**
- ❑ **D. Rapid-sequence intravenous pyelogram**
- ❑ **E. ASO titer**

Key Concept/Objective: To understand that patients with nephrotic syndrome are at risk for thrombosis of the renal vein

It is estimated that 10% to 40% of patients with nephrotic syndrome will develop arterial or venous thromboembolism. Urinary losses of antithrombin III are thought to contribute to the pathogenesis of this complication. Renal vein thrombosis is most commonly found in membranous nephropathy, where it may occur in up to 50% of patients. Some authors recommend the use of prophylactic low-dose warfarin when the plasma albumin concentration is less than 2 g/dl. The diagnosis of renal vein thrombosis is best made via Doppler ultrasonography. The urinary protein-to-creatinine ratio of 3.9 is consistent with 3.9 g of protein a day and is in the nephrotic range. *(Answer: A—Renal ultrasound and duplex scan)*

22. A 36-year-old hypertensive man develops macroscopic hematuria 24 hours after the onset of pharyngitis. The patient's brother had a history of poststreptococcal glomerulonephritis at age 6 after a streptococcal infection of the throat.

What is the most likely explanation for this patient's hematuria?

❑ **A. Poststreptococcal glomerulonephritis**

❑ **B. Glomerulosclerosis**

❑ **C. IgA nephropathy**

❑ **D. Henoch-Schonlein purpura (HSP)**

❑ **E. Renal vein thrombosis**

Key Concept/Objective: To understand the relation between hematuria and mucosal infections in patients with IgA nephropathy

Patients with IgA nephropathy typically present with nephritic-like symptoms that derive from deposition of IgA in the glomeruli. It is the leading cause of glomerulonephritis worldwide. The male-to-female ratio is 3:1. The classic presentation in up to 50% of patients with IgA nephropathy is episodic macroscopic hematuria within 24 hours of a mucosal infection of the upper respiratory tract. The majority of the rest of patients with IgA nephropathy present with persistent asymptomatic microscopic hematuria. This differs from the hematuria of poststreptococcal glomerulonephritis, which is delayed by 2 to 3 weeks following pharyngitis. The macroscopic hematuria usually resolves within days. *(Answer: C—IgA nephropathy)*

For more information, see Shankland SJ: 10 Nephrology: V Glomerular Diseases. ACP Medicine Online (www.acpmedicine.com). Dale DC, Federman DD, Eds. WebMD Inc., New York, September 2004

Acute Renal Failure

23. A 25-year-old woman presents to your clinic with fatigue of 1 week's duration. She thinks there was blood in her urine on two occasions after excessive exercise. Physical examination is unremarkable except for some mild muscle tenderness. Urinalysis is positive for 3+ blood. The blood urea nitrogen (BUN) level is 18 mg/dl, and the creatinine level is 1.1 mg/dl.

What is the most likely cause of this patient's symptoms?

❑ **A. Postinfectious glomerulonephritis**

❑ **B. Myoglobinuria caused by rhabdomyolysis**

❑ **C. IgA nephropathy**

❑ **D. Wegener granulomatosis**

Key Concept/Objective: To know the signs and symptoms of rhabdomyolysis

Over the past 50 years, our understanding of rhabdomyolysis has significantly broadened. The most common causes are trauma or other disorders that lead to muscle injury; excessive muscle activity, as occurs during seizures or strenuous exercise; use of medications; and electrolyte disorders. Recent increased use of HMG-CoA (3-hydroxy-3-methylglutaryl coenzyme A) reductase inhibitors (statins) has been associated with greater incidence of rhabdomyolysis. Diagnosis is made by symptoms of muscle pain, dark-brown urine without red cells on urinalysis, and elevated creatine kinase levels. Approximately 30% of patients develop acute renal failure (ARF) and other electrolyte imbalances; in these patients, early diagnosis and treatment are the keys to minimizing ARF. In patients who are acutely ill, volume repletion and close monitoring of urine output are imperative. Although, in the past, alkalinization was a mainstay in the treatment of rhabdomyolysis, it is no longer considered mandatory; in some studies, use of urinary alkalinization was not found to be superior to use of saline. *(Answer: B—Myoglobinuria caused by rhabdomyolysis)*

24. A 53-year-old woman presented to the emergency department with a cough, fever, and yellow sputum production; she had been experiencing these symptoms for 1 week. On physical examination, crackles were heard in the left lower and middle lung zones, and the patient experienced pain on inspiration. Laboratory results were as follows: Na, 128 mEq/L; K, 2.8 mEq/L; BUN, 25 mg/dl; creatinine, 1.1 mg/dl. A chest radiograph showed a consolidation in the left lower lobe. The patient was admitted and treated with I.V. antibiotics. On the day after admission, her blood pressure dropped to 90/75 mm Hg, and she became confused. After I.V. administration of normal saline, the blood pressure increased to 105/70 mm Hg and there was improvement in the patient's mental status. A repeat chest radiograph showed continued consolidation in the left lower lobe and progression in the right middle lobe. The patient's temperature was 103.2° F (39.5° C). Gentamicin was added. Six hours later, the patient's creatinine level is 2.1 mg/dl, and her BUN is 32 mg/dl.

What is the most likely cause of the increase in this patient's creatinine level?

- ❑ **A. IgA nephropathy**
- ❑ **B. Gentamicin nephrotoxicity**
- ❑ **C. Acute tubular necrosis (ATN) caused by hypotension**
- ❑ **D. Syndrome of inappropriate antidiuretic hormone (SIADH) associated with pneumonia**

Key Concept/Objective: To be able to differentiate aminoglycoside toxicity from hypotension-induced ATN

In the hospitalized patient, ATN is the most common cause of ARF. However, in most ARF patients, multiple insults complicate the clinical picture. Common contributing factors include sepsis and nephrotoxins in addition to the usual prerenal and postrenal azotemia. Determining the actual cause among various possible causes of ARF is often difficult. In this patient, sepsis, hypotension, and nephrotoxins may have contributed to the ARF. ATN from hypotension is the most likely cause, given the time and rapidity of onset. If her BUN and creatinine levels had risen a week later, aminoglycoside toxicity would have been a likely cause; however, 6 hours is too short an interval for this patient's ARF to have been caused by aminoglycoside toxicity. IgA nephropathy can occur rapidly; however, it is more likely to occur over a period of weeks than hours. Severe SIADH could potentially complicate the clinical picture over time. *(Answer: C—Acute tubular necrosis [ATN] caused by hypotension)*

25. A 24-year-old African-American woman comes to your office with complaints of fatigue, wrist and knee pain, and progressive lower extremity edema. She first noticed these symptoms 2 months ago; before then, she had been in good health. On physical examination, her blood pressure is elevated to 185/105 mm Hg, she has no fever, and her heart rate and respiratory rate are normal. Results of cardiovascular, lung, and abdominal examinations are normal. All her joints are normal, and no redness, warmth, or effusions are noted. You corroborate pitting edema up to her midshin bilaterally. Laboratory results are as follows: creatinine, 3.5 mg/dl; BUN, 56 mg/dl. The levels of all the electrolytes are normal.

Which of the following results of urinalysis would be most consistent with this patient's clinical picture?

- ❑ **A. Moderate number of hyaline and finely granular casts**
- ❑ **B. Presence of moderate to severe proteinuria (3+ to 4+), red blood cells (RBCs), and RBC casts**
- ❑ **C. Dipstick is positive for blood with few or no RBCs**
- ❑ **D. Dirty-brown granular casts and granular epithelial cells, both free and in casts**
- ❑ **E. Relatively normal results with no cells or few cells and no casts**

Key Concept/Objective: To understand the value of microscopic examination of the urine in determining the etiology of ARF

Urinalysis can provide invaluable information for patients with ARF. Prompt processing of the specimen is of paramount importance. Patients with myoglobinuria or hemo-

globinuria characteristically have positive findings on dipstick testing for blood and an absence of RBCs on microscopic examination of the urine. For patients with postrenal azotemia and those with hepatorenal syndrome, findings on urinalysis are relatively benign, and there is an absence of casts and cells. Patients with prerenal azotemia demonstrate hyaline and finely granular casts unless their condition has progressed to ATN. In patients with ATN, regardless of the etiology (renal or prerenal), the urine sediment has characteristic dirty-brown granular casts and both free renal epithelial cells and epithelial cell casts. This patient is likely to have proliferative glomerulonephritis; the urine sediment of such patients exhibits significant proteinuria, RBCs, and RBC casts. The differential diagnosis for proliferative glomerulonephritis includes connective tissue diseases, systemic vasculitis, postinfectious glomerulonephritis, and other diseases. *(Answer: B—Presence of moderate to severe proteinuria [3+ to 4+], red blood cells [RBCs], and RBC casts)*

For more information, see Shaver MJ, Shah SV: 10 Nephrology: VI Acute Renal Failure. ACP Medicine Online (www.acpmedicine.com). Dale DC, Federman DD, Eds. WebMD Inc., New York, June 2002

Vascular Diseases of the Kidney

26. A 32-year-old woman presents to you after a recent hospital admission for flash pulmonary edema. She was diagnosed with hypertension several months ago. Her blood pressure remains poorly controlled despite compliance with a regimen of hydrochlorothiazide, amlodipine, and metoprolol. She denies having headache and palpitation. Her physical examination is remarkable for a blood pressure of 204/106 mm Hg in the left arm and bilateral abdominal bruits. You consider the diagnosis of renal artery stenosis (RAS) secondary to fibromuscular dysplasia (FMD).

Which of the following statements regarding RAS and FMD is true?

- ❑ A. **Renal ultrasonography should be the first step in the evaluation of RAS because a finding of symmetrical kidneys precludes the need for further testing**
- ❑ B. **Angioplasty with stenting has become the most common method of managing FMD associated with hypertension and renal insufficiency; this procedure completely cures more then 50% of patients with hypertension and improves renal function in over one third**
- ❑ C. **The segmental nature of medial fibroplasia, the most common subtype of FMD, results in the classic so-called beads-on-a-string appearance in the proximal third of the main renal artery**
- ❑ D. **Surgical repair of aneurysms is required if their diameter is greater than 1.5 cm or if the patient has uncontrolled hypertension or is pregnant**

Key Concept/Objective: To understand the diagnosis and treatment of FMD

Medial fibroplasia, the most common subtype of FMD, is characterized by a predominance of fibrotic material in the media, with sparing of the intima and adventitia. It affects the distal two thirds of the main renal artery and its branches. In patients with a compatible clinical picture, evaluation for RAS starts with renal ultrasonography to measure kidney size. If there is a large discrepancy in kidney sizes (i.e., > 2 cm in the longitudinal axis), significant arterial stenosis is or was likely. Even if the ultrasound scan shows that the kidneys are equal in size, further diagnostic testing is required. The choice of procedures is determined by the level of renal function: patients with a serum creatinine level below 2 mg/dl should undergo renography; those with a serum creatinine above 2 mg/dl should undergo magnetic resonance angiography (MRA). The gold standard for the diagnosis of RAS remains a renal arteriogram. Percutaneous intervention has been the standard of care, but large comparative trials are not feasible, given the relative rarity of these conditions. Angioplasty and stenting completely cure hypertension in about 22% of patients. Surgical repair of aneurysms (the "beads" seen on arteriography)

is required if their diameter is greater than 1.5 cm; it is also required if the patient has uncontrolled hypertension or is pregnant. *(Answer: D—Surgical repair of aneurysms is required if their diameter is greater than 1.5 cm or if the patient has uncontrolled hypertension or is pregnant)*

27. A 58-year-old man known to have nephrotic syndrome presents to the emergency department. For several days, he has been experiencing low back pain and for the past several hours, he has been experiencing hematuria and shortness of breath. The patient is tachypneic, with an oxygen saturation of 92% on 4 L of oxygen via nasal cannula. A CT angiogram reveals pulmonary thromboembolism.

For this patient, which of the following statements regarding renal vein thrombosis (RVT) is true?

- ❑ **A. RVT is most frequently associated with idiopathic and secondary membranous nephropathy; of these patients, 30% may have RVT**
- ❑ **B. In addition to acute lower back pain and hematuria, most patients present with some degree of renal insufficiency**
- ❑ **C. Doppler ultrasonography is the most common modality used in the diagnosis of RVT**
- ❑ **D. For patients with RVT, a 6-month course of warfarin is indicated**

Key Concept/Objective: To understand the prevalence, clinical presentation, diagnostic modalities, and treatment of RVT

RVT has been most frequently associated with idiopathic and secondary membranous nephropathy; 30% of these patients may have RVT. Pulmonary embolism may develop in up to 30% of patients with RVT, although alarmingly, the vast majority of these patients are asymptomatic. The classic clinical presentation of RVT is acute lower back pain and gross hematuria. Patients typically do not have renal insufficiency or hypertension. RVT can be diagnosed by computed tomography, magnetic resonance imaging, and contrast venography. Doppler ultrasound imaging is notoriously operator dependent and therefore should not be used for the diagnosis of RVT. Anticoagulation with warfarin is indicated for patients with RVT. The therapeutic goal is an INR of 2 to 3. The appropriate duration of therapy is likely lifelong. *(Answer: A—RVT is most frequently associated with idiopathic and secondary membranous nephropathy; of these patients, 30% may have RVT)*

28. A 48-year-old white man with no significant medical history presents to your office with fever, weight loss, malaise, and arthralgia. He has had these symptoms for several months. Over the past few weeks, he has developed a purplish rash over his lower extremities and several sores on his toes. He is afebrile, but his blood pressure is 187/92 mm Hg and his heart rate is 97 beats/min. Livedo reticularis and digital ischemia are noted on examination. Laboratory results are significant for a potassium level of 3.2 mEq/L, a blood urea nitrogen (BUN) value of 28 mg/dl, and a creatinine level of 2.3 mg/dl.

Which of the following statements regarding polyarteritis nodosa (PAN) is true?

- ❑ **A. Serologic tests for PAN are diagnostic; most patients exhibit a positive enzyme-linked immunosorbent assay (ELISA) titer to antibodies against serine protease 3 and myeloperoxidase**
- ❑ **B. The pathogenesis of PAN is unclear, although there appears to be an association with hepatitis C infection**
- ❑ **C. ACE inhibitors and angiotensin receptor blockers (ARBs) should be used cautiously in patients with PAN because renal involvement may produce a functional equivalent of RAS**
- ❑ **D. In approximately 90% of patients with PAN, remission is achieved with high-dose steroids**

Key Concept/Objective: To understand the pathogenesis, diagnostic criteria, and treatment of PAN

The pathogenesis of PAN is unclear. There appears to be an association with hepatitis B viral infection. The diagnosis of PAN is made by demonstration of the characteristic

lesion in an artery. Serologic tests are not diagnostic in PAN, but low-titer antibodies to rheumatoid factor and nuclear antigen may be present. Immunofluorescence antibody staining for cytoplasmic and perinuclear antineutrophil cytoplasmic autoantibodies (ANCAs) may be positive, but the more specific test—serum ELISA titers for antibodies against both serine protease 3 (PR3) and myeloperoxidase—is negative. If left untreated, patients with PAN have a poor prognosis. In such cases, patients are at risk for ischemia of numerous organ systems; the major causes of morbidity and mortality include renal failure, mesenteric ischemia, and cerebrovascular disease. Corticosteroids and cytotoxic agents have been the mainstays of therapy for idiopathic PAN, although the optimal therapy remains unknown. Approximately 50% of patients with idiopathic PAN achieve remission with high-dose steroids (e.g., prednisone, 1 mg/kg/day) for 3 to 6 months. Cyclophosphamide, either intravenous (0.6 g/m^2) or oral (2 mg/kg/day), for up to 1 year is used in patients whose disease does not respond to steroids or in patients who are at risk for serious complications. ACE inhibitors and ARBs should be used cautiously in patients with PAN, because renal involvement may produce a functional equivalent of classic renal artery stenosis. *(Answer: C—ACE inhibitors and angiotensin receptor blockers [ARBs] should be used cautiously in patients with PAN because renal involvement may produce a functional equivalent of RAS)*

29. A 54-year-old man presents with a 4-day history of low-grade fever and confusion. He was previously healthy. His physical examination is significant for pallor and ecchymoses. Laboratory studies reveal a hemoglobin of 7.6 g/dl, a WBC of 8,200/µl, and a platelet count of 12,000/µl. The peripheral blood smear shows schistocytes and a decreased number of platelets.

For this patient, which of the following statements regarding thrombotic microangiopathies (TMAs) is true?

- ❑ A. **When plasma activity of metalloprotease (ADAMTS-13) is elevated, von Willebrand antigens predominate; those antigens bind to platelets and cause aggregation and thrombi in the small vessels**
- ❑ B. **A presumptive diagnosis of thrombotic thrombocytopenic purpura (TTP) is often based on the presence of thrombocytopenia, schistocytes, and prolonged prothrombin time (PT) and partial thromboplastin time (PTT)**
- ❑ C. **Hemolytic-uremic syndrome (HUS) is characterized by platelet aggregation and the presence of large von Willebrand multimers**
- ❑ D. **The clinical presentation of antiphospholipid syndrome (APS) generally comprises a single thrombotic event in the arterial system**

Key Concept/Objective: To understand the pathogenesis and clinical presentations of the various thrombotic microangiopathies

The classic TMAs include TTP and HUS. The critical role of ADAMTS-13 (a disintegrin and metalloprotease with thrombospondin type 1 motif) in the pathogenesis of TTP has emerged in the past 10 years. ADAMTS-13, which is found on the surface of endothelial cells, normally cleaves large multimers of the von Willebrand antigen as they are secreted by the cell. These large multimers bind more efficiently than the cleaved von Willebrand antigen to platelets (at the Iba component of platelet glycoprotein Ib/IX/V vWA receptor). Plasma ADAMTS activity must be severely depressed for TTP to develop. The level of ADAMTS-13 plasma activity is modestly depressed in patients with liver disease, disseminated cancer, chronic metabolic and inflammatory conditions, and pregnancy, as well as in newborns. When plasma activity of ADAMTS-13 falls to less than 5% of normal, these large von Willebrand antigens predominate, bind to platelets, and cause aggregation and thrombi in small vessels. Although TTP is often defined by the classic pentad of findings, a presumptive diagnosis can often be based on a triad of laboratory observations: thrombocytopenia, schistocytes, and elevated serum lactate dehydrogenase (from shredded erythrocytes). Conditions other than TMA may also be difficult to distinguish from TTP. HUS is defined as a TMA that occurs after exposure to *Escherichia coli* 0157:H7 or other enteropathogenic serotypes of *E. coli*, *Shigella dysenteriae*, and, occasionally, some other enteropathogenic organism. Systemically, Shiga tox-

ins produced by the bacteria play two key roles in the development of thrombi composed of platelets and von Willebrand antigen. First, they impair the secretion of ADAMTS-13 through an unspecified mechanism, resulting in large von Willebrand multimers. Second, they activate platelet adherence via the glycoprotein Ibα component of glycoprotein Ib/Ix/V1 and V2, which may then promote von Willebrand antigen and platelet aggregation. The clinical presentation of APS most often comprises a single thrombotic event in either the arterial or the venous system. Deep vein thrombosis of the lower extremities is the most common occurrence. *(Answer: C—Hemolytic-uremic syndrome [HUS] is characterized by platelet aggregation and the presence of large von Willebrand multimers)*

30. A 49-year-old man reports coughing up 2 to 4 oz of blood several times in the past few weeks. He has a history of chronic nasal congestion and sinus infections. On review of systems, he reports worsening fatigue, mild fevers to 100° F (37.8° C), cough, dyspnea, and a 10-lb weight loss over the past 3 to 4 months. He works as a manager for a grocery store chain, has never used I.V. drugs, and has been monogamous with his wife over the 10 years they have been married. His blood pressure is 130/80 mm Hg. A chest examination reveals scattered rales, and his skin is without rash. Laboratory test results are as follows: HCT, 33; WBC, 12, with normal differential; ESR, 98; creatinine, 2; BUN, 30; antineutrophilic cytoplasmic antibodies are present in a cytoplasmic staining distribution. Urinalysis shows moderate hemoglobin and protein levels, microscopic exam of the urine shows red cell casts, and sputum cultures are negative for acid-fast bacilli and bacteria. Thoracoscopic lung biopsy reveals necrotizing granulomas.

What is the most likely diagnosis for this patient?

- ❑ **A. Sarcoidosis**
- ❑ **B. Tuberculosis**
- ❑ **C. Polyarteritis nodosa**
- ❑ **D. Goodpasture syndrome**
- ❑ **E. Wegener granulomatosis**

Key Concept/Objective: To know the characteristic presentation of Wegener granulomatosis and the specificity of a positive cANCA test result for this disorder

Wegener granulomatosis classically occurs in middle-aged adults as a pulmonary renal syndrome with hemoptysis, pulmonary infiltrates, and glomerulonephritis with red cell casts. In addition, antineutrophilic antibodies are present in over 90% of patients with Wegener granulomatosis and are a relatively specific indication of Wegener granulomatosis when present in a cytoplasmic staining distribution. Lung biopsy that shows necrotizing granulomas is diagnostic. Sarcoidosis and TB cause noncaseating granulomas, not necrotizing granulomas in lung tissue. Sarcoidosis usually causes pulmonary fibrosis, bronchiectasis, and cavitation, along with mediastinal adenopathy. Renal sarcoidosis usually causes renal insufficiency through hypercalcemia or tubular dysfunction from granulomatous interstitial nephritis. Although pulmonary TB may [illegible] the lung or appears in a miliary pattern on chest x-ray. Furthermore, TB involving the kidneys more likely causes significant pyuria. Classic polyarteritis does not involve the lungs and is characterized by a perinuclear, not cytoplasmic, ANCA staining pattern. Goodpasture syndrome is a pulmonary renal syndrome with a presentation similar to that of Wegener granulomatosis, but in Goodpasture syndrome, ANCA test results are negative. *(Answer: E—Wegener granulomatosis)*

31. ***What treatment would be most appropriate for the patient described in Question 30?***

- ❑ **A. Prednisone**
- ❑ **B. Azathioprine**
- ❑ **C. Four-drug therapy for TB**
- ❑ **D. Trimethoprim-sulfamethoxazole**
- ❑ **E. Cyclophosphamide plus prednisone**

Key Concept/Objective: To know that the appropriate treatment of Wegener granulomatosis is cyclophosphamide in combination with prednisone

Early treatment with the combination of cyclophosphamide and prednisone is the most effective way to prevent rapid progression to renal failure in patients with Wegener granulomatosis. This combination can also induce remission in up to 75% of patients. Prednisone may cause temporary clinical improvement but rarely results in remission. Neither azathiaprine nor four-drug TB therapy would be useful against Wegener granulomatosis. In patients with Wegener granulomatosis who are in remission, trimethoprim-sulfamethoxazole is used to prevent relapse of disease; it is not used in patients with active disease. *(Answer: E—Cyclophosphamide plus prednisone)*

32. A 44-year-old woman reports severe right calf pain, which has been worsening over the past week. She occasionally takes acetaminophen and occasionally uses alcohol but does not use cigarettes or I.V. drugs; she has had a monogamous relationship with a female partner for 8 years. She has been feeling under the weather for several months, with fatigue, unintentional weight loss of 8 lb, and postprandial abdominal discomfort. She denies having cough, dyspnea, hemoptysis, chest pain, change in bowel habits, urinary symptoms, or rash. On examination, the patient's temperature is 99.8° F (37.7° C), her blood pressure is 160/100 mm Hg, and there are abrasions on her right knee and palm from a recent fall. On neurologic examination, the patient has marked weakness of right foot dorsiflexion. Skin examination reveals livedo reticularis over the patient's back and lower extremities. Urinalysis results are normal, ESR is 87, creatinine is 1.9, rheumatoid factor and antinuclear antibody test results are negative, and chest x-ray is normal.

What is the most likely diagnosis for this patient?

- ❑ **A. Microscopic polyarteritis**
- ❑ **B. Polyarteritis nodosa**
- ❑ **C. Sarcoidosis**
- ❑ **D. Cholesterol embolism**
- ❑ **E. Systemic lupus erythematosus**

Key Concept/Objective: To know the presentation of polyarteritis nodosa

Both polyarteritis nodosa and microscopic polyarteritis can cause neurologic deficits, livedo, renal compromise, and systemic symptoms of fatigue, fever, and weight loss. However, because polyarteritis nodosa affects larger vessels, it can cause downstream glomerular ischemia, thereby activating the renin-angiotensin system and raising blood pressure without causing an active urine sediment. Microscopic polyarteritis, on the other hand, affects smaller vessels, causing glomerular necrosis and the resulting active urine sediment of red cell casts and protein, without raising blood pressure. Although sarcoidosis can cause nerve and renal injury as well as systemic symptoms, sarcoidosis is unlikely to be the cause of this patient's symptoms because 90% of patients with sarcoidosis have pulmonary involvement. Cholesterol emboli can cause livedo and pain in the legs or abdomen, although it should not cause a footdrop. It is usually seen in patients with significant atherosclerotic disease or risk factors for atherosclerosis who have recently undergone an invasive angiographic procedure. Lupus could explain the systemic symptoms, the neurologic deficit, and livedo, although it is unlikely with a negative antinuclear antibody test result. *(Answer: B—Polyarteritis nodosa)*

33. ***For which of the following tests would a positive result be diagnostic for the condition of the patient in Question 32?***

- ❑ **A. Angiography**
- ❑ **B. Renal biopsy**
- ❑ **C. ANCA**
- ❑ **D. Electromyography**
- ❑ **E. Abdominal CT scan**

Key Concept/Objective: To know that renal or celiac angiographic findings can be diagnostic of polyarteritis nodosa when microaneurysms are present

Celiac or renal angiographic findings of microaneurysms and irregular, segmental constriction of the larger vessels with tapering and occlusion of smaller intrarenal arteries are diagnostic of classic polyarteritis nodosa. In the absence of active urine sediment, renal biopsy is unlikely to be diagnostic. In addition, because the findings associated with the vasculitides often overlap, renal biopsy findings are not usually diagnostic. Abdominal CT scanning is not sensitive enough to pick up the microaneurysms of polyarteritis nodosa. ANCA with a perinuclear staining pattern is more likely to be present in microscopic polyarteritis than in the classic form of polyarteritis nodosa. Electromyopathy can assist in determining whether nerve damage is axonal or demyelinating, although it is rarely diagnostic. *(Answer: A—Angiography)*

34. A 21-year-old college student reports abdominal pain, bilateral ankle and knee pain, bloody urine, and a worsening rash that began on his lower legs and has spread to his trunk. He denies having had any recent infectious exposures or infections; he also denies using I.V. drugs and having any sexual contacts. On examination, the patient is afebrile, his blood pressure is 120/80 mm Hg, and his pulse is 76 beats/min. Skin examination reveals raised, indurated, purple coalescing papules on his anterior shins, lower legs, and abdomen. Urinalysis shows moderate levels of hemoglobin and protein with red blood cell casts on microscopic examination. Stool guaiac results are positive; CBC is normal, with a normal WBC differential; creatinine is 0.8; and the results of testing for antinuclear antibodies, cryoglobulins, rheumatoid factor, and hepatitis antibodies are negative. Skin biopsy results reveal an intense neutrophilic infiltrate surrounding dermal blood vessels, confirming leukocytoclastic vasculitis.

Which of the following is most likely to be true about this man's condition?

- ❑ **A. Renal biopsy is diagnostic for Henoch-Schonlein purpura**
- ❑ **B. Polyclonal IgG deposits on skin biopsy confirm Henoch-Schonlein purpura**
- ❑ **C. Empirical treatment for gonococcal infection should be started**
- ❑ **D. The extent of renal involvement is the most important prognostic factor**
- ❑ **E. Prednisone and cyclophosphamide therapy should be started as soon as possible**

Key Concept/Objective: To know the diagnosis and prognosis of Henoch-Schonlein purpura

Henoch-Schonlein purpura is diagnosed on the basis of the classic tetrad of skin rash, abdominal pain, arthralgias and arthritis, and glomerulonephritis. The extent of renal involvement is the most important prognostic factor in Henoch-Schonlein purpura. Renal biopsy results are not diagnostic of Henoch-Schonlein purpura, as such results can be identical with the results obtained in cases of IgA nephropathy with IgA deposition in the mesangium and in cases involving severe crescent formation. Skin biopsy results also show IgA (not IgG) deposition on immunofluorescence. This patient does not have any risk factors or signs of sepsis; if there is any suspicion that gonococcal or rickettsial infection is causing the palpable purpura, empirical therapy should be started immediately. Most cases of Henoch-Schonlein purpura resolve spontaneously, although prednisone and cyclophosphamide should be considered for use in the few patients with acute renal failure. *(Answer: D—The extent of renal involvement is the most important prognostic factor)*

For more information, see Kshirsager A, Falk RJ: 10 Nephrology: VII Vascular Diseases of the Kidney. ACP Medicine Online (www.acpmedicine.com). Dale DC, Federman DD, Eds. WebMD Inc., New York, December 2004

Tubulointerstitial Diseases

35. A 67-year-old black man with a history of tobacco abuse and ethanol abuse is admitted for gradually worsening esophageal dysphagia complicated by a 1-day history of shortness of breath, productive cough, and fever. On examination, the patient has a temperature of 101.5° F (38.6° C); he is tachypneic and has signs of consolidation in his right posterior lung field. Chest radiography reveals a right lower lobe infiltrate consistent with aspiration pneumonia. He is placed on piperacillin-tazobactam and oxygen, and he gradually improves. By hospital day 3, he experiences defervescence, but on hospital day 10 he is noted to again have a fever (100.8° F [38.2° C]). In addition, the patient has a rash, and peripheral blood eosinophilia and acute renal insufficiency are present.

Which of the following statements concerning this patient's condition is most correct?

- ❑ **A. This patient will likely progress to end-stage renal disease**
- ❑ **B. Standard of care would include stopping the piperacillin-tazobactam and starting high-dose I.V. solumedrol**
- ❑ **C. Another β-lactam antibiotic can be safely substituted for piperacillin**
- ❑ **D. Urinalysis will most likely reveal sterile pyuria, mild proteinuria, and hematuria**
- ❑ **E. Most patients with this disorder become oligoanuric**

Key Concept/Objective: To understand the clinical manifestations and management of acute interstitial nephritis (AIN)

Virtually all β-lactam antibiotics (i.e., penicillins and cephalosporins) can produce AIN. It usually occurs after several weeks of high-dose antibiotic therapy. Classically, patients exhibit a triad of hypersensitivity reactions: rash, fever, and eosinophilia. The secondary fever associated with AIN usually occurs after defervescence from the original infectious disease and during the onset of the allergic reaction. Urinary findings in patients with AIN include the nonspecific findings of sterile pyuria and mild proteinuria, as well as the more significant finding of hematuria, which in some patients may be gross. Eosinophils may be found in the urine sediment on Wright or Hansel staining in over 75% of cases. The pathogenesis of β-lactam-associated AIN remains unknown. The disease is not dose related and occurs in only a small number of the millions of people taking β-lactam drugs each year. It can recur or be exacerbated on rechallenge with a second β-lactam drug. β-Lactam-associated AIN is treated by discontinuing the drug and avoiding other β-lactam antibiotics. Most patients regain renal function, and many regain baseline renal function. Only a minority of patients with AIN are oliguric. The use of corticosteroids to treat renal failure associated with AIN remains controversial. No randomized, controlled trials have yet proved that corticosteroid therapy has any advantages over discontinuance of medication. *(Answer: D—Urinalysis will most likely reveal sterile pyuria, mild proteinuria, and hematuria)*

36. A 65-year-old man with hypertension and reflux disease presents to your office for routine follow-up. He has no complaints. Laboratory data reveal an increased serum potassium level of 5.8 mEq/L. On questioning, you learn that the patient has a history of hesitancy, dribbling, and a decrease in the urinary stream.

Which of the following statements pertaining to renal interstitial damage from physical factors is false?

- ❑ **A. For patients with vesicoureteral reflux, medical therapy is unhelpful, and surgical intervention should be recommended immediately**
- ❑ **B. In patients older than 60 years, the most common causes of obstructive uropathy are benign prostatic hypertrophy and prostatic or gynecologic malignancies**
- ❑ **C. Ultrasonography is the diagnostic test of choice for obstructive nephropathy**
- ❑ **D. Before diagnosing a patient as having vesicoureteral reflux disease, any urinary tract infection should be treated if present, and a repeat voiding cystourethrogram should be performed**

Key Concept/Objective: To know that vesicoureteral reflux can cause chronic tubulointerstitial damage, known as reflux nephropathy

Vesicoureteral reflux can cause chronic tubulointerstitial damage, known as reflux nephropathy. When infection is present, even low-pressure refluxed urine that reaches the kidney can produce chronic interstitial inflammation and scarring. Presenting features can include such signs of urinary tract infection as back or flank pain, fever, and dysuria. Hypertension, when present, is often associated with high levels of renin, which may derive from the segmental areas of scarred parenchyma. Patients often have a urinary concentrating defect, leading to nocturia and polyuria. Reflux is demonstrated with a voiding cystourethrogram. Because urinary tract infection may be associated with reflux, it is best to wait several weeks after treating a urinary tract infection before trying to diagnose reflux nephropathy. Treatment of low-grade reflux is medical: long-term antibiotic therapy is used to sterilize the urine and prevent reinfection. Many persons with mild reflux undergo spontaneous remission with time. More severe reflux may require surgical intervention, although most comparative studies have not found an advantage for surgical intervention over medical therapy. Obstructive nephropathy may produce chronic interstitial damage, especially when the obstruction is partial or intermittent and longstanding. In persons older than 60 years, benign prostatic hypertrophy and prostatic and gynecologic cancers are common etiologies. The pathologic findings show dilatation of the collecting ducts and distal tubules. Ultrasonography usually shows dilatation of the urinary collecting system and hydronephrosis. Treatment consists of relieving the obstruction. *(Answer: A—For patients with vesicoureteral reflux, medical therapy is unhelpful, and surgical intervention should be recommended immediately)*

37. A 38-year-old man comes to your office for evaluation of a urinalysis that revealed proteinuria. Further evaluation demonstrated proteinuria in the nonnephrotic range and a creatinine level of 1.8 mg/dl. The patient has celiac disease with steatorrhea, which was diagnosed many years ago. You suspect he has chronic interstitial nephritis that is associated with celiac disease.

Which of the following scenarios is NOT associated with tubulointerstitial nephritis?

❑ A. **A patient who several years ago underwent stomach bypass surgery for morbid obesity**

❑ B. **A 35-year-old woman who has non-Hodgkin lymphoma with bulky disease and is 2 days post chemotherapy**

❑ C. **A patient with vitamin D deficiency who presents with tetany and paresthesias**

❑ D. **A 68-year-old man with hypertension who ingested moonshine for 40 years**

Key Concept/Objective: To understand the metabolic disturbances that can produce renal tubulointerstitial abnormalities, as well as environmental factors that can cause renal damage

Oxalic acid is a dicarboxylic end product of metabolism that is removed from the body only by renal excretion. Precipitation of calcium oxalate can produce nephrolithiasis, acute renal failure, or chronic tubulointerstitial damage. Patients with steatorrhea from various intestinal diseases—including celiac disease, Crohn disease, Wilson disease, and chronic pancreatitis—or from small bowel resection or bypass operations for obesity may hyperabsorb oxalate from the large bowel. The pathogenesis of oxalate hyperabsorption involves the abnormal binding of intraluminal gut calcium to fats, which frees more oxalate for absorption. In addition, the solubilizing effect of bile acids on the large bowel permits greater absorption of oxalate. The result can be nephrolithiasis, acute renal insufficiency, or chronic tubulointerstitial damage. Hyperuricemia and hyperuricosuria can lead to uric acid and acute oliguric renal failure from urate deposition. These conditions occur after massive release of uric acid, as occurs in the tumor lysis syndrome or chronic renal failure. Hypercalcemia and hypercalciuria can also produce a number of adverse renal effects. Hypercalcemia may lead to chronic tubulointerstitial damage. Chronic elevations of the calcium level can lead to calcium salt deposition in the tubules and interstitial regions; such depositions are associated with chronic interstitial inflammation, tubular atrophy, and fibrosis. Two heavy metals—lead and cadmium—clearly produce tubulointerstitial damage. Exposure to lead can occur from the ingestion of lead-based paints, the ingestion of beverages stored in crystal decanters

made with lead, the ingestion of moonshine whiskey made in a lead-containing still, the manufacture or destruction of lead batteries, or the ingestion of lead-containing aerosols in the workplace. *(Answer: C—A patient with vitamin D deficiency who presents with tetany and paresthesias)*

38. A 56-year-old black man presents with bone pain, anemia, hypercalcemia, and renal insufficiency. Bone marrow biopsy indicates a diagnosis of multiple myeloma.

Which of the following mechanisms does NOT classically cause renal damage in patients with multiple myeloma?

- ❑ **A. Excessive filtration of Bence-Jones proteins, causing direct tubular cell damage**
- ❑ **B. Renal artery thrombosis associated with tubular atrophy**
- ❑ **C. Hyperuricemia from urate overproduction or lysis of plasma cells, causing precipitation of urate crystals**
- ❑ **D. The suppression of humoral immunity, leading to urinary tract infections that cause chronic tubulointerstitial nephritis**
- ❑ **E. Hypercalcemia leading to calcium salt deposition in the kidneys**

Key Concept/Objective: To understand the different mechanisms of renal damage in patients with multiple myeloma

Renal insufficiency and acute renal failure are common and significant contributors to morbidity and mortality in patients with multiple myeloma. Clinical indications that a patient with unexplained renal disease has multiple myeloma include (1) low-level proteinuria, as seen on urinary dipstick measurement, in conjunction with high-level proteinuria, as seen on 24-hour quantitative measurement (the dipstick primarily detects albumin, not Bence-Jones protein), (2) a low anion gap (caused by the cationic charge on some monoclonal immunoglobulins), (3) hypercalcemia in the presence of renal failure and a high serum phosphate level, and (4) anemia that is out of proportion to the degree of renal insufficiency. A common manifestation of myeloma is renal insufficiency, present in more than 50% of patients. Excessive production and filtration of monoclonal light chains (Bence-Jones protein) can cause direct tubular cell damage, as well as tubular obstruction by casts. Dysproteinemias can also be associated with tubulointerstitial precipitation of urate crystals, caused by urate overproduction or lysis of plasma cells. In addition, the tubulointerstitial area can be damaged by deposition of calcium salt crystals as a result of hypercalciuria from lytic bone lesions and calcium-mobilizing humoral factors. Upper and lower urinary tract infections, from suppression of normal humoral immunity, are also common in patients with myeloma and can cause acute and chronic tubulointerstitial damage. *(Answer: B—Renal artery thrombosis associated with tubular atrophy)*

For more information, see Appel GB: 10 Nephrology: VIII Tubulointerstitial Diseases. ACP Medicine Online (www.acpmedicine.com). Dale DC, Federman DD, Eds. WebMD Inc., New York, January 2004

Chronic Renal Failure and Dialysis

39. A 48-year-old black woman visits your office as a new patient. Her only known medical problems are diabetes and hypertension. She was diagnosed with each illness about 15 years ago. She has no history of kidney disease. She reports her glycosylated hemoglobin (HgA_{1c}) level is typically 7% to 8%, and her average blood pressure is 150/88 mm Hg. Her current drug therapy consists of an angiotensin-converting enzyme (ACE) inhibitor, a calcium channel blocker, and a sulfonylurea. Laboratory studies reveal normocytic anemia, a creatinine level of 2.7 mg/dl, and 3+ protein on urinalysis. Other results are normal.

Which of the following statements regarding chronic renal failure (CRF) is false?

- ❑ **A. The incidence of new cardiovascular disease is the same for those with reduced kidney function as for those with normal kidney function**

❑ B. **Anemia is directly related to azotemia and is usually evident once the serum creatinine level exceeds 3 mg/dl**

❑ C. **Like the older preparations, the newer cyclooxygenase-2 (COX-2) nonsteroidal anti-inflammatory drugs (NSAIDs) have an adverse effect on renal function**

❑ D. **The decline in hematocrit is largely the result of a reduction in the production of erythropoietin by the kidney**

Key Concept/Objective: To know the clinical findings associated with CRF and the adverse effect of NSAIDs on renal function

There appears to be a surfeit of cardiovascular disease in persons with impaired kidney function. An analysis by the United States Renal Data System of patients older than 67 years showed that the incidence of new cardiovascular disease was more than 50% greater in those with reduced kidney function, as compared with those having normal kidney function. Anemia is directly related to azotemia and is usually evident once the serum creatinine level exceeds 3 mg/dl. Studies in patients with CRF have shown an inverse correlation of hematocrit with azotemia. This decline in the hematocrit is largely the result of a reduction in the production of erythropoietin by the kidney. Several general therapeutic measures can slow the progressive loss of renal function in CRF. Use of nephrotoxins must be avoided—especially NSAIDs, which may impair renal function because of their effects on prostaglandin synthesis. Patient education on this topic is important, because NSAIDs such as ibuprofen and naproxen are available without prescription. The newer COX-2 NSAIDs also reduce kidney function. *(Answer: A—The incidence of new cardiovascular disease is the same for those with reduced kidney function as for those with normal kidney function)*

40. A 61-year-old man with progressive hypertensive renal disease visits your office for a routine follow-up visit. You have followed this patient for many years. The patient reports that he has become progressively fatigued over the past few weeks, and his exercise tolerance is failing. He also reports that he has developed persistent, generalized itching. A 24-hour urine collection reveals that his creatinine clearance is stable at 15 ml/min. His blood urea nitrogen (BUN) level is 90 mg/dl, and his creatinine level is 8.5 mg/dl. A nephrologist recently referred the patient to a vascular surgeon for hemodialysis vascular access. He states that his nephrologist has advised that he initiate hemodialysis therapy as soon as his vascular access is placed and matured.

Which of the following statements regarding end-stage renal disease (ESRD) and hemodialysis is false?

❑ A. **Infection is second only to cardiovascular disease as a cause of death in patients with ESRD**

❑ B. **Most deaths caused by infection in patients with ESRD are the result of pneumonia**

❑ C. **Of the devices for gaining circulatory access, indwelling catheters carry the most risk for infection**

❑ D. ***S. aureus* and *S. epidermidis* are the most commonly identified agents in infections related to dialysis vascular access**

Key Concept/Objective: To understand that indwelling vascular catheters are a prominent source of fatal infection in patients with ESRD

ESRD patients are at risk for infection, which is second only to cardiovascular disease as a cause of death in these patients. A recent longitudinal cohort study of ESRD patients identified low serum albumin levels and use of devices such as central venous catheters and artificial arteriovenous fistulas as major risk factors for septicemia. Most deaths caused by infection are related to colonization of devices used to gain temporary access to the circulatory system, such as temporary dialysis catheters; pulmonary and intra-abdominal infections may also occur. Of the devices for gaining circulatory access, indwelling catheters carry the most risk, polytetrafluoroethylene arteriovenous grafts

carry somewhat less risk, and native arteriovenous fistulas are least likely to become infected. *S. aureus* and *S. epidermidis* are the most commonly identified infectious agents; both may cause septicemia and complications such as endocarditis and septic arthritis. Empirical treatment of either bacteremia or an infection at the site of circulatory access thus requires use of an agent that is effective against staphylococci. *(Answer: B—Most deaths caused by infection in patients with ESRD are the result of pneumonia)*

41. A 68-year-old man with chronic renal failure secondary to type 2 diabetes mellitus presents with hematemesis. Initial laboratory values indicate a hematocrit of 23%, platelet count of 267,000/mm^3, BUN of 126 mg/dl, and creatinine of 10.6 mg/dl. A decision is made to transfuse the patient with 2 units of packed red blood cells and to arrange for upper endoscopy. In addition, preparations are made for temporary access to initiate hemodialysis.

What other therapy would be most likely to minimize bleeding in this patient?

- ❑ **A. Platelet transfusion**
- ❑ **B. Desmopressin I.V.**
- ❑ **C. Vitamin K I.M.**
- ❑ **D. Protamine I.V.**
- ❑ **E. Octreotide I.V.**

Key Concept/Objective: To be able to recognize the bleeding diathesis of ESRD and understand its management

This patient presents with acute bleeding and compromised renal function. The renal dysfunction has a negative impact on platelet function. Desmopressin appears to help with platelet function. As there is generally an adequate platelet count, platelet transfusion does not have much impact. Vitamin K is used to help reverse problems with the extrinsic clotting cascade. Protamine is used to help reverse the effects of heparin, and octreotide is used for variceal bleeding. Estrogen is also used occasionally for uremic bleeding. *(Answer: B—Desmopressin I.V.)*

42. A 54-year-old woman with ESRD on hemodialysis presents with a traumatic fracture of the humerus. An orthopedic consultation recommends an open reduction and internal fixation to be performed the following day.

Which of the following medications should most be avoided for this patient?

- ❑ **A. Acetaminophen**
- ❑ **B. Morphine sulfate**
- ❑ **C. Meperidine**
- ❑ **D. Hydromorphone**
- ❑ **E. Oxycodone**

Key Concept/Objective: To appreciate the need to choose medications carefully for the patient with ESRD

This patient requires postoperative pain management. Most narcotics are metabolized primarily by the liver, but the metabolites of meperidine can accumulate, especially in the setting of compromised renal function. This leads to an increased risk of seizure. Therefore, alternative narcotic (and nonnarcotic) analgesics should be used and the doses monitored closely. *(Answer: C—Meperidine)*

43. A 58-year-old woman presents to discuss potential hemodialysis. She has had progressive renal failure secondary to polycystic kidney disease and awaits renal transplantation.

Which of the following metabolic abnormalities would most likely be present in this patient?

❑ A. Metabolic acidosis

❑ B. Hypokalemia

❑ C. Hypophosphatemia

❑ D. Hypercalcemia

❑ E. Metabolic alkalosis

Key Concept/Objective: To be able to recognize common metabolic abnormalities in chronic renal failure

A number of metabolic abnormalities can occur in the setting of chronic renal failure. Potassium levels tend to climb because of decreased excretion. Phosphate levels also rise because of the reduction in urine output. The fall in calcium levels is caused by many factors, including decreased intestinal absorption, decreased hydroxylation of vitamin D, increased levels of PTH (with decreased sensitivity), and, at times, decreased intake. Typically, the acid-base disorder is that of metabolic acidosis. This is related to decreased ammonia secretion and inability to excrete titratable acid. There may also be type IV renal tubular acidosis or hyporeninemic hypoaldosteronism (most commonly occurring in diabetic patients). *(Answer: A—Metabolic acidosis)*

44. A 61-year-old man on chronic hemodialysis undergoes elective hip replacement. In the recovery room, telemetry reveals numerous premature ventricular complexes. An electrocardiogram reveals a prolonged PR interval, a widened QRS complex, and peaking of the T waves.

Which of the following is the most appropriate intravenous intervention for this patient?

❑ A. Magnesium

❑ B. Calcium

❑ C. Potassium

❑ D. Phosphate

❑ E. Heparin

Key Concept/Objective: To be able to recognize hyperkalemia and to understand its association with renal failure

This patient presents with classic electrocardiographic signs of hyperkalemia. The most appropriate first step is the infusion of intravenous calcium, which will help stabilize the myocardium. Other potential interventions include infusions of glucose/insulin, dialysis, albuterol nebulizer, polystyrene resins, and sodium bicarbonate. *(Answer: B—Calcium)*

45. A 68-year-old woman presents with progressive renal failure secondary to hypertension. On routine laboratory screening, she is found to have a calcium level of 7.8 and an albumin level of 4.2.

Which of the following is contributing to this patient's calcium level?

❑ A. Enhanced intestinal calcium absorption

❑ B. Low levels of circulating parathyroid hormone (PTH)

❑ C. Hypophosphatemia

❑ D. Decreased vitamin D hydroxylation

❑ E. Decreased fecal calcium

Key Concept/Objective: To be able to recognize the abnormalities in calcium management in the patient with ESRD

Calcium homeostasis is dramatically altered in the patient with ESRD. There is decreased intestinal absorption in the small intestine. The combination of low calcium levels and elevated phosphate levels leads to an increase in PTH. The kidney itself is no longer able to adequately hydroxylate vitamin D. This combination of factors leads to

a worsening in bone health. Critical interventions include keeping phosphate levels down, assuring adequate calcium ingestion, and, if necessary, replacing hydroxylated vitamin D. *(Answer: D—Decreased vitamin D hydroxylation)*

For more information, see Cohen EP: 10 Nephrology: X Chronic Renal Failure and Dialysis. ACP Medicine Online (www.acpmedicine.com). Dale DC, Federman DD, Eds. WebMD Inc., New York, August 2004

Renal Transplantation

46. A 66-year-old man with diabetes mellitus, hypertension, and chronic kidney disease presents for a routine follow-up visit. Despite good control of his hypertension (blood pressure, 124/72 mm Hg) and diabetes (hemoglobin A_{1c} level, 7.0%), the patient's creatinine level continues to slowly increase (Cr, 3.7 mg/dl). The patient is concerned about the long-term implications of his kidney disease and would like more information regarding his ultimate treatment options.

For this patient, which of the following statements is true?

- ❑ **A. Kidney transplantation results in an improvement in quality of life but a decrease in long-term survival**
- ❑ **B. Being older than 65 years precludes this patient from being considered as a kidney transplant recipient**
- ❑ **C. Kidney transplant recipients initially have an increase in mortality, but they have an overall improvement in long-term survival**
- ❑ **D. Quality of life is similar for dialysis patients and transplantation patients**

Key Concept/Objective: To be able to counsel patients who are considering kidney transplantation

Continued improvement in outcomes has made transplantation the treatment of choice for patients with end-stage renal disease. Unlike dialysis patients, transplantation patients have a documented improvement in quality of life and a comparatively high rate of return to employment. A study of more than 220,000 patients showed that long-term survival of patients who received a renal transplant was superior to that of patients who either remained on the transplantation waiting list or continued with long-term dialysis. Patients who underwent transplantation had an initial increase in mortality related to the surgical procedure; however, this initial risk was rapidly eclipsed by the improved long-term survival of transplant recipients. Most transplantation programs offer transplants to medically appropriate recipients regardless of age. Data show that older transplant recipients have excellent survival rates after renal transplantation and may in fact have a lower incidence of episodes of acute rejection than younger recipients. *(Answer: C—Kidney transplant recipients initially have an increase in mortality, but they have an overall improvement in long-term survival)*

47. The condition of the patient in Question 46 worsens over the next few years, and he undergoes renal transplantation from a living, nonrelated donor. He is started on an immunosuppressant regimen consisting of prednisone, cyclosporine, and mycophenolate mofetil. As his primary care provider, you continue to follow the patient for his hypertension and diabetes, which remain well controlled.

For this patient, which of the following statement is true?

- ❑ **A. The leading cause of death in kidney transplant recipients is opportunistic infection secondary to immunosuppressive therapy**
- ❑ **B. Recurrent glomerular kidney disease is the most common cause of graft loss**
- ❑ **C. Nephrotoxicity is the most common side effect of mycophenolate mofetil**
- ❑ **D. There is a direct correlation between systolic blood pressure and graft half-life; goal systolic blood pressure should be 130 mm Hg or less**

Key Concept/Objective: To understand the complications following renal transplantation

The leading cause of death in transplant recipients, as in the general population, is cardiovascular disease. The three most important causes of allograft dysfunction are recurrent glomerular kidney disease, acute rejection, and chronic allograft nephropathy. Although recurrent kidney disease can occur and, in selected cases, may result in progressive loss of renal function, it is much less likely to occur than acute rejection or chronic allograft nephropathy. Long-term studies show that chronic rejection remains the single most important cause of graft loss. Antimetabolites such as mycophenolate mofetil are an important part of immunosuppressive strategies, largely because they have no demonstrable nephrotoxicity and little effect on blood pressure, cholesterol levels, or glycemic control. *(Answer: D—There is a direct correlation between systolic blood pressure and graft half-life; goal systolic blood pressure should be 130 mm Hg or less)*

48. A 56-year-old woman presents to your clinic for follow-up visit after undergoing renal transplantation 3 months ago. She has been experiencing increasing symptoms of shortness of breath and has had fevers of up to 101° F (38.3° C). You admit her to the hospital and initiate a work-up of her symptoms. Cytomegalovirus (CMV) serologies are positive, and you initiate treatment.

Which of the following interventions could have decreased the likelihood of this patient developing her illness and could have decreased the severity of her illness?

- ❑ **A. Intravenous ganciclovir during pretransplant evaluation**
- ❑ **B. Prophylactic ganciclovir at time of transplantation and for 12 weeks thereafter**
- ❑ **C. Trimethoprim-sulfamethoxazole daily for 3 to 6 months**
- ❑ **D. Amoxicillin-clavulanate, 875 mg p.o., b.i.d.**

Key Concept/Objective: To understand the spectrum of infection in the posttransplantation period

Because of immunosuppressive therapy, patients who receive transplants are at risk for acquiring a variety of infections. Infectious agents vary relative to the time of transplantation. The first month after transplantation is characterized by infections that are related to the hospitalization. In this period, urinary tract infections, bacteremia caused by gram-positive cocci, and hospital-acquired pneumonias are common. After the first month and up to 6 months after transplantation, the most common infections are related to immunosuppressive therapy. Opportunistic infections such as CMV, EBV, *Pneumocystis carinii* infection, and diverse fungal infections predominate. After 6 months, when immunosuppressive therapy is less intense, common infections become prevalent; these include community-acquired pneumonia and cellulitis. CMV is one of the most important posttransplantation infections; it can present as a systemic viral illness, pneumonia, or gastrointestinal disease. Patients can develop primary infection as a result of receiving an organ from a seropositive donor or through reactivation of latent virus. It has been shown that prophylactic oral ganciclovir therapy, started at the time of transplantation and continued for 12 weeks, decreases the incidence and severity of CMV disease. *(Answer: B—Prophylactic ganciclovir at time of transplantation and for 12 weeks thereafter)*

49. A 47-year-old man who recently received a renal transplant and was started on steroids, cyclosporine, and mycophenolate mofetil presents for routine follow-up. On physical examination, his blood pressure is noted to be 189/96 mm Hg.

Which of the following statements regarding hypertension and renal transplantation is true?

- ❑ **A. Hypertension is a rare posttransplantation complication**
- ❑ **B. Mycophenolate mofetil can cause vasoconstriction and worsen hypertension**
- ❑ **C. Graft dysfunction causes worsening of hypotension**
- ❑ **D. Cyclosporine commonly induces a volume-dependent form of hypertension**

Key Concept/Objective: To understand the relationship between immunosuppressive medications and hypertension

With the goal of graft survival in mind, the long-term follow-up of patients undergoing renal transplantation should focus on management of the major causes of morbidity and mortality. Cardiovascular disease, specifically hypertension, is one of the most common posttransplantation complications, affecting 80% to 90% of these patients. The etiology of hypertension in this population is multifactorial but includes diseased native kidneys, use of immunosuppressive medications, graft dysfunction, and, rarely, transplant renal artery stenosis. Although calcineurin inhibitors are the cornerstones of immunosuppression, as a class, these agents commonly cause hypertension. Specifically, cyclosporine causes direct vasoconstriction and induces preglomerular vasoconstriction, resulting in a volume-dependent form of high blood pressure. Other classes of immunosuppressants that cause hypertension are corticosteroids and TOR (target of rapamycin) inhibitors. Antimetabolites, however, such as azathioprine and mycophenolate mofetil, are important in immunosuppressive agents because of their lack of nephrotoxicity and because they have little effect on blood pressure. *(Answer: D—Cyclosporine commonly induces a volume-dependent form of hypertension)*

50. A 43-year-old woman with end-stage renal disease (ESRD) presents to your clinic for renal transplant evaluation. She has focal segmental glomerular sclerosis and has been doing well for some time on hemodialysis, but she is concerned about "losing the transplanted kidney" because of her original disease.

Which of the following statements regarding recurrence and graft loss associated with her primary renal disease is false?

❑ **A. Primary glomerular diseases frequently recur and are commonly associated with graft loss**

❑ **B. Lupus nephritis rarely recurs after transplantation**

❑ **C. Type II membranoproliferative glomerulosclerosis has a high recurrence rate, but only one fifth of those patients have graft loss**

❑ **D. Patients with Alport syndrome can develop anti-glomerular basement membrane (anti-GBM) disease in the allograft**

Key Concept/Objective: To understand the risk of disease recurrence in patients with primary glomerular disease

The recurrence rates of different primary renal diseases vary. Primary glomerular diseases frequently recur in the transplanted kidney; however, graft loss secondary to recurrence is uncommon. The patients who are at greatest risk of graft loss are those in whom renal function deteriorated rapidly and aggressively. In these patients, transplantation may be relatively contraindicated. Lupus nephritis, anti-GBM disease, and membranous nephropathy have low recurrence rates and are rarely associated with graft loss. Type II membranoproliferative disease has a high recurrence rate (80% to 90%); however, it too is associated with a low incidence of graft loss. Patients with Alport syndrome can develop anti-GBM disease in the allograft, although this is uncommon, and Alport syndrome is not a contraindication to transplantation. *(Answer: A—Primary glomerular diseases frequently recur and are commonly associated with graft loss)*

51. A 39-year-old black woman with ESRD secondary to membranous nephropathy presents to your clinic for routine follow-up. She underwent renal transplantation 3 months ago and is doing well on a regimen of steroids, sirolimus, and cyclosporine. On reviewing results of routine laboratory studies, you note that her total cholesterol level is elevated to 246 mg/dl.

Which of the following statements is true regarding the treatment of this patient's hyperlipidemia?

❑ **A. Her immunosuppresion is unrelated to the elevated cholesterol level**

❑ **B. Her hyperlipidemia is likely characterized by a low level of low-density lipoprotein (LDL) but a high level of high-density lipoprotein (HDL)**

❑ C. Diet and exercise will be sufficient to control her lipid abnormalities

❑ D. Her lipid abnormalities will probably improve within 6 months after transplantation

Key Concept/Objective: To understand the treatment of the patient with coexisting diseases

Of the cardiovascular diseases that affect the renal transplant population, hyperlipidemia is one of the most common. The presence of hyperlipidemia is an important factor for both patient survival and graft survival. If left untreated, arteriosclerosis can occur in the graft as a form of vasculopathy and can lead to tubulointerstitial ischemia, scarring, and fibrosis. Posttransplantation hyperlipidemia is characterized by an increase in total cholesterol and an increase in LDL and very low density lipoprotein levels. Although the etiology of posttransplantation hyperlipidemia is not clear, there is a relationship between hyperlipidemia and the use of immunosuppressive medications, specifically corticosteroids, cyclosporine, and sirolimus. Although the majority of lipid abnormalities resolve within 6 months posttransplantation secondary to a reduction in the doses of immunosuppressant agents, elevations in lipid levels need to be treated aggressively. Usually, dietary measures will not control these lipid abnormalities, and statins are needed for adequate control. Fibrates and nicotinic acid may also be necessary to control refractory lipid levels. In patients with coexisting diabetes, tight glycemic control is essential to good management of hyperlipidemia. *(Answer: D—Her lipid abnormalities will probably improve within 6 months after transplantation)*

For more information, see Klassen DK, Weir MR: 10 Nephrology: XI Renal Transplantation. ACP Medicine Online (www.acpmedicine.com). Dale DC, Federman DD, Eds. WebMD Inc., New York, December 2004

Benign Prostatic Hyperplasia

52. A 63-year-old man presents to your primary care clinic with a complaint of nocturia. He gets up to urinate two or three times a night and is having trouble getting a restful night's sleep. Review of symptoms is otherwise negative. Physical examination reveals a large, homogeneous prostate. Laboratory work effectively rules out diabetes mellitus.

Which of the following statements regarding the pathophysiology of benign prostatic hyperplasia (BPH) is true?

❑ A. The hyperplastic process of BPH begins in the peripheral zones and can eventually compress the urethra

❑ B. Only one type of alpha$_2$-adrenergic receptor has been identified in the lower urinary tract

❑ C. Type 1 5α-reductase isoenzyme converts testosterone to dihydrotestosterone preferentially in the prostate

❑ D. Peptide growth factors such as fibroblast growth factors, insulinlike growth factors, and epidermal growth factors are felt to be the local forces that determine prostate growth

Key Concept/Objective: To understand the basic pathophysiology involved in BPH

BPH involves hyperplasia of both the epithelial and the stromal compartments. The hyperplastic process begins in the periurethral and transition zones of the prostate; in contrast, prostate cancer preferentially develops in the peripheral zones. At least three types of alpha$_2$-adrenergic receptors have been identified in the lower urinary tract. The type 1 5α-reductase isoenzyme has low activity in the prostate and is expressed predominantly in the skin and liver. The pathophysiologic mechanisms underlying the development and progression of BPH are incompletely understood. Clearly, BPH involves prolonged exposure of the prostate gland to androgens. In the prostate, interactions between epithelial and stromal cells and the extracellular matrix, mediated primarily by locally produced (intrinsic) growth factors, appear important. These peptide

growth factors, which include fibroblast growth factors, insulinlike growth factors, and epidermal growth factors, are felt to be the local forces that determine prostate growth. *(Answer: D—Peptide growth factors such as fibroblast growth factors, insulinlike growth factors, and epidermal growth factors are felt to be the local forces that determine prostate growth)*

53. A 57-year-old man presents for evaluation of urinary frequency. He has had this problem for 2 years. On review of symptoms, the patient also reports occasional hesitancy and dribbling. Results of physical examination, including digital rectal examination, are normal.

Which of the following statements regarding the diagnosis of BPH is false?

- ❑ **A. Systemic diseases that can mimic BPH include diabetes, heart failure, and hyperparathyroidism**
- ❑ **B. It is important to ask about over-the-counter medications because they can contain anticholinergic and sympathomimetic agents that can cause or exacerbate symptoms**
- ❑ **C. Abdominal and pelvic ultrasound are indicated in the initial workup of BPH**
- ❑ **D. A urinalysis is a part of the workup of BPH to screen for hematuria or infection**

Key Concept/Objective: To understand the differential diagnosis and diagnostic workup of BPH

Symptoms of bladder emptying in men with BPH include straining, hesitancy, intermittency, a weak stream, terminal dribbling, and a sensation of incomplete emptying. Bladder filling symptoms include daytime frequency, nocturia, urgency, and urge incontinence. The physician should look for evidence of systemic diseases that can present with lower urinary tract symptoms, particularly urinary frequency and nocturia. Examples of such diseases include diabetes, heart failure, and hyperparathyroidism. Routine tests performed on men with lower urinary tract symptoms should generally include a urinalysis to screen for hematuria and infection. Pyuria suggests infection, either primary or superimposed on bladder outlet obstruction. Microscopic hematuria may indicate simply that the prostate is enlarged and vascular, but it should prompt further evaluation for genitourinary malignancy. Upper urinary tract imaging (by ultrasonography, computed tomography, or intravenous pyelography) and urethrocystoscopy are not indicated for routine cases of lower urinary tract symptoms attributable to BPH. *(Answer: C—Abdominal and pelvic ultrasound are indicated in the initial workup of BPH)*

54. A patient of yours whom you follow for BPH, hypertension, and osteoarthritis presents to your office. He has had symptoms of BPH for 3 years now, but over the past 2 to 3 months, his symptoms of hesitancy and straining have worsened to the point that he wishes to pursue therapy.

Which of the following statements regarding the medical management of BPH is true?

- ❑ **A. Alpha$_1$-adrenergic blockers work primarily through relaxation of the detrusor muscle of the bladder**
- ❑ **B. Alpha$_1$-adrenergic blockers reduce prostate size and lower prostate-specific antigen (PSA) levels**
- ❑ **C. The 5α-reductase inhibitors reduce prostate size and lower PSA levels**
- ❑ **D. Alpha blockers offer the same symptom relief as do 5α-reductase inhibitors**

Key Concept/Objective: To understand the medical management of BPH

Alpha$_1$-adrenergic blockers work primarily through relaxation of prostatic smooth muscle and relief of the dynamic component of bladder outlet obstruction. However, additional mechanisms have been proposed, including increased apoptosis of prostatic cells. Alpha blockers neither reduce prostate size nor lower PSA levels. Their onset of action is relatively rapid, although most alpha blockers require dose titration to achieve

a maximal therapeutic effect while minimizing side effects. The 5α-reductase inhibitors currently available for the treatment of BPH are finasteride and dutasteride. Finasteride selectively and irreversibly binds with the type 2 5α-reductase isoenzyme, which predominates in the prostate and thereby blocks conversion of testosterone to dihydrotestosterone (DHT), the dominant intraprostatic androgen. This agent lowers serum DHT by about 70% and intraprostatic DHT to an even greater degree. Dutasteride is a dual 5α-reductase inhibitor; it blocks both type 1 and type 2 isoenzymes and lowers serum DHT by about 90%. Men who take finasteride at the recommended dose of 5 mg daily or dutasteride at 0.5 mg daily can expect a 20% to 25% reduction in prostate size over the first year of therapy, accompanied by about a 50% reduction in PSA level. *(Answer: C—The 5α-reductase inhibitors reduce prostate size and lower PSA levels)*

55. A 61-year-old man presents for a follow-up visit for BPH. He has been taking an $alpha_1$-adrenergic blocker for 4 years now; he is currently taking the maximum dose. His symptoms have continued to progress, and he wishes to be referred to a urologist for surgical intervention.

Which of the following statements regarding the surgical treatment of BPH is false?

- ❑ **A. Retrograde ejaculation is a common outcome of transurethral prostatectomy (TURP)**
- ❑ **B. Open prostatectomy remains the gold standard for relieving symptoms and reducing the risk of complications for men with BPH**
- ❑ **C. Acute urinary retention does not always require surgery and can be managed with bladder rest via catheter drainage**
- ❑ **D. Symptom reduction is higher in patients who undergo TURP than in patients placed on watchful waiting**

Key Concept/Objective: To understand the surgical options for patients with BPH

TURP remains the gold standard for relieving symptoms and reducing the risk of complications for men with BPH. TURP involves resecting the central adenoma of the hyperplastic prostate transurethrally under direct visualization using a resectoscope with an electrified cutting loop. Retrograde ejaculation is a common outcome of TURP, occurring in the majority of cases. Acute urinary retention used to be considered an absolute indication for surgery. However, small case series have documented that up to half of men with acute retention have a successful voiding trial after a period of bladder rest via catheter drainage, and most of the men who experience success will continue to void, at least over the next 6 months. *(Answer: B—Open prostatectomy remains the gold standard for relieving symptoms and reducing the risk of complications for men with BPH)*

56. ***In which of the following patients with symptoms of lower urinary tract dysfunction would it be appropriate to begin an empirical trial of medications for BPH without further testing (other than physical examination)?***

- ❑ **A. A 60-year-old man with long-standing hypertension who has nocturia of new onset and intermittent shortness of breath at night**
- ❑ **B. A 58-year-old man who complains of weak stream, lower abdominal discomfort, and gross hematuria of 2 months' duration**
- ❑ **C. A 55-year-old man who describes symptoms of weak stream and intermittent straining to urinate, which he has been experiencing for 3 to 4 months**
- ❑ **D. An obese 35-year-old man with nocturia of recent onset, daytime urinary frequency, and increased thirst**
- ❑ **E. A 72-year-old man with dysuria of 2 days' duration**

Key Concept/Objective: To understand the need to assess for other clinical disorders in patients who present with urinary symptoms similar to BPH

The lower urinary tract symptoms seen in patients with BPH result from bladder outlet obstruction. Typical symptoms of BPH with bladder outlet obstruction are related to impaired bladder emptying (e.g., straining, hesitancy, intermittency, weak stream, terminal dribbling, and incomplete emptying) and bladder irritation/detrussor instability (e.g., daytime frequency, nocturia, urgency, and urge incontinence). In a middle-aged or elderly man with typical symptoms and a confirmatory examination, a presumptive diagnosis of BPH can be made. However, the physician must always be aware of other causes of lower urinary tract symptoms, and an appropriate workup should be carried out. Such causes include congestive heart failure (especially when urinary changes accompany edema, orthopnea, or paroxysmal nocturnal dyspnea), diabetes mellitus, urinary tract infection, and prostatitis. Although patients with BPH may have some hematuria, other diagnoses (including upper urinary tract disease and bladder cancer) should always be ruled out before gross hematuria is attributed to BPH. In a man with dysuria of sudden onset, urinary tract infection or prostatitis is more likely than BPH. *(Answer: C—A 55-year-old man who describes symptoms of weak stream and intermittent straining to urinate, which he has been experiencing for 3 to 4 months)*

57. A 75-year-old man with a history of mild cognitive impairment is brought to the emergency department because of altered mental status. His wife reports that 1 week ago, he developed nasal congestion and cough, for which he was given an over-the-counter cold medicine/decongestant. Five days ago, he began to complain of difficulty urinating. She states that he was spending an increasing amount of time in the bathroom, yet after leaving the bathroom he would complain that he still had to urinate. He became incontinent of small amounts of blood-tinged urine last night and complained of lower abdominal pain and nausea. On the morning of presentation, he was difficult to arouse and was "not making sense." Physical examination reveals an ill-appearing elderly man who is disoriented. There is a palpable suprapubic mass that is tender to palpation. Rectal examination reveals a symmetrically enlarged prostate gland. Initial laboratory results include a blood urea nitrogen (BUN) level of 68 and a serum creatinine level of 11 mg/dl. After a Foley catheter is passed with some difficulty, urine output measures approximately 2.0 L within 30 minutes.

Which of the following statements regarding this patient is false?

- ❑ A. **An ultrasound examination of the kidneys and ureters is likely to reveal significant hydronephrosis**
- ❑ B. **Sympathomimetic agents such as decongestants may exacerbate obstructive symptoms in patients with BPH**
- ❑ C. **Antihistamines with anticholinergic properties may exacerbate obstructive symptoms in patients with BPH and should be avoided**
- ❑ D. **The only reasonable approach to managing this patient involves TURP before discharge**
- ❑ E. **The patient's incontinence is likely the result of overflow from an obstructed bladder**

Key Concept/Objective: To recognize obstructive uropathy as a potential consequence of BPH and understand the treatment options

This patient has developed severe urinary outflow tract obstruction, resulting in acute renal failure. In patients with BPH, over-the-counter cold and allergy medicines should generally be avoided because the sympathomimetic and anticholinergic agents contained in them can worsen obstructive symptoms. This patient's severe outflow obstruction resulted in significant urinary retention. With very large bladder volumes, the pressure in the bladder may eventually overcome the resistance at the bladder neck and result in overflow incontinence, as seen in this patient. It is very likely that in this patient, initial upper urinary tract studies would show significant hydronephrosis. It is crucial to recognize such outflow tract obstruction and to relieve it promptly with bladder catheterization, if possible. Acute urinary retention was formerly considered an absolute indication for surgical intervention, but several studies have shown that after a period of bladder rest through catheter drainage combined with medical therapy, up to half of patients will achieve successful voiding. Given the clear precipitating factor

involved in the urinary retention seen in this patient, bladder rest and medical therapy with a subsequent voiding trial would be appropriate therapy. *(Answer: D—The only reasonable approach to managing this patient involves TURP before discharge)*

58. You have been following a 50-year-old man with BPH in clinic for the past 6 months. He had been bothered only slightly by symptoms of mild urinary hesitancy and occasional frequency. Today, however, he complains that since his last visit, his symptoms of straining, hesitancy, dribbling, incomplete emptying, and urinary frequency have been gradually worsening. On review of this patient's international prostate symptom score (IPSS), you note that his self-reported score of symptoms within the past month totals 15, reflecting moderate symptoms. After further discussion with the patient, you decide to start treatment with terazosin.

Which of the following statements regarding the use of alpha-adrenergic blockers for the treatment of lower urinary tract symptoms of BPH is true?

- ❑ **A. Long-term treatment with alpha-adrenergic blockers has been shown to result in a decrease in prostate size**
- ❑ **B. Treatment with alpha-adrenergic blockers can lower the PSA level, thereby altering the cutoff value at which one would be concerned about cancer**
- ❑ **C. Alpha-adrenergic blockers induce relaxation of prostatic smooth muscle and may relieve the dynamic component of bladder outlet obstruction**
- ❑ **D. Terazosin can usually be initiated at a dose of 10 mg, given before bedtime; a majority of men will achieve notable symptom relief at this dosage**
- ❑ **E. Studies have shown that alpha-adrenergic blockers are significantly less effective than the 5α-reductase inhibitor finasteride in reducing BPH symptom scores**

Key Concept/Objective: To understand the important aspects of drug therapy for BPH

Alpha-adrenergic blockers are among the mainstays of medical therapy for symptoms of BPH. In the absence of complications, the decision to initiate medical therapy depends in large part on the degree to which the patient is bothered by lower urinary tract symptoms. Symptom scores such as those based on the American Urology Association Symptom Index or IPSS can gauge severity of symptoms and help guide treatment decisions. Alpha-adrenergic blockers work by binding to alpha$_1$-adrenoceptors in the tissue of the bladder neck and reducing neuromuscular tone. They do not, however, have any impact on prostate size or PSA levels (in contrast to finasteride, which lowers PSA levels). Side effects of alpha-adrenergic blockers include orthostatic hypotension, dizziness, and asthenia. Most physicians initiate terazosin at a dose of 1 mg at bedtime for several days to avoid "first-dose" hypotension. The average effective dose of terazosin is closer to 10 mg; the dose should be gradually titrated up to this level in the absence of limiting side effects. Finasteride works by blocking the conversion of testosterone to dihydrotestosterone, which is a mitogen for prostatic tissue growth. Although this therapy may result in an actual decrease in prostate size, the average reduction in symptoms, as reflected in the IPSS, has been much more modest than that achieved with alpha-adrenergic blockers (total score reduction of 2 to 3 points for finasteride, versus 6 to 8 points for alpha-adrenergic blockers). *(Answer: C—Alpha-adrenergic blockers induce relaxation of prostatic smooth muscle and may relieve the dynamic component of bladder outlet obstruction)*

For more information, see Barry MJ: 10 Nephrology: XIII Benign Prostatic Hyperplasia. ACP Medicine Online (www.acpmedicine.com). Dale DC, Federman DD, Eds. WebMD Inc., New York, September 2004

SECTION 11

NEUROLOGY

The Dizzy Patient

1. A 50-year-old man presents to your clinic complaining of ringing in his right ear and of feeling as if the room is spinning around him. The latter symptom lasts for hours at a time. His wife points out that he is also losing his hearing. You suspect that he is suffering from Meniere syndrome.

Which of the following statements about Meniere syndrome is false?

- ❑ **A. Meniere syndrome is characterized by tinnitus, vertigo, and hearing loss**
- ❑ **B. Patients suffering from Meniere syndrome can have sudden attacks, during which they fall to the ground**
- ❑ **C. Episodes of vertigo and deafness in Meniere syndrome can last for hours to a day**
- ❑ **D. The deafness associated with Meniere syndrome begins with an inability to hear low-frequency sounds and later progresses to involve higher frequency sounds**

Key Concept/Objective: To be familiar with the presentation of Meniere syndrome

Although episodes of vertigo associated with Meniere syndrome usually last from hours to a day, deafness is constant after it develops. The deafness is characterized initially by a compromised ability to hear low-frequency sounds. Meniere syndrome is the result of excessive production and decreased absorption of inner ear endolymphatic fluid, resulting in endolymphatic hydrops. Patients usually complain of unilateral attacks of tinnitus (some have bilateral attacks), vertigo, and fullness in an ear. Deafness develops over time. Tumarkin otolithic crisis is a sudden spell of falling to the ground associated with Meniere syndrome. Meniere syndrome can be associated with nausea and vomiting. *(Answer: C—Episodes of vertigo and deafness in Meniere syndrome can last for hours to a day)*

2. A 52-year-old patient is diagnosed with Meniere syndrome. She has experienced several episodes of vertigo and now has right ear deafness. She has responded well to oral meclizine for the vertigo and to antiemetics for the associated vomiting. She wants to know if there are ways to avoid having similar attacks in the future, as this last one was particularly disabling.

Which of the following is not a long-term treatment for Meniere syndrome?

- ❑ **A. Salt restriction**
- ❑ **B. The Epley maneuver**
- ❑ **C. Diuretics**
- ❑ **D. Weight loss**

Key Concept/Objective: To know the treatment options for Meniere syndrome

Meniere syndrome is the result of increased levels of endolymphatic fluid. Treatments include salt restriction, diuretics, and weight loss. During attacks, vestibular suppressants and antiemetics can be useful for symptom relief. Refractory cases can be treated with sur-

gical endolymphatic shunting, labyrinthectomy, and vestibular neurectomy. The Epley maneuver is intended to dislodge otoconia from the semicircular canal system and is therefore useful in the treatment of benign paroxysmal positioning vertigo (BPPV). *(Answer: B—The Epley maneuver)*

3. A 66-year-old man presents to the emergency department complaining of nausea, vomiting, dizziness, and unsteadiness on his feet. The onset of these symptoms was acute. He states he has had a few similar episodes during the past month; each episode lasted a few hours. His medical history is notable for hypertension, hyperlipidemia, and coronary artery disease. He continues to smoke cigarettes despite his difficulties with heart disease.

The treatment of this patient should include which of the following measures?

- ❑ A. **Performance of the Epley maneuver**
- ❑ B. **Administration of vestibular suppressants**
- ❑ C. **Reassurance and the prescription of a salt-restricted diet**
- ❑ D. **A thorough neurologic examination and consideration of neurovascular imaging**

Key Concept/Objective: To be able to recognize patients at risk for vertebrobasilar insufficiency and to understand the need to search for this disorder in such patients presenting with vertigo

Episodes of vertigo in middle-aged patients should prompt consideration of vertebrobasilar insufficiency as a cause. The vertigo can represent transient ischemic attacks, which are warning signs of possible vertebrobasilar occlusion, a life-threatening condition. One should have even more concern about this condition in those with known risk factors for vascular disease or those with established vascular disease. Diagnosis often requires magnetic resonance angiography, a conventional angiogram, or both. This patient's episodes are very much a cause of concern, given his medical history and the recent onset of multiple attacks. Positive findings on neurologic examination would be even more compelling. *(Answer: D—A thorough neurologic examination and consideration of neurovascular imaging)*

4. A 30-year-old woman presents to the emergency department complaining of the room "moving all around her," nausea, and one episode of emesis. She states she was well until the week before, when she had a cold. Nasal congestion, a nonproductive cough, and a runny nose characterized the latter. She has no previous medical problems. Examination is notable only for torsional-horizontal nystagmus and difficulty with balance. You suspect she has vestibular neuritis.

Which of the following statements regarding vestibular neuritis is false?

- ❑ A. **It is commonly associated with upper respiratory tract infection**
- ❑ B. **It is rare**
- ❑ C. **It usually lasts from days to weeks**
- ❑ D. **It can be treated with vestibular suppressants during the first few days of the illness**

Key Concept/Objective: To understand the presentation and clinical features of vestibular neuritis

Vestibular neuritis is quite common, second only to BPPV as a cause of vertigo in most dizziness clinics. It is frequently associated with an upper respiratory tract infection and usually lasts from days to weeks. In most patients, symptoms improve within 1 to 2 days, and resolution occurs within 6 weeks of onset. The characteristic physical finding is torsional and horizontal nystagmus, with the slow component being toward the affected side. During the early phase of the illness, vestibular suppressants such as meclizine and diazepam can be useful in treating symptoms of vertigo. However, these agents should not be used for prolonged periods, because they may hinder the development of central compensation. Vertigo should be considered in the diagnosis of patients presenting with symptoms and signs consistent with vestibular neuritis, especially in the setting of diabetes or hypertension. Hearing is uniformly preserved. *(Answer: B—It is rare)*

For more information, see Solomon S, Frohman EM: 11 Neurology: I The Dizzy Patient. ACP Medicine Online (www.acpmedicine.com). Dale DC, Federman DD, Eds. WebMD Inc., New York, March 2005

Diseases of the Peripheral Nervous System

5. A 38-year-old white man presents to clinic with a complaint of sharp, "lightning-like" pain in both feet. He has had no recent trauma. His problem has been slowly progressing, and he is very concerned that this disorder will lead to disability. You suspect a peripheral neuropathy.

Which of the following statements regarding peripheral neuropathy is false?

- ❑ **A. A peripheral nerve disease can manifest as a dysfunction of motor, sensory, or autonomic systems**
- ❑ **B. Nerve conduction studies can provide support for a diagnosis of neuropathy and are a relatively objective way to follow the course of the disease**
- ❑ **C. Complete pain relief should be the goal when using medications to treat neuropathic pain**
- ❑ **D. Drugs used to treat neuropathic pain include tricyclics, carbamazepine, and gabapentin**

Key Concept/Objective: To understand the diagnosis and treatment of peripheral nervous system diseases

Peripheral nervous system disorders produce combinations of motor, sensory, and autonomic symptoms. These symptoms are primarily determined by the class of nerve fibers affected (e.g., motor or sensory fibers) and by the location of the lesions, rather than by the etiology of the process. Neurophysiologic testing (especially nerve conduction studies) can be considered a routine part of the evaluation of any patient with polyneuropathy. Nerve biopsy is best reserved for patients with disabling neurologic symptoms and signs. Nerve conduction studies can provide support for a diagnosis of neuropathy and are a relatively objective way to follow the course of the disease. These studies may also allow a clinician to infer whether a disease is affecting primarily axons or their myelin sheaths—an important distinction in the differential diagnosis of polyneuropathy. Needle electromyography is a complementary investigation that is usually performed at the same time as nerve conduction studies. In a patient with peripheral neuropathy, electromyography is helpful in detecting small degrees of axon loss that may go undetected by nerve conduction studies. The symptoms of neuropathy may be treatable even if the cause of the neuropathy is untreatable or unknown. With simple measures, many patients can have meaningful relief of symptoms. Medications can be useful in the management of neuropathic pain, but the goals of therapy should be realistic. Complete pain relief is unlikely. Therefore, the aim of therapy should be to make the pain more tolerable without adding intolerable side effects of medication. Of the many drugs that can be tried for neuropathic pain, tricyclics (especially amitriptyline) and carbamazepine are still most frequently used, although gabapentin is increasingly used as a first-line agent. *(Answer: C—Complete pain relief should be the goal when using medications to treat neuropathic pain)*

6. A 32-year-old woman presents to the emergency department with a complaint of weakness. Yesterday, she noticed some prickling paresthesias in her feet. Today, when she awoke, she noticed weakness in both legs; this weakness has rapidly worsened. You admit her to the hospital with a presumptive diagnosis of Guillain-Barré syndrome (GBS).

Which of the following statements regarding GBS is true?

- ❑ **A. Another name for GBS is chronic inflammatory demyelinating polyneuropathy**
- ❑ **B. The fundamental pathologic event in GBS is the stripping of myelin from axons by macrophages, which occurs in a patchy fashion throughout the peripheral nervous system**

❑ C. **Several studies have proved that there is a link between a preceding *Shigella* dysentery infection and GBS**

❑ D. **A cardinal feature of GBS is the asymmetrical pattern of involvement**

Key Concept/Objective: To understand the pathophysiology and clinical presentation of GBS

GBS, or acute inflammatory demyelinating polyradiculoneuropathy, is the most common cause of acute generalized paralysis in the Western world. Chronic inflammatory demyelinating polyradiculoneuropathy is an immune-mediated neuropathy whose onset is insidious, with symptoms and signs developing over weeks to months. In contrast, the initial course of GBS is rapid. Most often, the first symptom of GBS is prickling paresthesia, beginning in the feet and spreading proximally hour by hour. Weakness is noticed some hours to a few days later. Some patients have only motor symptoms without sensory symptoms. Classically, symptoms begin symmetrically in the distal limbs and proceed proximally (so-called ascending paralysis). Nerve conduction studies provide evidence of a demyelinating process affecting spinal roots and peripheral nerves (a demyelinating polyradiculoneuropathy). The fundamental pathologic event in GBS is the stripping of myelin from axons by macrophages, which occurs in a patchy fashion throughout the peripheral nervous system. A cascade of events involving cell-mediated and humoral immune mechanisms is assumed to be activated, and lymphocytic inflammatory infiltrates are often found in nerves and nerve roots by biopsy or at autopsy. Studies of the pathogenesis of GBS have focused on the potential roles of antecedent *Campylobacter jejuni* infection and the production of antiganglioside autoantibodies, both of which occur in a large number of patients with GBS. *(Answer: B—The fundamental pathologic event in GBS is the stripping of myelin from axons by macrophages, which occurs in a patchy fashion throughout the peripheral nervous system)*

7. A 68-year-old African-American patient with type 2 diabetes mellitus presents to clinic for a 6-month follow-up visit. His daily capillary blood glucose level has been ranging from 160 to 190 mg/dl, and he has not been adhering to his diet. His major complaint today is a burning pain in both feet. On foot examination, you discover a 1 cm ulcer on the plantar surface of the left foot and a loss of light touch sensation in both feet. You make a diagnosis of diabetic polyneuropathy.

Which of the following statements regarding diabetic polyneuropathy is false?

❑ A. **There is a strong correlation between the presence of diabetic polyneuropathy, retinopathy, and nephropathy**

❑ B. **Autonomic diabetic neuropathy can occur and cause orthostatic hypotension, impaired gastrointestinal motility, or blunting of the sympathetic response to hypoglycemia**

❑ C. **The classic distribution for diabetic polyneuropathy is the glove-and-stocking distribution**

❑ D. **The severity of the polyneuropathy correlates more closely with the duration of diabetes than the degree of hyperglycemia (mean glycosylated hemoglobin)**

Key Concept/Objective: To understand the clinical presentation of diabetic polyneuropathy

Peripheral neuropathy is common in patients with diabetes mellitus. Of the various types of diabetic neuropathy, by far the most common is a distal, symmetrical sensorimotor neuropathy, commonly referred to as diabetic polyneuropathy. In one prospective, population-based study of Americans of mainly northern European ancestry, diabetic polyneuropathy was found in 54% of patients with type 1 diabetes mellitus and in 45% of patients with type 2 diabetes mellitus. However, symptomatic polyneuropathy occurred in only 15% of the cohort, and none of the patients had disabling neurologic deficits. The severity of the polyneuropathy correlated more closely with the degree of hyperglycemia (mean glycosylated hemoglobin) than with the duration of diabetes. In this study and other large studies, the prevalence of diabetic polyneuropathy increased with the duration of diabetes, and a strong correlation existed between the presence of diabetic polyneuropathy,

retinopathy, and nephropathy. An important practical corollary of these observations is that a diagnosis of diabetic polyneuropathy in a patient with newly diagnosed diabetes but without other diabetic complications is likely to be incorrect. Diabetic polyneuropathy has the classic so-called glove-and-stocking distribution of symptoms, usually a combination of sensory loss and an unpleasant feeling of numbness or burning. Sensory loss in the feet and fingers and mild weakness in the feet and ankles are typical. Diabetic polyneuropathy can be expected to worsen slowly over years. The other varieties of diabetic neuropathy usually occur on a background of diabetic polyneuropathy. Some degree of diabetic autonomic neuropathy is found in most patients with diabetic polyneuropathy, although in some patients, the autonomic symptoms and signs predominate. Orthostatic hypotension, impaired gastrointestinal motility (including gastroparesis), and blunting of the sympathetically mediated warning symptoms of hypoglycemia are important management problems. *(Answer: D—The severity of the polyneuropathy correlates more closely with the duration of diabetes than the degree of hyperglycemia [mean glycosylated hemoglobin])*

8. A 49-year-old man presents to the emergency department with abrupt onset of right facial weakness. He experienced a respiratory infection 2 weeks ago and has had a dull ache behind the right ear for 2 days. This morning while shaving, he noticed a drooping of the right side of his face. Neurologic examination reveals a neuropathy of cranial nerve VII, with complete paralysis of the right upper face and forehead. Hearing, taste, and sensation are normal, and the other cranial nerves are functioning normally. No rash or shingles lesions are noted.

Which of the following clinical features seen in this patient suggests a poorer prognosis and would prompt more aggressive medical treatment (e.g., prednisone and acyclovir)?

- ❑ **A. Age younger than 60 years**
- ❑ **B. Normal hearing**
- ❑ **C. Normal taste**
- ❑ **D. Complete paralysis**
- ❑ **E. Abrupt onset of symptoms**

Key Concept/Objective: To be able to recognize and manage acute Bell palsy and to know the features that are associated with a poor prognosis and that suggest the need for early medical therapy

This patient has acute, idiopathic, facial neuropathy (Bell palsy). The abrupt onset of unilateral facial weakness with lower motor neuron (forehead) involvement preceded by pain behind the ear is classic. Over 80% of patients eventually recover fully. A course of corticosteroids and acyclovir may hasten recovery and is appropriate for patients with clinical features portending a poorer prognosis. Such features include severe (complete) paralysis, older age, hyperacusis, altered taste, and electromyographic evidence of axonal degeneration. Recent evidence implicates HSV type 1 infection in many patients, and trials of facial nerve decompression have not demonstrated efficacy. *(Answer: D—Complete paralysis)*

9. A 68-year-old diabetic man presents to the office for evaluation of double vision and right retro-orbital headache. Neurologic examination reveals right ptosis. The eye is deviated laterally and inferiorly. The right pupil is not dilated and reacts normally to light and accommodation. The patient has decreased sensation in his feet to pin and light touch, but the rest of the examination results are normal.

Which of the following is indicated for this patient at this time?

- ❑ **A. Cranial CT**
- ❑ **B. Magnetic resonance angiography**
- ❑ **C. Cerebral angiography**
- ❑ **D. Neurosurgical consultation**
- ❑ **E. Reassurance and no further evaluation at this time**

Key Concept/Objective: To be able to recognize oculomotor (third cranial nerve) paralysis and to understand the causes and implications of pupil-sparing third nerve palsy

This diabetic patient has developed an isolated third-nerve palsy. The presenting symptoms are fairly typical: the sudden development of ptosis with a "down-and-out eye" and a retro-orbital headache. The major consideration in the differential diagnosis is a mass lesion along the course of the third cranial nerve, particularly an aneurysm in the circle of Willis. The absence of pupillary paralysis (pupil-sparing third-nerve palsy) seen in elderly, hypertensive, and especially diabetic patients points to a putative microvascular lesion of the third cranial nerve. The finding of pupillary sparing can be distinguished at the bedside and can obviate the need for expensive neuroradiologic imaging in most cases, though such investigation is still advised in young patients who are without hypertension or diabetes. *(Answer: E—Reassurance and no further evaluation at this time)*

10. A 52-year-old man presented to the urgent care center 2 weeks ago with severe left shoulder pain. He was diagnosed with bursitis and treated with NSAIDs. The pain has gradually improved, but the patient has scheduled an office visit because he is concerned about weakness of the left arm. On examination, the patient has full passive range of motion of the arm and shoulder without pain. Marked atrophy and weakness are noted in the left deltoid and shoulder girdle muscles. Biceps and triceps reflexes are absent. The remainder of the examination is unremarkable.

Which of the following is the most likely diagnosis for this patient?

- ❑ **A. Thoracic outlet syndrome**
- ❑ **B. Brachial plexitis (Parsonage-Turner syndrome)**
- ❑ **C. Rotator cuff tear**
- ❑ **D. Spinal cord tumor**
- ❑ **E. Lacunar infarction**

Key Concept/Objective: To be able to recognize the syndrome of brachial plexus neuropathy (Parsonage-Turner syndrome)

Patients with Parsonage-Turner syndrome present with severe shoulder pain (frequently confused with bursitis) evolving to weakness of the muscles of the shoulder girdle, arm, or hand. This uncommon condition, also known as brachial plexitis or neuralgic amyotrophy (amyotrophy refers to wasting of muscle after denervation), appears to be an inflammatory peripheral neuropathy with causalgic pain. Affected patients are usually young or middle-aged men. It may also be seen in patients who are recovering from serious illness. Gradual, spontaneous recovery generally occurs; no specific therapy has been shown to be efficacious. Other less common causes of brachial plexopathy are irradiation (usually involving the upper plexus, cervical roots 5 through 7), trauma (as might be caused by the arm being jerked upwards or downwards), and malignant infiltration (usually involving cervical root 8 through thoracic root 1). Lumbosacral plexopathies are less common and are usually caused by diabetic neuropathy, malignant infiltration, or retroperitoneal hemorrhage. *(Answer: B—Brachial plexitis [Parsonage-Turner syndrome])*

11. A 72-year-old man has experienced numbness of his hands and feet for at least 5 years. Several times recently, he has tripped over the right foot. There is no history of diabetes, alcoholism, or other medical illness. He takes no medications or vitamin preparations. Examination reveals reduced pinprick and light-touch sensation in a stocking-and-glove distribution, which is worse in the feet than the hands. He has bilateral pes cavus and bilateral footdrop, which is worse on the right side. Chest x-ray, hematology group, chemistry panel, sedimentation rate, hemoglobin A_{1c} level, antinuclear antibody assay, and protein electrophoresis results are all normal or negative. Electromyography (EMG) shows primarily axonal degeneration of motor and sensory nerves of the lower and upper extremities.

Which of the following is most likely to identify the cause of this patient's neuropathy?

- ❑ **A. Family history and examination of suspect family members**
- ❑ **B. Screening of the urine for heavy metal**
- ❑ **C. Nerve biopsy**
- ❑ **D. Assessment of vitamin B_{12} levels**
- ❑ **E. Liver function tests, including GGT**

Key Concept/Objective: To understand the causes and evaluation of symmetrical polyneuropathy

Middle-aged or older patients with mild, nondisabling, slowly progressive polyneuropathy frequently have no identifiable etiology on routine examination and laboratory testing. In the absence of diabetes, alcohol abuse, medications, or other systemic illness, more extensive studies (e.g., screening of urine for heavy metals, fat aspiration for amyloid, sural nerve biopsy) rarely reveal an etiology. Many of these patients in fact suffer from inherited polyneuropathy. They frequently are asymptomatic for years, then develop numbness (prickling or pins-and-needles sensation suggests an acquired cause). The routine family history usually is negative. However, specific questioning about relatives with foot deformities or who need special shoes, braces, or gait-assist devices may be revealing. Neurologic evaluation of first-degree relatives who might be affected is more cost-effective than additional laboratory tests. *(Answer: A—Family history and examination of suspect family members)*

12. A 34-year-old woman presents to the emergency department complaining of a "pins-and-needles" sensation in her feet and legs, which began yesterday. Initially, this sensation involved only her feet, but it has gradually moved up to involve her ankles, calves, and thighs. She has had difficulty walking for the past few hours. She recalls a recent episode of bloody diarrhea, but otherwise she has been in good health. On examination, there is weakness of the foot and leg muscles in a symmetrical distribution. Deep tendon reflexes are absent at the knees and ankles. Plantar reflex is flexor. Fasciculations are not seen. Inconsistent results are obtained on sensory exam. Cranial nerves are intact. The rest of the physical exam is normal. CSF examination is normal except for an elevated protein level.

Which of the following is the most likely diagnosis for this patient?

- ❑ A. Botulism
- ❑ B. Motor neuron disease
- ❑ C. GBS
- ❑ D. Poliomyelitis
- ❑ E. Acute HIV infection

Key Concept: To understand the diagnosis of Guillain-Barré syndrome

Inflammatory demyelinating polyradiculoneuropathy is the most common variant of the GBS. The disease incidence is approximately 1 case per million population per month. Antecedent infections with viruses, mycoplasmas, or *Campylobacter jejuni* occur in one half to two thirds of patients. Patients typically present with paresthesias in the feet, which progress proximally. Pain is common early in the course of illness. An areflexic motor paralysis and an acellular increase in total protein levels in the CSF develop in most patients within 1 week. Paralysis can progress rapidly; early diagnosis facilitates early hospitalization for appropriate nursing and medical care. Up to one third of patients require ventilatory support. Complete or near-complete recovery is the rule in 85% of patients. Early in the course of disease, many patients are misdiagnosed as having anxiety disorder, as malingering, or as having other psychiatric illness. Careful neurologic examination and early neurologic consultation in suspect cases are advised. Early cranial nerve involvement would suggest botulism, myasthenia gravis, or the Miller-Fisher variant of GBS. Muscle cramps, normal sensation, fasciculations, and preserved or hyperactive deep tendon reflexes characterize motor neuron disease (e.g., ALS). Poliomyelitis was the major consideration in the differential diagnosis before the development of the polio vaccine, but it is now rare. A GBS-like syndrome with CSF pleocytosis can occur early in acute HIV infection. *(Answer: C—GBS)*

For more information, see Chalk CH, Dyck PJ: 11 Neurology: II Diseases of the Peripheral Nervous System. ACP Medicine Online (www.acpmedicine.com). Dale DC, Federman DD, Eds. WebMD Inc., New York, August 2004

Diseases of Muscle and the Neuromuscular Junction

13. A 46-year-old man presents with difficulties of gait and weakness of the face, neck, and hands. On examination, the patient has a "hatchet-face" appearance, with obvious wasting of the temporalis and masseter muscles. Bilateral eyelid ptosis without extraocular weakness is noted. There is prominent neck flexion but not extension, weakness, and atrophy. Interosseous atrophy and a bilateral footdrop are noted. The patient has prominent frontal baldness and testicular atrophy. When asked to grip the examiner's hand, the patient has difficulty relaxing the grip quickly. Percussion of the thenar eminence leads to slow relaxation. The serum creatine phosphokinse (CPK) level is normal.

Which of the following is the most likely diagnosis for this patient?

❑ **A. Becker muscular dystrophy**
❑ **B. Duchenne muscular dystrophy**
❑ **C. Autosomal recessive sarcoglycanopathy**
❑ **D. Autosomal dominant fascioscapulohumeral dystrophy**
❑ **E. Myotonic dystrophy (MD)**

Key Concept/Objective: To know the clinical signs and symptoms of MD

This patient likely has MD, the most common muscular dystrophy in adults. MD is an autosomal dominant disorder; patients present with a unique constellation of clinical features: ptosis, temporal and masseter atrophy, atrophy of the sternocleidomastoid muscles (with sparing of other posterior neck muscles), atrophy of distal musculature, dysarthria, and dysphagia. Myotonia (the inability to quickly relax a firm hand grip) should be specifically sought; its presence is characteristic. Most patients have disorders of the cardiac conduction system. Other features include frontal baldness, testicular atrophy, cataracts, mild mental dysfunction, GI motility disorders, and hypersomnia. The CPK level is normal or only mildly increased. EMG is diagnostic, revealing myotonic discharges. *(Answer: E—Myotonic dystrophy [MD])*

14. A 60-year-old woman is referred to you for a preanesthetic medical evaluation before elective total knee arthroplasty. Her degenerative joint disease of the knees has led to severe pain at rest and while walking, and conservative treatment measures have failed. Otherwise, she has been in good health and takes no medications. The patient has been told that no one in her family should undergo anesthesia with halothane, because her father developed a high fever and died during a cholecystectomy.

What is the most appropriate step to take next in the care of this patient?

❑ **A. Proceed with surgery; no additional precautions are needed**
❑ **B. Proceed with surgery but alert the anesthesiologist to avoid halothane anesthetics**
❑ **C. Proceed with surgery; administer I.V. dantrolene if fever develops**
❑ **D. Cancel surgery and refer for caffeine-halothane contraction test**
❑ **E. Cancel surgery and advise against any elective surgical procedure**

Key Concept/Objective: To be able to recognize malignant hyperthermia and to understand the most appropriate screening measures for patients suspected of having this disease

Malignant hyperthermia is an autosomal dominant disorder caused by a defect on chromosome 19q13, leading to a mutation of the ryanodine receptor (*RyR*) gene. Mutations of *RyR* cause accelerated calcium release from the sarcoplasmic reticulum during general anesthesia with compounds such as halothane, ether, and succinylcholine. This leads to a rapid increase in metabolism, dramatic elevations of body temperature, acidosis, muscle rigidity, myoglobinuria, and death. A careful family history may give clues to the diagnosis and should prompt referral for a muscle biopsy and in vitro caffeine-halothane contraction testing. Patients with malignant hyperthermia can usually safely undergo anesthesia with nitrous oxide, thiopental, and nonpolarizing muscle relaxants. I.V. dantrolene is effective if administered early in the disease course, but patients who develop the syndrome still have a 7% mortality. *(Answer: D—Cancel surgery and refer for caffeine-halothane contraction test)*

15. A 24-year-old Asian man presents to the emergency department with an attack of profound weakness after a meal with friends. He reports that for several years he has had similar episodes after exercise and large meals.

Which of the following diagnostic tests should be performed immediately for this patient?

- ❑ A. **Testing for acetylcholine receptor antibodies**
- ❑ B. **Assessment of serum potassium level**
- ❑ C. **Assessment of serum thyroxine level**
- ❑ D. **EMG**
- ❑ E. **Assessment of urinary aldosterone level**

Key Concept/Objective: To know the diagnosis of periodic paralysis

Both hyperkalemic and hypokalemic periodic paralysis are characterized by an abnormal serum potassium level at the time of symptom occurrence. However, the potassium levels can be normal between attacks, and thus, measurement of serum potassium during the period in which symptoms occur is the most important step to take next in treating this patient. Hyperkalemic periodic paralysis is caused by a defect of the sodium channel, precipitated by rest following exercise, stress, potassium administration, and the ingesting of certain foods. Hypokalemic periodic paralysis is caused by a defect in the calcium channel and is precipitated by the partaking of meals high in carbohydrates, rest following exercise, and excitement. If the potassium level is found to be low during attacks, secondary causes of hypokalemia (diuretics, hyperaldosteronism, laxatives, etc.) or thyrotoxicosis (especially in patients of Asian descent) should be sought. A serum potassium level that is elevated without apparent cause is suggestive of hyperkalemic periodic paralysis. *(Answer: B—Assessment of serum potassium level)*

16. A 25-year-old woman presents for evaluation of progressive muscle weakness and fatigability for the past 9 months. She has otherwise been healthy and takes no medication except oral contraceptives. The weakness involves her face, neck, and arms. The weakness is worse toward the end of the day and after repetitive activity. Her symptoms improve somewhat with sleep or rest. On examination, bilateral ptosis and extraocular muscle weakness are noted, particularly on upward and lateral gaze. Attempts at forced smiling produce a snarling expression. She has prominent neck muscle weakness. Her speech has a nasal quality. Moderate weakness is evident on upper-extremity muscle testing. Deep tendon reflexes and plantar reflexes are normal. Routine laboratory examinations, including CBC, chemistry panel, and thyroid function testing, are normal.

What is the most likely cause of this patient's symptoms?

- ❑ A. **Motor neuron disease**
- ❑ B. **Lambert-Eaton myasthenic syndrome**
- ❑ C. **Myasthenia gravis**
- ❑ D. **Congenital myasthenia**
- ❑ E. **Polymyositis**

Key Concept/Objective: To be able to diagnose myasthenia gravis and to distinguish it from other myasthenic and myopathic syndromes

Primary care physicians should suspect myasthenia gravis in patients who have progressive skeletal muscle weakness and fatigability. The illness typically presents in young women or older men as weakness of the eyelids and extraocular muscles, which leads to ptosis and diplopia. Patients develop weakness of the neck extensors and bulbar weakness that leads to dysarthria and dysphagia. Proximal weakness may present as progressive weakness experienced when climbing stairs or rising from a chair. Some patients complain of weakness combing their hair. Fluctuation of symptoms and fatigue with activity are characteristic. Deep tendon reflexes and the plantar reflex are normal. The presence of antibodies against the acetylcholine receptor and a positive EMG are diagnostic. Lambert-Eaton myasthenic syndrome is frequently associated with small cell lung cancer; its symptoms are ptosis, diplopia, fatigability, and muscle weakness. Features distinguishing it from myasthenia gravis include hyporeflexia, autonomic dysfunction, and an increase in mus-

cle strength after several seconds of maximal effort. Congenital myasthenia presents in infancy, childhood, or, occasionally, young adulthood. Motor neuron disease can present as muscle aches, weakness, and fatigue. The first manifestation may be asymmetrical distal weakness, with progressive wasting and atrophy of muscles or difficulty with chewing, swallowing, and moving the face and tongue. Fasciculation, caused by spontaneous twitching of motor units, is characteristic. With prominent corticospinal involvement, hyperactivity of the deep tendon reflexes is found. *(Answer: C—Myasthenia gravis)*

For more information, see Dalakas MC: 11 Neurology: III Diseases of Muscle and the Neuromuscular Junction. ACP Medicine Online (www.acpmedicine.com). Dale DC, Federman DD, Eds. WebMD Inc., New York, March 2005

Cerebrovascular Disorders

17. A 72-year-old man presents to the emergency department for evaluation. He is accompanied by his wife, who provides a history of his present illness. The patient was in his usual state of health until 1 hour ago, when he lost the use of his right arm and leg after sliding out of his chair. He is being treated for hypertension, diabetes, and dyslipidemia, all of which have been under moderately good control for many years. On physical examination, the patient has a dense paresis of his right upper and lower extremities. His language is unintelligible, and he is near mute. Intravenous fluids are started, serum is collected, and he is urgently transferred to radiology.

Which of the following statements regarding diagnosis of and therapy for acute ischemic stroke is true?

- ❑ **A. The brain should first be imaged with noncontrast CT**
- ❑ **B. Anticoagulation should be the initial medical therapy for most ischemic stroke patients**
- ❑ **C. The use of recombinant tissue plasminogen activator (rt-PA) for ischemic stroke should occur within 6 hours of symptom onset**
- ❑ **D. Heparin should not be used for prophylaxis of deep vein thrombosis in patients with ischemic stroke**

Key Concept/Objective: To understand the treatment of acute ischemic stroke

Noncontrast CT reliably distinguishes acute intracerebral hemorrhage from ischemia. This distinction is critical because the management of hemorrhagic stroke is substantially different from that of ischemic stroke. Anticoagulation is commonly used in the acute setting to prevent progressive or recurrent thromboembolic events. Nevertheless, the efficacy and safety of anticoagulation for this purpose are not well established, and its role in clinical [illegible] treated with anticoagulation. Aspirin is recommended as initial therapy for most acute stroke patients. However, aspirin should be withheld for at least 24 hours after administration of thrombolytics. Although the FDA has approved the use of intravenous rt-PA for acute ischemic stroke up to 3 hours after the onset of symptoms, physicians should strive to treat patients as quickly as possible, because earlier therapy is associated with better outcomes. Prophylaxis for deep vein thrombosis should be instituted early with heparin. For patients in whom heparin is contraindicated (e.g., patients with acute hemorrhage), pneumatic compression stockings are employed. *(Answer: A—The brain should first be imaged with noncontrast CT)*

18. A 44-year-old black man is brought by ambulance to the emergency department for evaluation. He was found earlier by his wife, who states that he was in his usual state of health when he went to bed the previous day. This morning, the patient awoke with severe headache; he was excessively groggy, and his speech was slurred. His wife called an ambulance. His only known medical problem is hypertension, for which he takes a thiazide diuretic. On physical examination, the patient's blood pressure is 210/140 mm Hg. He is arousable to pain and loud voice only, and he is combative and confused. The patient is treated with topical nitroglycerin. Serum is collected, and he is urgently transferred to radiology.

Which of the following statements regarding hemorrhagic stroke is true?

- ❑ A. **Blood pressure should be normalized rapidly in patients with intracranial hemorrhage**
- ❑ B. **Though hypertension is a clear risk factor for intracerebral hemorrhage (ICH), it is not known to increase the risk of aneurysmal rupture**
- ❑ C. **In ICH, the volume of hemorrhage and the level of consciousness are the two most powerful predictors of outcome**
- ❑ D. **Beta blockers have been shown to improve outcome in subarachnoid hemorrhage**

Key Concept/Objective: To understand the therapy for hemorrhagic stroke

ICH volume and consciousness level are the two most powerful predictors of outcome in ICH. Observations suggest that about one third of ICHs expand in the first 24 hours. Some investigators have juxtaposed this fact with a need to lower blood pressure in acute ICH. No trial has demonstrated that this action is necessary. The American Heart Association guidelines recommend only that mean arterial blood pressure be kept lower than 130 mm Hg in patients with a history of hypertension. Hypertension and cigarette smoking are clear risk factors for aneurysmal rupture. A family history of subarachnoid hemorrhage in first-degree relatives is also a risk factor for aneurysm rupture (about 4%), but routine screening is not recommended. Because it has been shown to improve outcome, nimodipine, a calcium channel blocker, is begun on the first day and continued for 21 days. *(Answer: C—In ICH, the volume of hemorrhage and the level of consciousness are the two most powerful predictors of outcome)*

19. A 73-year-old woman comes to the emergency department with a sudden onset of confusion, as described by her family. The patient was well and in her usual state of health until this event. She had no loss of consciousness or focal neurologic findings. She is independent in her activities of daily living. Her medical history is unremarkable except for a remote history of hypertension, and she is currently taking no medications. Her examination reveals a blood pressure of 140/84 mm Hg, a heart rate of 108 beats/min, and a temperature of 98.6° F (37° C). Her neck reveals no bruits, and her heart examination reveals an irregular rhythm without murmurs or extra sounds. Neurologic examination shows her to be alert and in no acute distress. Cranial nerve, sensory, motor, cerebellar, and reflex examinations are normal. Mental status examination reveals an intact ability to follow commands and verbal fluency but difficulty in associating meaning with words.

Which of the following is the most likely explanation of this patient's symptoms?

- ❑ A. **Acute ischemia to the left temporal lobe**
- ❑ B. **Acute infectious process**
- ❑ C. **Acute ischemia to the brain stem**
- ❑ D. **Central nervous system neoplasia**
- ❑ E. **Acute lacunar infarct of the basal ganglia**

Key Concept/Objective: To understand the pathogenesis of acute expressive aphasia and that expressive aphasia in the absence of other neurologic findings may be mistaken for confusion

This patient presents with what the family described as an acute confusional episode, but on examination by the medical team, she was noted to be able to follow commands. Her past history is essentially unremarkable, and she is on no medications and has no convincing evidence of a systemic or local infectious process. The major findings on her clinical examination are probable atrial fibrillation and expressive aphasia in the absence of other neurologic symptoms. This patient has almost assuredly experienced a thromboembolism to the speech area of the left temporal lobe, caused by her atrial fibrillation. *(Answer: A—Acute ischemia to the left temporal lobe)*

20. An 85-year-old man presents to the emergency department after being found with a diminished level of consciousness and dense left facial and left upper extremity paresis. Examination reveals a blood pressure of 162/90 mm Hg and a normal heart rate and rhythm. His physical examination confirms the above findings. Carotid Doppler examination reveals minimal atherosclerotic narrowing. An echocardiogram reveals minimal left ventricular hypertrophy and no intra-atrial or intraventricular thrombus. Serologic studies reveal a normal sedimentation rate of 32 mm/hr, a positive rapid plasma reagin (RPR) agglutination test at a titer of 1:8, and a positive fluorescent treponemal antibody (FTA) test.

What is the best step to take next in the management of this patient?

- ❑ **A. Begin high-dose intravenous penicillin therapy**
- ❑ **B. Obtain cerebrospinal fluid for VDRL (Venereal Disease Research Laboratories) test**
- ❑ **C. Obtain a CT scan of the head**
- ❑ **D. Begin aspirin therapy**
- ❑ **E. Begin antihypertensive therapy**

Key Concept/Objective: To understand that an imaging study of the brain is necessary in the acute phase of a cerebrovascular accident (CVA) to differentiate an intracerebral bleed from thrombosis

This patient was found to have a dense hemifacial and left upper extremity hemiparesis. His examination and ancillary studies failed to reveal an obvious arterial or cardiac source of an embolism. His elevated blood pressure is a normal finding in the acute phases of a CVA and generally should not be specifically treated unless (1) the patient is a candidate for thrombolytic therapy; (2) it is after hemorrhagic conversion of the infarct; (3) the patient has an aortic dissection; or (4) the patient has hypertensive encephalopathy. This patient had a positive RPR and FTA, which suggests a prior syphilitic infection and raises the possibility that his CVA was caused by meningovascular syphilis. However, before treatment is begun or the diagnosis is confirmed with a lumbar puncture, a head imaging study is necessary to exclude hemorrhage as the etiology of his symptoms. *(Answer: C—Obtain a CT scan of the head)*

21. A 32-year-old woman presents with a sudden onset of right-sided hemiparesis and headache. She has no history of cardiovascular or neurologic disease and was well before the onset of her symptoms. She uses no tobacco, alcohol, or illicit drugs. Her examination reveals a normal blood pressure and pulse. Her neck examination reveals no bruits. Her heart and lung examinations are normal, and her neurologic examination confirms the above findings. Laboratory studies reveal a sedimentation rate of 20 mm/hr, a normal comprehensive profile, and a negative urinary drug screen. Antinuclear antibody test was positive at 1:40 dilution, and her anti-dsDNA (double-stranded DNA) was negative. Imaging studies of her brain reveal acute ischemic transformation of her left temporal-parietal region.

What is the best step to take next in the management of this patient?

- ❑ **A. Biopsy of the temporal artery**
- ❑ **B. Visual evoked potentials**
- ❑ **C. Spinal fluid examination for oligoclonal bands**
- ❑ **D. Carotid duplex examination**
- ❑ **E. Administration of high-dose intravenous corticosteroids**

Key Concept/Objective: To know that carotid dissection is a cause of acute CVA in young adults

This is a case of a CVA occurring in a young, otherwise healthy female. In such cases, illicit drug use should be considered as a potential contributing factor, but in this case, it is essentially ruled out by the lack of confirmatory history or urinary drug screen. A vasculitis, perhaps secondary to a systemic process such as SLE, should be considered. This patient's sedimentation rate is normal, and her ANA is nonspecific and low. However, the absence of any illness preceding the onset of her symptoms decreases the probability of a systemic inflammatory process. Visual evoked potentials and CSF analysis would be recommended if multiple sclerosis were a serious possibility. This patient has a single CNS lesion in the distribution of a major cerebral vessel (middle cerebral artery) and no other findings on her imaging study that suggest multiple independent CNS lesions. In young

adults, carotid artery dissection needs to be considered in the differential diagnosis of CVA. Dissection may be diagnosed noninvasively with ultrasonography. *(Answer: D—Carotid duplex examination)*

22. A 49-year-old man presents to the emergency department with acute onset of severe headache, photophobia, and decreased level of consciousness. His mother had a subarachnoid hemorrhage at 54 years of age. He has no personal history of hypertension, vascular disease, or elevated cholesterol levels. His examination reveals a blood pressure of 148/84 mm Hg and mild nuchal rigidity. A CT scan of the head fails to reveal an abnormality.

What is the best step to take next in the management of this patient?

- ❑ **A. Cerebral angiography**
- ❑ **B. Beginning oral nimodipine**
- ❑ **C. Lumbar puncture**
- ❑ **D. Electroencephalogram**
- ❑ **E. Carotid Doppler examination**

Key Concept/Objective: To understand that CT scanning of the brain is not 100% sensitive in excluding subarachnoid hemorrhage (SAH)

This patient presents with many of the classic findings of acute subarachnoid hemorrhage, including the sudden onset of a severe headache, diminished level of consciousness, and nuchal rigidity. Family history of aneurysm is present in about 4% of patients with SAH. Establishing the diagnosis early is necessary to improve long-term morbidity and mortality. It is important to note that CT scanning of the head is not 100% sensitive in excluding this "high-stakes" entity. In the presence of clinical suspicion and a negative imaging study, a lumbar puncture is necessary to look for the presence of xanthochromia and RBCs. *(Answer: C—Lumbar puncture)*

23. A 55-year-old man presents to the emergency department with sudden onset of tachycardia and lightheadedness. He has had no previous episodes of similar symptoms. He has a history of hypertension controlled with amlodipine. He is otherwise healthy. His examination reveals a blood pressure of 132/82 mm Hg and an irregular heart rate of 120 beats/min. His lung examination is normal, and his cardiac examination reveals an irregular rhythm, with no obvious murmur or extra sounds and S_1 having variable intensity. An ECG reveals atrial fibrillation and left axis deviation. The chest x-ray is normal. An echocardiogram reveals normal left ventricular systolic and diastolic function and no thrombus or valvular abnormalities. TSH is 3.3.

Which of the following drugs would you give this patient to minimize the long-term risk of thromboembolism?

- ❑ **A. Intravenous heparin**
- ❑ **B. Oral warfarin**
- ❑ **C. Aspirin**
- ❑ **D. Ticlopidine**
- ❑ **E. Low-molecular-weight heparin**

Key Concept/Objective: To understand that patients younger than 65 years who are without risk factors are at low risk for thromboembolism from atrial fibrillation

Risk factors such as hypertension, diabetes, previous CVA/TIA, and poor LV function, along with older age (> 65 years), are associated with a yearly risk of thromboembolism from atrial fibrillation of approximately 5%. This risk can be decreased to approximately 1% with warfarin and 2% to 3% with aspirin. The risk of thromboembolism is 1% without therapy in patients without risk factors and younger than 65 years. This patient has a history of controlled hypertension and has a normal echocardiogram, which decreases the probability that his hypertension has caused end-organ complications. He has no other risk factors

for thromboembolism caused by his atrial fibrillation and likely has "lone atrial fibrillation." In such patients, warfarin is not necessary, and aspirin may be a logical alternative in the absence of contraindications. Ticlopidine or newer antiplatelet agents may be of benefit when aspirin has failed. In addition, converting patients to sinus rhythm: either with electrical cardioversion or chemically: is a desirable outcome in such situations. Finally, agents to control ventricular rate (beta blockers, diltiazem, or digoxin) should be considered in this patient. *(Answer: C—Aspirin)*

For more information, see Morgenstern LB, Kasner SE: 11 Neurology: IV Cerebrovascular Disorders. ACP Medicine Online (www.acpmedicine.com). Dale DC, Federman DD, Eds. WebMD Inc., New York, October 2004

Traumatic Brain Injury

24. A 24-year-old man is brought to the emergency department by the emergency medical service (EMS). He suffered head trauma 20 minutes ago while playing football. Immediately after the event, he lost consciousness for 3 minutes and then woke up mildly confused. He complains of a moderate frontal headache. On physical examination, the patient's vital signs are stable, his Glasgow Coma Scale (GCS) score is 15, and he has no focal signs on neurologic examination.

What interventions would be appropriate in the treatment of this patient?

- ❑ **A. Continue with observation and repeated neurologic examinations; repeat assessment with the GCS periodically; and consider imaging with a CT scan to rule out contusions**
- ❑ **B. Continue with observation and repeated neurologic examinations; repeat assessment with the GCS periodically; and obtain an MRI**
- ❑ **C. Admit the patient for prolonged observation; obtain a CT scan to rule out contusions; and start I.V. mannitol for brain edema**
- ❑ **D. Admit the patient to the ICU; obtain an MRI; and consider intraventricular monitoring of intracranial pressure (ICP)**

Key Concept/Objective: To understand the appropriate treatment of mild traumatic brain injury (MTBI)

With an incidence of 180 per 100,000 people, MTBI is more common than any other neurologic diagnosis except migraine. MTBI is defined as any traumatic brain injury/concussion with loss of consciousness of 0 to 30 minutes, a GCS score of 13 to 15 on admission, posttraumatic amnesia or confusion lasting less than 24 hours, and no evidence of contusion or hematoma on CT. Although the emergency department evaluation and management of MTBI is controversial, the principal concern is with identifying evolving surgical lesions such as hematomas and contusions. In addition to history and examination, CT has become the mainstay of evaluation. Prolonged or deteriorating mental status or the presence of neurologic signs or other risk factors are still indications for CT scanning, observation, or both after MTBI. MRI promises to be very useful in the long-term management of moderate and severe TBI, as well as in the documentation of brain pathology in patients with milder injury. However, it is often impractical and not cost-effective in the acute setting. This patient has MTBI, and observation for a few hours and possibly a CT scan to rule out contusions are appropriate. He does not have severe enough trauma to warrant admission or invasive monitoring of his ICP. *(Answer: A—Continue with observation and repeated neurologic examinations; repeat assessment with the GCS periodically; and consider imaging with a CT scan to rule out contusions)*

25. A 46-year-old woman is brought to the emergency department by EMS after being involved in a car accident. She was a passenger in the back seat of the car. The accident involved frontal impact, with the car moving at 50 mph. The patient was not wearing a seatbelt. The driver says she has not been awake since the accident, which occurred 30 minutes ago. On admission, the patient's vital signs are as follows: blood pressure, 100/60 mm Hg; heart rate, 78 beats/min; respiratory rate, 8 breaths/min; GCS score, 7. A CT scan shows a frontal epidural hematoma with mass effect.

How would you treat this patient?

- ❑ **A. Intubate the patient, administer hyperventilation to a carbon dioxide tension (P_{CO_2}) of 25 to 35 mm Hg, induce a barbiturate coma, and admit the patient to the ICU for further evaluation**
- ❑ **B. Intubate the patient, administer hyperventilation to a P_{CO_2} of 25 to 35 mm Hg, and ask for emergent neurosurgery consult for evacuation of the hematoma**
- ❑ **C. Intubate the patient, administer hyperventilation to a P_{CO_2} of 25 to 35 mm Hg, admit to ICU for close observation, and consult neurosurgery for intraventricular ICP monitoring**
- ❑ **D. Admit to ICU for further evaluation and start mannitol and steroids**

Key Concept/Objective: To understand the treatment of severe head injury

In patients with severe brain injury, the first priority should be cardiopulmonary resuscitation. Comatose patients with TBI are often hypoxic or hypercapnic, even though ventilation may appear to be normal. Patients who are in a coma (GCS score of less than 8) should undergo gentle hyperventilation via intubation until a P_{CO_2} of about 35 mm Hg is achieved. Short-term hyperventilation to levels of about 25 mm Hg can be lifesaving in the patient with impending herniation. Subdural and epidural hematomas should be evacuated promptly when associated with a significant mass effect, because it has been shown that there is a significant poorer outcome with surgical delays of greater than 4 hours. The literature supports a standard recommendation that corticosteroids should not be used for neuroprotection or control of ICP in patients with severe TBI. *(Answer: B—Intubate the patient, administer hyperventilation to a P_{CO_2} of 25 to 35 mm Hg, and ask for emergent neurosurgery consult for evacuation of the hematoma)*

26. A 22-year-old man is transferred to your hospital from a local hospital, where he presented 3 hours ago with closed head trauma. He lost consciousness for 10 minutes. At the first hospital where he was taken, he was given pain medications, and a CT scan was performed; the CT scan was negative. The patient is awake and complains only of moderate headache. His physical examination is unremarkable. The family is concerned about the development of seizures in the future, because they had a relative who had that problem.

What would you recommend regarding prophylaxis for seizures in this patient?

- ❑ **A. Phenytoin for 1 to 2 weeks**
- ❑ **B Carbamazepine for 6 months**
- ❑ **C. Obtain an electroencephalogram; if it is abnormal, start phenytoin**
- ❑ **D. Do not start any antiseizure medication at this time**

Key Concept/Objective: To understand the evaluation of the risk of posttraumatic epilepsy

The risk of epilepsy in patients with closed-head injury is relatively small: 2% to 5% in all patients and about 10% to 20% in patients with severe closed-head injury. A higher incidence of seizures has been seen in patients with depressed skull fractures (15%), hematomas (31%), and penetrating brain wounds (50%). This patient has a mild, closed injury, and he is at very low risk for developing seizures. Because most patients who develop posttraumatic epilepsy in the first week after injury will have recurrent seizures for some time, anticonvulsant therapy is indicated in documented cases. Controlled, randomized studies have shown that the use of phenytoin, phenobarbital, carbamazepine, and valproate do not prevent the development of posttraumatic epilepsy beyond the first week after injury. It is recommended as a standard of care that these medications should not be used to prevent posttraumatic epilepsy in patients who have not had a seizure. *(Answer: D—Do not start any antiseizure medication at this time)*

27. A 44-year-old woman presents to your clinic complaining of persistent problems since being in a car accident 2 years ago. At the time of the accident she suffered moderate head trauma, which required admission to a hospital for 3 days. Since then, she has felt as if she is not the same person. She has had problems with her husband, and she feels sad all the time. She also has lost interest in social activities, and she has lost 12 lb. Her thought process seems slow since the accident. Her physical examination is unremarkable.

What is the most likely diagnosis, and how would you treat this patient's symptoms?

- ❑ **A. The patient probably has a personality disorder; she should not have sequelae from accidents of this nature; refer for psychotherapy**
- ❑ **B. The patient probably has an undisclosed substance abuse problem; refer to psychiatry**
- ❑ **C. The patient probably has neuropsychiatric sequelae from the accident; educate her about the possible sequelae, and start a selective serotonin reuptake inhibitor (SSRI) for depression**
- ❑ **D. The patient probably has major depression, but it is unlikely that this depression is related to the accident; start an SSRI**

Key Concept/Objective: To understand neuropsychiatric sequelae of head trauma

The neuropsychiatric sequelae of brain injury, both socially and in the workplace, are well appreciated. Neurologic abnormalities may not be as distressing to the patient or the patient's family as personality changes and inappropriate behavior. Suitable treatment of neurobehavioral sequelae will often decrease patient and caregiver distress and markedly improve overall outcome. The SSRIs are favored because they are safe and easy to administer. Other common neuropsychiatric sequelae are irritability, aggression, attention deficits, seizures, memory problems, and posttraumatic stress disorder. *(Answer: C—The patient probably has neuropsychiatric sequelae from the accident; educate her about the possible sequelae, and start a selective serotonin reuptake inhibitor [SSRI] for depression)*

For more information, see Salazar AM: 11 Neurology: V Traumatic Brain Injury. ACP Medicine Online (www.acpmedicine.com). Dale DC, Federman DD, Eds. WebMD Inc., New York, April 2003

Neoplastic Disorders

28. A 43-year-old African-American man with known HIV disease presents to the emergency department with a 2-week history of progressive, frontal headache and associated blurry vision. Two days before admission, he developed generalized tonic-clonic seizures. The patient denies having fever, chills, or weight loss. He occasionally uses alcohol and has smoked two packs of cigarettes a day for 25 years; he admits to having used intravenous drugs in the remote past. Physical examination reveals right homonymous hemianopsia and generalized brisk deep tendon reflexes. External ocular movements are intact. Papilledema is not present, nor does the patient have any motor or sensory defects. A firm, nodular, right supraclavicular lymph node measuring 2 cm is noted. The patient's laboratory results are as follows: Hb, 9.5 g/dl; Hct, 28%; renal function test results are normal; liver function test results are normal, with the exception of an albumin value of 3.0 g/dl; LDH, 365 mg/dl; $CD4^+$ T cell count, 260 cells/µl; viral load, 45,000 copies/ml; serum cryptoccocal antigen is negative. Chest radiography reveals widening of the mediastinum, and right paratracheal adenopathy is present. An abrupt cutoff of the right main-stem bronchus is noted. MRI of the head shows large right parietal and right occipital lesions with ring enhancement and significant surrounding edema. No midline shift is noted. Multiple contrast-enhancing ring lesions are observed in the bilateral frontal lobes. CT of the chest shows a large mediastinal mass encroaching on the right mainstem bronchus. A speculated mass measuring 2 cm is also noted at the right upper lobe.

Which of the following diagnoses is most likely?

- ❑ **A. Primary CNS tumor**
- ❑ **B. Primary CNS lymphoma**
- ❑ **C Metastatic lung cancer**
- ❑ **D. Cryptoccocal meningitis**
- ❑ **E. Metastatic prostate cancer**

Key Concept/Objective: To understand the relationship of immunosuppression with the risk of malignancy

This patient has HIV disease with poor control of viral burden. However, his CD4 count is relatively preserved. As such, he is at negligible risk for a number of opportunistic infections, including primary CNS lymphoma and toxoplasmosis. He is still at risk for cryptoccocal disease; however, a negative serum antigen coupled with the presence of extensive intrathoracic disease makes this diagnosis very unlikely.

Primary CNS tumors are much less common than metastatic disease to the CNS. Astrocytomas and oligodendrogliomas more commonly present as infiltrating lesions. Meningiomas arise from the dura mater and are almost always solitary masses. Acoustic neuromas can be single or bilateral, but they affect the eighth cranial nerve.

The radiologic characteristics in this patient favor the diagnosis of metastases to the CNS. Tumors that frequently metastasize to the CNS include tumors of the breast and lung and melanomas. Prostate cancer almost never metastasizes to the brain. The presence of extensive intrathoracic disease, the history of tobacco exposure, and the MRI pattern support the diagnosis of lung carcinoma. *(Answer: C—Metastatic lung cancer)*

29. A 55-year-old white woman with known breast cancer that was treated 10 years ago with mastectomy comes for evaluation of rhythmic movement of the right arm. These episodes occurred on three occasions over the past 2 weeks; each episode lasted 5 to 10 minutes. No loss of consciousness or incontinence of the bladder or bowel was associated with the episodes. The patient denies having headache, blurry vision, or diplopia. Her family notes that the patient seems less prone to engage in conversation and seems to be sleeping more than usual. No nausea or vomiting is noted. On examination, the right breast is normal. A prosthesis of the left breast is noted; otherwise, the physical examination is unremarkable. No axillary or supraclavicular adenopathy is noted. The patient's neurologic function is intact. MRI shows a 2 cm mass adjacent to the frontal lobe. The lesion exhibits the same density as the surrounding brain parenchyma. Minimal edema is noted. No other lesions are appreciated.

Which of the following is the most likely diagnosis?

- ❑ A. **Metastatic disease from breast cancer**
- ❑ B. **Astrocytoma**
- ❑ C. **Oligodendroglioma**
- ❑ D. **Schwannoma**
- ❑ E. **Meningioma**

Key Concept/Objective: To understand the relationship between meningioma and breast cancer and the radiologic characteristics of different CNS tumors

Breast cancer is known to metastasize to the CNS. As with other metastatic tumors, breast cancer tends to produce multiple lesions that are most commonly located at the junction of the white matter and gray matter. These lesions are characteristically surrounded by a significant amount of edema; occasionally, the edematous area is out of proportion with the size of the metastasis. In this patient, the amount of time that has elapsed since her mastectomy makes this possibility unlikely, although tumor recurrence after 10 years has been reported.

Both astrocytomas and oligodendrogliomas are tumors situated within the brain parenchyma. Both types tend to present as solitary masses without clearly defined margins. Edema, although frequently present, is less significant than the cerebral edema associated with metastatic disease.

Schwannomas occur in the cranium or peripheral nerves. Schwann cells produce myelin, which accounts for why these tumors are adjacent to nerves. Schwannomas of the eighth cranial nerve are known as acoustic neuromas. They usually present with unilateral deafness, unilateral tinnitus, or both. When they occur bilaterally, they are always associated with type 2 neurofibromatosis, a disease caused by a deletion of the tumor suppressor gene located in the short arm of chromosome 22. In this patient, the location of the tumor and the absence of deafness and tinnitus effectively exclude this diagnosis.

Meningiomas arise from the dura and the arachnoid villa of intracranial and spinal spaces. These are slow-growing tumors; patients usually present with either symptoms of

a space-occupying lesion or seizures of new onset. Radiologically, these tumors are characterized by their extraparenchymal location and the fact that they have a density similar to that of surrounding brain tissue. Of interest, women with breast cancer are known to have an increased incidence of meningiomas. Prognosis of meningiomas is in general excellent; surgical excision tends to be curative. Meningiomas that are difficult to excise completely (e.g., those located at the base of the brain) or that have anaplastic features are more likely to recur. For such patients, postsurgical radiation therapy is recommended. *(Answer: A—Metastatic disease from breast cancer)*

30. A 45-year-old white woman presents to the office for evaluation; she has been having difficulty speaking and her gait has been unsteady. Both symptoms were first noted 1 month ago and have progressed since then. The patient has not experienced fever, chills, headache, diplopia, or weight loss. The patient does not have a history of alcohol abuse, and she denies having numbness, tingling, or any weakness. Physical examination reveals ataxia of both upper extremities and both lower extremities. Ataxic gait is noted. All laboratory tests are normal. No masses are identified on chest x-ray. MRI of the head shows no evidence of cerebellar lesions, hemorrhage, or atrophy.

Which of the following antibodies are most likely to be present in the serum of this patient?

- ❑ **A. Anti-Hu**
- ❑ **B. Anti-Yo**
- ❑ **C. Anti-MAG**
- ❑ **D. Antibody against acetylcholine receptor**

Key Concept/Objective: To understand the relationship between symptoms of primary malignancy and the diagnosis of paraneoplastic syndrome and to understand the clinical characteristics of cerebellar degeneration

This case illustrates how the indirect manifestations of primary malignancies can precede the direct manifestations of those malignancies. Such disorders are known as paraneoplastic syndromes. Examples of such manifestations include deep vein thrombosis, nephritic syndrome, polycythemia, and neurologic manifestations. Certain tumor antigens are similar to native antigens. Antibodies to the malignant tumor cross-react with native antigen, giving rise to these clinical syndromes. It is well recognized that paraneoplastic syndromes can precede by weeks to months the clinical presentation of the underlying primary malignancy. As such, awareness of these syndromes is of great importance, and maintaining a high index of suspicion could lead to an earlier diagnosis.

Patients with Lambert-Eaton syndrome present with weakness. The symptoms get better during the day (unlike the symptoms of myasthenia), and repetitive use of the affected limb increases the strength of that limb. An antibody against the acetylcholine receptor is responsible for this paraneoplastic syndrome. Small cell carcinoma is most often found to be the underlying tumor.

The peripheral nervous system is affected by two different sets of antibodies. Both peripheral neuropathies are predominantly sensory. In patients with lymphoma and Waldenström disease, myelin-associated glycoprotein antibodies (anti-MAG) are produced. Anti-Hu antibodies are found in patients with peripheral neuropathy and encephalomyelitis associated with small cell carcinoma of the lung.

This patient has clear cerebellar signs and symptoms. A main characteristic that points toward a paraneoplastic syndrome is the bilateral nature of the findings. Furthermore, cerebellar changes in imaging were detected several months after the onset of symptoms. Patients with cerebellar tumors tend to present with unilateral signs and symptoms and abnormal neuroimaging studies. Cerebellar hemorrhage presents in a more acute manner. Alcohol abuse is associated with bilateral findings, although truncal ataxia frequently dominates the clinical picture. MRI usually demonstrates severe atrophy. The fact that this patient does not use alcohol and the normal findings on MRI argue strongly against this diagnosis. Because of the clear relationship between ovarian cancer and paraneoplastic cerebellar degeneration, this patient should undergo evaluation for this malignancy. *(Answer: B—Anti-Yo)*

For more information, see Posner JB: 11 Neurology: VI Neoplastic Disorders. ACP Medicine Online (www.acpmedicine.com). Dale DC, Federman DD, Eds. WebMD Inc., New York, August 2001

Anoxic, Metabolic, and Toxic Encephalopathies

31. A 45-year-old man with a history of hypertension and alcohol abuse and dependence presented to the emergency department with confusion. The patient was oriented only to person and was easily distracted. Results of physical examination were as follows: temperature, 99.2° F (37.3° C); heart rate, 88 beats/min; blood pressure, 143/88 mm Hg; and respiratory rate, 16 breaths/min. On questioning, the patient was confused and mildly agitated. The remainder of the physical examination was largely unrevealing; there were no signs of chronic liver disease and no focal neurologic findings. Laboratory evaluation was significant for a serum sodium level of 112 mEq/L and a normal serum ammonia level. The patient was admitted for further evaluation, and 3% NaCl was initiated to correct his hyponatremia. The following day, the serum sodium level was 135 mEq/L. After showing initial clinical improvement in alertness and cognition, the patient's clinical status declined on hospital day 4. He has become obtunded and has developed flaccid quadraparesis and extensor plantar responses.

Which of the following conditions most likely accounts for the change in this patient's status?

- ❑ **A. Portosystemic encephalopathy**
- ❑ **B. Wernicke-Korsakoff syndrome**
- ❑ **C. Central pontine myelinolysis**
- ❑ **D. Delirium tremens**

Key Concept/Objective: To understand that rapid correction of hyponatremia can lead to central pontine myelinolysis

Hyponatremia and hypernatremia have several causes. Rapid changes in serum sodium concentration can cause encephalopathy because the osmotic equilibrium between the cerebral spinal fluid and other body fluids is altered. Disturbances of cognition and arousal occur and may lead to coma. Associated features include myoclonus, asterixis, tremulousness, and seizures. Seizures often respond poorly to anticonvulsant medication unless the associated metabolic disturbance has been corrected. Focal motor deficits (e.g., hemiparesis) can occur with hyponatremia in the absence of any structural lesion or can occur with hypernatremia as a result of intracerebral or subdural hemorrhage related to osmotically caused brain shrinkage, with secondary tearing of blood vessels. Hyponatremia should be corrected at a rate not exceeding 12 mEq/L/day because rapid correction of hyponatremia leads to central pontine myelinolysis. Central pontine myelinolysis may obscure or follow improvement in hyponatremic encephalopathy. The pathologic hallmark of the disorder is breakdown and loss of myelin in the anterior pons and other brain stem regions, which may be visualized by magnetic resonance imaging. The disorder is associated with alcoholism, electrolyte disturbances, malignant disease, and malnutrition, and it relates particularly to the rapid correction of hyponatremia. *(Answer: C—Central pontine myelinolysis)*

32. A 78-year-old woman is transported to the emergency department after being "found down" by a family member. Upon arrival at the emergency department, the patient is pulseless and apneic. A "code 10" is called, and advanced cardiac life support is initiated. Chest compressions are performed, and the patient is intubated and oxygenated with 100% fraction of inspired oxygen (F_IO_2). Cardiac monitoring reveals asystole. Pharmacologic therapy with epinephrine and atropine is administered. After the second round of epinephrine and atropine, the patient regains a pulse. She is transferred to the medical intensive care unit for further care. You are concerned about the possibility of anoxic-ischemic encephalopathy secondary to circulatory arrest.

Which of the following statements regarding anoxic-ischemic encephalopathy is accurate?

- ❑ **A. In the mature nervous system, white matter is generally more vulnerable to ischemia than gray matter**

❑ B. **In the mature nervous system, the brain stem is more vulnerable to ischemia than the cerebral cortex**

❑ C. **The persistent vegetative state is characterized by the return of the sleep-wake cycle, but wakefulness is without awareness**

❑ D. **Brain death is defined as the loss of all cerebral activity for at least 48 hours**

Key Concept/Objective: To understand the characteristics of the persistent vegetative state and the definition of brain death

The persistent vegetative state is characterized by the return of sleep-wake cycles and of various reflex activities, but wakefulness is without awareness. Recent studies have indicated that the minimally conscious state, which is characterized by inconsistent but clearly discernible behavior of consciousness, can be distinguished from coma and a vegetative state by the presence of behavioral conditions not found in either of those two conditions; this distinction is important because outcome appears to be different in minimally conscious patients. Brain death is defined as the loss of all cerebral activity, including activity of the cerebral cortex and brain stem, for at least 6 hours if confirmed by electroencephalographic evidence of electrocerebral inactivity or for 24 hours without a confirmatory electroencephalogram. *(Answer: C—The persistent vegetative state is characterized by the return of the sleep-wake cycle, but wakefulness is without awareness)*

33. A 68-year-old woman with a history of alcohol abuse and dependence presents to the primary care clinic for evaluation of confusion. The patient is accompanied by her daughter, who is concerned about her mother's forgetfulness and who feels that her mother has been "making things up." Physical examination is significant for nystagmus, ophthalmoplegia, and ataxic gait. On the basis of the physical examination and a history of confabulation, you make the diagnosis of Wernicke encephalopathy.

A deficiency of which of the following is responsible for this condition?

❑ A. **Vitamin B_{12} (cyanocobalamin)**

❑ B. **Folic acid**

❑ C. **Niacin**

❑ D. **Thiamine (vitamin B_1)**

Key Concept/Objective: To understand that thiamine (vitamin B_1) deficiency is responsible for Wernicke encephalopathy

Thiamine (vitamin B_1) deficiency is responsible for the hallmark features of Wernicke encephalopathy. These features include ophthalmoplegia, gait ataxia, and the [illegible]fusional states. Pathologic changes occur in characteristic regions of the brain stem, especially in the mamillary bodies and thalamus. Diffusion-weighted magnetic resonance imaging may show signal changes in these characteristic midline locations. As with Wernicke encephalopathy, Korsakoff encephalopathy is attributed to thiamine deficiency, though the precise pathophysiology is unknown. Selective disturbance of memory is the predominant clinical abnormality in Korsakoff encephalopathy. Thiamine replacement therapy rarely leads to improvement. There is marked impairment of recent memory and difficulty in incorporating new memories, though immediate recall is intact. Patients are unaware of any deficit and often confabulate. Other cognitive abnormalities are found less often. The disorder is common in chronic alcoholics, often occurring in association with Wernicke encephalopathy. The pathologic changes are similar in distribution to those in Wernicke encephalopathy. *(Answer: D—Thiamine [vitamin B_1])*

For more information, see Aminoff MJ: 11 Neurology: VII Anoxic, Metabolic, and Toxic Encephalopathies. ACP Medicine Online (www.acpmedicine.com). Dale DC, Federman DD, Eds. WebMD Inc., New York, January 2003

Headache

34. A 25-year-old woman comes to your clinic complaining of headaches. She's been having unilateral headaches for about a year, at a rate of approximately two to three episodes a month. The headaches last for 6 to 8 hours, are pulsating, and are accompanied by nausea, vomiting, and photophobia. She also has been experiencing some rhinorrhea with the headaches. The pain is moderate in intensity and gets worse with routine physical activity. She usually gets relief by taking over-the-counter ibuprofen. Her medical history is positive for sinus allergies. She has a family history of headaches. Her physical examination, including a neurologic examination, is unremarkable. She has heard on the news that headaches can be a sign of a tumor, and she is concerned about this possibility.

On the basis of this patient's history and physical examination, what is the most likely diagnosis, and how would you evaluate her?

- ❑ A. **Tension-type headache; further workup is not indicated at this time**
- ❑ B. **Sinus headache; obtain a sinus computed tomographic scan**
- ❑ C. **Migraine without aura; no further workup is indicated at this time**
- ❑ D. **Migraine without aura; magnetic resonance imaging is indicated to rule out intracranial pathology**

Key Concept/Objective: To understand the clinical characteristics and evaluation of migraines

Migraine can occur with and without aura. According to International Headache Society criteria for migraine without aura, the duration of untreated or unsuccessfully treated episodes ranges from 4 to 72 hours. The headaches are associated with at least two of the following pain characteristics: unilateral location, pulsating quality, moderate or severe intensity, and aggravation by routine physical activity. The pain is accompanied by at least one of the following symptoms: nausea with or without vomiting, photophobia, and phonophobia. Forty-five percent of migraineurs have at least one autonomic symptom (i.e., lacrimation, eye redness, or rhinorrhea) during an attack; these symptoms can lead to confusion of migraine with sinus headaches. Tension-type headaches are usually nonpulsating, last from 30 minutes to 7 days, are mild or moderate in severity, and are bilateral in location. There should be no nausea or vomiting; either photophobia or phonophobia may be present, but not both. The vast majority of patients require no diagnostic testing at all; they can be diagnosed accurately on the basis of a detailed history and a physical examination. *(Answer: C—Migraine without aura; no further workup is indicated at this time)*

35. A 38-year-old man with a 15-year history of migraine presents to your clinic complaining of worsening headaches. He has been taking ibuprofen. The headaches are unilateral and are accompanied by nausea, vomiting, and photophobia. In the past, the patient obtained relief with ibuprofen, but over the past few months, the headaches have failed to respond to this medication. The only change in the characteristics of the headaches is that they have increased in frequency. He used to have two or three attacks a week, and now he has headaches 5 or 6 days a week. His physical examination is unremarkable.

What is the most likely explanation of this patient's worsening headaches, and how would you treat these headaches?

- ❑ A. **Misdiagnosed tension-type headaches; start a tricyclic antidepressant as a prophylactic agent**
- ❑ B. **Worsening migraines; start triptans**
- ❑ C. **Brain tumor; obtain imaging studies and refer to neurosurgery**
- ❑ D. **Chronic daily headache (CDH) from a transformed migraine; stop short-acting nonsteroidal anti-inflammatory drugs (NSAIDs) (e.g., ibuprofen)**

Key Concept/Objective: To understand CDH

CDH has a frequency of 15 or more days a month. CDH includes four different headache types: transformed migraine, chronic tension-type headache, hemicrania continua, and

new drug persistent headache. Transformed migraine, with or without medication overuse, is a complication of intermittent migraine that usually occurs by 20 to 30 years of age. In 80% of patients, there is a gradual transformation from episodic migraine to CDH that may be associated with analgesic overuse and psychological factors. Migraine characteristics are present to a significant degree. Migraineurs are particularly susceptible to rebound headaches, which can occur with frequent use of symptomatic medications, including acetaminophen, aspirin, caffeine, NSAIDs with short half-lives, butalbital, ergotamine, opiates, and triptans. In the treatment of these patients, these medications should be discontinued. Usually the headaches improve within 9 days. A migraine-preventive medication can also be started. Two strategies that can be used during this withdrawal period are the use of steroids and, alternatively, a combination of tizanidine and an NSAID with a long half-life. Chronic tension-type headache presents with a frequency of 15 or more a month for at least 6 months. The pain characteristics are the same as for episodic tension-type headaches. The possibility of a brain tumor is less likely in this patient, given the similarity of his current headaches to his previous headaches, the temporal progression, and the presence of a more likely explanation. *(Answer: D—Chronic daily headache [CDH] from a transformed migraine; stop short-acting nonsteroidal anti-inflammatory drugs [NSAIDs] [e.g., ibuprofen])*

36. A 48-year-old man presents to a walk-in clinic complaining of headaches. The headaches are unilateral, located behind his right eye; they are constant, severe, and are of rapid onset. The patient notes that the headaches are accompanied by right-sided nasal congestion. The headaches usually last for 30 to 40 minutes. The headaches started 3 or 4 weeks ago, and he has two or three attacks a day. The patient does not have a history of headaches. At this time, the headache is 8/10 in severity. The patient has a medical history of hypertension, for which he takes an angiotensin-converting enzyme (ACE) inhibitor. On physical examination, the patient's blood pressure is 150/78 mm Hg; right-sided ptosis, miosis, and conjunctival injection are present. The rest of the examination is normal.

What is the most likely diagnosis for this patient, and how would you approach the diagnosis?

- ❑ **A. Cluster headaches; consider obtaining an imaging study to evaluate for secondary headaches**
- ❑ **B. Hypertension; increase dosage of blood pressure medications**
- ❑ **C. Posterior communicating artery aneurysm; get an urgent cerebral angiography**
- ❑ **D. ACE inhibitor–induced headache; stop use of the ACE inhibitor**

Key Concept/Objective: To know the clinical manifestations of cluster headaches

Cluster headaches are an uncommon headache type that occurs in only about 0.4% of the general population. Cluster headaches are five times more common in males. This condition is marked by periods of recurrent headaches (one to eight a day) interspersed with periods of remission. Cluster headaches are unilateral and severe. The most common types of pain are orbital, retroorbital, temporal, supraorbital, and infraorbital. The headache may alternate sides. Cluster headaches have a rapid onset, with peak intensity in 5 to 10 minutes, and are usually of short duration, lasting 30 to 45 minutes. Autonomic symptoms are present in over 97% of the cases. Lacrimation and conjunctival injection are each present in 80% of the cases, and ipsilateral congestion is present in 74%. A partial Horner syndrome is present in 65% of the cases. Cluster headaches can usually be diagnosed on the basis of the clinical criteria alone. Neuroimaging, preferably MRI, may be considered in cases with the following features: a pattern of clusterlike headache not conforming to the clinical criteria; age of onset older than 40 years; a progressive pattern of headaches; chronic cluster headache; and any focal neurologic deficit other than Horner syndrome. A posterior communicating artery aneurysm can cause a subarachnoid hemorrhage and pupillary changes characteristic of third-nerve palsy (i.e., midriasis with ptosis); it would not cause miosis. Mild to moderate hypertension does not usually cause headache. ACE inhibitors can cause headaches in some patients; however, in this patient, this possibility seems less likely than cluster headaches. *(Answer: A—Cluster headaches; consider obtaining an imaging study to evaluate for secondary headaches)*

37. You are asked to evaluate a 25-year-old woman for headaches. Her symptoms started 2 months ago with daily frontal bilateral headaches. The headaches are pulsatile and continuous. She also complains of occasional blurred vision. She has no significant medical history. She takes over-the-counter acetaminophen for her headaches. On physical examination, her blood pressure is 120/76 mm Hg. She weighs 200 lb, and she is 5 ft 2 in tall. Her fundoscopic examination shows papilledema. The rest of her examination is normal. You are concerned about her symptoms and order an MRI, which shows no significant abnormalities.

What should be your next step in the management of this patient?

❑ **A. Perform a lumbar puncture**

❑ **B. Start a triptan**

❑ **C. Start indomethacin**

❑ **D. Start a beta blocker as prophylaxis for migraines**

Key Concept/Objective: To recognize the manifestations of pseudotumor cerebri

Pseudotumor cerebri, also known as idiopathic intracranial hypertension, is a disorder of unknown etiology. Onset usually occurs in persons between the ages of 11 and 58 years. Ninety percent are young, obese women. Headache is present in 75% or more of patients, papilledema in 95%, cranial nerve VI palsy in 25%, transient visual obscurations in 70%, visual loss in 30%, and roaring noises in 70%. The headaches are usually pulsatile, continuous, and daily; they can be unilateral or bilateral, with a bifrontotemporal location being the most common. Nausea is present in 60% of cases, and vomiting is present in 40%. The diagnosis of pseudotumor cerebri is one of exclusion, because there are many other causes of papilledema. Testing includes a scan of the brain; MRI is the test of choice. If the brain scan is negative, a lumbar puncture should be obtained. The opening pressure is usually elevated and the cerebrospinal fluid analysis is normal, except for a low CSF protein level in some patients. Treatments include weight loss and diuretics to decrease the CSF production. *(Answer: A—Perform a lumbar puncture)*

For more information, see Evans RW: 11 Neurology: VIII Headache. ACP Medicine Online (www.acpmedicine.com). Dale DC, Federman DD, Eds. WebMD Inc., New York, April 2003

Demyelinating Diseases

38. A 54-year-old man comes to the hospital complaining of left arm weakness of 3 days' duration. He has no significant medical history. He takes no medications and denies using alcohol or tobacco. His physical examination is unremarkable except that his motor examination shows 3/5 strength in the left upper extremity. Results of the neurologic examination are within normal limits. MRIs of the brain are obtained. T_2-weighted MRI shows a single hyperintense white matter lesion on the right hemisphere; the lesion is hypointense on T_1-weighted MRI.

On the basis of this patient's symptoms and imaging studies, which of the following would be the most appropriate step to take next in his management?

❑ **A. Start glatiramer for treatment of multiple sclerosis (MS)**

❑ **B. Start interferon beta for treatment of MS**

❑ **C. Perform a lumbar puncture, obtain a spinal MRI, and assess evoked responses**

❑ **D. Start mitoxantrone to prevent progression of symptoms**

Key Concept/Objective: To understand the diagnosis of MS

The diagnosis of MS is based on clinical signs and symptoms, MRI findings, and other laboratory tests. The diagnosis of MS requires evidence of dissemination of lesions in time and space and the careful exclusion of other causes. The patient should have had more than one episode of neurologic dysfunction and should have evidence of white matter lesions

in more than one part of the CNS. MRI is the single most useful laboratory test in the diagnosis of MS. Although MRI is extremely sensitive in detecting white matter lesions in patients with MS, it is not very specific. Many other diseases produce white matter lesions. Therefore, MRI findings should never be used as the sole basis for the diagnosis. The most characteristic abnormality of the CFS in MS is the presence of intrathecal synthesis of immunoglobulins of restricted heterogeneity, which is demonstrated by the presence of oligoclonal immunoglobulin bands. Evoked responses are a useful marker of subclinical MS and can be used in support of the diagnosis of MS. Interferon beta, glatiramer, and mitoxantrone have been used in MS; however, the specific indications for treatment with these agents are not met in this case. *(Answer: C—Perform a lumbar puncture, obtain a spinal MRI, and assess evoked responses)*

39. A 40-year-old woman with a history of MS presents to clinic with numbness in her left arm and weakness in her right leg. She was diagnosed 2 years ago after having an episode of left leg weakness. She has experienced mild, persistent weakness since then. She had optic neuritis 3 years ago. Her physical examination is remarkable for severe left arm weakness and increased deep tendon reflexes of the left arm. The left leg shows mild weakness and increased reflexes. She has decreased sensation in the right leg. MRI shows multiple white matter lesions.

On the basis of this patient's history and symptoms, which of the following would be the most appropriate therapeutic regimen?

- ❑ **A. Short-term steroids**
- ❑ **B. Long-term mitoxantrone**
- ❑ **C. Long-term steroids**
- ❑ **D. Long-term glatiramer or interferon beta and short-term steroids**

Key Concept/Objective: To understand therapy for MS

In MS, the management of acute relapses varies with the severity of the presenting symptoms and signs. High-dose corticosteroid therapy is indicated for exacerbations that adversely affect the patient's function. A short, tapering course of corticosteroids may be given afterward. In the past few years, three different medications that affect the long-term clinical course of MS have been approved: interferon beta-1b, interferon beta-1a, and glatiramer acetate (previously known as copolymer-1). These drugs reduce the frequency of attacks and limit the accumulation of fixed lesions on MRI. In patients with relapsing-remitting MS, these agents may delay the accumulation of disability. The choice of which agent to use depends on the particular patient. Patients who are maintained on these therapies can expect an 18% to 50% reduction in attack frequency. Best responses with any of the available drugs appear to result from initiation of treatment relatively early in the disease course. Mitoxantrone currently has a role for selected patients with very active disease; it is approved for the treatment of aggressive relapsing and secondary progressive MS. Its significant side effects limit its use. *(Answer: D—Long-term glatiramer or interferon beta and short-term steroids)*

40. A 26-year-old woman is evaluated for decreased vision and eye pain. Her symptoms started 2 days ago with pain in her right eye with ocular movements. Over the past 24 hours, she has experienced a decrease in central vision in her right eye. She has no significant medical history. Physical examination shows decreased central vision and pain on ocular movement of the right eye. There is an afferent pupillary defect on the right. Results of fundoscopic examination are normal. The rest of her examination is unremarkable. MRIs of the brain and spinal cord are consistent with optic neuritis on the right; there are two white matter lesions in the periventricular area.

On the basis of this patient's presentation and MRI findings, which of the following statements is most accurate?

- ❑ **A. The patient has MS and should be started on steroids and glatiramer**
- ❑ **B. The patient has optic neuritis; she is at significant risk for developing MS in the future**

❑ C. **The patient has optic neuritis; she is at no risk of progressing to MS in the future**

❑ D. **The patient has MS; she should be started on mitoxantrone**

Key Concept/Objective: To know the association between optic neuritis and MS

Optic neuritis is an acute inflammatory optic neuropathy. The cardinal symptoms are unilateral vision loss and retrobulbar pain with eye movement. Treatment with intravenous methylprednisolone followed by oral prednisone hastens recovery of vision. Even without treatment, almost all patients begin to recover vision within 4 weeks. The relationship of optic neuritis to MS is controversial. Some regard optic neuritis as a distinct entity, but others consider it part of the clinical continuum of MS. More than half of all patients with MS have optic neuritis at some time during the course of disease. Of patients who present with optic neuritis and who have no other neurologic deficit, almost 40% have one or more ovoid periventricular lesions on brain MRI; clinically definite MS eventually develops in 60%. Patients with completely normal results on MRI and comprehensive CSF evaluation seldom progress to MS. *(Answer: B—The patient has optic neuritis; she is at significant risk for developing MS in the future)*

41. A 44-year-old man comes to the hospital complaining of progressive lower extremity weakness and decreased sensation. He has been experiencing these symptoms for 5 days. He also complains of having difficulties with bowel movements and urination. He recalls having an upper respiratory infection 1 or 2 weeks ago. His physical examination is remarkable for decreased sensation starting at the level of T10, symmetrical severe lower extremity weakness, urinary retention, and decreased rectal tone. The muscle tone and deep tendon reflexes in his lower extremities are diminished. T_2-weighted MRI of the spinal cord shows a hyperintense lesion that involves the majority of the cross-sectional area of the cord; the lesion extends from T6 to L3. No cord compression is seen. MRI of the brain is normal.

Of the following, which is the most likely diagnosis?

❑ A. **Devic disease**

❑ B. **Acute disseminated encephalomyelitis**

❑ C. **Transverse myelitis**

❑ D. **MS**

Key Concept/Objective: To be able to recognize transverse myelitis

Acute transverse myelitis is a syndrome of spinal cord dysfunction. It has a rapid onset; it may occur after infection or vaccination or it may occur with no discernible precipitant. It may also be the initial presentation of MS. Symptoms include paraparesis, which is initially flaccid and then spastic; loss of sensation with a sensory level in the trunk; and bowel and bladder dysfunction. The thoracic cord is most often affected. MRI is extremely helpful for excluding other structural lesions and for confirming the presence of an intramedullary lesion, which is typically hyperintense in T_2-weighted imaging. No treatment has proven to be beneficial, but corticosteroids are often used. Neuromyelitis optica is also known as Devic disease. It is characterized by the simultaneous or sequential involvement of the optic nerves and spinal cord; it often has a malignant course. Acute disseminated encephalomyelitis is a monophasic syndrome that is usually preceded by a viral exanthema, an upper respiratory infection, or vaccination. Onset is rapid and is characterized by meningeal signs, headache, seizures, and altered mental status. The neurologic deficits include hemiplegia, paraplegia, sensory loss, vision loss, and transverse myelitis. In this patient, the lack of multiple lesions and the monophasic nature of the disease make the diagnosis of MS less likely. *(Answer: C—Transverse myelitis)*

42. A 43-year-old woman with a 14-year history of MS with lower-extremity spasticity presents with increased spasticity, mild confusion, abdominal discomfort, and a temperature of 100° F (37.8° C).

Which of the following choices best combines medical indication and favorable cost-benefit ratio?

❑ A. **Urodynamic study**

- ❑ B. **Abdominal CT scan**
- ❑ C. **MRI scan of the lumbosacral spine**
- ❑ D. **Brain MRI**
- ❑ E. **Urinalysis**

Key Concept/Objective: To understand the frequency of UTIs in women with MS and how acute UTI can mimic relapse of acute MS

Bladder dysfunction is common in patients with MS; in women especially, bladder dysfunction often results in UTIs. Because of loss of sensation, the infections may not cause dysuria but may instead cause more global deterioration of neurologic function, mimicking an acute relapse. Lower limb spasticity in particular may accompany urinary retention with overflow incontinence. In this patient, as in others who appear to have acute relapse, a urinalysis should be part of the evaluation. A formal urodynamic study will define the specific pattern of dysfunction and help determine appropriate therapy. *(Answer: E—Urinalysis)*

43. A 30-year-old woman presents with vision loss in the left eye and pain behind the left eye with eye movement. Ophthalmologic consultation reveals optic neuritis. Brain MRI and comprehensive CSF examination are normal.

Which of the following statements is true for this patient?

- ❑ A. **Treatment with high-dose methylprednisolone will result in improved visual retention at 1 year**
- ❑ B. **This patient has a high likelihood of progression to definite MS within 2 years**
- ❑ C. **Without treatment, this patient has a high likelihood of progressive unilateral visual loss**
- ❑ D. **It is unlikely that this patient will progress to MS**
- ❑ E. **Optic neuritis is distinct from MS**

Key Concept/Objective: To understand the relation between optic neuritis and multiple sclerosis

Although more than half of all patients with MS have optic neuritis at some time, patients with optic neuritis who have completely normal results on MRI scanning and comprehensive CSF examination seldom progress to MS. Whether optic neuritis is a distinct clinical entity or part of a continuum with MS is controversial. Treatment of optic neuritis may result in hastened benefit, but even without treatment, most patients begin to recover vision within 4 weeks. *(Answer: D—It is unlikely that this patient will progress to MS)*

44. A 45-year-old man presents with paresthesias in his feet and mild ataxia. He has an uneventful medical history and has never used alcohol. On physical examination, he has decreased proprioception and vibratory sensation in the lower extremities. Routine laboratory studies show a macrocytic anemia.

Which test should be ordered next for this patient?

- ❑ A. **Serum cobalamin**
- ❑ B. **CSF immunoglobulin electrophoresis**
- ❑ C. **Visual evoked potentials**
- ❑ D. **Serum folate**
- ❑ E. **Brain MRI**

Key Concept/Objective: To understand the neurologic consequences of vitamin B_{12} deficiency

In addition to causing a macrocytic anemia, vitamin B_{12} deficiency results in axonal demyelination, especially in the dorsal and lateral columns of the spinal cord. This leads to the common presenting symptoms of peripheral paresthesias, ascending sensory loss, and sensory ataxia. More severe and prolonged deficiency can result in memory loss and

confusion. Folate deficiency can result in macrocytic anemia but does not cause the neurologic complications of B_{12} deficiency. *(Answer: A—Serum cobalamin)*

For more information, see Linsey JW, Wolinsky JS: 11 Neurology: IX Demyelinating Diseases. ACP Medicine Online (www.acpmedicine.com). Dale DC, Federman DD, Eds. WebMD Inc., New York, July 2003

Inherited Ataxias

45. The parents of a 16-year-old boy bring him to you with concerns about alcohol use. He has been experiencing slurring of speech and was twice sent home from school for falling in gym class. He reports generalized fatigue and dizziness with exercise. He denies using alcohol or drugs. The patient's maternal uncle developed difficulty walking at a young age but died in an accident before a diagnosis was made. On examination, the patient has impaired proprioception, a staggering gait, and extensor plantar response. He has a laterally displaced sustained point of maximal impulse.

What is the most likely diagnosis for this patient?

- ❑ A. **Ataxia-telangiectasia**
- ❑ B. **Friedreich ataxia**
- ❑ C. **Neuroblastoma**
- ❑ D. **Chiari-Arnold deformity**
- ❑ E. **Episodic ataxia type 2**

Key Concept/Objective: To know the presenting features of Friedreich ataxia

Friedreich ataxia is the most common recessively inherited ataxia. Patients often present before the age of 25 years with ataxia. Other symptoms can include dysarthria, vision problems, weakness, and dysphagia. Physical examination reveals loss of deep tendon reflexes, poor proprioception, weakness, and extensor plantar response. Phenotypic variation is not uncommon, and some patients have preserved or brisk deep tendon reflexes. Between 30% and 50% of patients develop symptomatic heart disease, including hypertrophic cardiomyopathy. *(Answer: B—Friedreich ataxia)*

For more information, see Subramony SH: 11 Neurology: X Inherited Ataxias. ACP Medicine Online (www.acpmedicine.com). Dale DC, Federman DD, Eds. WebMD Inc., New York, February 2004

Alzheimer Disease and Other Dementing Illnesses

46. A 79-year-old man comes to establish primary care. He is accompanied by his daughter. He has been in very good health for most of his life. His only medication is a beta blocker, which he has been been taking for moderate hypertension. He has undergone all screening examinations appropriate for his age. Over the past several months, he underwent evaluation for possible onset of dementia. The patient and his daughter agree that the patient's memory has been worsening over the past 1 to 2 years. He easily recalls events of his childhood, but he is not able to tell you what he ate for his morning meal. He had been an avid outdoorsman, but he had to give up outdoor activities because he recently got lost in the woods for several hours. The family seeks your opinion and further workup.

Which of the following statements regarding Alzheimer disease (AD) is true?

- ❑ A. **AD is histopathologically defined by neurofibrillary tangles and neuritic plaques in the cerebral cortex**
- ❑ B. **The definition of AD requires impairment in only one area of cognitive function**
- ❑ C. **The pivotal cognitive finding in AD is retrograde amnesia**

❑ D. **The prevalence of AD is approximately 1% of the United States population older than 65 years**

Key Concept/Objective: To understand the general clinical features of AD

AD is histopathologically defined by neurofibrillary tangles and neuritic plaques in the cerebral cortex. The definition of dementia requires impairment in more than one area of cognitive function. In the dementia syndrome of AD, in addition to anterograde amnesia, there must be impairment in at least one of the following: language, abstract reasoning, executive function, or visuospatial processing. The pivotal cognitive finding in AD is anterograde amnesia, which represents an inability to learn new things. Persons with anterograde amnesia typically cannot keep track of the date, remember recent conversations, or remember where they set something down, and they often repeat themselves in conversation. The prevalence of AD is approximately 8% of the United States population older than 65 years. *(Answer: A—AD is histopathologically defined by neurofibrillary tangles and neuritic plaques in the cerebral cortex)*

47. An 80-year-old male patient of yours with AD is brought to your office by his daughter. According to the daughter, the patient's functional status has been declining rapidly. She states that along with worsening memory, the patient has become tearful, and she feels he is hallucinating. He had been stable for the past year while receiving donepezil therapy. The patient's functional decline and tearfulness, as well as occasional severe confusion with combativeness, are causing severe stress for both the patient and the household. The patient's daughter asks if there are further medication options for the patient.

Which of the following statements regarding primary and secondary therapies for AD is true?

❑ A. **The cholinesterase inhibitors, such as donepezil, have shown promise as a cure for AD**

❑ B. **The cholinesterase inhibitors are the only class of agents available for the primary treatment of AD**

❑ C. **Treatment of depression associated with AD should be pursued as aggressively as in patients without dementia**

❑ D. **For treatment of anxiety and agitation in AD, short-acting benzodiazepines and typical antipsychotics are generally recommended**

Key Concept/Objective: To know the appropriate primary and secondary therapies for AD

The cholinesterase inhibitors donepezil, galantamine, and rivastigmine have been approved by the Food and Drug Administration for the treatment of AD. Clinical trials with each of these agents have shown that long-term use results in modest stabilization of cognitive and functional status for approximately 6 to 12 months, compared with no treatment. Vitamin E is often recommended for patients with AD on the basis of a study of 2 years' duration. The glutamate modulator memantine has also been approved by the FDA for the treatment of AD. This agent is a noncompetitive receptor antagonist of *N*-methyl-D-aspartate. Several clinical trials have reported positive results with memantine in the treatment of moderate to severe dementia. Treatment of depression or anxiety in patients with AD should be pursued as aggressively as in patients without AD, with adherence to the best practices of geriatric pharmacology. Depression frequently coexists with AD and contributes to morbidity and loss of function. Treatment of anxiety presents somewhat more of a challenge in AD patients, because the agents commonly used in younger patients, the benzodiazepines, have distinctly unwanted side effects in AD patients. Drugs such as lorazepam and alprazolam can increase confusion in AD patients. The longer-acting agent clonazepam may be a better choice. Buspirone is another alternative for the treatment of anxiety in AD patients. Treatment of agitation generally requires antipsychotics. Quetiapine has the significant advantage of being much less likely to induce extrapyramidal signs than both newer and older agents. *(Answer: C—Treatment of depression associated with AD should be pursued as aggressively as in patients without dementia)*

48. A 69-year-old female patient whom you have been treating for many years for hypertension and dyslipidemia comes for a routine appointment. Both her hypertension and dyslipidemia have been difficult to control. She has been hospitalized on several occasions over the past few years for likely transient ischemic attacks (TIA). Her most recent TIA occurred 18 months ago. She has been on aspirin therapy for many years. Today she complains that her "mind wanders." On questioning, she reports that her short-term memory and her ability to learn new information have declined over the past several months. She believes she has "hardening of the arteries."

Which of the following statements regarding vascular dementia (VaD) is true?

- ❑ A. **The National Institute of Neurological Disorders and Stroke–Association Internationale pour la Recherche et l'Enseignement en Neurosciences (NINDS-AIREN) criteria for the diagnosis of VaD are highly sensitive**
- ❑ B. **Though lacking sensitivity, the NINDS-AIREN criteria for the diagnosis of VaD are highly specific**
- ❑ C. **As described in NINDS-AIREN criteria, the onset of all cases of VaD occurs within a 3-month period following a stroke**
- ❑ D. **VaD and AD are roughly equal in prevalence**

Key Concept/Objective: To know the diagnostic criteria and prevalence of VaD

The essence of the NINDS-AIREN criteria is that (1) the onset or worsening of dementia occurred within 3 months after a clinical stroke; (2) imaging studies show evidence of bilateral infarcts in cortical regions, basal ganglia, thalamus, or white matter; and (3) neurologic examination shows focal neurologic deficits. All three criteria are required for the diagnosis. Clinical-pathologic correlation studies have shown that this definition is quite specific, meaning that patients who meet these criteria are highly likely to have VaD pathologically. However, the NINDS-AIREN criteria are very insensitive, failing to diagnose the majority of patients who prove to have VaD at autopsy. VaD may also begin insidiously, because there is a substantial percentage of VaD cases that appear to result from the accumulation of a series of so-called silent or covert infarcts. Patients in this group do not meet the diagnostic criterion of dementia temporally linked to stroke, but they do have brain infarcts, best visible with MRI. VaD is approximately one tenth to one fifth as common as AD in prevalence and incidence. *(Answer: B—Though lacking sensitivity, the NINDS-AIREN criteria for the diagnosis of VaD are highly specific)*

49. An 84-year-old man presents to your office with his live-in son. His son states that his father has become progressively forgetful over the past several months. He now has difficulty remembering to complete even simple daily tasks. He also states that his father has become physically slowed over the same period. His father now walks slowly and with a wider-than-usual gait. In addition, he falls several times a month. The son also notes that for several years, his father has talked in his sleep and that he has "nightmares" almost every night. He is concerned that his father has "old-timer's" disease, and he seeks your opinion.

Which of the following statements regarding dementia with Lewy bodies (DLB) is true?

- ❑ A. **The clinical presentation of DLB is identical to that of AD**
- ❑ B. **The parkinsonism of DLB is consistently severe**
- ❑ C. **As with AD, the patient with DLB has no changes in level of arousal**
- ❑ D. **The rapid eye movement sleep behavior disorder (RBD) is highly specific for DLB**

Key Concept/Objective: To know the clinical distinction of DLB and AD

The term DLB is in vogue as a label for patients who have spontaneous (i.e., not drug-induced) parkinsonism, dementia, and often symptoms of disordered arousal. The cognitive disorder of DLB can closely resemble AD, but in many patients, there are some notable differences. These differences in DLB include a slightly less prominent deficit in learning and memory and more prominent difficulties with visuospatial functions, performance on timed tasks, and executive functions. The parkinsonism in DLB can range from a relatively isolated gait instability with frequent falling to a typical pattern of Parkinson disease

with rest tremor, rigidity, bradykinesia, and postural instability. Patients with DLB often experience marked fluctuations in their alertness and level of arousal from one day to the next. They often sleep excessively. In RBD, patients engage in dream enactment, thrashing about in bed or talking in their sleep. RBD can often precede the dementia and the movement disorder by years and is highly specific for DLB. *(Answer: D—The rapid eye movement sleep behavior disorder [RBD] is highly specific for DLB)*

50. A 72-year-old woman is referred to you for evaluation of 2 to 3 years of gradual memory loss. Although she clearly has significant difficulties with memory and slowed speech, she seems surprisingly apathetic toward her condition. She has hypertension and mild osteopenia but is otherwise healthy; she has no history of head trauma. Her only medication is 12.5 mg of hydrochlorothiazide once daily. Her Mini-Mental State Exam (MMSE) score is 21/30; her neurologic exam is normal. Neuropsychological testing confirms cognitive dysfunction. Laboratory evaluation for other causes of dementia is negative.

Which of the following is the most appropriate diagnosis for this patient?

- ❑ **A. Definite Alzheimer disease**
- ❑ **B. Probable Alzheimer disease**
- ❑ **C. Progressive supranuclear palsy**
- ❑ **D. Normal-pressure (communicating) hydrocephalus**
- ❑ **E. Polypharmacy**

Key Concept/Objective: To know the diagnostic criteria for Alzheimer disease

This patient has at least two areas of cognitive dysfunction (memory and speech), confirmed by neuropsychological testing. She has no evidence of other disorders, such as the motor dysfunction expected with progressive supranuclear palsy or the ataxia and incontinence associated with normal-pressure hydrocephalus. It is unlikely that a low dose of hydrochlorothiazide would be responsible for significant cognitive dysfunction, particularly in the absence of laboratory abnormalities. The patient meets criteria for probable Alzheimer disease. The diagnosis of definite Alzheimer disease requires evidence of pathologic changes in brain tissue from either biopsy or autopsy specimens. *(Answer: B—Probable Alzheimer disease)*

51. A 65-year-old man is brought in by his family for evaluation of altered cognitive function. The family members say that he is "normal" midday but sleeps poorly and frequently wanders about the house at night. When the patient is questioned about this, he seems confused and says that he has no recollection of these events. He is being treated for depression and has no other medical problems. Current medications include amitriptyline, 100 mg at bedtime, with 1 mg of lorazepam as needed for sleep. His MMSE score is 26/30; his neurologic examination is normal. Laboratory evaluation for other causes of dementia is negative.

Which of the following is the most appropriate diagnosis for this patient?

- ❑ **A. Definite Alzheimer disease**
- ❑ **B. Probable Alzheimer disease**
- ❑ **C. Huntington disease**
- ❑ **D. Normal-pressure (communicating) hydrocephalus**
- ❑ **E. Polypharmacy**

Key Concept/Objective: To recognize medications as a common cause of "dementia"

This patient presents with a history of sleep disturbance with nocturnal disorientation. Although this is common in dementia syndromes, this patient is on two medications that often cause cognitive dysfunction: amitriptyline (a tricyclic antidepressant with anticholinergic activity) and lorazepam (a benzodiazepine). These medications should be changed or discontinued before considering the diagnosis of a primary dementia syndrome. *(Answer: E—Polypharmacy)*

52. A 78-year-old man comes in with his family to discuss the fact that he does not seem to be thinking as clearly as he once did. His family says that he frequently takes a long time to respond to simple questions and does not participate in conversations as he used to. He has a history of prostate cancer, status 5 years' postradiotherapy. He takes 325 mg of aspirin once a day. Speaking to him, you notice that he does take a long time to answer, although his answers are usually appropriate. His speech is slowed and noticeably slurred. His MMSE score is 23/30. The neurologic examination is remarkable for expressionless facies and halting, unsteady gait. Laboratory evaluation for other causes of dementia is negative.

Which of the following is the most appropriate diagnosis for this patient?

- ❑ **A. Definite Alzheimer disease**
- ❑ **B. Probable Alzheimer disease**
- ❑ **C. Progressive supranuclear palsy (PSP)**
- ❑ **D. Pick disease**
- ❑ **E. Depression**

Key Concept/Objective: To be able to recognize evidence of subcortical dementia

Motor dysfunction is typical of the subcortical dementias, of which PSP is the only one listed among the available answers. PSP often presents with parkinsonian symptoms, typically with prominent dysarthria and dysphagia. *(Answer: C—Progressive supranuclear palsy [PSP])*

53. A 28-year-old man wishes to have genetic testing for Alzheimer disease because his mother and maternal grandfather both died of the disease in their early 60s. He has one child, age 5.

Before genetic testing, what should this patient be told is the risk of transmission of the gene to his child if his test is positive?

- ❑ A. 13%
- ❑ B. 25%
- ❑ C. 33%
- ❑ D. 50%
- ❑ E. 100%

Key Concept/Objective: To understand autosomal dominant mutations causing Alzheimer disease and the implications for genetic counseling

The patient's history is strongly suggestive of autosomal dominant inheritance of early-onset Alzheimer disease. If he is tested for APP or PS1, he should be advised that a positive test in his case indicates a 50% risk of transmission of the gene to his children. *(Answer: D—50%)*

For more information, see Knopman DS: 11 Neurology: XI Alzheimer Disease and Other Major Dementing Illnesses. ACP Medicine Online (www.acpmedicine.com). Dale DC, Federman DD, Eds. WebMD Inc., New York, May 2004

Epilepsy

54. A 22-year-old woman comes to your clinic after being seen in a local emergency department 1 week ago, when she presented with seizures. She denies having any previous episodes. She does not remember the episode, which was witnessed by her mother. The mother relates that she noticed that the patient had a blank stare and then, after a few seconds, she started moving her hands repetitively, "like she was washing them." During this episode, the patient did not respond to any commands; it lasted approximately 1 minute. After this episode, the patient remained confused for about 10 minutes. The patient's physical examination is unremarkable.

On the basis of clinical presentation, how would you classify this patient's seizure?

❑ A. Myoclonic seizure

❑ B. Absence seizure

❑ C. Complex partial seizure

❑ D. Tonic-clonic seizure

Key Concept/Objective: To understand the major classification of seizures

The International League Against Epilepsy has classified epileptic seizures on the basis of the clinical presentation and electroencephalographic criteria. The classification divides seizures into three major categories: partial, generalized, and unclassified. Partial seizures are described as either simple or complex, depending on whether consciousness remains intact or is impaired during the seizure. Simple partial seizures can be motor, sensory, autonomic, or psychic. Complex partial seizures usually begin with arrest of motion and a blank stare. Automatisms, oroalimentary behavior, or verbal utterances may occur initially or during the seizure. Most spells last only a few minutes. At the termination of the seizure, the patient may be momentarily confused, fatigued, or disoriented. Generalized seizures cause a spectrum of behavior from the nonconvulsive pattern of simple absence seizure through myoclonus to the fully developed generalized tonic-clonic seizure. Absence seizures are brief, usually lasting 10 seconds or less; the seizures are not preceded by an aura or followed by postictal effects, which helps differentiate them from complex partial seizures. Myoclonus consists of brief jerks or contractions of a specific muscle or group of muscles. Atonic seizures involve a sudden loss of postural tone. Convulsions are the most common types of generalized seizures; they are characterized by loss of consciousness associated with apnea and violent contractions of the musculature of the trunk and extremities. *(Answer: C—Complex partial seizure)*

55. A 46-year-old diabetic man is started on insulin therapy for poorly controlled diabetes. After 2 weeks, he has a generalized tonic-clonic seizure and is brought to the emergency department by the emergency medical service. He was found in the field to have a blood sugar level of 25 mg/dl. He received a dose of 50% dextrose in water (D50W) and lorazepam, which resulted in resolution of the seizure. When you examine the patient in the emergency department, he still has mild confusion. His physical examination shows a tongue laceration; otherwise, the examination is normal. An imaging study of the brain is obtained, and the results are normal. Over the next several hours, the patient regains normal mental function.

What is the best step to take next in the treatment of this patient?

❑ A. Refer the patient to a neurologist

❑ B. Reevaluate the management of his diabetes

❑ C. Obtain a sleep-deprived electroencephalogram

❑ D. Start an antiepileptic drug

Key Concept/Objective: To understand the differential diagnosis of epilepsy

Although sudden alterations in neurologic function are characteristic of seizures, sudden alterations also occur when intracranial structures are deprived of glucose or oxygen. Although a simple syncope usually does not cause any motor activity, prolonged interruption of cerebral perfusion may cause convulsive movements or even tonic-clonic seizures. Sensory or motor dysfunction may be caused by transient ischemia. Seizures may occur with embolic strokes. Metabolic disease, particularly disease related to glucose metabolism that requires regulation of blood sugar concentration with insulin therapy, may be associated with episodes of hypoglycemia. Both focal and generalized seizures can be manifestations of hypoglycemia or of hyperosmolar states. Lumbar puncture should be performed if the patient is febrile or has altered cognitive function. To prevent complications from lumbar puncture, the clinician must first exclude the presence of an intracranial mass or increased intracranial pressure. This patient developed symptomatic hypoglycemia with a secondary tonic-clonic seizure, which resolved with correction of the hypoglycemia. No further treatment and evaluation for a seizure disorder is warranted. However, reevaluation of the management of the diabetes is of paramount importance. *(Answer: B—Reevaluate the management of his diabetes)*

56. A 14-year-old boy with a history of juvenile myoclonic epilepsy is seen for recurrent seizures. His disease was very well controlled in the past with valproate, and he was seizure-free for 18 months. During the past 2 months, the patient has had eight seizures, which the patient's father describes as being different from his usual myoclonic jerks and generalized tonic-clonic seizures. These seizures are different each time; they last from 20 to 45 minutes. His physical examination is unremarkable.

On the basis of this patient's clinical picture, what would be the most likely cause of these seizures?

- ❑ A. **Progression of juvenile myoclonic epilepsy**
- ❑ B. **Intracranial mass**
- ❑ C. **Valproate toxicity**
- ❑ D. **Nonepileptic seizure**

Key Concept/Objective: To recognize the clinical picture of nonepileptic seizures

Approximately 20% of patients admitted to epilepsy monitoring units for diagnostic evaluation have episodic behavioral alterations that are not caused by physiologic dysfunction of the brain. In the past, these alterations were called pseudoseizures; currently, the preferred term for such seizures is nonepileptic seizures. Use of this term tends to help the patients understand their problem and facilitates referral for behavioral therapy. An important clue to the diagnosis of nonepileptic seizures is that they are periodic events that tend not to be stereotyped. Both patients and observers report varied behaviors with each event. Another clue is the prolonged duration. Nonepileptic seizures may last 30 minutes to several hours—longer than typical seizures. Patients with both nonepileptic seizures and epilepsy pose a challenging problem; this combination is occasionally found in patients undergoing assessment in epilepsy monitoring units. Treatment of nonepileptic seizures requires behavioral intervention. If both disorders are found, treatment of epilepsy needs to be continued in parallel with behavioral therapy. *(Answer: D—Nonepileptic seizure)*

57. A 44-year-old woman is admitted to the hospital with pneumonia. She has a medical history of epilepsy, for which she has been receiving phenytoin for the past 10 years. Her last seizure occurred 14 months ago. She reports having fever, cough, and shortness of breath, but she denies having any neurologic symptoms. Her physical examination shows increased breath sounds at the right base, consistent with pneumonia. Her neurologic examination, including gait, is normal. The patient is started on antibiotics. In the emergency department, the patient's phenytoin level was assessed; results show the phenytoin level to be elevated at 25 µg/ml (normal, 10 to 20 µg/ml).

Which of the following would be the most appropriate way to address this patient's elevated phenytoin level?

- ❑ A. **Continue the same regimen of phenytoin for now**
- ❑ B. **Hold the next dose of phenytoin, then restart the previous regimen of phenytoin**
- ❑ C. **Hold phenytoin, assess the patient's phenytoin levels daily until they are subtherapeutic, then restart phenytoin**
- ❑ D. **Hold phenytoin, then restart before discharge and follow the patient's phenytoin levels periodically to make sure they are therapeutic**

Key Concept/Objective: To recognize the general principles of epilepsy drug therapy

Antiepileptic drug (AED) treatment should be directed at both controlling seizures and, when possible, correcting the underlying disease or disorder. AEDs may be used only briefly, if at all, in patients who have had a single seizure or a few seizures resulting from a transient disorder. Patients who have recurrent seizures should be treated with AEDs. Treatment with AEDs should follow certain basic principles. Therapy should be started with a single agent. Seizure control should be achieved, if possible, by increasing the dosage of this agent. If seizure control cannot be achieved with the first medication, an alternative agent should be considered. Monotherapy can control seizures in about 60% of

the patients with newly diagnosed epilepsy. The use of two or more AEDs should be avoided if possible, but drug combinations may be useful when monotherapy fails. Drug selection should be guided by the patient's seizure type and epilepsy syndrome classification in concert with the mechanisms of action and side effects. Changes in dosage should be guided by the patient's clinical response rather than by drug levels; inadequate seizure control indicates the need for increasing the dose, and toxicity indicates the need to lower the dosage. Monitoring of levels is usually not necessary for patients who tolerate their medication well and have adequate seizure control. In some circumstances, the monitoring of drug levels may be useful in determining prescription compliance or to explain changes in seizure control or drug toxicity. This patient's seizures are adequately controlled, and there are no clinical symptoms or signs of toxicity; therefore, changes in the dosage are not indicated, and phenytoin levels should not be followed. *(Answer: A—Continue the same regimen of phenytoin for now)*

For more information, see Wheless JW: 11 Neurology: XII Epilepsy. ACP Medicine Online (www.acpmedicine.com). Dale DC, Federman DD, Eds. WebMD Inc., New York, May 2003

Disorders of Sleep

58. A 48-year-old man presents to your clinic complaining of excessive daytime somnolence. His symptoms started 2 years ago. They have slowly progressed to the point where he falls asleep frequently throughout the day. The patient also reports having early morning headaches. He has tried taking naps during the day, without relief of his somnolence. His physical examination is significant for obesity and hypertension.

Which of the following tests would provide the most helpful information for the diagnosis and treatment of this patient?

❑ A. Overnight polysomnography (PSG)

❑ B. Multiple Sleep Latency Test (MSLT)

❑ C. Actigraphy

❑ D. Magnetic resonance imaging of the brain

Key Concept/Objective: To understand the tests used to evaluate sleep disorders

The two most important laboratory tests for sleep disorders are the all-night PSG study and the MSLT. This patient's presentation is consistent with obstructive sleep apnea syndrome (OSAS); the best diagnostic test for OSAS is PSG, because it provides both diagnostic and therapeutic information. The all-night PSG study simultaneously records several physiologic variables by use of electroencephalography (EEG), electromyography (EMG), electrooculography (EOG), electrocardiography, airflow at the nose and mouth, respiratory effort, and oxygen saturation. Such studies are important in confirming a diagnosis of excessive daytime somnolence [illegible] hypoxemia, and sleep fragmentation. Overnight PSG determines the optimal pressure for continuous positive airway pressure (CPAP)—a treatment for OSAS—and is also helpful for supporting the diagnosis of narcolepsy and the parasomnias. Overnight PSG with simultaneous video recording can confirm rapid eye movement (REM) sleep behavior disorder and is particularly useful for the documentation of unusual movements and behavior during nighttime sleep in patients with parasomnias and nocturnal seizures. The MSLT is essential in documenting pathologic sleepiness (sleep-onset latency of less than 5 minutes) and in diagnosing narcolepsy; the presence of two sleep-onset REMs with four or five naps and pathologic sleepiness strongly suggest narcolepsy. Another important laboratory test for assessing sleep disorders is actigraphy. This technique utilizes an actigraph worn on the wrist or ankle to record acceleration or deceleration of body movements, which indirectly indicates sleep-wakefulness. Actigraphy employed for days or weeks is a useful laboratory test in patients with insomnia and circadian rhythm sleep disorders, as well as in some patients with prolonged daytime sleepiness. Actigraphy is not the test of choice for patients with suspected OSAS. Magnetic resonance imaging studies and other neuroimaging techniques should be performed to exclude structural neurologic lesions if indicated; MRI will not make a diagnosis of a sleep disorder, but it can detect lesions associated with sleep disorders. *(Answer: A—Overnight polysomnography [PSG])*

59. A 19-year-old man is being evaluated for excessive somnolence. His symptoms appeared a few months ago, when he started to experience an irresistible desire to sleep during the day; he would then sleep for 20 or 30 minutes. He also reports having vivid hallucinations when falling asleep at night. His physical examination is unremarkable.

Which of the following is likely to be found in this patient?

- ❑ **A. Delta waves that occupy more than 50% of sleep during a daytime nap**
- ❑ **B. Excess of hypocretin in the hypothalamus**
- ❑ **C. Seizure activity on electroencephalography**
- ❑ **D. Hypocretin deficiency**

Key Concept/Objective: To understand the pathophysiology of narcolepsy

This patient likely has narcolepsy. Narcolepsy is a disorder of unknown etiology. A strong association exists between narcolepsy and the presence of the DR-15 subtype of DR2 and the DQB1*0602 subtype of DQw1 haplotypes. The most exciting recent development in our understanding of narcolepsy is the documentation of an abnormality in the hypocretin neurons in the lateral hypothalamus. Human narcolepsy-cataplexy can be considered a hypocretin (orexin) deficiency syndrome. Four lines of evidence can be cited in support of hypocretin abnormality in narcolepsy: (1) induction of narcolepsy-like symptoms after mutation of the hypocretin receptor 2 gene in dogs and after preprohypocretin knockout in mice; (2) decreased hypocretin 1 levels in the cerebrospinal fluid of narcolepsy-cataplexy patients; (3) postmortem documentation of a decrease in the number of hypocretin neurons in narcoleptic brains; and (4) preprohypocretin gene mutation in a child with severe narcolepsy associated with a generalized absence of hypocretin peptides in the brain. In narcolepsy, REM sleep is seen during attacks. Delta waves that occupy more than 50% of sleep are seen in stage IV non-REM sleep. *(Answer: D—Hypocretin deficiency)*

60. A 56-year-old woman is being evaluated for insomnia of recent onset. For the past 2 months, she has been waking up at 3:00 A.M. every morning and has been having difficulty returning to sleep. She denies having difficulty falling asleep at bedtime. Review of systems is significant for poor appetite and weight loss. The physical examination is unremarkable.

Which of the following interventions is the most appropriate in the treatment of this patient?

- ❑ **A. Start a benzodiazepine at bedtime**
- ❑ **B. Establish sleep-hygiene measures**
- ❑ **C. Start a sedative-antidepressant**
- ❑ **D. Start melatonin at bedtime**

Key Concept/Objective: To understand the treatment of insomnia

Insomnia may occur at any age. The patient may complain of difficulty initiating or maintaining sleep or of awakening early in the morning and being unable to go back to sleep. Insomnia may be associated with a variety of medical, psychiatric, and neurologic illnesses or may be drug or alcohol induced. Insomnia is most commonly caused by psychiatric or psychophysiologic disorders, depression and anxiety being among the most important. Early morning awakening is a characteristic finding in depression. In some cases, no cause of the insomnia is found; this disorder is termed idiopathic, or primary, insomnia and is a lifelong condition. For transient insomnia or insomnia of short duration, treatment with sedative-hypnotics (e.g., zolpidem) or short- or intermediate-acting benzodiazepines for a few nights to a few weeks is appropriate. Hypnotic medications should not be used for chronic insomnia. The best treatment for patients with chronic insomnia consists of a combination of sleep-hygiene measures (e.g., setting fixed times for retiring and awakening; avoiding caffeinated beverages, tobacco, and alcohol before retiring; and regular exercise, preferably undertaken 4 to 6 hours before bedtime), stimulus-control therapy, sleep restriction, relaxation training, and other psychological treatments. Sedative-antidepressants should be used for insomnia associated with depression. Melatonin has been found to be useful in some persons with jet lag and shift-work sleep disorders and in patients with non–24-hour circadian rhythm disorders. *(Answer: C—Start a sedative-antidepressant)*

61. A 53-year-old man who is otherwise healthy presents with excessive daytime somnolence. The patient has been increasingly fatigued during the day for the past several years and is now experiencing an overwhelming need for a nap during the day. He typically goes to bed around 9:45 P.M. and awakens at 6:00 A.M. He does not feel refreshed upon awakening in the morning. He takes no medications and does not use alcohol. He sleeps alone and has no unusual awakenings during the night. He has been told that he snores at night. He occasionally experiences early-morning headache. His body mass index is 24. The rest of his exam is normal.

What should be the next step in the management of this patient's condition?

- ❑ A. **Referral to an ENT specialist for uvulopalatopharyngoplasty**
- ❑ B. **Therapeutic trial of modafinil**
- ❑ C. **Therapeutic trial of clonazepam**
- ❑ D. **All-night polysomnography**
- ❑ E. **Weight loss**

Key Concept/Objective: To understand the treatment approaches for a patient suspected of having obstructive sleep apnea syndrome (OSAS)

This patient has excessive daytime somnolence. This may result from decreased sleep quantity, OSAS, narcolepsy, or sleep disturbance caused by restless leg syndrome. Excessive daytime somnolence caused by OSAS is commonly associated with an airway obstruction. Respiration may be disturbed during normal sleep because of an increase in upper airway resistance. This increase occurs as a result of the loss of muscle tone in the upper airways during sleep. Ventilatory responses are also decreased during sleep. Most healthy people have brief periods of apnea. Although excessive body weight is a risk factor for OSAS, approximately 30% of patients who have OSAS have normal body weight. For the decrease in respiration to be considered pathologic, the sleep apnea or hypopnea must last for at least 10 seconds, and these episodes must occur at a rate of at least five times per hour of sleep. The diagnosis is suggested by the patient's history and is confirmed by sleep study. *(Answer: D—All-night polysomnography)*

62. A 52-year-old man presents with fatigue that has been increasing for the past 9 months. He describes an inability to stay awake during the midafternoon hours. He has symptoms of mild benign prostatic hyperplasia with 2 awakenings during the night to urinate. He is generally able to fall back asleep at those times, but he experiences early-morning awakenings with some difficulty in returning to sleep at that time. He has a history of chronic hepatitis B infection but has had no signs of cirrhosis or liver dysfunction for the past 10 years. He has a history of alcohol dependence, which has been in remission for the past 12 years. He consumes three cups of caffeinated products during the morning hours. He is an architect and professor at a community college and works long hours in his own consulting business. He describes his mood as average but has noted a decreased interest in his hobbies. His examination is unremarkable.

What should be the next step in managing this patient's fatigue?

- ❑ A. **Liver biopsy**
- ❑ B. **Michigan Alcoholism Screening Test**
- ❑ C. **An evening dose of an alpha$_1$-adrenergic blocking agent**
- ❑ D. **A trial of an antidepressant**
- ❑ E. **A trial of a benzodiazepine**

Key Concept/Objective: To understand that depression is a common cause of insomnia

There are several potential causes of this patient's insomnia. First, although the urinary symptoms he is experiencing may interfere with sustained and refreshing sleep, he relates no difficulty in returning to sleep after urinating. Second, alcohol use is known to be a contributing factor in decreasing sleep effectiveness. Although this remains a possibility in this case, the 12-year history of abstinence should be taken at face value unless other data emerge that suggest alcohol relapse. Chronic hepatitis B infection can be a factor in pro-

ducing fatigue, but more evidence of progressive disease would be needed to implicate this as a cause of his problems. Excessive caffeine use may be a contributing factor here, but caffeine typically impedes sleep initiation rather than causes early-morning awakenings. The most likely explanation for this patient's current fatigue is masked depression, in which mood disturbance is not a prominent feature but anhedonia and insomnia are. The use of benzodiazepines generally should be avoided in patients with a history of alcohol dependence. *(Answer: D—A trial of an antidepressant)*

63. A 12-year-old boy is seen for evaluation of several episodes of confusion and inappropriate behavior in the middle of the night. The patient has no symptoms during the day and is able to return to sleep after these nocturnal episodes. He is healthy, takes no medications, and is progressing well in school; family support is strong. His exam is unremarkable.

Which of the following is the most likely explanation for this patient's problem?

❑ A. **Partial arousal disorder**

❑ B. **Somnambulism**

❑ C. **Pavor nocturnus**

❑ D. **Psychological stress**

❑ E. **Drug withdrawal**

Key Concept/Objective: To understand the classification of partial arousal disorders

Partial arousal disorders include confusional arousals, sleepwalking (somnambulism), and sleep terrors (pavor nocturnus). These conditions are a subset of the parasomnias: disorders that occur during the sleep-wake transitions and during partial arousals. Parasomnias are characterized by abnormal movements or behaviors that intrude into sleep without disturbing sleep architecture. An overnight sleep study with simultaneous video recording can confirm unusual movements or behavior during nighttime sleep in patients with parasomnias. This patient has confusional arousals, which are characterized clinically by mild automatic and inappropriate behavior and confusion; they occur during slow-wave sleep. Most partial arousal disorders are benign. Sleepwalking is common in children between 5 and 12 years of age; most episodes last 10 minutes or less. There is a high probability that patients with sleepwalking have a family history of sleepwalking. Many patients with sleep terrors also have sleepwalking episodes. *(Answer: A—Partial arousal disorder)*

64. A 17-year-old woman presents to her primary care physician complaining of excessive tiredness. This has become increasingly serious for her over the past year. She has had difficulty staying awake in class. She falls asleep easily at night and generally is in bed at 10:00 P.M. and awakens at 6:30 A.M. She is an above-average student, uses no recreational drugs or alcohol, and is not sexually active. She denies having depressive symptoms. Her family history is unremarkable. Her body weight, complete blood count, and TSH level are normal.

What should be the next step in this patient's workup?

❑ A. **Multiple Sleep Latency Test**

❑ B. **Trial of antidepressants**

❑ C. **Urine drug screen**

❑ D. **Serum cortisol**

❑ E. **Assessment of serum free T_3 level**

Key Concept/Objective: To understand the presentation of narcolepsy without cataplexy

Narcoplepsy is characterized by "sleep attacks" and cataplexy. The narcoleptic attacks begin between ages 15 and 25 years, and the prevalence of this disorder is higher in patients with a family history of narcolepsy. The cause is unknown. The manifestations include an irresistible urge to fall asleep at inappropriate times; attacks last less than 30 minutes. Most patients experience cataplexy (a transient loss of muscle tone) after several

years of narcolepsy. Narcolepsy becomes less severe with age. Multiple sleep-onset latency testing can be useful in diagnosing narcolepsy (sleep-onset latency refers to time to unconsciousness after attempting sleep; normal is about 5 minutes). A finding of sleep-onset latency of less than five minutes with REM sleep occurring in two out of five nap studies supports the diagnosis of narcolepsy. *(Answer: A—Multiple Sleep Latency Test)*

65. A 52-year-old man presents with increasing fatigue of 2 years' duration. He has a history of mild hypertension without end-organ changes, which is being treated with a diuretic. He occasionally awakens with headaches. He naps during the day for about 30 minutes when he can and almost always falls asleep while watching the news after work. He uses no alcohol and does not smoke. His exam is remarkable for a body mass index of 29. His blood pressure is 142/88 mm Hg. The rest of his exam is normal. Serum electrolytes are remarkable for a potassium level of 3.5, and TSH is normal.

Which of the following is the most likely cause of this patient's fatigue?

- ❑ **A. Hypokalemia**
- ❑ **B. Deconditioning**
- ❑ **C. Medication side effect**
- ❑ **D. Sleep disturbance**
- ❑ **E. Cerebrovascular disease**

Key Concept/Objective: To understand the presenting complaints of patients with excessive daytime somnolence

Patients with excessive daytime somnolence (EDS) commonly awaken in the morning not feeling refreshed. Insufficient sleep is among the most common causes of EDS. Others include obstructive and central sleep apnea, narcolepsy, and periodic limb movements. These patients commonly have a decreased sleep-onset latency, fatigue upon awakening, and urges to sleep during the day. History-taking should be directed at sleep patterns, drug and alcohol use, and psychiatric illness. If an obvious cause of sleep disturbance is not found during the clinical exam, a sleep study can help identify such causes as obstructive sleep apnea, restless leg syndrome, and periodic limb movement in sleep. *(Answer: D—Sleep disturbance)*

For more information, see Chokroverty S: 11 Neurology: XIII Disorders of Sleep. ACP Medicine Online (www.acpmedicine.com). Dale DC, Federman DD, Eds. WebMD Inc., New York, October 2003

Pain

66. Complaints of pain are among the most common reasons for patients to visit a health care professional. New pain complaints account for close to 40 million physician visits annually in the United States.

Which of the following statements regarding pain is false?

- ❑ **A. Chronic pain, in contrast to acute pain, does not warn the patient of bodily injury and serves no useful function**
- ❑ **B. Neuropathic pain is caused by injury to the peripheral nervous system or CNS and can occur chronically without ongoing damage**
- ❑ **C. Between one third and one half of cancer patients report pain that cannot be controlled with analgesics**
- ❑ **D. Treatment of chronic pain should not be undertaken unless physical examination reveals demonstrable pathology, such as neurologic changes or signs of duress (e.g., tachycardia)**
- ❑ **E. Inquiries about psychosocial and financial factors related to pain are an important part of an initial pain evaluation**

Key Concept/Objective: To understand that chronic pain is common and to know the basic tenets of the management of chronic pain

Pain is a subjective experience, and its expression is unique to each patient. Often there is little objective evidence with which to assess the source or intensity of pain. Thus, one of the most important aspects of the patient-physician relationship regarding the treatment of chronic pain is trust: the physician is obligated to rely on the patient's self-reports of pain; to do otherwise may be unethical. Pain is a complex process that involves biologic and psychosocial factors. It can be classified as somatic (involving activation of nociceptors in cutaneous and deep musculoskeletal tissues), visceral (resulting from abnormal forces on thoracic, abdominal, and pelvic viscera), and neuropathic (resulting from injury to the peripheral nervous system or the CNS). Pain complaints are extremely common in patients with chronic disease, such as cancer and AIDS; over three fourths of such patients report pain symptoms. Unfortunately, a large percentage of patients with terminal cancer have pain that is inadequately controlled. A detailed financial and psychosocial history is of paramount importance because of the multifactorial nature of pain. *(Answer: D—Treatment of chronic pain should not be undertaken unless physical examination reveals demonstrable pathology, such as neurologic changes or signs of duress [e.g., tachycardia])*

67. A 50-year-old diabetic woman has diabetic nephropathy and neuropathy that involves her lower extremities. She complains of paresthesias and chronic lancinating pains in the feet. She has received treatment with several nonsteroidal anti-inflammatory drugs (NSAIDs), and for the past 6 months she has been taking a combination of acetaminophen and codeine. Despite this, she has persistent symptoms. Her pain has limited her ability to perform her job, which requires spending long periods of time on her feet.

Which of the following is the most appropriate option for treating this patient's chronic pain?

- ❑ A. **Substitution of oral meperidine for her current analgesic regimen**
- ❑ B. **Addition of an adjuvant analgesic such as gabapentin or a tricyclic antidepressant to her regimen**
- ❑ C. **Immediate discontinuance of opioid medication and referral to physical therapy**
- ❑ D. **The addition of high-dose ibuprofen three times daily to her current regimen**

Key Concept/Objective: To understand the use of adjuvant medications for the treatment of neuropathic pain

Neuropathic pain is common in patients with diabetic neuropathy and in those who have had shingles (postherpetic neuralgia). The pain is often described as a constant, dull ache; superimposed episodes of burning or electric shock–like sensations are common. Several studies have demonstrated the efficacy of both tricyclic antidepressants and gabapentin in the treatment of neuropathic pain related to these conditions. These medications are often used as first-line agents in the treatment of neuropathy and are also useful as adjuncts to opioids in this setting. Oral meperidine is generally not recommended for chronic use because of the potential for the buildup of toxic metabolites. Chronic narcotic medications should not be abruptly discontinued because of the potential for withdrawal symptoms. The administration of high-dose NSAIDs would not be the appropriate step to take next in the treatment of this patient with nephropathy, given their effects on renal blood flow. *(Answer: B—Addition of an adjuvant analgesic such as gabapentin or a tricyclic antidepressant to her regimen)*

68. You are caring for a 67-year-old man with widely metastatic small cell carcinoma of the lung who was diagnosed 4 months ago. He suffers from chronic pain secondary to bony metastases. His pain regimen includes sustained-release morphine, which he takes twice daily, and fast-acting morphine for breakthrough episodes of pain. Your nurse reports that the patient has called the office to request an increase in his pain medicines. He feels that they are not as effective as they were previously. His wife reports that he is afraid to take additional doses beyond what is prescribed for fear of being "hooked on them."

Which of the following is the patient experiencing with regard to his pain medications?

- ❑ A. **Addiction**
- ❑ B. **Pseudoaddiction**

❑ C. **Tolerance**

❑ D. **Substance abuse**

❑ E. **Drug resistance**

Key Concept/Objective: To understand the differences between addiction and physical dependence

This patient is experiencing the expected physiologic results of long-term opioid use: physical dependence and tolerance. Physical dependence is a state of adaptation that is manifested by specific withdrawal symptoms that occur with abrupt discontinuance of the drug. Tolerance is a physiologic state resulting from regular use of the drug. For patients experiencing tolerance, an increased dose is needed to produce the same effect as the original dose, or a reduced effect is observed with a constant dose. Addiction is a neurobehavioral syndrome influenced by genetic and environmental factors. It results in psychological dependence on the use of substances for their psychic effects. It is characterized by compulsive use despite harm and impaired control over drug use. Pseudoaddiction is a pattern of behavior in which a patient who is receiving inadequate pain medication seeks drugs for pain. This drug-seeking behavior can be mistaken for addiction. *(Answer: C—Tolerance)*

69. A 35-year-old patient comes to your office for a follow-up visit after experiencing a clavicle fracture. He has a history of cerebral palsy with moderate cognitive dysfunction and a seizure disorder. He lives in a group home. One week ago, he had a generalized tonic-clonic seizure that resulted in a fall, at which time he injured his right clavicle. His clavicle injury is being treated conservatively with a sling. His caretakers have brought him to clinic with reports that he has become more withdrawn and is eating and sleeping poorly. Although communication with the patient regarding his specific symptoms is difficult, there is concern that he may be in significant pain. Using a face pain-rating scale, you are able to elicit a complaint of pain from the patient that rates 6 on a scale of 10.

Which of the following is the most appropriate pharmacologic intervention for treatment of this patient's pain?

❑ A. **Tramadol, 50 mg p.o. every 6 hours as needed**

❑ B. **Amitriptyline, 25 mg p.o. at bedtime, with titration to 100 mg over the next 2 weeks**

❑ C. **Combination acetaminophen 300 mg/codeine 30 mg, 1 to 2 tablets every 4 to 6 hours as needed, plus a stool softener**

❑ D. **Meperidine, 50 mg I.M. in clinic, followed by 50 mg p.o. every 4 hours as needed, plus a stool softener**

❑ E. **Prednisone at an initial dosage of 60 mg a day, tapering to discontinuance over the next 2 weeks**

Key Concept/Objective: To understand which analgesic medications can lower seizure threshold

The assessment and treatment of pain in patients with cognitive impairment can be challenging. Treatment of any patient must take into account any comorbid conditions, and pharmacologic therapy must be initiated carefully, with attention given to possible adverse effects. In this patient with a known seizure disorder, a combination of acetaminophen and codeine is a safe choice for short-term treatment of pain. Tramadol, a nonnarcotic analgesic that binds to mu opiate receptors in the CNS and causes inhibition of ascending pain pathways, is contraindicated in this patient because it tends to make seizures worse. Similarly, tricyclic antidepressants and the opioid analgesic meperidine can induce seizures and thus would not be the best initial choice for this patient. Although corticosteroids are potent anti-inflammatories that are useful adjuncts in certain conditions, their use here would be unlikely to give symptomatic relief. *(Answer: C—Combination acetaminophen 300 mg/codeine 30 mg, 1 to 2 tablets every 4 to 6 hours as needed, plus a stool softener)*

For more information, see Galer B, Gammaitoni A, Alvarez NA: 11 Neurology: XIV Pain. ACP Medicine Online (www.acpmedicine.com). Dale DC, Federman DD, Eds. WebMD Inc., New York, May 2002

Parkinson Disease and Other Movement Disorders

70. A 67-year-old woman comes to your office accompanied by her family. She has a history of multiple falls, which have been increasing over the past 6 months. She says that she feels unsteady almost all the time, is frequently light-headed, and has difficulty walking. On examination, she has bradykinesia, mild cogwheeling of both upper extremities, a blood pressure drop of 25 mm Hg on standing with no change in pulse, and an ataxic gait.

Which of the following is the most likely diagnosis for this patient?

- ❑ **A. Parkinson disease**
- ❑ **B. Wilson disease**
- ❑ **C. Multiple systems atrophy**
- ❑ **D. Huntington disease**
- ❑ **E. Progressive supranuclear palsy**

Key Concept/Objective: To be able to recognize the symptoms of different parkinsonian disorders

Bradykinesia could occur in patients with Parkinson disease, multiple systems atrophy, or progressive supranuclear palsy. Parkinson disease is sometimes accompanied by autonomic insufficiency in its later stages, but this patient presents with only mild motor symptoms. The combination of parkinsonism, autonomic insufficiency, and ataxia is strongly suggestive of multiple systems atrophy. *(Answer: C—Multiple systems atrophy)*

71. A 35-year-old man is referred to your clinic for evaluation of early-onset Parkinson disease. His symptoms began approximately 2 years ago with tremor and difficulty speaking. These symptoms have progressed to the degree that he has become severely depressed and unable to work. His family history is remarkable for mental illness and alcoholism, and his maternal grandfather had cirrhosis of the liver. There is no history of Parkinson disease in his family. On examination, the patient has a mild resting tremor and uneven gait but no bradykinesia. As you speak with him, he is quite dysarthric and occasionally manifests writhing facial and neck movements. When asked if these are voluntary, he becomes angry, then tearful, and then says that God is punishing him with these movements.

Which of the following is the most appropriate step to take next in the management of this patient?

- ❑ **A. MRI of the brain**
- ❑ **B. Trial of therapy with carbidopa-levodopa**
- ❑ **C. Trial of therapy with risperidone**
- ❑ **D. Measurement of 24-hour urinary copper excretion**
- ❑ **E. Trial of therapy with sertraline**

Key Concept/Objective: To know the symptoms of Wilson disease

This young patient presents with tremor, prominent dysarthria, and facial dystonias. The latter two symptoms are atypical of Parkinson disease and should lead to consideration of other possibilities. The psychiatric symptoms of irritability, depression, and delusions of reference are suggestive of Wilson disease, for which a 24-hour urinary copper excretion test would be diagnostic. Initial therapy consists of antiabsorptive therapy followed by chelation with penicillamine. Unfortunately, neurologic symptoms often do not improve with chelation. *(Answer: D—Measurement of 24-hour urinary copper excretion)*

72. A 68-year-old man presents to your office for evaluation of tremor. He has had this problem for 3 years and it is beginning to affect his work. He has difficulty writing and has begun to notice wavering in his voice when dictating letters (now his preferred method of correspondence). He denies having any history of regular alcohol consumption but keeps a bottle of scotch in his desk because it "steadies his nerves" before important meetings. On examination, he has a relatively fast tremor of the right hand that is enhanced significantly with finger-to-nose testing. His voice has a shaky, quivering quality. His gait is normal, but his handwriting is very difficult to read because of shaking when he writes.

Which of the following medications is most likely to help this patient?

- ❑ A. **Carbidopa-levodopa**
- ❑ B. **Valproic acid**
- ❑ C. **Selegiline**
- ❑ D. **Amitriptyline**
- ❑ E. **Propranolol**

Key Concept/Objective: To be able to distinguish the clinical presentation and treatment of essential tremor from those of other movement disorders

This patient's fast tremor that increases with intention and involves his voice is most likely caused by essential tremor. Parkinson symptoms typically decrease with intention, and although it can involve facial and jaw muscles, the disease usually spares phonation. Alcohol consumption often briefly suppresses symptoms of essential tremor, and beta blockers can prove to be helpful in long-term therapy. Essential tremor does not typically respond to antiparkinsonian agents, and tricyclic antidepressants or valproate can worsen the problem. *(Answer: E—Propranolol)*

73. A 27-year-old patient of yours comes in because her 48-year-old father has been diagnosed with Huntington disease. She wants to know what this means for her risk of getting the disease.

What is the best thing to tell this patient?

- ❑ A. **She is a carrier of the gene for Huntington disease, but she is unlikely to get the disease herself unless it runs in her mother's family**
- ❑ B. **There is a 50% chance that she has inherited the gene for Huntington disease, but if she has, she is unlikely to show symptoms until she is in her 50s or 60s**
- ❑ C. **There is a 50% chance that she has inherited the gene for Huntington disease, but fewer than half of the people with the gene develop the disease, so her odds are not too bad**
- ❑ D. **There is a 50% chance that she has inherited the gene for Huntington disease; if she has, she is likely to show symptoms at a younger age than did her father**
- ❑ E. **She may have inherited the gene for Huntington disease, but it usually only manifests in men because it is on the X chromosome**

Key Concept/Objective: To understand the genetics of Huntington disease and the implications for families of affected patients

Huntington disease is an autosomal dominant disorder that manifests anticipation (i.e., a tendency toward earlier onset in subsequent generations). The genotype manifests when an area of glutamine (CAG) repeats on chromosome 4 exceeds 40 repetitions of the CAG codon. These repeats tend to increase in subsequent generations, a phenomenon that correlates with onset of the disease. It is a disease characterized by very high penetrance: almost all patients with the genotype develop Huntington disease. For this reason, genetic testing of asymptomatic family members is an ethically complex and difficult proposition. With regard to the alternative answers to this question, choice A characterizes autosomal recessive inheritance; choice B characterizes autosomal dominant inheritance with negative anticipation; choice C characterizes autosomal dominant inheritance with low penetrance; and choice E characterizes X-linked recessive inheritance. *(Answer: D—There is a 50% chance that she has inherited the gene for Huntington disease; if she has, she is likely to show symptoms at a younger age than did her father)*

For more information, see Juncos JL, DeLong MR: 11 Neurology: XV Parkinson Disease and Other Movement Disorders. ACP Medicine Online (www.acpmedicine.com). Dale DC, Federman DD, Eds. WebMD Inc., New York, April 2005

Acute Viral Central Nervous System Diseases

74. A 26-year-old elementary schoolteacher presents to the emergency department for evaluation of headache and neck stiffness. Vital signs are as follows: temperature, 100.8° F (38.2° C); heart rate, 92 mm Hg; blood pressure, 124/78 mm Hg; and respiratory rate, 14 breaths/min. On physical examination, the patient is noted to have an erythematous, maculopapular rash. The remainder of the physical examination, including neurologic examination, is unremarkable. A lumbar puncture is performed to evaluate for meningitis.

Which of the following cerebrospinal fluid findings is NOT characteristic of viral meningitis?

- ❑ **A. A protein level of 245 mg/dl**
- ❑ **B. A white blood cell (WBC) count of 80 cells/mm^3**
- ❑ **C. A glucose level of 60 mg/dl**
- ❑ **D. Clear cerebrospinal fluid (CSF)**

Key Concept/Objective: To know the typical CSF findings of viral meningitis

Careful examination of the CSF is the mainstay of diagnosis of viral meningitis or encephalitis. Characteristically, the CSF is clear and features a predominantly mononuclear pleocytosis and normal glucose content. Initially, the CSF may contain polymorphonuclear leukocytes. The CSF cell count is usually below 100 cells/mm^3; it may be higher with enteroviral infections, however, and the CSF may contain thousands of mononuclear cells after mumps and lymphocytic choriomeningitis (LCM) virus infections. The CSF protein concentration is usually normal or mildly elevated (not markedly elevated, as seen in this patient). Bacteria are not found on Gram stain, and CSF cultures are sterile. A mild depression in the CSF glucose content develops in approximately one third of patients with meningitis caused by mumps or LCM virus; this drop in CSF glucose level occurs less often after enterovirus infection. In rare instances, the CSF glucose content is depressed in patients with aseptic meningitis caused by herpes simplex virus (HSV) or varicella-zoster virus (VZV). *(Answer: A—A protein level of 245 mg/dl)*

75. A 32-year-old man presents to the emergency department with fever, headache, and neck stiffness. Lumbar puncture reveals clear CSF with a marked lymphocytic pleocytosis, a slightly elevated protein level, and a normal glucose level. Gram stain and India ink did not reveal any organisms on culture. A presumptive diagnosis of viral meningitis is made on the basis of CSF findings. On reviewing the patient's medical records, you discover that he has been evaluated for similar symptoms on multiple occasions in the past. Lumbar punctures performed at these visits have revealed CSF findings similar to those observed on this visit.

Which of the following viruses is most likely responsible for this patient's recurrent episodes of viral meningitis?

- ❑ **A. VZV**
- ❑ **B. HSV-1**
- ❑ **C. Echovirus**
- ❑ **D. HSV-2**

Key Concept/Objective: To know that HSV-2 is the primary cause of benign recurrent lymphocytic meningitis

HSV-2 aseptic meningitis is the main neurologic complication of HSV-2 infection. HSV-2 causes genital herpes. In the United States, HSV-2 is the third most common cause of aseptic meningitis, accounting for approximately 5% of all cases. Unlike viral meningitides that have a seasonal association, HSV-2 meningitis occurs at any time of year. The typical symptoms and signs are headache, fever, stiff neck, and a marked lymphocytic pleocytosis in the CSF. Meningitis may be preceded by genital or pelvic pain, and the astute clinician who suspects HSV-2 meningitis will ask about recent symptoms of pelvic inflammatory disease or associated penile or scrotal pain. The workup for suspected HSV-2 menin-

gitis should include a careful search for vesicular lesions over the external genitalia and a pelvic examination for lesions in the vagina or on the cervix. Polymerase chain reaction has revealed that the primary agent causing benign recurrent lymphocytic meningitis is HSV-2. Occasionally, HSV-1 is the culprit, as evidenced by the detection by PCR of HSV-1 DNA in the CSF of patients with benign recurrent lymphocytic meningitis. HSV-2 meningitis is self-limited; treatment with acyclovir is not required. *(Answer: D—HSV-2)*

76. A 72-year-old man presents to a primary care clinic for the evaluation of a painful rash on the right side of his face. Physical examination reveals a vesicular eruption in the maxillary distribution of the trigeminal nerve. The patient is diagnosed with zoster and treated with famciclovir.

Which of the following neurologic sequelae is most likely to develop in this patient in the weeks or months following this episode?

- ❑ **A. Ramsay Hunt syndrome**
- ❑ **B. Viral meningitis**
- ❑ **C. Left-sided hemiparesis**
- ❑ **D. Viral encephalitis**

Key Concept/Objective: To understand the CNS sequelae of zoster infection and to recognize that unifocal VZV vasculopathy presents with focal neurologic findings

The salient feature of VZV unifocal vasculopathy is an acute focal deficit that develops weeks or months after the development of herpes zoster in a contralateral pattern of trigeminal distribution. Stroke results from a necrotizing arteritis, primarily of large cerebral arteries. One comprehensive review showed that most patients with large vessel vasculopathy were older than 60 years and that there was no sex bias. The mean onset of neurologic disease was 7 weeks, and the longest interval between the onset of herpes zoster and the onset of neurologic disease was 6 months. Transient ischemic attacks and mental symptoms were common. Twenty-five percent of patients died. The majority of patients had CSF pleocytosis, usually fewer than 100 cells/mm^3 (predominantly mononuclear), oligoclonal bands, and increased CSF IgG. Besides contralateral hemiplegia, ipsilateral central retinal artery occlusion and posterior circulation involvement have been described. There is no definitive treatment for large vessel herpes zoster vasculopathy. Nevertheless, because productive virus infection is found in arteries, patients should receive intravenous acyclovir (to kill persistent replicating virus) and steroids (for their anti-inflammatory effect). Overall, the neurologic features of VZV vasculopathy are protean. Neurologic disease often occurs months after zoster and sometimes in patients who have no history of zoster rash. Magnetic resonance imaging, cerebral angiography, and examination of CSF with virologic analysis are needed to confirm the diagnosis. When VZV vasculopathy develops months after zoster, antiviral treatment is often effective. *(Answer: C—Left-sided hemiparesis)*

77. A 62-year-old woman presents to the emergency department for the evaluation of a seizure. The patient is lethargic and confused. Her husband reports she has epilepsy and that she has been complaining of headache for the past 3 days. He also states that the patient has been somewhat confused. On physical examination, the patient is noted to have a low-grade fever. The remainder of her vital signs are stable, and her examination is otherwise unrevealing. A head CT scan reveals a hypodense lesion in the right medial temporal region. A lumbar puncture is performed, revealing an elevated opening pressure, mononuclear pleocytosis, and moderate red blood cells (RBCs).

Which of the following viruses is most likely responsible for this patient's clinical picture?

- ❑ **A. VZV**
- ❑ **B. HSV-1**
- ❑ **C. Cytomegalovirus (CMV)**
- ❑ **D. HSV-2**

Key Concept/Objective: To know the characteristic clinical features of HSV-1 encephalitis

Unlike most viral encephalitides, HSV-1 encephalitis is focal. HSV replication in the medial temporal lobe and orbital surface of the frontal lobe, with accompanying inflammation, produces the characteristic clinical picture. Fever, headache, lethargy, irritability, and confusion are typical symptoms. Seizures (major motor, complex partial, focal, and even absence attacks) affect approximately 40% of patients. If the dominant temporal lobe is involved, aphasia and focal motor or sensory deficits develop. The CSF is usually abnormal in HSV encephalitis. The CSF opening pressure is often elevated and may be very high if there is brain swelling and impending temporal lobe herniation. Clinicians usually perform the CSF examination in the first few days of illness, before there is significant brain swelling, to decrease the potential for herniation after lumbar puncture. The electroencephalogram (EEG) and imaging studies may demonstrate features highly suggestive of HSV encephalitis, often obviating the need for subsequent lumbar punctures. CSF pleocytosis is observed in more than 90% of patients, although its absence at initial evaluation does not rule out HSV encephalitis. The CSF cell count ranges from 4 to 755 cells/mm^3, and more than 200 cells/mm^3 may be present weeks after the onset of disease. The predominant cell type is mononuclear. Although RBCs are unusual in other viral encephalitides, in HSV encephalitis they are often present in the CSF, which may also be xanthochromic; this presumably reflects the hemorrhagic nature of brain lesions. Instead of attributing the presence of RBCs in CSF to a so-called traumatic tap, the astute clinician may use this finding to support the presumptive diagnosis of HSV encephalitis. The majority of patients with HSV encephalitis have elevated CSF protein and IgG indexes. In rare instances, hypoglycorrhachia occurs. Increased levels of antibody to HSV, suggestive of recent infection, may be found in serum and CSF; increased anti-HSV antibody ratios of CSF and serum may help in making the diagnosis of HSV encephalitis. Unfortunately, increased antibody titers are not usually detected until 2 weeks or longer after the onset of disease; thus, their practical value lies more in retrospective presumptive diagnosis than in identifying acute encephalitis. PCR detection of HSV-1 DNA in the CSF is both sensitive and specific and has become the gold standard in suspected cases of HSV encephalitis. Nonetheless, clinicians should be aware that PCR may be negative for HSV in the first few days of illness with HSV encephalitis. *(Answer: B—HSV-1)*

For more information, see Gilden DH: 11 Neurology: XVI Acute Viral Central Nervous System Diseases. ACP Medicine Online (www.acpmedicine.com). Dale DC, Federman DD, Eds. WebMD Inc., New York, March 2003

Central Nervous System Diseases Due to Slow Viruses and Prions

78. A 34-year-old man was found to be HIV seropositive 4 years ago. He refused antiretroviral therapy. He began having headaches and low-grade fevers 1 month ago. Previously, his friends noted no change in his functioning, personality, or thinking, but now, he is becoming progressively more confused and has difficulty caring for himself. On examination, the patient's temperature is 100° F (37.8° C). He is sleepy but arouses easily. He has no nuchal rigidity. A mental status examination shows diminished cognitive ability. There are no focal motor or sensory findings. A magnetic resonance imaging study shows global cortical atrophy, no ventricular enlargement, and no focal lesions.

What is the most likely diagnosis in this case?

- ❑ A. **Toxoplasmosis**
- ❑ B. **Progressive multifocal leukoencephalopathy (PML)**
- ❑ C. **Central nervous system lymphoma**
- ❑ D. **HIV dementia complex**
- ❑ E. **Cryptococcal meningitis**

Key Concept/Objective: To understand that because multiple CNS diseases can occur with HIV infection, HIV dementia remains a diagnosis of exclusion

Toxoplasmosis presents with fever, headache, focal exam findings, and multiple ring-enhancing brain lesions on imaging studies. PML presents with focal deficits on exam

without alteration in consciousness and with multiple white matter lesions on T_2-weighted MRI images. CNS lymphoma presents with focal neurologic deficits, headache, and one to a few focal brain lesions on radiographic studies. HIV dementia is associated with a slower progression of personality changes, dementia, and unsteady gait. Cortical atrophy and ventricular enlargement are commonly seen on MRI, but the findings are not diagnostic. Atrophy can be seen in patients with AIDS who otherwise would exhibit only subtle findings on formal psychological testing. Cryptococcal meningitis is an opportunistic infection presenting with fever, headache with or without nuchal rigidity, and confusion. *(Answer: E—Cryptococcal meningitis)*

79. A 42-year-old woman from Florida prevents for evaluation. Four years ago, she developed leg numbness, constipation, and urinary incontinence developed, and she became wheelchair-bound 12 months ago. Skin examination reveals scattered red-brown maculopapular lesions. Neurologic examination reveals decreased pinprick sensation at the thoracic level, paraplegia, increased leg muscle tone, brisk leg reflexes, and Babinski signs. Serologic tests for Lyme disease, syphilis, and HIV are negative. Skin biopsy reveals lymphoid infiltrates within the epidermis. MRI reveals areas of T_2-weighted increased signal intensity and atrophy in the thoracic spinal cord.

What is the most likely diagnosis for this patient?

❑ **A. HIV vacuolar myelopathy**

❑ **B. Poliomyelitis**

❑ **C. Human T cell lymphotropic virus type I (HTLV-I)–associated myelopathy (HAM)**

❑ **D. Multiple sclerosis**

❑ **E. PML**

Key Concept/Objective: To understand the need to consider a retroviral cause for a myelopathy that can mimic multiple sclerosis

PML is a disease of brain white matter presenting with motor and vision findings and eventual dementia. HIV involvement of the cord does occur, but this patient has no serologic evidence for HIV infection. Poliomyelitis involves the anterior horn cells of the cord, causing a flaccid paralysis with absent reflexes rather than spastic paraparesis. Radiologic findings can be similar in HAM and multiple sclerosis. Both diseases can cause elevated IgG and oligoclonal bands in the CSF. Although HAM is reported mainly in Japan, the Caribbean region, and Central America, it does occur in the southeastern United States. HTLV-I can also cause a T cell lymphoma/leukemia, and although it is rare to have the neurologic and hematopoietic complications occur at the same time, this patient's skin biopsy is characteristic of a cutaneous lymphoma. Serology testing should be done to confirm HTLV-I infection. *(Answer: C—Human T cell lymphotropic virus type I (HTLV-I)–associated myelopathy [HAM])*

80. A 54-year-old beef farmer was visiting this country on an extended visit. For a period of 2 months he experienced difficulty reading, and his relatives took him to the hospital for evaluation. On examination, the patient was agitated; he had memory impairment, and a left homonymous defect was noted on visual-field testing. He was admitted to the hospital, and 1 week later he developed ataxia and myoclonic jerks of the hands. CT scan and MRI were negative. An EEG showed triphasic wave forms. One month later, he was barely responsive, with severe generalized myoclonic jerks, and he died shortly afterward. A review of patient history revealed that five years ago, two animals in his beef herd developed mad cow disease. There is no family history of a similar neurologic disorder. He underwent no surgeries or blood transfusions.

This patient most likely had which form of transmittable spongiform encephalopathy?

❑ **A. Kuru**

❑ **B. Sporadic Creutzfeldt-Jakob disease (CJD)**

❑ **C. Gerstmann-Strussler-Scheinker disease (GSS)**

❑ D. Scrapie

❑ E. Variant Creutzfeldt-Jakob disease (vCJD)

Key Concept/Objective: To be familiar with the characteristics of the variety of transmittable spongiform encephalopathies

Kuru previously was the disease associated with cannibalism in New Guinea but no longer occurs. Scrapie is the spongiform encephalopathy that occurs in sheep. GSS is a human spongiform encephalopathy, transmitted as an autosomal dominant trait, that presents with ataxia followed by dementia. Variant CJD is believed to be the accidental transmission to humans of the agent of bovine spongiform encephalopathy (mad cow disease). It differs from CJD in that it occurs in younger patients. Patients present with psychiatric disturbances; dementia develops much later. Patients with CJD lack characteristic EEG findings and have a longer survival time. This patient had classic findings of CJD: visual changes, dementia, ataxia, myoclonic jerks, a characteristic EEG study, and rapid progression to death. It was the sporadic rather than the genetic or iatrogenic form. *(Answer: B—Sporadic Creutzfeldt-Jakob disease [CJD])*

81. ***What is the pathogenetic mechanism for the disease of the patient in Question 80?***

❑ A. Secretion of neurotoxins from microglia chronically infected with a retrovirus

❑ B. Oligodendroglial cytolysis caused by a papovavirus

❑ C. CD8+ T cell attack on neuroglial cells minimally infected with a retrovirus

❑ D. Misfolding of a protease-resistant protein causing plaques in the brain

❑ E. Mutation in the matrix protein of a virus causing viral persistence

Key Concept/Objective: To be familiar with theories of pathogenesis for CNS diseases caused by slow viruses and similar agents

Spongiform encephalopathies are caused by prions: proteins that, when abnormal, precipitate as crystals, yielding plaques and spongiform degeneration. HIV dementia is thought to be caused by injury to neurons by toxins secreted from HIV-infected microglia. HTLV-I–associated myelopathy is thought to be the result of autoimmune attack by CD8+ T cells on HTLV-I–infected glial cells. Lysis of cells that produce myelin (oligodendrocytes) by reactivated JC virus, a papovavirus, is the cause of progressive multifocal leukoencephalopathy. Subacute sclerosing panencephalitis (SSPE) is a late CNS disease caused by the measles virus containing mutated protein, perhaps accounting for viral persistence in the presence of an appropriate host-humoral response. *(Answer: D—Misfolding of a protease-resistant protein causing plaques in the brain)*

82. An HIV-seropositive 36-year-old woman presents with progressive right-sided weakness and right inferior quadrantanopia. MRI reveals hypointense T_1-weighted lesions without gadolinium enhancement and with hyperintense T_2-weighted lesions involving the left frontoparietal and occipital white matter. Biopsy shows areas of demyelination, large atypical astrocytes with bizarre nuclei, and oligodendrocytes with enlarged nuclei, some with displacement of the chromatin by an intranuclear basophilic process.

What is the most appropriate therapy for this patient at this time?

❑ A. Ethambutol, rifabutin, and clarithromycin

❑ B. Aggressive therapy for HIV

❑ C. Pyrimethamine and sulfadiazine

❑ D. Cytarabine

❑ E. Radiation therapy

Key Concept/Objective: To understand the findings of progressive multifocal leukoencephalopathy (PML) and current thought regarding its therapy

This patient has a classic presentation and studies for PML. On MRI, the lack of contrast enhancement is typical for PML, as distinct from toxoplasmosis, lymphoma, or astrocytoma. Bizarre cells are seen on biopsy but do not indicate the presence of a malignancy. The intranuclear inclusions in the oligodendrocytes are typical for PML. There are no proven therapies of benefit in managing PML, although it is believed that partial reversal of the immunodeficient state may be responsible for transient improvement. Cytarabine, a cancer drug, was thought to be of benefit in isolated case reports, but controlled studies in AIDS patients have not borne this out. The patient does not have toxoplasmosis requiring pyrimethamine and sulfadiazine, nor does she have *Mycobacterium avium* complex infection requiring ethambutol, rifabutin, and clarithromycin or CNS malignancy requiring radiation. *(Answer: B—Aggressive therapy for HIV)*

83. A 62-year-old man weighing 70 kg presents with a 2-day history of fever, headache, increasing confusion, and a single generalized seizure. On examination, he has a temperature of 102° F (38.9° C), is drowsy and confused, has no nuchal rigidity, and has an upgoing right plantar reflex. CT scan is normal, but a T_2-weighted MRI scan shows increased signal intensity in the left temporal lobe. Peripheral WBC is normal, as are the serum electrolytes. Lumbar puncture reveals an opening pressure of 250 mm H_2O; clear cerebrospinal fluid with protein 100 mg/dl; glucose, 70 mg/dl, with simultaneous blood glucose 120 mg/dl; 40 WBC/mm^3, predominantly mononuclear; and 850 RBC/mm^3. Gram stain of the fluid shows no organisms.

Which of the following test is likely to be most helpful in confirming your clinical diagnosis at this point?

- ❑ A. **CSF for viral tissue culture**
- ❑ B. **CSF for polymerase chain reaction (PCR) detection of viral DNA**
- ❑ C. **CSF for viral antibody detection**
- ❑ D. **EEG**
- ❑ E. **Brain biopsy for pathology and viral tissue culture**

Key Concept/Objective: To understand the tests to confirm the diagnosis of HSV-1 encephalitis

A rapid neurologic deterioration, seizure, fevers, focal examination and radiographic findings, and mononuclear CSF pleocytosis with increased RBCs are enough for a clinical diagnosis of HSV encephalitis. PCR detection of HSV-1 DNA in the CSF has become the gold standard to confirm suspected cases of HSV encephalitis. Although CSF viral cultures are performed, they have a very low yield. CSF viral antibody levels can be detected after 2 or more weeks of illness. EEG findings usually show generalized slowing early and may later develop more characteristic periodic sharp-wave and slow-wave complexes. With focal temporal lobe involvement on MRI, an EEG in this case would add little. Brain biopsy for culture and pathology was the previously recommended confirmatory test. It is not as sensitive as the PCR studies and carries greater risks. *(Answer: B—CSF for polymerase chain reaction [PCR] detection of viral DNA)*

84. ***Which of the following treatment regimens would you now begin for the patient in Question 83?***

- ❑ A. **Acyclovir, 700 mg I.V., q. 8 hr, and maintenance I.V. fluids at a rate of 150 ml/hr**
- ❑ B. **Acyclovir, 700 mg I.V., q. 8 hr, maintenance I.V. fluids at 150 ml/hr, and phenytoin**
- ❑ C. **Acyclovir, 700 mg I.V., q. 8 hr, and maintenance I.V. fluids at 50 ml/hr**
- ❑ D. **Acyclovir, 700 mg I.V., q. 8 hr, maintenance I.V. fluids at 50 ml/hr, and phenytoin**
- ❑ E. **Ganciclovir, 350 mg I.V., q. 12 hr, and maintenance I.V. fluids at 150 ml/hr**

Key Concept/Objective: To understand the treatment of HSV encephalitis

The earlier the initiation of antiviral therapy in HSV encephalitis, the better is the outcome. Treatment should not be withheld pending confirmatory results of diagnostic testing. The drug to use is acyclovir, 10 mg/kg I.V., every 8 hours, for at least 10 days. Ganciclovir is the drug to use if the patient has CMV encephalitis. Because the patient has already had a generalized seizure, he should be started on anticonvulsants, which should be continued for at least several months after the acute illness, should the patient survive. There are no controlled studies to support the use of prophylactic anticonvulsants, had the patient not had seizures. Cerebral edema is a significant concern in patients with HSV encephalitis. Fluids should be reduced to approximately 50% of usual maintenance levels. *(Answer: D—Acyclovir, 700 mg I.V., q. 8 hr, maintenance I.V. fluids at 50 ml/hr, and phenytoin)*

85. A 15-year-old boy lives adjacent to a swampy region of Florida. He presents with worsening stupor after 3 days of fevers, headache, nausea, and vomiting. On examination, the patient has a temperature of 101° F (38.3° C). He is disoriented with marked lethargy. There is no nuchal rigidity and no focal neurologic findings. Initial laboratory studies show a leukocytosis of 14,500 cells/mm³ and mild hyponatremia. Results of CSF analysis are as follows: 370 WBC/mm³, with 70% neutrophils; protein, 95 mg/dl; glucose, 68 mg/dl, with simultaneous serum glucose, 110 mg/dl. T_2-weighted MRI images reveal increased signal intensity in the basal ganglia and thalami.

Which of the following statements regarding this patient's disease is true?

- ❑ **A. The disease spreads primarily via the fecal-oral route**
- ❑ **B. Neutrophilic CSF pleocytosis is distinctly unusual early in the course of this disease**
- ❑ **C. Using sentinel chickens to detect viral infection is important in controlling outbreaks**
- ❑ **E. The mortality from this disease is less than 20%**
- ❑ **E. The disease is caused by an arenavirus**

Key Concept/Objective: To be familiar with the presentation of an arboviral encephalitis and the means to detect the mosquito vectors

Rapid alteration in mental status associated with fevers should raise suspicion for viral encephalitis. Of the various types of viral encephalitides, Eastern equine encephalitis (EEE), in a recent review, was found to have distinctive basal ganglion and thalamus involvement on MRI scan. It is one of the arboviral (arthropod-borne) encephalitides and is spread by mosquito bite rather than a fecal-oral route. Neutrophilic CSF pleocytosis would not be unusual early in the course of any acute viral CNS infection and is common in EEE. The mortality is 35% to 50%. Control of outbreaks comes from monitoring and controlling the mosquito vectors. Presence of the virus in swampy habitats can be detected by recovering virus from mosquitoes or by measuring serum antibodies in wild passerine birds or caged sentinel birds (chickens). EEE is caused by an alphavirus. The arenaviruses are endemic in rodents, with lymphocytic choriomeningitis virus being most common in the United States. *(Answer: C—Using sentinel chickens to detect viral infection is important in controlling outbreaks)*

86. A 59-year-old woman from Missouri has a 20-year history of systemic lupus erythematosus, for which she is taking corticosteroids. One day before admission, the patient started taking ibuprofen for a flare in arthralgias. The next day, she was found obtunded and confused. She has a temperature of 100.2° F (37.9° C); she can be aroused but she cannot follow simple commands. The rest of the examination is normal. Chest x-ray, complete blood count, and urinalysis are normal. CSF analysis shows 400 WBC/mm³, with 51% monocytes, normal glucose, slightly elevated protein, and negative Gram stain for bacteria. Without therapy, she becomes fully alert and afebrile within 24 hours. At this point, she relates that she had two identical episodes within the past 5 years, each after ibuprofen use.

What is the most likely diagnosis for this patient?

- ❑ **A. Recurrent enteroviral aseptic meningitis**
- ❑ **B. Systemic lupus erythematosus cerebritis**

- ❑ C. **Recurrent herpes simplex aseptic meningitis**
- ❑ D. **Ibuprofen hypersensitivity**
- ❑ E. **St. Louis encephalitis**

Key Concept/Objective: To be aware that both infectious and noninfectious processes can present as an aseptic meningitis or meningoencephalitis syndrome

The patient has evidence of CNS inflammation with a mononuclear CSF pleocytosis. Enteroviruses commonly cause acute viral meningitis, but recurrent acute infections would be very unlikely. St. Louis encephalitis—the other "SLE"—is an arboviral encephalitis that would neither resolve clinically within 24 hours nor recur. Mollaret recurrent meningitis might have a herpesvirus origin, but there is a more likely explanation in this patient. Cerebritis can be part of active systemic lupus erythematosus, but rapid resolution and no other manifestations of active disease argue against the diagnosis. Nonsteroidal anti-inflammatory drugs can cause a meningoencephalitis, especially in patients with underlying collagen vascular diseases. Three identical episodes occurring immediately after the use of ibuprofen, with rapid improvement after its removal, argue for this diagnosis. *(Answer: D—Ibuprofen hypersensitivity)*

87. Eight weeks ago, a 26-year-old woman with Hodgkin disease developed a zosteriform eruption of the left periorbital and left forehead regions. The skin lesions resolved, and apart from episodic neuralgic pains, the patient was doing well until today, when she experienced the sudden development of right hemiplegia. On examination, the patient is awake, afebrile, and aphasic; residual small scabs are noted on the left side of the face, and she has a dense right hemiplegia.

For this patient, which of the following diagnostic test results is most likely?

- ❑ A. **Increased left frontal and temporal lobe intensity on T_2-weighted MRI scan images**
- ❑ B. **Isolation of CMV from the buffy coat of the blood**
- ❑ C. **Bilateral large and small ischemic infarcts of the white and gray matter on CT scan**
- ❑ D. **Mononuclear pleocytosis and presence of HSV-1 antibody in the CSF**
- ❑ E. **Beading of the left middle cerebral artery on angiography**

Key Concept/Objective: To understand that a vasculopathy (granulomatous arteritis) can occur as a late complication of localized varicella-zoster infection

This patient has just developed a sudden, severe contralateral hemiplegia in relation to the site of the recent localized varicella-zoster ophthalmicus. It is caused by a vasculopathy or granulomatous arteritis, which can occur weeks to months after a local infection. The presentation is that of a stroke in the left middle cerebral artery distribution. Radiographic scans would show a middle cerebral artery distribution defect rather than the bilateral ischemic white and gray matter infarcts characteristic of herpes zoster encephalitis. Angiography would show segmental changes involving the large arteries, described as beading. Left temporal and frontal lobe involvement on MRI is seen with herpes simplex encephalitis. CMV in the buffy coat indicates active cytomegalovirus in the blood and would not explain the neurologic complication of post–varicella-zoster infection. Mononuclear pleocytosis is likely to be present but not HSV-1 antibody, which is the antibody found in herpes simplex encephalitis. *(Answer: E—Beading of the left middle cerebral artery on angiography)*

88. A 38-year-old man with AIDS who has been followed in clinic for 5 years is brought in by his partner/caregiver, who has concerns that the patient is showing signs of forgetfulness, inability to concentrate, and loss of ability to perform tasks requiring higher function, such as paying bills and making phone calls. The partner states that he first noticed changes in the patient about a year ago, but the cognitive decline has become more noticeable in the past few months. He has also noticed that the patient has developed a slight tremor and mild unsteadiness of gait. Examination reveals a thin man with oral thrush who has psychomotor slowing and appears apathetic. On neurologic examination, there is a slight intention tremor and difficulty with rapid, alternating movements; other symptoms are nonfocal, and the muscle tone is normal. On the Mini-Mental State Examination, the patient scores 22 out of 30 (when the patient took this examination on his initial visit to the clinic 5 years ago, he scored 29 out of 30). A lumbar puncture is performed; the opening pressure is 11 cm H_2O, and the cerebrospinal fluid is normal except for a mildly elevated protein level. Gram stain and India ink smear are negative. Magnetic resonance imaging of the brain shows only cerebral atrophy.

Which of the following is the most likely diagnosis for this patient?

- ❑ **A. Toxoplasmosis**
- ❑ **B. HIV dementia**
- ❑ **C. Cryptococcal meningitis**
- ❑ **D. Alzheimer dementia**
- ❑ **E. Parkinson disease**

Key Concept/Objective: To be able to recognize the clinical features of HIV dementia

This patient most likely has HIV dementia (HIVD, also called AIDS dementia complex), a disorder of the central nervous system caused by a primary effect of the HIV virus. Before the development of highly active antiretroviral therapy (HAART), HIVD developed in up to 30% of HIV-infected patients. The pathogenesis is not completely understood but is thought to result from the effects of neurotoxins secreted from chronically infected microglia. HIVD generally occurs in the later stages of HIV infection and can present initially as mild cognitive impairment. Presentation is consistent with a subcortical dementia: in addition to loss of memory and language function, patients may demonstrate generalized psychomotor slowing, apathy, ataxia, and even paralysis. The diagnosis depends on the exclusion of other reversible causes of dementia and altered mental status in the patient with AIDS. In this patient, MRI did not reveal ring-enhancing lesions, which would have suggested toxoplasmosis. A normal opening pressure and negative India ink smear, although not completely ruling out cryptococcal meningitis, would certainly make it less likely. The subcortical features in this patient would not be typical of Alzheimer dementia, and the absence of rigidity makes Parkinson disease less likely than HIVD. HAART may improve HIVD. *(Answer: B—HIV dementia)*

89. A 60-year-old woman is admitted to the hospital from the emergency department because the family is no longer able to care for her at home. The patient has diet-controlled diabetes and had been doing well, but the family now describes mental deterioration, which has been progressing over the past 3 to 4 months. The patient first demonstrated forgetfulness and subsequently developed sleep difficulties, mood swings, and progressively poorer judgment and loss of short-term memory. The family has been struck by the rapidity of the changes in the patient in the past month. At the time of admission, the patient is awake but minimally responsive and has completely lost the ability to perform basic activities of daily living. Examination is significant for frequent myoclonic jerks, which are especially prominent when the patient is startled. She is unable to follow commands, but strength and sensation appear intact. She is markedly ataxic and ambulates only with assistance. The results of CT of the head are normal, as are the results of lumbar puncture.

Which of the following statements regarding the likely diagnosis in this patient is false?

- ❑ **A. The disease is uniformly progressive and fatal**
- ❑ **B. Detection of the abnormal 14-3-3 protein in the CSF can help support what is often a difficult diagnosis**
- ❑ **C. T_2-weighted MRI of the brain may show hyperintensity in the basal ganglia and thalamus**
- ❑ **D. In the past, use of cadaveric dural grafts and human pituitary hormones was associated with iatrogenic cases of the disease**
- ❑ **E. The majority of cases are either inherited or transfusion-associated**

Key Concept/Objective: To understand the clinical features of Creutzfeldt-Jakob Disease (CJD)

This patient has several of the hallmarks of CJD, a rare, transmissible spongiform encephalopathy thought to be caused by the accumulation of an abnormal form of an endogenous protein (prion) in the CNS. There are several recognized forms, including sporadic (which make up the majority of cases), familial, iatrogenic, and variant forms. CJD is uniformly fatal. The most striking finding is a progressive dementia that occurs over weeks to months (as compared to Alzheimer dementia, which progresses over years). Myoclonic jerking, especially with startle, is an important physical finding: its presence in association with dementia of unclear etiology should strongly suggest the possibility of CJD. Other clinical findings may include signs of pyramidal tract involvement, muscle atrophy, cerebellar ataxia, and seizures. There is no gold standard test for diagnosis, but typical findings on MRI of hyperintensity of the basal ganglia and the presence of the abnormal 14-3-3 protein in CSF can support the diagnosis. Diagnostic criteria have been proposed; these include, in addition to the clinical features described, the finding of typical loss of neurons, gliosis, or spongiform degeneration in histopathologic specimens of brain tissue, as well as the demonstration of transmission of neurodegenerative disease from brain specimens to animals. Although cannibalism and the use of cadaveric human tissues such as dural grafts and pituitary hormones pose a risk of spreading the disease, there has been no definitive evidence of spread of prion disease through blood products. *(Answer: E—The majority of cases are either inherited or transfusion-associated)*

90. A 29-year-old Hispanic woman with HIV presents to the emergency department with gait difficulties and visual disturbances; these symptoms have persisted for several weeks. Her medical history includes previous episodes of oral thrush and *Pneumocystis carinii* pneumonia, and she is not currently receiving antiretroviral therapy because of problems with compliance. Recently, the patient was found to have a $CD4^+$ T cell count of 75 cells/mm^3. On examination, the patient has an appreciable visual-field defect (left homonymous quadrantic defect) and an ataxic gait. After admission to the hospital, an MRI of the brain is performed; this MRI reveals multiple coalescent areas of demyelination in the subcortical white matter of the left occipital lobe and the cerebellum. Results of CSF examination are normal, and toxoplasmosis titers are normal. You suspect that the patient may have progressive PML.

Which of the following statements regarding PML is false?

- ❑ A. **PCR analysis of CSF for the presence of JC virus material has been used to confirm the diagnosis**
- ❑ B. **HAART may result in improvement and remission of PML**
- ❑ C. **PML is most often a manifestation of early HIV disease**
- ❑ D. **PML is an opportunistic infection involving reactivation of latent JC virus in the CNS**

Key Concept/Objective: To understand the manifestations and diagnosis of PML

PML is a disease of white matter seen primarily in immunosuppressed patients; it characteristically follows a protracted course. PML is associated with multifocal neurologic defects, which may include motor deterioration, loss of vision, incontinence, aphasia, and sensory defects. Mental-status changes may or may not be present. The disease is caused by reactivation of latent human papillomavirus JC in the CNS and is thus an opportunistic infection. The disease is typically a late manifestation of HIV disease; it occurs in 1% to 5% of HIV-infected persons. The diagnosis should be considered in any person with immunodeficiency who presents with a subacute, progressive illness involving motor function and cognition. Other considerations in the differential diagnosis for this patient include toxoplasmosis infection, CNS lymphoma, and other CNS infections, such as tuberculosis and neurocysticercosis. MRI findings of multiple, nonenhancing white matter lesions that tend to coalesce are typical. These lesions have a predilection for the occipital and parietal lobes. The definitive diagnosis has previously been established only by brain biopsy, but PCR techniques for the detection of JC virus DNA material in the CSF have been used with increasing success (the reported sensitivity and specificity of these techniques are greater than 90%). Improved outcomes in AIDS patients with PML have been reported with the use of HAART. *(Answer: C—PML is most often a manifestation of early HIV disease)*

91. A woman comes to your clinic with concerns about mad cow disease (bovine spongiform encephalopathy [BSE]). She has heard media reports of infected cattle in other countries and of the possible risk of a similar disease spreading to people. She wants to know if it is safe for her and her children to consume beef and dairy products in the United States.

Which of the following statements about new-variant Creutzfeldt-Jakob disease (nvCJD) is false?

❑ **A. Compared to CJD, nvCJD typically develops in younger adults**

❑ **B. The agent of disease is thought to be a protein, or prion, which is spread by the consumption of animal protein products**

❑ **C. There have been documented cases in the United States**

❑ **D. There is currently minimal risk of acquiring the disease from consumption of milk or beef in the United States**

Key Concept/Objective: To understand the epidemiology of BSE and its association with nvCJD

BSE is a spongiform encephalopathy that has occurred primarily in the United Kingdom and is associated with the consumption (by cows) of protein supplements derived from ruminant tissue. There have been substantial efforts to reduce the incidence of BSE by banning the feeding of such ruminant-derived tissue to cattle and by the disposal of potentially infected herds. There is evidence that nvCJD may represent bovine-to-human spread of BSE in the United Kingdom. nvCJD typically affects younger adults (mean age at onset, 29 years), causing the typical rapidly progressive cognitive decline seen with CJD. Unlike the sporadic or familial forms of CJD, patients with nvCJD have shown prominent sensory disturbances and psychiatric symptoms. Current epidemiologic evidence suggests that the United Kingdom epidemic will be less widespread than initially thought. There have been no documented cases of BSE or nvCJD in the United States. Thus, the patient can be reassured that dairy products and beef are in general safe to consume. *(Answer: C—There have been documented cases in the United States)*

92. During a regular office visit, a clinic patient raises concerns about her 12-year-old son's receiving a booster dose of the mumps-measles-rubella (MMR) vaccine. She read on the Internet about a variant form of measles that can result in an incurable degenerative neurologic disease. She is strongly considering not allowing him to receive the booster, and she wants your opinion. You inform her that the disease she is describing, subacute sclerosing panencephalitis (SSPE), is a rare condition that develops years after exposure to measles.

Which of the following statements would you include in your discussion with this patient?

❑ **A. SSPE is no longer a concern because the MMR vaccine that is currently used is a killed-virus vaccine, not a live-virus vaccine**

❑ **B. You agree that she should not allow her son to complete his MMR series because the risk of developing SSPE is greater than the threat of measles or mumps**

❑ **C. The rate of development of SSPE is 10 times less after vaccination than after having measles infection**

❑ **D. SSPE typically develops 7 to 10 years after measles and occurs in about 1 in 500 people infected with measles**

Key Concept/Objective: To be able to recognize SSPE, a rare but deadly complication of measles infection

SSPE is a rare sequela of measles infection, occurring in approximately 1 in 100,000 persons infected with measles virus. The disease is characterized by CNS deterioration, which progresses from personality changes and lethargy to myoclonus, dementia, decorticate rigidity, and death. The typical patient with SSPE is younger than 20 years and develops the disease 7 to 10 years after infection with measles. The risk of developing SSPE is at least ten times less after vaccination with live virus than it is after contracting wild-type measles infection. The MMR vaccine is a live-virus vaccine, but given the very small risk of serious

sequelae compared to the risk of the adverse effects of actual measles or mumps infection, completion of the immunization series should be advised. *(Answer: C—The rate of development of SSPE is 10 times less after vaccination than after having measles infection)*

For more information, see González-Scarano F: 11 Neurology: XVII Central Nervous System Diseases Due to Slow Viruses and Prions. ACP Medicine Online (www.acpmedicine.com). Dale DC, Federman DD, Eds. WebMD Inc., New York, June 2002

SECTION 12

ONCOLOGY

Cancer Epidemiology and Prevention

1. A 25-year-old white woman presents to your clinic for a routine examination. She is feeling well, but she is unhappy about the fact that she has gained 10 lb since graduating from college. She attributes the weight gain to her new investment banking job. Her job is highly stressful, and she reports that her company's office culture revolves around "happy hour." She denies using tobacco, but she frequents smoky bars. On physical examination, the patient appears well nourished; her body mass index is 25. The examination is otherwise unremarkable.

Which of the following statements regarding primary cancer prevention is true?

❑ A. **In nonsmokers, long-term passive exposure to tobacco smoke is associated with a significantly increased risk of lung cancer**

❑ B. **A diet that includes antioxidant supplements, such as β-carotene, reduces the risk of lung cancer**

❑ C. **Stress reduction has been proved to decrease the incidence of gastric cancer associated with gastric ulcers**

❑ D. **Annual Papanicolaou smears have reduced the incidence of adenocarcinoma of the vagina**

Key Concept/Objective: To understand the factors that increase the risk of cancer

Long-term exposure to environmental tobacco smoke (passive smoking) has been associated with a 30% increase in the risk of lung cancer in nonsmokers. β-Carotene has been associated with an increase in the risk of lung cancer. *Helicobacter pylori*, not stress, is the causal agent in gastric cancer. Papanicolaou smears are used for the secondary prevention of cervical cancer. *(Answer: A—In nonsmokers, long-term passive exposure to tobacco smoke is associated with a significantly increased risk of lung cancer)*

2. During a routine office visit, a 49-year-old woman of Ashkenazi Jewish descent expresses concern about her risk of cancer. She reports that her younger sister has just been diagnosed with breast cancer. In addition, the patient tells you that her father was recently found to have an adenomatous polyp on colonoscopy. Her mother died in an automobile accident at an early age; she was otherwise healthy.

Which of the following statements about factors that predispose to cancer is true?

❑ A. **The retinoblastoma gene (*Rb-1*) is inherited in an autosomal recessive pattern**

❑ B. **Familial colon cancer has been linked to germline mutations in DNA repair genes such as *MSH2, MLH1, MSH6, PMS1,* and *PMS2***

❑ C. **Hereditary breast cancer resulting from mutations in the *BRCA1* and *BRCA2* genes account for the majority of all breast cancers in Ashkenazi Jews**

❑ D. **Major susceptibility loci for hereditary prostate cancer has been mapped to the Y chromosome**

Key Concept/Objective: To understand that genetic alterations underlie the transformation of a normal cell to a cancerous cell

Approximately one third of retinoblastomas occur in an autosomal dominant pattern with high penetrance. In contrast, familial colon cancer without multiple polyposis may be caused by germline mutations in one of the DNA repair genes: *MSH2, MLH1, MSH6, PMS1,* or *PMS2. BRCA1* and *BRCA2* account for most of the hereditary breast cancers in young women; carriers of *BRCA1* are also predisposed to ovarian cancer of early onset. Hereditary prostate cancer, which accounts for 5% to 10% of all cases, is primarily associated with disease of early onset. Major susceptibility loci for hereditary prostate cancer were recently mapped to chromosome 1 and the X chromosome. *(Answer: B—Familial colon cancer has been linked to germline mutations in DNA repair genes such as* MSH2, MLH1, MSH6, PMS1, *and* PMS2*)*

For more information, see Neugut AI, Li FP: 12 Oncology: I Cancer Epidemiology and Prevention. ACP Medicine Online (www.acpmedicine.com). Dale DC, Federman DD, Eds. WebMD Inc., New York, November 2004

Molecular Genetics of Cancer

3. A 51-year-old male patient recently presented with splenomegaly and weight loss. He was diagnosed as having chronic myelogenous leukemia (CML). He has done some reading on his own and is inquisitive about the etiology of this cancer.

Which of the following statements regarding the molecular genetics of CML is false?

- ❑ A. **The chromosomal translocation in CML involves the c-*myc* gene**
- ❑ B. **Philadelphia chromosome is associated with CML**
- ❑ C. **The accelerated or blast phase of CML is often associated with duplication of the Philadelphia chromosome**
- ❑ D. **Imatinib mesylate is directed against the tyrosine kinase produced by the Philadelphia chromosome and is therefore used in the treatment of CML**

Key Concept/Objective: To understand the molecular genetics of CML

The first specific chromosomal translocation identified in human cancer was the Philadelphia chromosome, which underlies CML. The fusion of chromosomes 9 and 22 leads to the joining of two unrelated genes, the c-*abl* gene, which encodes a tyrosine kinase and is located on chromosome 9, and the gene *bcr* (for breakpoint recombination), located on chromosome 22. A chimeric protein with novel transforming properties is formed from this specific chromosomal rearrangement. The accelerated or blast phase of CML is often associated with duplication of the Philadelphia chromosome, suggesting that increased copies of this aberrant gene confer a dose-dependent transforming effect. The recent discovery of an effective inhibitor of the bcr-abl kinase, imatinib mesylate (formerly STI571), has led to dramatic responses in CML and has revolutionized treatment of this leukemia. In Burkitt lymphoma, the chromosomal locus containing the c-*myc* gene is rearranged such that the upstream negative regulatory regions (i.e., regions located to the 5' side of a gene) of c-*myc* are lost; expression of the gene is directed by the strong immunoglobulin heavy-chain enhancer, which is constitutively active in B cells. Deregulation of c-*myc* expression in these cells is thus a potent force driving cellular proliferation. *(Answer: A—The chromosomal translocation in CML involves the* c-myc *gene)*

4. A 31-year-old female patient comes to your office with concerns about her family being "predisposed" to cancer. She says that her son was recently diagnosed with retinoblastoma. She wants to know if future children will also develop cancer.

Which of the following statements regarding the Knudson model of human cancer genetics is false?

- ❑ A. **Children with familial tumors have inherited an initial genetic hit (i.e., a distinct genetic alteration) and require only one additional, rate-limiting genetic hit to initiate tumorigenesis**
- ❑ B. **Tumor suppressor gene mutations are gain-of-function mutations; they are dominant mutations**

❑ C. **Both retinoblastoma and Wilms tumor follow the Knudson model of human cancer genetics**

❑ D. **Children with sporadic tumors need to acquire two independent genetic hits within the same cell**

Key Concept/Objective: To understand the Knudson model of human cancer genetics

Alfred Knudson proposed the model that now forms the foundation of human cancer genetics. The Knudson model predicts that children with familial tumors have inherited an initial genetic hit (i.e., a distinct genetic alteration) and require only one additional, rate-limiting genetic hit to initiate tumorigenesis. In contrast, children with sporadic tumors need to acquire two independent genetic hits within the same cell, an unlikely event that explains the less frequent, unilateral presentation and later onset of sporadic cancers. Subsequent genetic studies in two of the tumors studied by Knudson identified these so-called genetic hits as the sequential inactivation of the two alleles of a critical tumor suppressor gene: *RB1* in retinoblastoma and *WT1* in Wilms tumor. The Knudson model also explains the paradox that tumor suppressor gene mutations are loss-of-function or recessive mutations, yet familial cancer presents as an autosomal dominant trait. Although loss of a single allele of a tumor suppressor gene may be functionally silent in the presence of a normal second allele, the frequency of spontaneous mutations is sufficiently high to ensure that at least one cell within the target tissue is likely to lose the second allele and initiate malignant transformation. *(Answer: B—Tumor suppressor gene mutations are gain-of-function mutations; they are dominant mutations)*

5. A 57-year-old man presents to the hospital with generalized weakness, weight loss, and worsening constipation. He is found to be profoundly anemic. His stools test positive for occult blood. A colonoscopy is performed, and a large intraluminal mass is seen. Results of biopsy indicate adenocarcinoma of the colon.

Which of the following statements regarding* p53 *is false?

❑ A. ***p53* plays a critical role in the maintenance of genomic integrity and is known as the "guardian of the genome"**

❑ B. **Genetic injuries trigger the stabilization and activation of p53 protein**

❑ C. **p53 protein functions by repairing DNA molecules**

❑ D. **High levels of p53 protein in tumor specimens are commonly taken as evidence of a mutation in *p53***

Key Concept/Objective: To understand the basic principles of the p53 *genomic stability gene*

***p53* plays a critical role in the maintenance of genomic integrity—hence its popular designation as "guardian of the genome." The p53 protein is normally expressed at low levels in all cells. However, genetic injuries, such as those that occur through ionizing radiation, trigger the stabilization and activation of p53 protein. p53 functions as a transcription factor, directing expression of p21, an inhibitor of the cyclin-dependent kinases that regulate the cell cycle. Activation of p53 leads to arrest in the G1 phase of the cell cycle, enabling cells to repair DNA damage before proceeding into S phase and DNA replication. In other cells, activation of p53 causes activation of multiple effectors, leading to apoptosis—a suicide program in cells whose DNA may have been irreparably damaged. Not surprisingly, mutations of *p53* are common in human cancers, being demonstrable in about 50% of cases. Most mutations are amino acid substitutions within the DNA-binding domain of p53, resulting in its misfolding and binding to heat shock proteins. The rate of protein turnover is greatly slowed for these mutant p53 molecules. This explains the paradox that high levels of p53 protein in tumor specimens are commonly taken as evidence of a mutation in *p53*.** *(Answer: C—p53 protein functions by repairing DNA molecules)*

6. A 75-year-old woman presents with left flank pain, weight loss, and bilateral lower extremity edema. She is noted to have microscopic hematuria and erythrocytosis on laboratory evaluation. A CT scan of her abdomen and pelvis reveals a large left renal cell carcinoma with near total occlusion of the inferior vena cava by the tumor. It is known that certain tumor suppressor genes can undergo mutation and lead to cancer.

Which of the following statements regarding tumor suppressor genes is false?

❑ A. von Hippel-Lindau gene (*VHL*) is frequently mutated in adult renal cell cancers

❑ B. The *WT1* gene encodes a transcription regulator that is specifically expressed in podocytes of the developing glomerulus; mutations in *WT1* cause Wilms tumor, an embryonic kidney cancer

❑ C. *SMAD* genes, active in signaling by transforming growth factor–α (TGF-α), are mutated in pancreatic tumors

❑ D. The *APC* gene is a key target in breast cancer

Key Concept/Objective: To know the tumor suppressor gene mutations that are involved in common solid tumors

The identification of tumor suppressor genes implicated in cancer predisposition syndromes led to the discovery of key components of cellular differentiation pathways. The *WT1* gene encodes a transcription regulator that is specifically expressed in podocytes of the developing glomerulus. Mutations in *WT1* cause Wilms tumor, an embryonic kidney cancer. *VHL* is frequently mutated in adult renal cell cancers and in the germline of persons who have a syndrome that includes both benign and malignant vascular tumors. The VHL protein appears to be involved in the regulation of protein degradation pathways, particularly that of the transcription factor hypoxia-inducible factor. The *APC* gene is a key target in colorectal cancer: germline mutations cause familial polyposis coli, a syndrome characterized by the development of numerous colonic polyps that are at very high risk for malignant transformation; somatic mutations constitute the earliest step in the development of colorectal cancer. The *SMAD* genes, active in signaling by TGF-α, are mutated in pancreatic tumors. *(Answer: D—The* APC *gene is a key target in breast cancer)*

For more information, see Haber DA: 12 Oncology: II Molecular Genetics of Cancer. ACP Medicine Online (www.acpmedicine.com). Dale DC, Federman DD, Eds. WebMD Inc., New York, June 2004

Principles of Cancer Treatment

7. A 74-year-old woman presents to your office complaining of a breast mass. On physical examination, the patient is found to have a 2 × 3 cm mass in the right breast. A mammogram is obtained, and the results are suspicious for cancer. A fine-needle aspiration biopsy shows adenocarcinoma. As part of your evaluation before deciding the best therapy to offer, you wish to determine the stage of her malignancy.

What is the usual method for staging the majority of tumors?

❑ A. Tumor size, presence of comorbidities, and the involvement of lymph nodes

❑ B. Tumor size, involvement of lymph nodes, and the presence of metastasis

❑ C. Histology type, tumor size, the involvement of lymph nodes, and metastasis

❑ D. Performance status, involvement of lymph nodes, and metastasis

Key Concept/Objective: To understand tumor staging

Knowledge of the extent of the disease at the time of diagnosis (stage) is required to properly manage patients with cancer. Staging is based on three components: the size or depth of penetration of the tumor (T), the involvement of lymph nodes (N), and the presence or absence of metastases (M). The TNM staging system is now standard; its use is required not only for the management of cancer cases but also for the reporting of cancer cases to cooperative groups and many tumor registries. Within each TNM category, the extent of involvement correlates with prognosis and can help in deciding the appropriate treatment. Although there are few exceptions, the majority of tumors are staged on the basis of this

classification. Although the performance status and the presence of comorbidities are important factors that should be considered when deciding the best therapy for the patient, they are not part of the staging system. *(Answer: B—Tumor size, involvement of lymph nodes, and the presence of metastasis)*

8. A 37-year-old man is diagnosed with Hodgkin lymphoma after presenting with fever and lymphadenopathy. The patient is treated with a combination of doxorubicin, bleomycin, vincristine, and dacarbazine. After 3 days of treatment, the patient complains of mouth pain and diarrhea. His physical examination shows erythematous buccal mucosa.

Which of the following is the most likely pathogenesis of these complications?

- ❑ **A. Progression of his lymphoma**
- ❑ **B. Vitamin B_{12} deficiency**
- ❑ **C. *Clostridium difficile* colitis**
- ❑ **D. A side effect of the chemotherapy**

Key Concept/Objective: To understand the most common mechanisms of toxicity of antineoplastic drugs

Most antineoplastic drugs target proteins or nucleic acids that are common to both malignant and nonmalignant cells and thus have a narrow therapeutic index. In addition, antineoplastic drugs are usually administered at very high doses. Several toxicities are shared by many antineoplastic drugs. These include nausea and vomiting, mucositis and diarrhea, myelosuppression, alopecia, infertility, and increased risk of secondary malignancy. Nausea and vomiting result from local gastrointestinal effects as well as activation of the chemoreceptor trigger zone in the central nervous system. Mucositis and diarrhea are attributable to the relatively high proliferative rate of normal gastrointestinal tissues, which makes these tissues more susceptible to the cytotoxic effects of many chemotherapeutic regimens. Similar mechanisms result in chemotherapy-induced myelosuppression, alopecia, and infertility. Many chemotherapeutic agents are found to be mutagenic when tested in vitro. Moreover, epidemiologic studies of patients cured of a pediatric cancer have demonstrated that certain therapies are associated with a higher risk of secondary malignancies. *(Answer: D—A side effect of the chemotherapy)*

9. A 33-year-old woman is diagnosed with non-Hodgkin lymphoma. She is treated with chemotherapy and has a good initial response; however, after a few courses of therapy, she develops progressive disease. The oncologist considers drug resistance as the cause of this therapeutic failure and mentions the presence of P-glycoprotein as a possible mechanism.

Of the following, which best describes the mechanism of resistance associated with P-glycoprotein?

- ❑ **A. Induction of mutations of the receptor to which the antineoplastic drug binds**
- ❑ **B. Induction of angiogenesis**
- ❑ **C. Recognition of the antineoplastic drug and pumping of the drug to the extracellular space**
- ❑ **D. Induction of hepatic microsomes and an increase in the metabolic rates of different antineoplastic agents**

Key Concept/Objective: To understand the mechanisms of resistance to antineoplastic drugs

For an anticancer drug to kill a cancer cell, the drug must enter the bloodstream, be activated or escape inactivation by drug-metabolizing enzymes, and reach the target in its active form. The drug-drug-target interaction must then produce cell death. Resistance to anticancer therapy results from interference with one or more of these critical steps. Some of the factors affecting these steps are poor absorption or distribution of the drug; metabolism of the drug in the liver; decreased blood supply to the target organ; hypoxia; changes in the receptors; and mechanisms that block the intracellular accumulation of the drug. Multidrug resistance refers to the clinical and laboratory circumstance in which a tumor

is no longer susceptible to several chemotherapeutic drugs having different mechanisms or targets. P-glycoprotein is a member of the adenosine triphosphate (ATP)-binding cassette family. P-glycoprotein spans the plasma membrane and recognizes a broad spectrum of anticancer drugs. In the presence of ATP, P-glycoprotein pumps the drugs to the extracellular space, so that effective concentration at the intracellular target is never achieved. *(Answer: C—Recognition of the antineoplastic drug and pumping of the drug to the extracellular space)*

10. A 58-year-old man presents with hemoptysis and a weight loss of 5 kg over the past month. Chest x-ray shows a 1 cm nodule in the right upper lung, near the periphery. Biopsy confirms non–small cell lung cancer. Node sampling is negative, and no metastases are found. The patient smokes one pack of cigarettes a day but is willing to quit. His medical history includes chronic obstructive pulmonary disease, hypertension (well controlled with medications), and stable angina with a normal electrocardiogram. His FEV_1 is 700 ml.

Which of the following is the determining factor in the decision regarding whether or not to pursue curative therapy in this patient?

- ❑ **A. The size of the tumor**
- ❑ **B. The patient's node-negative status**
- ❑ **C. The patient's stable angina**
- ❑ **D. The fact that the patient smokes**
- ❑ **E. The patient's FEV_1 value**

Key Concept/Objective: To understand the rationale for palliative therapy versus curative therapy

This patient has a potentially curable tumor. It is small and distant from the mediastinum, and he has no positive lymph nodes or metastases (T1N0M0). Although he still smokes, he is willing to consider quitting, and smoking is not an absolute contraindication to curative surgery. His stable angina is also not a contraindication to surgery. However, his FEV_1 of less than 800 ml is below the lower limit for safe resection of the tumor. He would not have enough reserve lung capacity to survive the surgery. For this reason, therapy should be aimed at palliation. In general, the extent of involvement described by the TNM system correlates with prognosis. In addition to cancer prognosis, tolerability of therapy is crucial to decisions regarding palliation or goal of cure because aggressive therapy may be harmful to patients, as in this case. *(Answer: E—The patient's FEV_1 value)*

11. The patient in Question 10 wants your advice about the treatment options for his cancer. Clinical trials relevant to his condition are available. He is very well educated and wants to know which ones he should participate in. You tell him that there are several phase III trials available, and he asks what a phase III trial studies.

Which of the following is investigated in a phase III trial?

- ❑ **A. The maximum tolerated dose of an antineoplastic agent**
- ❑ **B. Efficacy of treatment as measured by changes in the size of tumors and time to progression**
- ❑ **C. Efficacy of treatment as measured by survival rates and quality of life**
- ❑ **D. Efficacy of a new active agent compared with that of the best available therapy**

Key Concept/Objective: To understand the phases of treatment trials

Phase I clinical trials identify the maximum tolerated dose of a new drug. Phase II clinical trials assess efficacy by use of change in tumor size, quality of life, disease-progression parameters, and survival. Phase III clinical trials compare a new chemotherapeutic agent with the best available therapy. *(Answer: D—Efficacy of a new active agent compared with that of the best available therapy)*

12. A 43-year-old woman presents with a 2 cm breast mass. Excision biopsy and node dissection reveal an aggressive carcinoma with 6 of 10 axillary nodes positive. Combination chemotherapy is recommended. The patient is concerned about combination therapy and wishes to have single-agent therapy.

You explain that combination chemotherapy is desirable because it does which of the following?

- ❑ **A. Reduces the risk of secondary malignancy**
- ❑ **B. Increases cure rates by decreasing the risk of cross-resistance**
- ❑ **C. Decreases resistance-conferring mutations by allowing larger doses of each agent to be given**
- ❑ **E. Eliminates the need for radiation therapy**
- ❑ **F. Decreases the risk of gastrointestinal side effects**

Key Concept/Objective: To understand the rationale for combination chemotherapy

The Goldie-Coldman model predicts drug resistance by use of cell number and the spontaneous cancer cell mutation rate. Even a tumor that is too small to be detected clinically has a significant chance of containing a cell with a resistance-conferring mutation. Although combination chemotherapy allows for reduction of the dosage of any one agent, it does not inherently reduce side effects or the risk of mutation-induced secondary malignancy or eliminate the need for radiation therapy (which reduces the risk of local recurrence). Finally, combination therapy does not allow for higher dosages. If anything, combination chemotherapy necessitates lower dosages of agents that have common toxicities. Combination chemotherapy attempts to address possible cross-resistance by employing different mechanisms, and nonoverlapping toxicities allow for effective dosing. *(Answer: B—Increases cure rates by decreasing the risk of cross-resistance)*

13. A 55-year-old man returns to the office 2 months into treatment for metastatic prostate cancer. His treatment includes prostatectomy, nilutamide, and radiation. He now reports tender, enlarged breasts, whitish nipple discharge, nausea, and diarrhea. He has no ill contacts and has recently returned from a trip to Arizona. He also reports that he has stopped drinking alcohol because it makes him feel ill. Examination results are as follows: temperature is 99.5° F (37.5° C); pulse, 88 beats/min; and blood pressure, 120/82 mm Hg. Breast examination confirms gynecomastia and galactorrhea. Abdominal examination shows mild tenderness in the lower abdomen without rebound. Rectal examination shows no masses, and the stool is heme-negative.

Which of the following is the best step to take next for this patient?

- ❑ **A. Determine serum prolactin and testosterone levels**
- ❑ **B. Order a mammogram**
- ❑ **C. Send stool sample to assess for enteric pathogens and ova and parasite**
- ❑ **D. Reassure the patient that these are common side effects of his chemotherapy**
- ❑ **E. Arrange for urgent head CT with contrast**

Key Concept/Objective: To know the common side effects of antiandrogenic chemotherapy

The common side effects of antiandrogenic chemotherapeutic agents such as nilutamide include nausea, diarrhea, and constipation. Hormonal effects include gynecomastia, galactorrhea, breast tenderness, hot flashes, and decreased facial hair. Idiosyncratic reactions associated with nilutamide include delayed dark-light adaptation, interstitial pneumonitis, and alcohol intolerance. Thus, in this case, the patient needs to be reassured that these are usual side effects of his regimen. *(Answer: D—Reassure the patient that these are common side effects of his chemotherapy)*

For more information, see Rubin EH, Hait WN: 12 Oncology: IV Principles of Cancer Treatment. ACP Medicine Online (www.acpmedicine.com). Dale DC, Federman DD, Eds. WebMD Inc., New York, May 2003

Colorectal Cancer

14. A 55-year-old white man presents to your primary care clinic for his annual physical examination. He underwent a colonoscopy 2 years ago, and an adenomatous polyp was removed. After the examination, the patient mentions that he has been reading about colon cancer and polyps in the news and wants to know his risk of having colon cancer.

Which of the following statements regarding the relationship between colon cancer and polyps is false?

- ❑ A. **Most colorectal cancers arise from preexisting adenomas**
- ❑ B. **Adenomatous polyps, as well as juvenile polyps, hamartomas, and inflammatory polyps, progress to colorectal carcinoma**
- ❑ C. **Larger polyps, especially those larger than 1 cm, are more likely to contain invasive carcinoma**
- ❑ D. **On the basis of histology, villous polyps are more likely to contain invasive carcinoma than are tubular polyps**
- ❑ E. **Fewer than 1% of adenomatous polyps become malignant**

Key Concept/Objective: To understand the relationship between various types of polyps and colorectal cancer

It is thought that most colorectal cancers arise from preexisting adenomas. Such potentially premalignant lesions should be distinguished from juvenile polyps, hamartomas, and inflammatory polyps, which are not thought to progress to colorectal cancer. Histologically, adenomatous polyps may be tubular, villous, or both (tubulovillous). The larger the adenoma, the greater the likelihood that a villous component will be present. Villous polyps are more likely to contain invasive carcinoma than are tubular polyps of the same size. Regardless of histologic class, large polyps—especially those larger than 1 cm in diameter—are more likely to contain invasive carcinoma. Fewer than 1% of adenomatous polyps ever become malignant. *(Answer: B—Adenomatous polyps, as well as juvenile polyps, hamartomas, and inflammatory polyps, progress to colorectal carcinoma)*

15. A 45-year-old woman presents to your office to establish primary care. While taking her medical history, you notice she has a strong family history of colon cancer occurring at a young age. You suspect hereditary nonpolyposis colorectal cancer (HNPCC).

Which of the following is NOT a part of the Amsterdam-2 criteria for identifying patients with HNPCC?

- ❑ A. **Histologically documented colorectal cancer (or other HNPCC-related tumor) in at least three relatives, one of whom is a first degree relative of the other two**
- ❑ B. **Cases of colorectal cancer in at least two successive generations of the family**
- ❑ C. **A family history of one or more cases of colorectal cancer diagnosed before 60 years of age**
- ❑ D. **Affected relatives must be on the same side of the family (maternal or paternal)**

Key Concept/Objective: To know the diagnostic criteria for HNPCC

HNPCC is an autosomal dominant disorder associated with an unusually high frequency of cancers in the proximal large bowel. The median age at which adenocarcinomas appear in HNPCC is less than 50 years, which is 10 to 15 years younger than the median age at which they appear in the general population. Also, families with HNPCC often include persons with multiple primary cancers; in women, an association between colorectal cancer and either endometrial or ovarian carcinoma is especially prominent. Several sets of selection criteria have been developed for identifying patients with this syndrome. The Amsterdam-2 criteria comprise the following: histologically documented colorectal cancer

(or other HNPCC-related tumor) in at least three relatives, one of whom is a first-degree relative of the other two; a family history of one or more cases of colorectal cancer diagnosed before 50 years of age; and cases of colorectal cancer in at least two successive generations of the family. Affected relatives should be on the same side of the family (maternal or paternal), familial adenomatous polyposis (FAP) must be excluded in colorectal cancer cases, and tumors must be pathologically verified. *(Answer: C—A family history of one or more cases of colorectal cancer diagnosed before 60 years of age)*

16. A 50-year-old black male patient returns to your office for follow-up for hypertension. His hypertension is well controlled with hydrochlorothiazide and an angiotensin-converting enzyme inhibitor. Because the patient is 50 years old, you talk about colorectal cancer screening measures.

Which of the following statements regarding colorectal cancer screening is false?

- ❑ A. A fecal occult blood test (FOBT) is equally useful at detecting adenomas and early-stage cancers
- ❑ B. A case-control study demonstrated a risk reduction of 70% for death from cancers within reach of the sigmoidoscope
- ❑ C. Colonoscopic polypectomy lowers the incidence of colorectal cancers by 50% to 90%, and the American Cancer Society currently recommends colonoscopy every 10 years, starting at age 50, for asymptomatic adults at average risk for colorectal cancer
- ❑ D. There has not been a formal trial of double-contrast barium enema (DCBE) as a screening test for colorectal neoplasia in a general population

Key Concept/Objective: To understand colorectal cancer screening tests

Screening and early detection (secondary prevention) are important in influencing the outcome in patients with colorectal neoplasia. Many deaths from colorectal cancers could probably be averted by appropriate use of screening. The rationale for screening for colorectal neoplasia is twofold: First, detection of adenomas and their removal will prevent subsequent development of colorectal cancer. Second, detection of localized, superficial tumors in asymptomatic individuals will increase the surgical cure rate. The rationale for screening for the presence of blood in the stool is that large adenomas and most cancers bleed intermittently. Annual testing may allow detection of disease that, although undetected on previous occasions, has not yet reached an advanced and perhaps incurable stage. Compared with endoscopic tests, FOBT detects relatively few adenomas; the principal benefit of an FOBT program is to increase detection of early-stage cancers. A case-control study demonstrated a risk reduction of 70% for death from cancers within reach of the sigmoidoscope; the data suggested that the benefit may last as long as 10 years. The effectiveness of colonoscopy has been demonstrated by several studies. Observational, case-control, and prospective, randomized trials have shown that colonoscopic polypectomy lowers the incidence of colorectal cancers by 50% to 90%. The American Cancer Society currently recommends colonoscopy every 10 years, starting at age 50, for asymptomatic adults at average risk for colorectal cancer. Repeat examinations at more frequent intervals are indicated for patients at increased or high risk. There has not been a formal trial of DCBE as a screening test for colorectal neoplasia in a general population. A comparison study in patients who have undergone colonoscopic polypectomy found colonoscopy to be a more effective method of surveillance than DCBE. *(Answer: A—A fecal occult blood test [FOBT] is equally useful at detecting adenomas and early-stage cancers)*

17. A 62-year-old black male patient is in the hospital for evaluation of anemia with associated fatigue and weight loss. He was found to be heme-positive on rectal examination, and a colonoscopy was performed. A mass was found in his ascending colon; biopsy revealed adenocarcinoma. A CT scan of his chest, abdomen, and pelvis revealed a 3 cm mass in his ascending colon; there were no liver lesions or other metastatic disease and no intraperitoneal lymphadenopathy. The patient was taken to surgery for resection. Surgical pathology revealed invasive adenocarcinoma extending into the serosa, but no lymph node involvement.

Which of the following statements regarding this patient's staging and prognosis is false?

❑ A. The patient has stage B disease because no lymph nodes are involved and no distant metastasis was found

❑ B. The fact that the patient's primary tumor was larger than 2 cm is a poor prognostic factor

❑ C. Because most recurrences after resection occur within 3 to 4 years, the cure rate is reasonably estimated by 5-year survival rates

❑ D. Postoperatively, the carcinoembryonic antigen (CEA) level may serve as a measure of the completeness of tumor resection

Key Concept/Objective: To understand the staging and prognosis of colorectal carcinoma

The prognosis for patients with adenocarcinoma of the colorectum is closely associated with the depth of tumor penetration into the bowel wall and the presence or absence of regional lymph node involvement and distant metastases. The Dukes system has been applied to the TNM classification method, in which T represents the depth of tumor penetration; N, the presence or absence of lymph node involvement; and M, the presence or absence of distant metastases. Stage A (T1N0M0) cancers are superficial lesions that do not penetrate the muscularis and do not involve regional lymph nodes. Stage B cancers penetrate more deeply into the bowel wall without lymph node involvement. Stage C cancers involve regional nodes. Stage D cancers have metastasized to liver, lung, bone, or other anatomically distant sites. Because most recurrences after resection occur within 3 to 4 years, the cure rate is reasonably estimated by 5-year survival rates. Although CEA is an imperfect tumor marker, it can provide useful information for the management of colorectal cancer patients if its limitations and attributes are understood. Postoperatively, the CEA level may serve as a measure of the completeness of tumor resection. If a preoperatively elevated CEA value does not fall to normal levels within 4 weeks (a period that is twice the plasma half-life of CEA) after surgery, the resection was probably incomplete or occult metastases are present. In contrast to the prognosis for patients with most other solid tumors, the prognosis for patients with colorectal cancer is not influenced by the size of the primary lesion when corrected for nodal involvement and histologic differentiation. *(Answer: B—The fact that the patient's primary tumor was larger than 2 cm is a poor prognostic factor)*

For more information, see Levin B: 12 Oncology: V Colorectal Cancer. ACP Medicine Online (www.acpmedicine.com). Dale DC, Federman DD, Eds. WebMD Inc., New York, February 2004

Pancreatic, Gastric, and Other Gastrointestinal Cancers

18. A 61-year-old black man presents to your clinic with a 6-month history of progressive esophageal dysphagia and weight loss. He has a history of hypertension and severe gastroesophageal reflux disease (GERD). He is admitted to the hospital, and an esophagogastroduodenoscopy (EGD) with biopsy is performed. The findings indicate a diagnosis of adenocarcinoma of the esophagus.

For this patient, which of the following statements regarding esophageal cancer is false?

❑ A. Proton pump inhibitors have been shown to stop the progression of Barrett esophagus to adenocarcinoma

❑ B. In the United States, the incidence of adenocarcinoma is increasing and the incidence of squamous cell carcinoma (SCC) is decreasing

❑ C. Barrett esophagus is a complication of chronic reflux disease and is associated with an increased risk of adenocarcinoma of the esophagus

❑ D. Staging of esophageal cancer can involve CT scanning of the chest, abdomen, and pelvis; endoscopic ultrasound (EUS); and PET scanning

❑ E. The mainstay of therapy for esophageal cancer is surgery

Key Concept/Objectives: To understand the risk factors, diagnosis, and treatment of esophageal adenocarcinoma

Esophageal cancer, which includes SCC and adenocarcinoma, is the ninth most common cancer worldwide. The annual rate of SCC of the esophagus per 100,000 population is declining, and the incidence of esophageal adenocarcinoma is rapidly increasing in the United States and other countries. GERD is a risk factor for esophageal adenocarcinoma. Barrett esophagus, a metaplastic change of the lining of the esophagus in which the normal squamous cell epithelium is replaced by columnar intestinal-type epithelium, is a complication of chronic reflux disease. It is associated with an increased risk of adenocarcinoma of the esophagus. Because GERD is a risk factor for esophageal adenocarcinoma and because Barrett esophagus is highly associated with the disease, there is increased clinical interest in pharmacologic, surgical, or endoscopic therapy to decrease the risk, as well as prevent the development, of adenocarcinoma of the esophagus. However, there is no evidence to suggest that proton pump inhibitors either stop the progression of Barrett esophagus to adenocarcinoma or lead to regression in the presence of metaplastic tissue. Once a diagnosis has been established and careful physical examination and routine blood tests have been performed, a CT scan of the chest, abdomen, and pelvis should be obtained to assess tumor extent, nodal involvement, and metastatic disease. However, CT scanning may underestimate the depth of tumor invasion and periesophageal lymph node involvement in up to 50% of cases. EUS has the advantage of being able to image distinct wall layers, thereby providing a representation of the depth of tumor invasion with an accuracy of up to 90% and detecting regional lymph node involvement with an accuracy of 75%. EUS also can detect local tumor recurrence at an early stage. EUS should be considered as a mandatory procedure for staging workup, especially for patients who are being considered for preoperative treatments. PET scanning has become widely available and may be an important tool for staging, with both a sensitivity and a specificity of approximately 90%. PET scanning is considered to be superior to CT scanning in the evaluation of distant metastases. Treatment options for esophageal cancer are based on the stage of the disease at presentation. Surgery remains the mainstay of treatment of esophageal cancer. It can be curative in persons with resectable local and locoregional disease. *(Answer: A—Proton pump inhibitors have been shown to stop the progression of Barrett esophagus to adenocarcinoma)*

19. A 68-year-old white man presents for evaluation of early satiety, mild epigastric pain, nausea, and weight loss. On examination, the patient is pale and thin. He has a palpable periumbilical lymph node. Rectal examination shows heme-positive brown stool. EGD reveals a large mass in the stomach, and biopsy is performed.

For this patient, which of the following statements regarding risk factors for gastric cancer is false?

- ❑ A. ***Helicobacter pylori*** **infection is a primary risk factor for gastric cancer**
- ❑ B. **Hereditary syndromes such as HNPCC, FAP, the Li-Fraumeni syndrome, and the Peutz-Jeghers syndrome are associated with gastric cancer**
- ❑ C. **Approximately 50% of gastric cancers involve familial clustering**
- ❑ D. **Salted, smoked, and dried foods that contain high concentrations of nitrates may be associated with the development of gastric cancer**

Key Concept/Objective: To understand the risk factors for gastric cancer

Gastric cancer is an aggressive neoplasm that has a marked variation in both incidence and mortality between different populations. A high incidence of gastric cancer is observed in Asia, South and Central America (Chile and Costa Rica), Eastern Europe, and the Middle East. Extensive research has identified factors and events that influence the initiation, promotion, and progression of stomach cancer. Gastric cancer is a disease of complex etiology involving multiple risk factors, including dietary, infectious, occupational, genetic, and preneoplastic factors. Salted, smoked, and dried foods contain high concentrations of nitrates, which are converted into carcinogenic nitrosamines and nitrites by anaerobic bacteria; diets rich in such foods may be associated with the development of gastric cancer. Infection with *Helicobacter pylori*, a gram-negative spiral bacterium, is a primary risk factor for gastric cancer. The first strong data came from three separate, nested case-control studies. The statistically significant relative risk ranged from 2.8 in a British population to 6.0 in a cohort of Japanese males living in Hawaii. *H. pylori* gastritis causes cell proliferation with increased risk of DNA damage, leading to inadequate repair and malignant transformation. Although most cases of gastric cancer appear to be sporadic, approximately 10%

of cases involve familial clustering. Other hereditary cancer syndromes in which gastric cancer may occur include HNPCC, FAP, the Li-Fraumeni syndrome, and the Peutz-Jeghers syndrome. *(Answer: C—Approximately 50% of gastric cancers involve familial clustering)*

20. A 63-year-old black man presents to the emergency department with abdominal pain, dizziness, and nausea. He reports that he has lost about 20 lb during the past month and a half and that his abdominal pain has just recently become severe. It is midepigastric, gnawing, and radiates to his back. Over the past 3 days, he has had polyuria, but nausea has prevented him from being able to stay hydrated. On examination, the patient is cachectic, has dry mucous membranes, and is orthostatic. His abdomen is tender in the midepigastric region, and there is no palpable mass. Results of laboratory studies are notable for an elevated glucose level of 630 mg/dl and mild renal insufficiency; pancreatic enzyme levels are normal. You diagnose the patient as having diabetes mellitus of new onset, but you are concerned that he may have an underlying pancreatic malignancy.

For this patient, which of the following statements regarding pancreatic cancer is false?

- ❑ A. **Pancreatic cancer is more common in males than in females and is more common in blacks than whites**
- ❑ B. **Tumor size is a very important predictor of resectability, with tumors larger than 4 cm having less than a 10% chance of being resectable and nonmetastatic**
- ❑ C. **EUS is the single most accurate test for imaging and staging pancreatic carcinoma**
- ❑ D. **Risk factors for pancreatic cancer include increasing age, tobacco smoking, chronic pancreatitis, and coffee ingestion**
- ❑ E. **Surgical resection is the only curative modality for pancreatic cancer**

Key Concept/Objectives: To understand the risk factors and initial workup for pancreatic cancer

Pancreatic cancer is the fourth leading cause of death from cancer in both males and females in the United States. Ninety-five percent of malignant pancreatic tumors are exocrine pancreatic cancers, two thirds of which occur in the pancreatic head and one third in the pancreatic body and tail; the remaining 5% of malignant lesions are mostly islet cell tumors. The incidence of pancreatic cancer is higher in males than in females and is higher in blacks than in whites. Tobacco smoking has been the most consistently demonstrated risk factor, implicated as a cause in roughly 30% of cases of pancreatic cancer. Age is also an extremely important determinant of risk. With increasing age, the risk of pancreatic cancer increases exponentially. Coffee and alcohol consumption do not seem to increase the risk of pancreatic cancer. Initial symptoms experienced by pancreatic cancer patients are insidious and relatively nonspecific (e.g., weight loss, anorexia, abdominal discomfort or pain, and nausea); this may delay the diagnosis for several months. Pain can be a presenting symptom and is usually associated with localized invasion of peripancreatic structures (e.g., splanchnic plexus and retroperitoneum), particularly from lesions located in the body or tail of the pancreas. Pain is typically described as gnawing and severe, radiating to the back and worsening in the supine position. The early diagnosis of a potentially resectable pancreatic cancer is extremely difficult because of nonspecific initial symptoms and poor sensitivity of noninvasive techniques such as CT and ultrasonography. EUS is the single most accurate test for imaging and staging pancreatic carcinoma and can clearly evaluate pancreatic mucosal, vascular, ductal, and parenchymal abnormalities, as well as lymph node metastases. Patients with clinical symptoms that may represent pancreatic cancer should have an initial standard CT scan or an abdominal ultrasound. If a pancreatic mass is suspected on one of these initial tests, further evaluation is necessary. If the tumor appears to be larger than 4 cm or appears unresectable, spiral CT with intravenous contrast and endoscopic retrograde cholangiopancreatography with fine-needle aspiration should be considered. On the basis of size alone, masses greater than 4 cm have less than a 10% chance of being resectable and nonmetastatic. Because surgical resection is the only curative modality for pancreatic cancer and because only 10% to 15% of patients present with resectable disease, the diagnosis, stage, and management are based on resectability. *(Answer: D—Risk factors for pancreatic cancer include increasing age, tobacco smoking, chronic pancreatitis, and coffee ingestion)*

21. A 46-year-old white man with a history of I.V. drug abuse and cirrhosis complicated by ascites presents with massive hematemesis. He is intubated in the emergency department and is treated with fluid resuscitation. Emergent EGD reveals esophageal varices, and band ligation is performed. The patient has never had portal hypertension before, so a workup is performed. It reveals a 4 cm mass in the liver. The serum α-fetoprotein level is checked and is found to be 440 ng/ml.

For this patient, which of the following statements regarding risk factors for hepatocellular carcinoma (HCC) is true?

❑ **A. Cirrhosis induced by hepatitis B virus (HBV) or hepatitis C virus (HCV), but not by alcoholism, is a risk factor for HCC**

❑ **B. The recent increase in incidence of HCC in the United States is most likely attributable to the increasing rates of HBV infection**

❑ **C. Hereditary hemochromatosis is not a risk factor for the development of HCC**

❑ **D. The presence of hepatitis infection and concomitant heavy alcohol consumption are synergistic in the development of HCC**

Key Concept/Objective: To understand the risk factors for HCC

HCC is the most common primary malignant tumor of the liver. It is the fifth most common malignancy in the world (564,000 cases a year) and the third-highest cause of cancer-related deaths worldwide. HCC is most often a complication of liver cirrhosis caused by chronic infection by HBV, HCV, or alcohol. The incidence of HCC in the United States has increased from 1.4 per 100,000 population for the period from 1976 through 1980 to 2.4 per 100,000 for the period from 1991 through 1995. This increase is considered to be primarily related to an increase in HCV infection. Hereditary hemochromatosis is also a risk factor for the development of HCC. Diabetes mellitus may be associated with HCC in patients with chronic HCV infection, and a significant synergy exists between heavy alcohol consumption, hepatitis virus infection (both HBV and HCV), and diabetes mellitus and the development of HCC. Patients with other metabolic disorders or conditions that may lead to cirrhosis (e.g., α_1-antitrypsin deficiency, type I glycogen storage disease, tyrosinemia, and even biliary atresia) are also at risk for developing HCC. Other risk factors include long-time ingestion of food contaminated with aflatoxins, metabolites of the mold *Aspergillus flavus*, exposure to oral contraceptives, and exogenous androgens. *(Answer: D—The presence of hepatitis infection and concomitant heavy alcohol consumption are synergistic in the development of HCC)*

For more information, see Sun W, Haller D: 12 Oncology: VI Pancreatic, Gastric, and Other Gastrointestinal Cancers. ACP Medicine Online (www.acpmedicine.com). Dale DC, Federman DD, Eds. WebMD Inc., New York, February 2004

Breast Cancer

22. A 40-year-old African-American woman presents to your clinic for an annual health examination. She has hypertension and hyperlipidemia, for which she takes hydrochlorothiazide and a statin, respectively. Otherwise, she is in good health, and she exercises regularly. Her main concern today is her risk of breast cancer. She has a close friend who was recently diagnosed with breast cancer, and she is now very worried that she might one day get it.

Which of the following statements regarding the risk factors for breast cancer is true?

❑ **A. Because of germline mutations of either *BRCA1* or *BRCA2*, the breast-ovarian cancer syndrome is inherited in an autosomal recessive fashion**

❑ **B. Reproductive risk factors include late menarche, early menopause, and increasing parity**

❑ **C. The diagnosis of breast cancer in first-degree relatives younger than 50 years is associated with a threefold to fourfold increased risk**

❑ **D. Women between the ages of 40 and 50 years are at greatest risk; 75% of all breast cancers are diagnosed in that age group**

Key Concept/Objective: To understand the risk factors for breast cancer

In first-degree relatives younger than 50 years, the diagnosis of breast cancer is associated with a threefold to fourfold increased risk. Several familial breast cancer syndromes and their associated molecular abnormalities have been identified. These include the breast-ovarian cancer syndrome, which is attributed to germline mutations in either of two breast cancer susceptibility genes, *BRCA1* and *BRCA2*. These mutations are inherited in an autosomal dominant fashion and can therefore be transmitted through both the maternal and the paternal lines. Reproductive risk factors include early menarche, late menopause, late first pregnancy, and nulliparity. All are felt to lead to a condition of prolonged estrogen exposure to the breast. *(Answer: C—The diagnosis of breast cancer in first-degree relatives younger than 50 years is associated with a threefold to fourfold increased risk)*

23. On clinical examination, a 54-year-old woman is noted to have a nontender mass in the upper outer quadrant of her left breast. There are no overlying skin changes, and there is no palpable adenopathy in the axilla. The other breast is without masses. A mammogram obtained 1 year ago was normal. You immediately set up an appointment for mammography, but your patient is obviously disturbed. She has several questions regarding the therapy for breast cancer.

Which of the following statements regarding breast cancer therapy is true?

- ❑ **A. For women with stage I or II breast cancer, the survival rate with breast conservation therapy involving lumpectomy and radiotherapy is identical to the survival rate with modified radical mastectomy**
- ❑ **B. Sentinel lymph node mapping is difficult to perform and offers no benefit to axillary lymph node dissection**
- ❑ **C. The benefit of tamoxifen is limited to 5 years, and therefore, the recommendation is to discontinue therapy after 5 years**
- ❑ **D. Aromatase inhibitors offer a viable alternative to tamoxifen therapy for premenopausal women**

Key Concept/Objective: To understand the basic principles of breast cancer therapy

Breast conservation therapy that involves lumpectomy with radiotherapy and modified radical mastectomy that involves removal of the breast and axillary nodes provide identical survival rates for women with stage I or II breast cancer. Sentinel lymph node mapping involves injection of a radioactive tracer, vital blue dye, or both into the area around the primary breast tumor. The injected substance tracks rapidly to the dominant axillary lymph node—the so-called sentinel lymph node. This node can be located by use of a small axillary incision and visual inspection or by use of a handheld counter. If the sentinel node is tumor free, the remaining lymph nodes are likely to be tumor free as well, and further axillary surgery can be avoided. The benefit of tamoxifen increases with the duration of treatment; the proportional reductions in 10-year recurrence and mortality were 47% and 26%, respectively, with 5-year regimens of tamoxifen therapy. The aromatase inhibitors specifically inhibit this conversion, leading to further estrogen deprivation in older women. Randomized trials have shown that the aromatase inhibitors (e.g., anastrozole, letrozole, and exemestane) provide efficacy similar or superior to that of tamoxifen, along with an acceptable side-effect profile for postmenopausal women with metastatic breast cancer. Given their mechanism of action, aromatase inhibitors should not be used for treatment in premenopausal women. *(Answer: A—For women with stage I or II breast cancer, the survival rate with breast conservation therapy involving lumpectomy and radiotherapy is identical to the survival rate with modified radical mastectomy)*

24. A 42-year-old woman presents for a routine health maintenance visit. She underwent menarche at age 13 and is still menstruating. She has never been pregnant. There is no history of breast cancer in her family. Several of her friends have recently been diagnosed with breast cancer, and she is concerned about developing it herself. She performs monthly breast self-examinations and has noted no abnormalities. On physical examination, her breasts are normal.

Which of the following statements regarding breast cancer screening is true?

❑ A. Yearly mammography improves survival
❑ B. Mammography will detect more than 95% of breast cancers
❑ C. The combination of clinical breast examination and mammography improves survival
❑ D. Mammography is recommended by several professional organizations but has not been shown to improve survival
❑ E. Screening for the *BRCA* gene mutations is recommended

Key Concept/Objective: To understand the recommended modalities in breast cancer screening

Screening modalities used for breast cancer include breast self-examination, clinical breast examination, and mammography. Breast self-examination is recommended by the American Cancer Society and other organizations despite the failure of a large clinical trial to show any benefit of self-examination over observation. The combination of clinical breast examinations and screening mammography in women 50 to 69 years of age has been shown to prolong survival; this approach resulted in a 25% to 30% decrease in mortality and is recommended by numerous advisory panels. In women 40 to 50 years of age who are at average risk, there is considerable controversy about the proper screening strategy because there has been no convincing evidence of survival benefit with clinical breast examinations and mammography. The clinical breast examination is an important part of screening because mammography does not detect 10% to 15% of breast cancers. Screening for the *BRCA1* and *BRCA2* mutations, which are seen in some families with a strong history of breast cancer, has not been rigorously investigated. In patients with no significant family history, this test would not be advisable. *(Answer: D—Mammography is recommended by several professional organizations but has not been shown to improve survival)*

25. A 59-year-old woman comes to your clinic wanting to know if there is anything she can do to decrease her risk of breast cancer. Two of her four sisters developed breast cancer while they were in their 50s. She experienced menarche at 12 years of age and menopause at 55 years of age. She had one child at 34 years of age. She underwent two breast biopsies for suspicious masses, which revealed normal breast tissue. Since she was 50 years of age, she has undergone yearly screening mammography, the results of which have been normal. Her breast examination reveals no masses, and there is no axillary lymphadenopathy.

Which of the following statements is false?

❑ A. Bilateral prophylactic mastectomy would reduce this patient's breast cancer risk by approximately 90%
❑ B. Treatment with daily tamoxifen for 5 years would reduce this patient's breast cancer risk by approximately 50%
❑ C. Lifestyle modifications, such as adherence to a low-fat diet, weight loss for obese patients, and smoking cessation, have been shown to reduce breast cancer risk
❑ D. Tamoxifen therapy is associated with an increased incidence of endometrial cancer and pulmonary embolism
❑ E. A clinical history that includes multiple benign breast biopsy results increases this patient's breast cancer risk

Key Concept/Objective: To understand the risk factors and the primary prevention strategies for breast cancer

Risk factors for the development of breast cancer include age, early menarche, late menopause, older age at first live birth or nulliparity, number of breast biopsies, number of first-degree relatives with breast cancer, and biopsies showing atypical hyperplasia. Women at high risk who received a 5-year course of tamoxifen were found to have 50% fewer diagnoses of breast cancer compared with women at comparable risk who did not receive tamoxifen. This therapy is associated with an increased risk of endometrial cancer and pulmonary embolism. Evidence from case series indicate that bilateral prophylactic mastectomy is associated with a greater than 90% reduction in the incidence of breast cancer. Prophylactic surgery has not been compared with aggressive screening in combination

with appropriate management of breast cancer and should be considered only for high-risk patients. Lifestyle modifications, such as adherence to a low-fat diet, weight loss for obese patients, and smoking cessation, have not been shown in prospective clinical trials to reduce breast cancer risk but are associated with decreased breast cancer risk in epidemiologic studies and are therefore recommended by some advisory groups. *(Answer: C—Lifestyle modifications, such as adherence to a low-fat diet, weight loss for obese patients, and smoking cessation, have been shown to reduce breast cancer risk)*

26. A 67-year-old woman returns to your clinic for follow-up. Two years ago, she was diagnosed with stage I breast cancer and treated with lumpectomy and radiation therapy. The tumor, 0.8 cm in its largest dimension, tested negative for estrogen and progesterone receptors. The patient's oncologist has asked you to conduct surveillance visits. The patient has no complaints. She denies having fevers, chills, weight loss, shortness of breath, or pain. She has been performing monthly breast self-examinations and has noted no changes or masses. On physical examination, she has a well-healed scar on her left breast with no other abnormalities. There are no breast masses palpable, and there is no axillary or supraclavicular lymphadenopathy. Bilateral mammograms are normal.

Which, if any, additional recommended surveillance studies should be conducted?

- ❑ **A. No additional studies are needed**
- ❑ **B. Complete blood count and liver function tests**
- ❑ **C. Complete blood count, liver function tests, and chest radiographs**
- ❑ **D. Complete blood count, liver function tests, chest radiographs, and tumor markers (CEA and CA 27.29)**
- ❑ **E. Bone scan and tumor markers (CEA and CA 27.29)**

Key Concept/Objective: To understand the follow-up surveillance of patients with early-stage breast cancer

Breast cancer is both a common and curable malignancy; increasingly, primary care physicians are being called upon to conduct follow-up surveillance for patients who have undergone treatment of breast cancer. The issue of which methods are appropriate for follow-up surveillance has been investigated in two randomized clinical trials. Both studies found that the standardized use of laboratory and diagnostic tests did not enhance survival or quality of life when compared with the use of tests chosen on the basis of individual patients' symptoms and clinical examination results. Recommended follow-up surveillance measures are patient education regarding symptoms of recurrence; regular history-taking and physical examinations; monthly breast self-examinations; annual mammography; and age-appropriate screening for other cancers. Routine use of complete blood counts, chemistry panels, tumor markers, chest x-rays, CT, or bone scans is not recommended. *(Answer: A—No additional studies are needed)*

27. A 54-year-old woman presents with a breast mass she discovered 2 days ago. She has been performing breast self-examinations monthly and noted a new mass in the upper outer quadrant of her left breast. She denies having any breast pain or nipple discharge. She has experienced no weight loss, headache, shortness of breath, or bony pain. On examination, she is found to have a 0.5 cm × 1 cm hard, mobile mass that is easily palpated. No skin abnormalities or other masses are detectable by palpation in either breast. There is no axillary or supraclavicular lymphadenopathy, and the remainder of a detailed physical examination is normal. A biopsy is performed of the patient's breast mass, which is found to have infiltrating ductal carcinoma. Results of a complete blood count, liver function tests, and metabolic panel are all within normal limits.

At this point, the interventions that would provide the best survival and least morbidity for this patient include which of the following?

- ❑ **A. Modified radical mastectomy**
- ❑ **B. Lumpectomy with axillary lymph node dissection**
- ❑ **C. Radiation therapy**

❑ D. **Modified radical mastectomy and radiation therapy**

❑ E. **Lumpectomy with axillary lymph node dissection and radiation therapy**

Key Concept/Objective: To understand the local treatment of early-stage breast cancer

The local management of early breast cancer has changed significantly in recent years, as breast-conservation therapy (BCT) has been shown to have survival rates identical to those of more extensive surgeries, such as radical mastectomy and modified radical mastectomy (MRM). In multiple clinical trials, a combination of lumpectomy and radiation therapy has yielded survival rates equivalent to those of MRM. Radiation therapy is a critical component of BCT because it reduces the recurrence rate from 40% to less than 10%. Axillary node dissection is important in diagnosis because positive nodes confer a worse prognosis and would prompt systemic chemotherapy. Sentinel node biopsy, in which the dominant axillary node is sampled and examined for tumor, is currently under investigation. If the sampled sentinel node is negative for tumor, the patient is spared the axillary node dissection and its morbidity. In general, BCT is preferred to MRM; MRM is indicated in cases in which radiation is contraindicated (such as in patients who have previously undergone breast irradiation or who are pregnant), in cases in which there is multifocal disease, or in cases in which there is strong patient preference. *(Answer: E—Lumpectomy with axillary lymph node dissection and radiation therapy)*

28. A 70-year-old woman presents for evaluation. Five years ago, she was diagnosed with stage II infiltrating ductal carcinoma of the right breast and was treated with lumpectomy and radiation. Over the past several weeks, she has experienced increasing fatigue and right upper quadrant pain. She denies having any bone pain. Physical examination reveals a hard, 3 cm palpable mass in the left breast (contralateral to her previous cancer); the examination is otherwise unremarkable. Results of laboratory testing include the following: AST, 78; ALT, 40; alkaline phosphatase, 200; total bilirubin, 1.3; and albumin, 3.0. CT of the abdomen shows three liver lesions that are consistent with metastases. Mammography reveals a spiculated mass in the left breast; a biopsy is performed, and the mass is found to be invasive ductal carcinoma that expresses both estrogen and progesterone receptors.

In this patient, first-line treatment should begin with which of the following?

❑ A. **Surgical resection of the breast nodule**

❑ B. **Radiation of the left breast**

❑ C. **Hormonal therapy**

❑ D. **High-dose chemotherapy with autologous stem cell transplantation**

❑ E. **Cytotoxic chemotherapy**

Key Concept/Objective: To understand the management of metastatic breast cancer

This patient presents with metastatic breast cancer. In such patients, the goal of treatment is not cure but palliation of symptoms and improved survival. The role of surgery in advanced disease is limited to situations such as the resection of a solitary chest wall nodule or orthopedic stabilization. Radiation therapy is used to palliate bony lesions or brain metastases. Endocrine therapy is the first-line treatment of hormone-responsive metastatic disease. In postmenopausal women, therapy is initiated with an antiestrogen and followed by aromatase inhibitors, progestins, and androgens or estrogens, in that order, if these therapies prove ineffective. If the patient's disease is unresponsive to hormonal therapy or is life-threatening, cytotoxic chemotherapy is initiated. Recent data have shown no advantage of CAF (cyclophosphamide, Adriamycin [doxorubicin], and fluorouracil) chemotherapy followed by high-dose alkylator therapy and stem cell support (autologous transplantation) as compared with CAF chemotherapy followed by CMF (cyclophosphamide, methotrexate, and fluorouracil) maintenance chemotherapy. *(Answer: C—Hormonal therapy)*

For more information, see Davidson NE: 12 Oncology: VII Breast Cancer. ACP Medicine Online (www.acpmedicine.com). Dale DC, Federman DD, Eds. WebMD Inc., New York, October 2004

Lung Cancer

29. A 44-year-old man comes to your clinic with questions about smoking cessation; he has smoked one and a half packs of cigarettes a day for the past 25 years. His father recently died of lung cancer, and your patient has decided to quit smoking. He wants to know about his risk of developing lung cancer.

Which of the following statements concerning the risk of this patient's developing lung cancer is true?

- ❑ **A. His risk would be no higher if he had smoked two packs a day than if he had smoked one pack a day**
- ❑ **B. If he does quit smoking now, in 20 years his risk of lung cancer will be the same as a man of the same age who never smoked**
- ❑ **C. With regard to his risk of lung cancer, it makes no difference whether he stops smoking now or in 10 years**
- ❑ **D. Even though he may quit smoking now, his risk of lung cancer will continue to rise with age**
- ❑ **E. When assessing risk of lung cancer, it does not matter at what age he started smoking**

Key Concept/Objective: To understand that age is a risk factor for the development of lung cancer and that, in former smokers, the risk of lung cancer increases with age

The following smoking factors have been identified as increasing lung cancer risk: aggregate amount of smoking; early onset of smoking; deeper inhalation; use of unfiltered cigarettes; high tar and nicotine content; and increasing age. A person who quits smoking does see a mortality benefit compared with someone of the same age who continues to smoke; however, the risk never returns to that of a lifelong nonsmoker. In addition, an American Cancer Society study showed that quitting at an earlier age (30 to 49 years) reduces risk more than quitting at a later age (50 to 64 years). *(Answer: D—Even though he may quit smoking now, his risk of lung cancer will continue to rise with age)*

30. A 52-year-old man comes to the office to ask if you know of any tests that will detect lung cancer at an early stage. He has a 45 pack-year history of smoking and continues to smoke.

For this patient, which of the following statements regarding screening for lung cancer is true?

- ❑ **A. Chest x-ray alone often fails to identify cancers that are potentially curable**
- ❑ **B. On the basis of best evidence, spiral computed tomography is currently the recommended screening tool**
- ❑ **C. Spiral CT combined with positron emission tomography (PET) has failed to detect early lung cancers**
- ❑ **D. There are no data to suggest that screening for lung cancer improves survival**

Key Concept/Objective: To understand that chest x-rays often miss curable cancers that are too small or indistinct to be detected

Clinical trails completed in the 1960s have shown the lack of efficacy of plain radiography as a screening tool for lung cancer. Spiral CT has been a promising technique, and at least one study has indicated a 5-year survival benefit to screening for lung cancer with spiral CT; however, other trials have failed to show any improvement in survival. The addition of PET scanning to CT of the chest has allowed the detection of early lung cancers in a few trials, but no randomized trials have been completed that have investigated the effect of the use of this combined diagnostic strategy on lung cancer mortality. There are currently insufficient data to allow an evidence-based recommendation regarding lung cancer screening with spiral CT, with or without the addition of PET scanning. *(Answer: A—Chest x-ray alone often fails to identify cancers that are potentially curable)*

31. A 63-year-old woman presents with a complaint of cough; the cough began 3 months ago. Evaluation further reveals a weight loss of 20 lb, left shoulder pain, generalized weakness, clubbing of the fingers, and loss of breath sounds in the left apex.

For this patient, which of the following statements regarding the clinical manifestations of lung cancer is false?

- ❑ A. **Cough is the most common symptom of a primary lung cancer**
- ❑ B. **Weight loss is not a specific symptom of lung cancer**
- ❑ C. **The left shoulder pain, if a manifestation of lung cancer, usually points to a tumor in the superior sulcus**
- ❑ D. **Clubbing is a paraneoplastic syndrome resulting from nail bed swelling and deformity**
- ❑ E. **Weakness may be the result of metastases or a paraneoplastic syndrome**

Key Concept/Objective: To know that clubbing is a common manifestation of lung cancer and that it arises from periosteal swelling of the distal phalanges

Cough is the most commonly reported symptom of a primary lung tumor. Weight loss, although cause of suspicion of lung cancer in this patient, may also be found in a variety of other illnesses, including other cancers, chronic infections, and collagen-vascular disorders. Shoulder and arm pain may be caused by a tumor of the superior sulcus involving the eighth cervical and first thoracic nerves. Weakness can arise from several mechanisms in lung cancer, including metastases, anemia, electrolyte disturbances, and Lambert-Eaton syndrome. *(Answer: D—Clubbing is a paraneoplastic syndrome resulting from nail bed swelling and deformity)*

32. A 62-year-old woman with a 65 pack-year history of smoking comes to your office complaining of blood-tinged sputum. She has also experienced weight loss of 20 lb and left-sided chest pain. Chest x-ray reveals a 4 cm opacity in the left lower lobe.

Which of the following statements regarding the evaluation and staging of a possible lung cancer in this patient is false?

- ❑ A. **CT of the chest is indicated; images should include the adrenal glands**
- ❑ B. **Staging of the cancer is more important than histologic type or degree of differentiation in determining prognosis**
- ❑ C. **Bone scanning is indicated to evaluate for bony metastases**
- ❑ D. **PET scanning, though not formally recommended at this point, may be helpful in identifying metastases, particularly those measuring more than 1 cm**
- ❑ E. **The procedure of choice for biopsy of most suspected peripheral lung cancers is thoracotomy**

Key Concept/Objective: To know that for most patients with peripheral lung masses, the procedure of choice for biopsy is video-assisted thoracoscopy (VATS) or needle biopsy

In the evaluation of a suspected lung cancer, the choice of biopsy technique depends on the site. If the lesion is centrally located or in the mediastinum, a bronchoscopy or mediastinoscopy is the procedure of choice; if the lesion is peripheral, VATS or CT-guided needle biopsy is preferred. If a metastatic site is identified, the patient should be offered the least invasive technique for diagnosis. Staging should include CT of the chest with visualization of the adrenals; CT of the head; and bone scanning. PET scanning is a promising technology and is being used in many centers; most data involve studies with lesions larger than 1 cm. The stage of the cancer is more important for prognosis than type or grade. *(Answer: E—The procedure of choice for biopsy of most suspected peripheral lung cancers is thoracotomy)*

For more information, see Crawford J: 12 Oncology: VIII Lung Cancer. ACP Medicine Online (www.acpmedicine.com). Dale DC, Federman DD, Eds. WebMD Inc., New York, February 2004

Prostate Cancer

33. A 65-year-old Chinese man comes to your indigent care clinic for routine health maintenance. He immigrated to the United States 35 years ago and works as a grocer. He has no complaints. Physical examination reveals poor dentition but is otherwise normal. Prostate examination reveals a smooth, normal-sized, symmetrical prostate. A lipid panel shows the LDL cholesterol level to be 95 mg/dl and the HDL cholesterol level to be 50 mg/dl. The prostate-specific antigen (PSA) level is 1.3 ng/ml.

Which of the following statements regarding this patient's risk of prostate cancer is true?

- ❑ **A. Advanced age is the most important risk factor for prostate cancer; most clinically detected prostate cancers are detected in the fifth and sixth decades of life**
- ❑ **B. Chinese men have a moderate risk of prostate cancer**
- ❑ **C. A diet high in red meat increases the risk of prostate cancer**
- ❑ **D. Men with low testosterone levels who develop prostate cancer are more likely to develop lower-grade prostate cancer**

Key Concept/Objective: To know that age, race, family history, diet, and hormone levels are important risk factors in the development of prostate cancer

Advancing age is the most obvious risk factor for prostate cancer; perhaps no other cancer is as age dependent. Most clinically detected prostate cancers are detected in the seventh and eighth decades of life. African Americans have the highest incidence of prostate cancer. The lowest incidence rates are in Japan and China. The dramatic differences between the Asian and Western diets possibly contribute to the significant difference in risk. Data from large cohort studies and case-control studies support the contentions that red meat, animal fat, and total fat consumption increase the risk of prostate cancer. In the Health Professionals Follow-up Study, men with lower testosterone levels who subsequently developed prostate cancer were more likely to develop higher-grade prostate cancer. *(Answer: C—A diet high in red meat increases the risk of prostate cancer)*

34. A 58-year-old white man presents to your clinic with a chief complaint of frequent urination. He awakes three or four times nightly to urinate. He denies having dysuria or hematuria. DRE reveals a smoothly enlarged prostate. Other results of the physical examination are normal. Results of a urinalysis are normal. The patient's PSA level is 4.0 ng/ml.

For this patient, which of the following statements regarding screening for prostate cancer is true?

- ❑ **A. Most cancers detected by DRE are confined to the prostate and are usually curable**
- ❑ **B. PSA is a glycoprotein with serine protease activity; it is a member of the kallikrein family and is produced only by malignant prostatic epithelial cells**
- ❑ **C. Biopsy of the prostate in men who have moderately elevated PSA levels (i.e., PSA of 4 to 10 ng/ml) usually reveals prostate cancer**
- ❑ **D. Prostate cancer is more likely when the total PSA level is high and the percentage of free PSA is low**

Key Concept/Objective: To understand that the goal of screening for prostate cancer is to detect organ-confined prostate cancer that is potentially curable

Optimal screening for prostate cancer combines use of the PSA test and the DRE. Historically, DRE was used to screen for prostate cancer. DRE is inadequate, however, because its interpretation is highly variable, many cancers are not palpable, and most cancers detectable by DRE are not organ confined and therefore are incurable. PSA, a glycoprotein with serine protease activity in the kallikrein family, is abundant in semen, where it dissolves seminal coagulum. Both normal and malignant prostatic epithelial cells produce PSA; production may actually be higher in normal cells than in malignant cells. A

problem with PSA-based screening is that an elevated PSA level lacks specificity. Despite the increased likelihood of prostate cancer in men with a moderately elevated serum PSA level (i.e., a level 4 to 10 ng/ml), biopsy usually reveals benign prostatic hyperplasia (BPH) rather than prostate cancer. Determination of the free PSA level (i.e., the percentage of PSA that is unbound to serum proteins) is also a potential means of distinguishing malignancy from benign hyperplasia. PSA derived from malignant epithelial cells tends to bind more avidly to serum proteins. Thus, in men with an elevated serum PSA level, cancer is more likely when the percentage of free PSA is low. *(Answer: D—Prostate cancer is more likely when the total PSA level is high and the percentage of free PSA is low)*

35. A 58-year-old white man with a PSA of 4.5 ng/ml and a normal DRE elects to undergo prostate biopsy to evaluate for prostate cancer. The biopsy is performed transrectally with ultrasound guidance, and multiple samples are obtained. The majority of tissue samples reveal BPH. However, one sample reveals prostate intraepithelial neoplasia (PIN).

For this patient, which of the following statements regarding the diagnosis of prostate cancer is true?

- ❑ **A. The most common prostate cancer is squamous epithelial cancer**
- ❑ **B. The most commonly used grading system for prostate cancer is the Gleason grading system**
- ❑ **C. PIN is a premalignant state; once diagnosed, further prostate biopsies are not indicated**
- ❑ **D. Clinical staging of prostate cancer relies on CT imaging and bone scanning to determine degree of metastatic disease**

Key Concept/Objective: To understand the role of multifactorial assessment in the diagnosis and stratification of patients with prostate cancer

The vast majority of prostate cancers are adenocarcinomas; small cell carcinomas, squamous cell carcinomas, and sarcomas are uncommon. The most commonly used grading system is the Gleason grading system, in which tumors are classified by the degree of disorganization of glandular structures. PIN represents a premalignant state; it is felt to predate true carcinoma and often coexists with carcinoma in the prostate gland. When biopsy reveals PIN but no actual cancer, further biopsies are warranted. The clinical stage of prostate cancer is based on the extent of disease assessed by palpation during DRE. Currently, prostate cancer is almost always diagnosed in men who have no radiographic evidence of metastases. The most clinically useful means of stratifying patients according to prognosis is through multifactorial staging—that is, through combined use of the clinical stage, the serum PSA level, and the Gleason score. *(Answer: B—The most commonly used grading system for prostate cancer is the Gleason grading system)*

36. A 76-year-old African-American man presents to the emergency department complaining of severe pain in the lower back and right hip. He reports that the pain has gotten gradually worse over the past month. He denies having other medical problems, and he has not seen a clinician for the past 10 years. He takes no medications. Results of physical examination are as follows: blood pressure, 130/60 mm Hg; heart rate, 88 beats/min; respiratory rate, 16 breaths/min; and temperature, 97.8° F (36.5° C). The lungs are clear. The cardiovascular examination is normal. The abdominal examination is benign with no organomegaly. Musculoskeletal examination reveals tenderness to palpation of the lumbar spine and right ischial tuberosity. Results of the neurologic examination are within normal limits. On DRE, the prostate is smooth and of normal size. Results of laboratory testing are as follows: WBC, 3,400 cells/mm^3; hematocrit, 42%; platelet count, 450,000 cells/mm^3. Bilirubin, aspartate aminotransferase (AST), and alanine aminotransferase (ALT) levels are normal, with an elevated alkaline phosphatase level of 240 mg/dl. The PSA level is 22 mg/dl.

For this patient, which of the following statements regarding the treatment of prostate cancer is true?

- ❑ **A. The only clear mortality benefit for radical prostatectomy is in patients with metastatic prostate cancer**

- ❑ B. External-beam radiation therapy may be preferable to radical prostatectomy for patients with localized prostate cancer because of the significantly decreased incidence of erectile dysfunction in patients treated with radiation
- ❑ C. The standard treatment for patients with advanced prostate cancer is androgen ablation
- ❑ D. Chemotherapy for hormone-resistant prostate cancer typically includes docetaxel plus prednisone; this treatment has been shown to improve quality of life but not decrease mortality

Key Concept/Objective: To understand the treatment of prostate cancer

In the United States, radical prostatectomy has been the standard treatment for prostate cancer and may offer the greatest chance of cancer control for patients with organ-confined prostate cancer. Radical prostatectomy is associated with urinary incontinence and erectile dysfunction; the frequency and severity of these side effects are a source of debate. In comparisons between radical prostatectomy and external-beam radiation therapy, men who undergo radical prostatectomy are more likely to have urinary incontinence or impotence, although significant decreases in sexual function are seen with both treatments; men who receive external-beam radiation therapy are more likely to suffer changes in bowel function. For patients with advanced prostate cancer, the standard initial treatment is androgen ablation, a therapeutic strategy that involves either lowering the production of testosterone or blocking its binding to the androgen receptor. Androgen ablation is achieved by a variety of strategies. Castration or diminishing testosterone production can be achieved surgically with orchiectomy or chemically with luteinizing hormone–releasing hormone agonists. Chemotherapy has a clear role in patients with hormone-refractory prostate cancer. Docetaxel plus prednisone is now the standard chemotherapy for men with metastatic prostate cancer. *(Answer: C—The standard treatment for patients with advanced prostate cancer is androgen ablation)*

37. A 65-year-old man attended a community-based health fair, where it was discovered that his PSA level was elevated; he was referred to your clinic. The patient states that he has always been healthy and that he has not seen a physician for years. On review of systems, he does note some frequency, hesitancy, and urgency of urination, which he has been experiencing for the past few years. DRE reveals a smooth, symmetrically enlarged prostate gland and brown guaiac-negative stool.

Which of the following is NOT associated with elevated PSA levels?

- ❑ A. Prostate cancer
- ❑ B. Benign prostatic hypertophy
- ❑ C. Urethritis
- ❑ D. Prostatitis

Key Concept/Objective: To know those conditions associated with elevated PSA levels

Screening for prostate cancer by use of PSA has led to an increase in the number of cases of prostate cancer diagnosed in recent years and has enhanced the ability to detect organ-confined prostate cancer. However, some prostate cancers do not produce sufficient amounts of PSA to result in elevations in PSA serum levels, and there are several other conditions that can lead to elevations in PSA levels. These conditions include BPH, prostatitis, seminal ejaculation, and genitourinary instrumentation. Uncomplicated urethritis cannot lead to an elevation in PSA level. *(Answer: C—Urethritis)*

38. A 58-year-old patient of yours is diagnosed with prostate cancer after PSA levels were found to be elevated. Transrectal ultrasonography-guided biopsy is performed, and it is determined that the patient has adenocarcinoma of the prostate, with a Gleason score of 8. He asks you about his prognosis and the likelihood that he will die of his prostate cancer.

Which of the following patients is most likely to die of prostate cancer?

- ❑ A. **A 40-year-old man with a Gleason score of 8**
- ❑ B. **A 40-year-old man with a Gleason score of 4**
- ❑ C. **A 75-year-old man with a Gleason score of 8**
- ❑ D. **A 75-year-old man with a Gleason score of 4**

Key Concept/Objective: To know the key prognostic factors for patients with prostate cancer

The Gleason grading system is the most commonly used method of classifying prostate cancers. Tumors are graded from 1 (least malignant) to 5 (most malignant) on the basis of histologic findings. The two most common patterns observed are then added together to give a composite score. The majority of tumors are classified as Gleason 6 or 7, with grades of 7 or more considered high grade. In the Connecticut Tumor Registry, the two most important determinants of mortality from prostate cancer were age and Gleason grade. The patients at highest risk of dying of prostate cancer are those younger than 74 years and those with Gleason scores of 7 or higher. *(Answer: A—A 40-year-old man with a Gleason score of 8)*

39. A 70-year-old patient has been seeing you for treatment of hypertension for several years. Recently, you referred him to a urologist after a prostatic nodule was discovered on DRE and his PSA level was found to be elevated. The urologist diagnosed the patient as having prostate cancer on the basis of the results of a biopsy. He has offered the patient the option of radical prostatectomy or external-beam radiation therapy. The patient asks you about the side effects of these treatments.

Which of the following statements is false?

- ❑ A. **Most patients undergoing radical prostatectomy will become impotent**
- ❑ B. **Erectile dysfunction occurs in a minority of patients undergoing external-beam radiation therapy**
- ❑ C. **Radical prostatectomy is more likely to produce urinary incontinence or impotence than is external-beam radiation therapy**
- ❑ D. **External-beam radiation therapy is more likely to result in a decline in bowel function than is radical prostatectomy**

Key Concept/Objective: To know the major adverse side effects of radical prostatectomy and external-beam radiation therapy

Adverse side effects are frequent and significant in patients undergoing radical prostatectomy and external-beam radiation therapy. It is important to consider these adverse effects when deciding on a course of treatment. Stress urinary incontinence and erectile dysfunction are frequent in those undergoing radical prostatectomy. In fact, most patients undergoing the procedure are rendered impotent. The rates of both of these adverse effects are higher in patients undergoing radical prostatectomy than in those who receive external-beam radiation therapy. However, erectile dysfunction still occurs in the majority of patients who undergo radiation therapy. In addition, a decline in bowel function is more common in patients receiving external-beam radiation therapy than in those who undergo radical prostatectomy. *(Answer: B—Erectile dysfunction occurs in a minority of patients undergoing external-beam radiation therapy)*

40. A 60-year-old man comes to you because he has heard there is a blood test for prostate cancer that he would like to be given. You explain that the decision to undergo screening for prostate cancer is not as simple as it might seem, and you want him to understand the screening process.

Which of the following statements should be included in your explanation to this patient?

- ❑ A. **Although one-time or repeated screening and aggressive treatment of prostate cancer may save lives and avert future cancer-related illness, we do not yet know this for certain**
- ❑ B. **The available tests for prostate cancer (PSA and DRE) will sometimes indicate cancer when there is none (false positives) and will sometimes fail to detect cancer when it is present (false negatives)**

- ❑ C. **A positive result on PSA or DRE will suggest that he should undergo invasive testing, such as transrectal ultrasound and prostate biopsy**
- ❑ D. **Should he be found to have prostate cancer, he will want to consider aggressive therapy, and there is a small but finite risk of early death and a significant risk of chronic illness, particularly with regard to sexual and urinary function**
- ❑ E. **All of the above**

Key Concept/Objective: To understand the uncertainty surrounding screening for prostate cancer, and be able to communicate that uncertainty intelligibly to patients

There is disagreement as to whether men should be screened for prostate cancer. It is important to understand that it is not yet known whether screening for prostate cancer will help men live longer and that significant morbidity and mortality have been associated with the diagnostic and therapeutic procedures involved in screening. These facts should be conveyed to the patient to help him make an informed decision. *(Answer: E—All of the above)*

41. A 65-year-old man who is otherwise in excellent health comes to you for a second opinion regarding therapy for his recently diagnosed prostate cancer. His records show that his cancer was diagnosed on the basis of a screening PSA level of 5.0; his DRE result at the time was negative. Transrectal ultrasound revealed no apparent tumor, but four of six random biopsy specimens tested positive for cancer. His Gleason score is 7.

What is this patient's risk of biochemical relapse (rising PSA) after local therapy?

- ❑ A. **Low, because his clinical tumor stage is T1c**
- ❑ B. **Low, because his clinical tumor stage is T1c and his PSA level is less than 10**
- ❑ C. **Intermediate, because his clinical tumor stage is T2b**
- ❑ D. **Intermediate, because his Gleason score is 7**
- ❑ E. **High, because a Gleason score of 7 indicates a high-grade tumor**

Key Concept/Objective: To understand the clinical staging of prostate cancer

Clinical staging is based on the means of diagnosis and the size and location of the tumor. This patient's tumor is stage T1c because it is not palpable and was found by biopsy after a positive PSA screening result. In such cases, risk of biochemical relapse (i.e., rising PSA level) is further assessed on the basis of clinical stage, PSA level, and Gleason score. Because this patient's Gleason score is 7, his risk category is intermediate, even though his PSA level and clinical stage are relatively low. This case highlights the point that the tumors of patients whose Gleason scores are greater than 6 should be considered high grade. *(Answer: D—Intermediate, because his Gleason score is 7)*

42. ***From your assessment of risk for the patient in Question 41, what is the best advice that you can give him about treatment?***

- ❑ A. **It is highly likely that his tumor is confined to the prostate, so radical prostatectomy, external-beam radiation, brachytherapy, and watchful waiting are all reasonable options**
- ❑ B. **There is about a 50% chance of recurrence in 5 years, so radical prostatectomy is of no benefit**
- ❑ C. **There is about a 50% chance of recurrence in 5 years, and radical prostatectomy is curative in 50% of patients with his profile**
- ❑ D. **There is conclusive evidence that external-beam radiation is superior to radical prostatectomy in patients with his profile**

❑ E. **It is very likely that his cancer has spread beyond the prostate, so the risks of radical prostatectomy are not justified; external-beam radiation with androgen ablation is a better choice**

Key Concept/Objective: To understand that treatment options for patients with clinically localized prostate cancer depend on the patient's risk of biochemical relapse

Because this patient is at intermediate risk, he has a 50% chance of relapse. Although this means that 50% of men with cancer of this stage will have clinically silent metastases, radical prostatectomy is curative in 50% of men in this risk group who undergo that procedure. There are as yet no data to suggest that prostatectomy or radiation therapy is of benefit with regard to mortality, and patients should be educated about the risks and benefits of both. *(Answer: C—There is about a 50% chance of recurrence in 5 years, and radical prostatectomy is curative in 50% of patients with his profile)*

43. The patient in Question 41 elects to undergo external-beam radiation. For 3 years, his PSA result is negative, then it rises to 2.8.

Which of the following treatment regimens has the best data to support it?

❑ A. **Salvage radical prostatectomy**

❑ B. **Salvage radical prostatectomy and either surgical castration or chemical castration with LHRH agonists**

❑ C. **Repeated external-beam radiation and either surgical castration or chemical castration with LHRH agonists**

❑ D. **Antiandrogens, such as flutamide, bicalutamide, and nilutamide, and either surgical castration or chemical castration with LHRH agonists**

❑ E. **Antiandrogens, such as flutamide, bicalutamide, and nilutamide**

Key Concept/Objective: To know the therapies available for advanced prostate cancer and which to select, given the patient's previous treatment

Because this patient initially underwent radiation therapy, he is not a candidate for salvage radical prostatectomy, because in such patients, the higher morbidity and mortality of the procedure outweigh the benefits. Neither would further radiation treatment be of benefit. From the available data, the best therapy would be to combine lowering of testosterone levels (which can be effected either surgically or through hormonal manipulation wih LHRH analogues) and treatment with antiandrogens, such as flutamide, bicalutamide, or nilutamide. *(Answer: D—Antiandrogens, such as flutamide, bicalutamide, and nilutamide, and either surgical castration or chemical castration with LHRH agonists)*

For more information, see Kantoff PW: 12 Oncology: IX Prostate Cancer. ACP Medicine Online (www.acpmedicine.com). Dale DC, Federman DD, Eds. WebMD Inc., New York, December 2004

Gynecologic Cancer

44. A 67-year-old nulliparous white woman presents to the clinic for evaluation of increasing abdominal girth and bloating; these symptoms have been occurring for several months and are associated with some abdominal discomfort. She previously underwent upper GI evaluation, the results of which were negative. She has not had a gynecologic examination for several years, but she denies having any vaginal bleeding or discharge. She also denies having any other relevant medical history, but her sister and her mother have breast cancer.

Which of the following gynecologic cancers is most likely for this patient?

❑ A. **Cervical cancer**

❑ B. **Uterine cancer**

❑ C. **Ovarian germ cell cancer**

❑ D. **Ovarian epithelial cell cancer**

❑ E. **Ovarian stromal cell cancer**

Key Concept/Objective: To know the common gynecologic cancer risk factors and clinical presentation

Epithelial ovarian cancer occurs at a mean age of 60 years in the United States and is the most lethal of gynecologic tract tumors. In approximately 70% of women, the tumor has spread beyond the pelvis by the time of diagnosis. Temporary suppression of menstrual function is associated with a decreased risk of epithelial ovarian cancer. Nulliparity is associated with an increased risk of ovarian cancer. Women with advanced disease often note a progressive increase in abdominal girth and bloating for several months before they are diagnosed. These symptoms are caused by malignant ascites. Because of the nonspecific nature of the abdominal complaints, which are related to the presence of ascites and omental disease, many patients initially undergo an upper GI tract evaluation for a possible ulcer before the true nature of the illness is recognized. Two familial syndromes are associated with an increased risk of ovarian cancer. A family history suggestive of a genetic predisposition may be found in as many as 10% of patients with ovarian cancer. The breast-ovarian cancer syndrome, as the name implies, occurs in families whose members may have breast, ovarian, or both types of cancers. Mutations in the *BRCA1* or *BRCA2* genes are responsible for this syndrome. Ovarian germ cell tumors are derived from the oocyte and often occur in women younger than 20 years. Ovarian stromal cell tumors are derived from supporting elements such as granulosa or theca cells, which are normally responsible for sex steroid production. These tumors are characterized by their ability to secrete estradiol. Postmenopausal women present with breast tenderness, vaginal bleeding, or both. Women with cervical and uterine cancers most commonly present with vaginal bleeding or a grossly visible cervical lesion. *(Answer: D—Ovarian epithelial cell cancer)*

45. A 72-year-old woman presents with vaginal bleeding of 2 weeks' duration. Her medical history is significant for right breast cancer, which was surgically cured and for which she takes tamoxifen. She has not had any other surgeries. Evaluation of this patient shows endometrial cancer.

Under which of the following circumstances is chemotherapy indicated for this patient?

❑ A. **After initial surgical intervention, the patient experiences rapidly progressive, symptomatic recurrence of the cancer**

❑ B. **The cancer involves either ovary on initial evaluation**

❑ C. **The cancer involves the uterus and cervix**

❑ D. **The cancer involves distant sites such as lung or bone**

❑ E. **All of the above**

Key Concept/Objective: To understand the evaluation and treatment of uterine cancer

For rapidly progressive, symptomatic recurrence of uterine cancer, platinum-based chemotherapy is a reasonable treatment. There is no proven survival advantage associated with the use of adjuvant hormonal therapy (e.g., progestational agents) or chemotherapy, although these modalities may be useful for the management of systemic relapse. If the endometrial biopsy establishes the presence of uterine cancer, surgery for definitive resection and staging is the next most common step in management. For patients who are not optimal surgical candidates, primary radiotherapy is an option that can produce long-term survival in selected patients. Postoperative pelvic radiotherapy is considered when certain features confer an increased risk of local pelvic failure. These features include (1) deeply invasive, high-grade, early stage lesions (e.g., stage IC, grade III), especially with lymphovascular involvement, as these features are associated with an approximately 20% risk of occult pelvic lymph node involvement, and (2) cervical involvement (i.e., stage II), which confers an increased risk of vaginal vault recurrence. The use of tamoxifen, a drug traditionally thought of as an estrogen antagonist, is also associated with an increased uterine cancer risk. This is in part caused by the tissue-specific action of tamoxifen, which has antagonistic effects on proliferation of breast epithelium but agonistic effects on bone mineral density, lipid metabolism, and endometrial proliferation. However, the benefits of

tamoxifen in the adjuvant breast cancer setting far outweigh the small risk of uterine cancer development. *(Answer: A—After initial surgical intervention, the patient experiences rapidly progressive, symptomatic recurrence of the cancer)*

46. A 50-year-old white woman with a history of fibrocystic breast disease and arthritis presents with abdominal pain of new onset. The patient describes the pain as an ache. The pain is mild and suprapubic and does not radiate. A urine dipstick evaluation performed in the clinic reveals that she has a urinary tract infection. The patient, however, is concerned that she may have ovarian cancer, because her mother died of ovarian cancer at age 59.

For this patient, which of the following statements is consistent with a diagnosis of ovarian cancer?

- ❑ A. **Approximately 30% of women present with advanced disease**
- ❑ B. **Patients with advanced disease commonly complain of a progressive increase in abdominal girth and bloating**
- ❑ C. **The primary lymphatic drainage site of ovarian cancer is the inguinal lymph nodes**
- ❑ D. **The most common paraneoplastic syndrome associated with ovarian cancer is hypercalcemia**

Key Concept/Objective: To understand the common clinical features of ovarian cancer

The ovary contains three distinct cell types, known as germ cells, stromal cells, and epithelial cells. The type of ovarian tumor that most commonly affects adult women, however, is derived from the epithelial cells that cover the ovarian surface. Epithelial ovarian cancer occurs at a mean age of 60 years in the United States and is the most lethal of gynecologic tract tumors. In approximately 70% of women, the tumor has spread beyond the pelvis by the time of diagnosis and cannot be completely resected at the time of exploratory laparotomy. Early-onset ovarian cancer that is restricted to the pelvis usually produces no signs or symptoms. Unfortunately, approximately 70% of women present with advanced disease that has extended beyond the pelvis to involve other areas, such as the upper abdomen (stage III) and the pleural space (stage IV). Women with advanced disease often note a progressive increase in abdominal girth and bloating for several months before they are diagnosed. These symptoms are caused by malignant ascites. The tumor can spread via the lymphatics to involve the para-aortic lymph node chain, which is the primary drainage site for the ovaries (as with the testes). In rare instances, patients may present with inguinal adenopathy as the first sign of disease. A large omental tumor cake can cause early satiety and weight loss as a result of gastric compression; however, weight loss is more commonly offset by the development of ascites. *(Answer: B—Patients with advanced disease commonly complain of a progressive increase in abdominal girth and bloating)*

47. A 65-year-old African-American woman presents with progressive increase in abdominal girth, bloating, and early satiety. A CT scan reveals a large left ovarian mass, ascites, and omental studding. The patient is sent for exploratory laparotomy and undergoes debulking. The tissue diagnosis is epithelial ovarian cancer.

For this patient, which of the following statements regarding the treatment of ovarian cancer is true?

- ❑ A. **Ovarian cancer relapse can be treated with the same chemotherapeutic drugs and has the same disease-free survival rate as those used for primary therapy**
- ❑ B. **All women with ovarian cancer, even low-risk stage I disease, derive benefit from postoperative adjuvant chemotherapy**
- ❑ C. **The mainstay of treatment for advanced-stage ovarian cancer is total abdominal hysterectomy with bilateral oophorectomy plus debulking and partial omentectomy, followed by a combination chemotherapy regimen containing a taxane and a platinum analogue**

❑ D. **Platinum compounds, such as carboplatin and cisplatin, exert their cytotoxic effects by binding to and stabilizing the tubulin polymer during mitotic spindle formation**

Key Concept/Objective: To understand the basic treatment for ovarian cancer

Exploratory laparotomy for evaluation of suspected ovarian cancer is typically performed with a vertical midline incision to provide adequate visualization of the upper abdomen. If the suspicion of epithelial ovarian cancer is confirmed by frozen section, a bilateral salpingo-oophorectomy and total abdominal hysterectomy are usually performed, along with a partial omentectomy. Other sites of tumor involvement are carefully evaluated with palpation and biopsy of the undersides of the diaphragm, the serosal surfaces of the bowel, and the paracolic gutters. The para-aortic lymph nodes are typically assessed when information about lymph node status would change patient management or when precise surgical staging is required to determine eligibility for protocol therapy. Finally, an attempt is made to remove as much tumor as possible at the time of initial surgery (debulking), because patients with residual tumor measuring less than 1 cm in diameter are more likely to respond to chemotherapy and have an improved survival rate. Some women with ovarian cancer have low-risk features that confer a 5-year survival rate of about 95%. Members of this low-risk group have stage IA or stage IB disease that is well-differentiated or moderately well-differentiated (i.e., grade I or II). These patients do not generally derive benefit from the use of postoperative adjuvant therapy. The goal of treatment of ovarian cancer relapse is palliation of symptoms. For patients with relapse detected only by the finding of an elevation of the CA-125 level, there is no convincing evidence that second-line, cytotoxic chemotherapy improves survival rate; however, it can compromise quality of life at a time when patients are feeling well. Platinum compounds, such as carboplatin and cisplatin, exert their cytotoxic effects by inducing DNA damage, primarily through the formation of intrastrand cross-links. *(Answer: C—The mainstay of treatment for advanced-stage ovarian cancer is total abdominal hysterectomy with bilateral oophorectomy plus debulking and partial omentectomy, followed by a combination chemotherapy regimen containing a taxane and a platinum analogue)*

48. A 45-year-old white woman presents to your clinic with postcoital bleeding. She has not had a Papanicolaou (Pap) smear or pelvic examination in 15 years, despite the fact that she has multiple risk factors for cervical cancer. A Pap smear and pelvic examination are performed, and you diagnose her as having cervical cancer.

For this patient, which of the following statements regarding cervical cancer is false?

❑ A. **Cervical cancer is associated with human papillomavirus (HPV)**

❑ B. **Risk factors for cervical cancer include multiple male sexual partners, sexual intercourse at an early age, and immunosuppression**

❑ C. **Cervical cancer staging is based entirely on clinical criteria**

❑ D. **Cervical cancer is a rapidly progressing malignancy**

Key Concept/Objective: To understand the basic risk factors for and clinical features of cervical cancer

Invasive cervical cancer is uncommon in developed countries, partly because of the effectiveness of Pap smear screening. Nevertheless, it is estimated that in the United States in 2001, cervical cancer affected 12,900 women and caused approximately 4,400 deaths. Part of the success of Pap smear screening is due to the fact that this approach typically detects premalignant lesions, as opposed to invasive cancer. This unique feature makes it possible to eradicate precursor lesions before the development of frankly invasive cancers. In addition, the interval of time between the development of a precursor lesion and the occurrence of invasive disease may be several years, thus allowing many opportunities for the detection and eradication of premalignant disease. Cervical cancer is typically a disease of women in their fifth and sixth decades, whereas premalignant cervical lesions are often discovered in women younger than 40 years. This rather large gap in the age distribution between precursor lesions and invasive cancer is indicative of a long latency period for

malignant transformation. Infection with HPV, most commonly subtypes 16, 18, 31, 33, and 35, is largely responsible for the development of precursor lesions and subsequent transformation to invasive disease. Not surprisingly, factors that predispose to transmission of this virus are associated with an increased risk of the development of cervical cancer. These high-risk factors are sexual intercourse at an early age, multiple male sexual partners, and male sexual partners who themselves have multiple partners. A history of smoking also confers a higher risk. Immunosuppression associated with either an underlying lymphoproliferative disorder such as Hodgkin disease or immunosuppressive drugs used in the prevention of allograft rejection also confers a higher risk of cervical cancer. In women with HIV infection, the immunosuppressive state associated with the infection increases the risk of development of cervical precursor lesions, although it is not clear whether the development of such lesions results in a higher incidence of invasive cervical disease. *(Answer: D—Cervical cancer is a rapidly progressing malignancy)*

For more information, see Cannistra SA: 12 Oncology: X Gynecologic Cancer. ACP Medicine Online (www.acpmedicine.com). Dale DC, Federman DD, Eds. WebMD Inc., New York, March 2004

Oncologic Emergencies

49. A 57-year-old woman with recently diagnosed stage IIIb squamous cell lung cancer presents to clinic with complaints of anorexia, fatigue, and diffuse abdominal discomfort. Additionally, her husband expresses concern that she has been more forgetful of late. Physical examination is largely unrevealing. Routine laboratory data are significant for a serum calcium level of 13.2 mg/dl. The patient is diagnosed with hypercalcemia of malignancy and is admitted to the hospital for management of this condition.

Which of the following treatments is contraindicated in patients with hypercalcemia of malignancy?

- ❑ A. **Thiazide diuretics**
- ❑ B. **Loop diuretics**
- ❑ C. **Infusion of I.V. normal saline**
- ❑ D. **Bisphosphonates**
- ❑ E. **Glucocorticoids**

Key Concept/Objective: To understand the management of hypercalcemia of malignancy

Hypercalcemia of malignancy occurs in 10% to 20% of patients with cancer at some time during their illness. The treatment of patients with hypercalcemia of malignancy includes volume and electrolyte repletion, inhibition of bone resorption, and treatment of the underlying malignancy. Extracellular volume deficits exist in all patients with symptomatic hypercalcemia of malignancy. The single most important and urgent treatment is the infusion of normal saline to correct the extracellular volume deficit, increase the glomerular filtration rate, and, secondarily, increase renal calcium excretion. Loop diuretics should not be used until after the volume deficit has been fully corrected. Loop diuretics cause calciuresis and therefore may be effective in acutely decreasing calcium levels after volume repletion. Thiazide diuretics decrease renal calcium excretion and should be specifically avoided. The bisphosphonates offer an improved and simplified treatment of hypercalcemia of malignancy. The bisphosphonates have a high affinity for areas of high bone turnover, such as areas of bony involvement with malignancy, where they block osteoclast attachment to bone matrix and osteoclast recruitment and differentiation. *(Answer: A—Thiazide diuretics)*

50. A 72-year-old man with prostate cancer presents to the emergency department complaining of back pain. On further questioning, the patient reports having difficulty with ambulation for the past week, but he denies having bladder or bowel dysfunction. Physical examination reveals focal midthoracic vertebral body tenderness to percussion, 4/5 strength in the bilateral lower extremities, and normal patellar reflexes bilaterally. While plans for further evaluation are being made, the patient is treated with I.V. dexamethasone because of concern for epidural spinal cord compression.

Which of the following imaging modalities of the spine is recommended to evaluate for this complication?

❑ **A. Plain films**

❑ **B. Radionuclide bone scan**

❑ **C. Myelography**

❑ **D. Gadolinium-enhanced MRI**

❑ **E. CT with contrast**

Key Concept/Objective: To know that the current recommendation for the radiographic evaluation of patients with possible epidural spinal cord compression is gadolinium-enhanced MRI

Epidural spinal cord compression should be suspected on the basis of the symptoms reported by the patient and the signs elicited by the physician on physical examination. Imaging of the spine provides the definitive diagnosis and the localization of the level of epidural spinal cord compression. Myelography, CT myelography, and gadolinium-enhanced MRI of the spine are the most sensitive and specific methods of evaluation. However, myelography is invasive and may be uncomfortable for the patient with severe bone pain; in addition, radiologists experienced in its interpretation may not be available. CT of the spine should not be performed, because its ability to scan the entire spinal axis efficiently and its sensitivity in identifying epidural disease are inferior to those of gadolinium-enhanced MRI. The current recommendation for the radiographic evaluation of patients with suspected epidural compression is gadolinium-enhanced MRI of the entire spinal axis. *(Answer: D—Gadolinium-enhanced MRI)*

51. A 63-year-old woman with no significant medical history presents to clinic with the report of facial swelling. Physical examination confirms the patient's report of facial swelling and reveals distention of the jugular veins. A chest radiograph reveals superior mediastinal widening when compared with an earlier radiograph. Subsequently, contrast-enhanced CT of the chest reveals mediastinal lymphadenopathy and external compression of the superior vena cava (SVC) by an enlarged node.

What is the most appropriate step to take next in the management of this patient?

❑ **A. Immediate initiation of mediastinal irradiation**

❑ **B. Fine-needle aspiration of an enlarged mediastinal lymph node**

❑ **C. Positron emission tomography**

❑ **D. Initiation of anticoagulation with warfarin**

❑ **E. Thoracic MRI**

Key Concept/Objective: To be aware that recent experience in adults suggests that SVC syndrome is not a true emergency and that histologic diagnosis should be quickly established and treatment promptly initiated

SVC syndrome is most commonly caused by extrinsic compression of the thin-walled, low-pressure SVC by a malignant mediastinal mass such as bronchogenic carcinoma (especially small cell lung cancer) and non-Hodgkin lymphoma. Before a histologic diagnosis is established, emergency treatment with mediastinal irradiation is only warranted in children and occasionally in adults who have mental status alteration, other life-threatening manifestations of increased intracranial pressure, cardiovascular collapse, or evidence of upper airway obstruction. In the absence of such conditions, as with this patient, the next step in the management of SVC syndrome should focus on efforts to obtain a histologic diagnosis of the underlying condition so that appropriate therapy may be initiated. Obtaining further radiologic studies will not assist in making a histologic diagnosis and are therefore not the most appropriate next step in the management of this patient. *(Answer: B—Fine-needle aspiration of an enlarged mediastinal lymph node)*

52. A 39-year-old woman with a history of T2N2M0 breast cancer presents with dyspnea that has been increasing over the past 3 days. She has no pleuritic chest pain. She received six cycles of chemotherapy with cyclophosphamide, doxorubicin, and fluorouracil; the chemotherapy ended 6 months ago. On examination, her blood pressure is 80/60 mm Hg and her pulse is 120 beats/min. Her jugular venous pressure is elevated to 10 cm, and her lungs are clear. She has trace edema in the lower extremities. Chest x-ray reveals cardiomegaly with no pleural effusions or infiltrates.

What is the most likely diagnosis for this patient?

- ❑ **A. Doxorubicin-induced cardiomyopathy**
- ❑ **B. Pericardial tamponade**
- ❑ **C. Pulmonary embolus**
- ❑ **D. Tension pneumothorax**
- ❑ **E. Superior vena cava syndrome**

Key Concept/Objective: To be able to recognize the typical signs and symptoms of pericardial tamponade

This patient presents with dyspnea, hypotension, and elevated neck veins. She does not have signs or x-ray findings of left ventricular failure. She has significant risk of malignant pericardial disease (T2N2M0 breast cancer). The most likely diagnosis is cardiac tamponade caused by malignant pericardial disease. She is at risk for doxorubicin-induced cardiomyopathy, but her physical examination and chest x-ray do not show evidence of left-sided heart failure. A pulmonary embolus could cause dyspnea, hypotension, and acute right heart failure. Her cardiomegaly is not consistent with an acute pulmonary embolus. Both doxorubicin-induced cardiomyopathy and pulmonary embolus are important considerations, though these are less likely in this patient than pericardial tamponade. An echocardiogram would be the most useful test to sort out these diagnostic possibilities. Tension pneumothorax and superior vena cava syndrome are unlikely because of the chest x-ray results. *(Answer: B—Pericardial tamponade)*

53. A 63-year-old woman with acute myeloid leukemia (AML) after chemotherapy presents for follow-up. She has been tired but is not having any fevers or bleeding. On examination, the patient is pale, with a grade II/VI systolic ejection murmur at the left sternal border. Laboratory test results are as follows: Hb, 8; HCT, 24; platelet count, 15,000; WBC, 1.8.

What would you recommend for this patient?

- ❑ **A. Platelet transfusions to maintain a platelet count greater than 20,000**
- ❑ **B. Platelet transfusions to maintain a platelet count greater than 50,000**
- ❑ **C. Platelet transfusion if patient has bleeding or if the platelet count drops below 10,000**
- ❑ **D. Platelet transfusion if patient experiences bleeding**

Key Concept/Objective: To understand the risks associated with platelet transfusions and the basis for recommending platelet transfusions in leukemia patients with thrombocytopenia

This patient has thrombocytopenia related to her AML, her chemotherapy, or both. Although the best time to intervene with platelet therapy is somewhat controversial, there is a growing consensus that treatment should be initiated if the platelet count is low and the patient is bleeding and that prophylactic platelet therapy should be started only when the count is below 10,000. *(Answer: C—Platelet transfusion if patient has bleeding or if the platelet count drops below 10,000)*

54. A 26-year-old woman with Hodgkin disease presents after her third cycle of chemotherapy. She had her last chemotherapy session 10 days ago. She does not have cough, pleuritic chest pain, or abdominal pain. Her temperature is 103.8° F (39.8° C); her pulse is 100 beats/min; her respiration rate is 18 breaths/min; her skin is without rashes; her chest is clear; she is without heart murmur; and her abdomen is soft. Chest x-ray shows no infiltrates. The WBC is 0.7 (200 neutrophils, 400 lymphocytes, 100 basophils).

What would you recommend next for this patient?

- ❑ A. **Blood, sputum, and urine cultures**
- ❑ B. **Blood, sputum, and urine cultures; begin amoxicillin-clavulanate**
- ❑ C. **Blood, sputum, and urine cultures; begin ceftriaxone**
- ❑ D. **Blood, sputum, and urine cultures; begin ceftazidime and tobramycin**
- ❑ E. **Blood, sputum, and urine cultures; begin granulocyte colony-stimulating factor**

Key Concept: To understand the approach to the treatment of patients with neutropenic fevers

This patient with chemotherapy-induced neutropenia has a fever, and her examination does not suggest a cause of this fever. She should receive antibiotics that provide coverage of gram-negative rods, including *Pseudomonas aeruginosa*, as well as gram-positive coverage. There is no one optimal treatment regimen. Studies have shown that monotherapy with imipenem and ceftazidime have been as effective as two-drug combinations. In this patient, amoxicillin-clavulanate would not provide broad enough coverage against gram-negative rods. Several studies have suggested that oral quinolone therapy may be an option in selected patients. Ceftriaxone would not offer *Pseudomonas* coverage. *(Answer: D—Blood, sputum, and urine cultures; begin ceftazidime and tobramycin)*

For more information, see Carlson RW: 12 Oncology: XII Oncologic Emergencies. ACP Medicine Online (www.acpmedicine.com). Dale DC, Federman DD, Eds. WebMD Inc., New York, December 2002

Sarcomas of Soft Tissue and Bone

55. A 40-year-old white woman presents to your office complaining of a painful, rapidly enlarging mass on her chest. The mass has been present for 1 month. She has a history of Hodgkin disease, for which she underwent radiotherapy 20 years ago. Biopsy reveals osteosarcoma.

Which of the following statements is true regarding this patient?

- ❑ A. **Sarcomas arising in radiation ports are more resistant to chemotherapy**
- ❑ B. **Her risk of developing a sarcoma after radiotherapy was 10%**
- ❑ C. **Her case is unusual in that most cases of sarcoma related to radiotherapy occur approximately 40 years after exposure to radiation**
- ❑ D. **The most common type of sarcoma associated with previous radiotherapy is not osteosarcoma but rather leiomyosarcoma**

Key Concept/Objective: To know that radiotherapy is a risk factor for sarcoma

Patients who have undergone radiotherapy are at increased risk for developing sarcoma. Sarcomas arising in radiation ports are more resistant to chemotherapy. The risk of a secondary sarcoma after radiation exposure is substantially less than 1%, and the patient is typically exposed to radiation 4 to 20 years before the development of sarcoma. Most radiation-associated sarcomas are osteosarcomas. *(Answer: A—Sarcomas arising in radiation ports are more resistant to chemotherapy)*

56. A 55-year-old man presents for evaluation of an enlarging mass in his left upper extremity. He first noticed the mass 3 months ago. It is painless, and the only reason he is concerned is because it continues to enlarge. Results of CT scanning and biopsy are consistent with soft tissue sarcoma.

Which of the following statements regarding this patient is true?

- ❑ A. **The grade of the tumor is based on the amount of necrosis seen on imaging**
- ❑ B. **His prognosis would be better if he had an intra-abdominal or retroperitoneal tumor**

❑ C. The 5-year survival rates for patients with sarcomas (excluding intra-abdominal and retroperitoneal sarcomas) are similar when corrected for grade, size, and depth

❑ D. Patients with high-grade tumors have an unusually poor prognosis, even when the tumors are less than 5 cm

Key Concept/Objective: To understand the basic principles regarding the grading and staging of sarcomas, as well as prognosis

Staging of sarcomas is based on tumor size, grade, and depth. The 5-year survival rates for patients with soft tissue sarcomas arising in different anatomic sites are similar when corrected for grade, size, and depth, except for intra-abdominal and retroperitoneal tumors, which tend to be large and to invade vital organs, even if they are low grade. Patients with low-grade, superficial tumors tend to do well if the tumors are adequately resected. Even patients with high-grade tumors have a good prognosis if the tumors are less than 5 cm in diameter. Tumor grade is based largely on the number of mitoses per high-powered field (magnification, 10×). *(Answer: C—The 5-year survival rates for patients with sarcomas [excluding intra-abdominal and retroperitoneal sarcomas] are similar when corrected for grade, size, and depth)*

57. A patient is referred to you by his dermatologist for evaluation of a soft tissue mass on his leg. You obtain an MRI of the primary lesion and a CT scan of the chest, because you are concerned about the possibility of soft tissue sarcoma. You recommend that an incisional biopsy be performed for definitive diagnosis. The patient wants to know how you would treat such a tumor.

Which of the following is true regarding the general treatment of soft tissue sarcomas?

❑ A. Soft tissue sarcomas are usually well encapsulated and are seen to have clear margins on resection

❑ B. Local control of soft tissue sarcomas consists of surgical resection, often with radiotherapy

❑ C. Chemotherapy is never indicated for soft tissue sarcomas

❑ D. The presence of necrosis on MRI suggests a low-grade sarcoma

Key Concept/Objective: To understand the basic principles of sarcoma therapy

The goals of the treatment of sarcomas are local and systemic control of the sarcoma; preservation of the extremity or organ function; and quality of life. Local control of a soft tissue sarcoma is generally achieved by surgical resection, which is often combined with radiotherapy. Low-grade tumors push aside contiguous structures, whereas high-grade tumors invade adjacent organs and have large areas of necrosis. Soft tissue sarcomas grow along histologic planes and are usually pseudoencapsulated (i.e., microscopic projections of tumor extend beyond the apparent tumor capsule). Any excision that merely "shells out" the apparently encapsulated tumor generally leaves behind microscopic residual tumor, resulting in regrowth of the tumor 80% of the time. Multimodality therapy, including chemotherapy, is routine therapy for osteosarcomas, rhabdomyosarcomas, and Ewing sarcoma. *(Answer: B—Local control of soft tissue sarcomas consists of surgical resection, often with radiotherapy)*

58. A 48-year-old black woman presents to your office for follow-up. She was recently admitted to the hospital for upper gastrointestinal bleeding. An esophagoduodenoscopy was performed. A mass was noted in her stomach, and a biopsy was performed. The pathology report identified a gastrointestinal stromal tumor (GIST).

Which of the following statements is true regarding GISTs?

❑ A. The prognosis is better when the tumor is in the small intestine than when it is in the stomach or esophagus

❑ B. GISTs have muscle markers similar to those of leiomyosarcomas, including muscle or Schwann cell (S-100) markers

❑ C. GISTs are only found in the stomach

- ❑ D. **GISTs express c-*kit* (a proto-oncogene that encodes transmembrane tyrosine kinase receptors) with a mutation that causes the receptor to be constitutively active; imatinib (Gleevec) has shown promise in the treatment of GISTs**

Key Concept/Objective: To understand GISTs

GISTs occur predominantly in middle-aged patients. Approximately 70% occur in the stomach, 20% occur in the small intestine, and less than 10% occur in the colon, esophagus, and rectum. Survival correlates with tumor location. The best prognoses are associated with tumors of the esophagus and stomach; the worst prognoses are associated with tumors occurring in the small intestine. GISTs frequently lack muscle and Schwann cell markers that are typical of leiomyosarcomas found in other anatomic sites. The proto-oncogene c-*kit* encodes a transmembrane tyrosine kinase receptor located on the long arm of chromosome 4. Mutations of c-*kit* cause the receptor to be activated constitutively without its ligand. Imatinib is an oral, relatively specific inhibitor of three tyrosine kinase receptors. It is used in the treatment of GISTs. *(Answer: D—GISTs express* c-kit *[a proto-oncogene that encodes transmembrane tyrosine kinase receptors] with a mutation that causes the receptor to be constitutively active; imatinib [Gleevec] has shown promise in the treatment of GISTs)*

For more information, see Raftopoulos H, Antman KH: 12 Oncology: XIII Sarcomas of Soft Tissue and Bone. ACP Medicine Online (www.acpmedicine.com). Dale DC, Federman DD, Eds. WebMD Inc., New York, November 2003

Bladder, Renal, and Testicular Cancer

59. A 60-year-old man presents to the walk-in clinic with fever and malaise of 3 days' duration. He was recently diagnosed with transitional cell bladder cancer after presenting with microscopic hematuria. Staging protocol found no evidence of metastatic disease. An endoscopic resection of the tumor showed superficial bladder cancer that was restricted to the bladder mucosa. After transurethral resection, the patient was started on weekly intravesical infusions of bacillus Calmette Guérin (BCG); he has received five such infusions so far. On physical examination, the patient has fever but is otherwise normal. He has had macroscopic hematuria for 2 days. A chest x-ray is normal.

Of the following, which is the most likely cause of this patient's symptoms?

- ❑ A. **Recurrent bladder cancer**
- ❑ B. **BCG infusion**
- ❑ C. **Early pneumonia**
- ❑ D. **Febrile neutropenia**

Key Concept/Objective: To know the possible side effects of BCG infusion

Superficial bladder cancer, which constitutes about 80% of incident cases, is restricted to the level of the bladder mucosa and lamina propria. For superficial bladder cancer, the initial treatment is careful and thorough endoscopic resection of the tumor or tumors. In patients at high risk for recurrence, BCG may be infused into the bladder through a catheter as an adjuvant to transurethral resection. The mechanism of action is incompletely understood, but it appears to be based on local immunologic response. Side effects of intravesical BCG include dysuria, urinary frequency, hematuria, and a flulike syndrome. More significantly, because BCG is an attenuated mycobacterium, it can produce local, regional, and systemic infections. Granulomatous infections can occur at extravesical sites, including the prostate, epididymis, testes, kidney, liver, and lungs. BCG sepsis is the most serious complication and can be life-threatening. Systemic involvement is treated with triple-antibiotic antituberculous therapy for 6 months. *(Answer: B—BCG infusion)*

60. A 30-year-old woman comes to your clinic complaining of right-side flank pain and macroscopic hematuria. You make a presumptive diagnosis of nephrolithiasis and order a CT scan, which shows no stones;

however, the report describes three masses in the right kidney, the largest measuring 5 × 4 cm; two masses are seen in the left kidney, the larger measuring 3 × 3 cm. A 3 × 3 cm pancreatic cyst is also found. You call your patient to discuss these CT findings, and you ask her about her family history. She says her sister had a brain tumor that caused her to have gait problems, and a brother had kidney cancer.

What is the most likely diagnosis for this patient?

- ❑ **A. Metastatic pancreatic cancer**
- ❑ **B. Familial papillary renal cell cancer**
- ❑ **C. Polycystic kidney disease with malignant transformation**
- ❑ **D. Von Hippel-Lindau (VHL) disease**

Key Concept/Objective: To know the manifestations of VHL disease

Most renal cell carcinomas occur sporadically, but about 4% of cases present in an inherited pattern. Such familial cancers include VHL disease and familial papillary renal cell cancers. Approximately 1.6% of renal cell cancers are part of the autosomal dominant VHL disease, which is also characterized by retinal and central nervous system hemangioblastoma, pheochromocytoma, and pancreatic cyst. Compared with sporadic cases, renal cell cancer in the VHL syndrome tends to be multifocal and bilateral and to appear at a younger age. This patient's age, the presence of a strong family history, and the findings on the CT scan make the likelihood of VHL disease very high. Polycystic kidney disease is not a risk factor for renal cell cancer. However, a threefold- to sixfold-higher incidence of renal cell cancer has been found in the chronic dialysis population as well as in renal transplant recipients, presumably because of the development of acquired cystic kidney disease. *(Answer: D—Von Hippel-Lindau [VHL] disease)*

61. A 25-year-old man comes to the clinic after finding a painless mass on his right testicle. He has no symptoms except for mild pain on the right flank and headache of new onset. The physical examination shows a 2 × 2 cm solid, hard mass on the right testicle. Physical examination shows no lymphadenopathy or other abnormalities. An ultrasound is obtained, which shows a mass on the right testicle consistent with a tumor. A chest x-ray shows multiple "cannonball" lesions in both lungs. A pelvic CT scan shows diffuse retroperitoneal lymphadenopathy. A magnetic resonance imaging scan of the brain also shows multiple masses consistent with metastatic disease.

On the basis of these findings and the overall prognosis, how would you approach this patient?

- ❑ **A. Refer to surgical oncology and radiation oncology for orchiectomy and radiotherapy**
- ❑ **B. Explain the bad prognosis of his extensive disease and refer to palliative care**
- ❑ **C. Refer to oncology to start chemotherapy**
- ❑ **D. Refer to surgical oncology and radiation oncology for orchiectomy with radical retroperitoneal lymph node dissection and radiotherapy**

Key Concept/Objective: To outline the management of metastatic testicular cancer

For testicular cancer patients with lymph node metastases measuring more than 5 cm in diameter and for those with visceral metastases (e.g., liver, lung, bone), the treatment of choice is systemic chemotherapy. The early combination of cisplatin, vinblastine, and bleomycin (the PVB regimen) produced cures in up to 70% of cases. Subsequently, a less toxic regimen, in which vinblastine was replaced by etoposide, was tested and shown to be equivalent to the PVB regimen. Metastatic diseases in the brain and liver, and possibly in bone, are associated with a worse prognosis. However, it must be emphasized that cure is possible in patients in the worst prognostic groups; even patients with brain metastases may be cured by aggressive multimodality treatment. Orchiectomy, radiotherapy, and radical retroperitoneal lymph node dissection are used in early stages of testicular cancer, when the disease is confined to the testicles or when the lymph node metastases are smaller than 5 cm. *(Answer: C—Refer to oncology to start chemotherapy)*

62. A 32-year-old man with a recently diagnosed metastatic seminoma is started on a regimen of cisplatin, vinblastin, and bleomycin. His initial human chorionic gonadotropin (hCG) level is 80 mIU/ml. One day after starting his chemotherapy, the hCG level rises to 100 mIU/ml, and the following day it is 130 mIU/ml.

On the basis of these laboratory findings, what would be the next step in the treatment of this patient?

- ❑ **A. Reaccess the hCG level in 3 or 4 days; you expect it to be decreased by then**
- ❑ **B. Consider switching the patient's regimen to cisplatin, etoposide, vinblastine, and bleomycin**
- ❑ **C. Ask the pathologist to reevaluate the biopsy, considering the possibility that the correct diagnosis is choriocarcinoma and not seminoma**
- ❑ **D. Change the regimen by alternating cisplatin, vincristine, methotrexate, and bleomycin with actinomycin D, cyclophosphamide, and etoposide**

Key Concept/Objective: To describe the usual response in testicular tumor markers to chemotherapy

About 30% of seminomas include syncytiotrophoblastic giant cells, and these may produce hCG. The circulating testicular tumor markers hCG and α-fetoprotein should be measured as part of the initial diagnostic workup and in the monitoring of therapy. The first specimen should be obtained before primary surgery. hCG has a half-life of 24 to 36 hours. Failure of a circulating marker to decline in accordance with normal half-life gradients after orchiectomy suggests the continuing release of the marker into the blood by occult metastatic disease. In patients with metastatic disease, during chemotherapy, the release of markers from dying cancer cells may result in a transient elevation of blood levels, after which they will decline according to half-life gradients. Thus, serial measurements should be taken to determine whether the patient is responding adequately to treatment. The other regimens listed among the choices have been used for patients with poor risk or who have previously undergone treatment for metastatic disease. An extremely high hCG level (i.e., one in the thousands) is typical in choriocarcinoma. *(Answer: A—Reaccess the hCG level in 3 or 4 days; you expect it to be decreased by then)*

For more information, see Raghavan D: 12 Oncology: XIV Bladder, Renal, and Testicular Cancer. ACP Medicine Online (www.acpmedicine.com). Dale DC, Federman DD, Eds. WebMD Inc., New York, May 2003

Chronic Lymphoid Leukemias and Plasma Cell Disorders

63. A 70-year-old woman presents for routine check up. She has hypertension that is well controlled on medication. She has no specific complaints but is fatigued. On physical examination, a few anterior cervical and axillary lymph nodes are found to measure 2 cm in diameter. Laboratory results are as follows: WBC, 106,000/μl, with a lymphocyte predominance; hematocrit, 39%; platelet count, 160,000/μl. Other laboratory results are normal. A CT scan of the abdomen reveals some periaortic lymphadenopathy. Flow cytometry of her peripheral blood reveals that most of the cells express CD20, CD23, and CD5 antigens.

What is the most appropriate treatment for this patient at this time?

- ❑ **A. Chlorambucil**
- ❑ **B. Intravenous γ-globulin (IVIG)**
- ❑ **C. Chlorambucil and prednisone**
- ❑ **D. Fludarabine**
- ❑ **E. Observation**

Key Concept/Objective: To know the appropriate therapy for CLL

CLL, a malignancy of the B cells, is the most common of all the leukemias. It generally affects older adults; it affects men more than women and is more common in Jewish peo-

ple of Eastern European descent. Patients are usually asymptomatic at the time of diagnosis; the lymphocytosis is usually noted on routine screening. The etiology of CLL is unknown. CLL is a clonal expansion of mature lymphocytes. Diagnosis can be confirmed by flow cytometry because CLL cells usually express normal CD19 and CD20 antigens, but they also express activation antigens CD5 and CD23. Disease staging is based on the Rai or the Binet classification system, and prognosis is related to the stage of the disease. Of the currently available therapies for CLL, none are curative, and no survival advantage has been shown with treatment of early stage disease at diagnosis. Therapy should therefore be initiated only when indicated by symptoms: fever, chills, weight loss, severe fatigue, bone marrow failure with anemia or thrombocytopenia, massive lymphadenopathy or hepatosplenomegaly, or recurrent infections. Although most patients with CLL have hypogammaglobulinemia, IVIG fails to protect patients from infections; it has no influence on survival and is not cost-effective. In this patient, who is otherwise doing well, there is no role for chemotherapy. *(Answer: E—Observation)*

64. ***Which of the following is NOT associated with chronic lymphocytic leukemia (CLL)?***

- ❑ A. Richter syndrome
- ❑ B. Hypogammaglobulinemia
- ❑ C. Increased risk of bacterial and fungal infection
- ❑ D. Chronic myelogenous leukemia (CML)
- ❑ E. Transformation to prolymphocytic leukemia (PLL)

Key Concept/Objective: To know the complications of CLL

CLL is a clinically heterogeneous disorder; survival is variable. Some patients live for years after diagnosis, and some die within months. The clinical course depends on the stage of disease at diagnosis; prognostic risk factors include male sex, black race, poor performance status, and older age. In addition, short lymphocyte doubling time is also predictive of poor outcome. In some patients with CLL, the clinical course is complicated by progressive conditions, secondary malignancies, immune abnormalities, and infections. Progressive conditions include Richter syndrome, in which patients develop worsening lymphadenopathy, hepatosplenomegaly, fever, abdominal pain, weight loss, and anemia. Patients who develop Richter syndrome do not respond well to therapy, and survival is short. PLL is the second most common transformation in CLL; however, most cases of PLL arise de novo. Compared with patients with de novo disease, patients with PLL that arises through transformation tend to be younger, and they have less marked lymphocytosis. Other transformations in CLL include acute lymphoblastic leukemia, multiple myeloma, and Hodgkin lymphoma. CML is not a known complication of CLL. *(Answer: D—Chronic myelogenous leukemia [CML])*

65. A 64-year-old man presents with fatigue and weakness. His physical examination is normal except for splenomegaly. A complete blood count reveals pancytopenia, with lymphocyte predominance and normal red cells. A bone marrow aspirate was dry. The bone marrow biopsy is pending.

Which of the following is the most likely diagnosis for this patient?

- ❑ A. CLL
- ❑ B. Hairy-cell leukemia (HCL)
- ❑ C. CML
- ❑ D. Multiple myeloma
- ❑ E. Myelofibrosis

Key Concept/Objective: To understand the diagnosis and differential diagnosis of HCL

HCL is a rare B cell neoplasm that most often occurs in older men. Patients usually present with symptoms related to impairment of the bone marrow, such as infections and bleeding, although they may be asymptomatic. The physical examination is usually only significant for splenomegaly; laboratory studies typically reveal pancytopenia. The bone

marrow aspirate is often dry secondary to fibrosis; biopsy may be needed to make the diagnosis. In this patient, CLL and CML are unlikely because of the leukopenia. Multiple myeloma is unlikely, given the dry marrow aspirate. Myelofibrosis is unlikely secondary to the normal red cell morphology. Treatment of HCL is indicated only if there is worsening splenomegaly or lymphadenopathy or if there are more than 20,000 hairy cells/µl. In the past, splenectomy was the treatment of choice; however, splenectomy is used less commonly today. Although splenectomy may improve symptoms, it does not affect the disease itself. The current treatment of choice is either cladribine or the purine analogue pentostatin; both of these agents have been shown to induce remission in 80% of patients, and the choice is based on physician preference. *(Answer: B—Hairy-cell leukemia [HCL])*

66. A 76-year-old man presents with back pain and malaise. Initial laboratory results are as follows: WBC, 3,000/µl; hematocrit, 28%; platelet count, 200,000/µl. Serum chemistries are otherwise normal. Serum protein electrophoresis (SPEP) reveals a monoclonal protein level of 3.8 g/dl; immunoelectrophoresis revealed these monoclonal proteins to be IgG-κ. Bone marrow evaluation reveals sheets of dysplastic plasma cells, and skeletal survey reveals osteolytic lesions in the skull and vertebrae.

In addition to melphalan and prednisone, which of the following would be best to add to this patient's regimen?

- ❑ **A. Granulocyte colony-stimulating factor (G-CSF)**
- ❑ **B. Doxorubicin**
- ❑ **C. Fludarabine**
- ❑ **D. Pamidronate**
- ❑ **E. Interferon alfa**

Key Concept/Objective: To understand the role of bisphosphonates in the treatment of multiple myeloma

This patient has most of the classic symptoms of multiple myeloma, including plasma cell infiltration of the bone marrow, osteolytic bone lesions, anemia, and an M protein level of greater than 3.5 g/dl on SPEP. Chemotherapy with melphalan and prednisone is a reasonable therapeutic option because this combination has been shown to have a higher response rate than monotherapy with either drug. In patients who have bone disease, pamidronate is added to provide protection against skeletal complications; this approach appears to improve quality of life and possibly provides a survival advantage. Therefore, current recommendations are to add bisphosphonates such as pamidronate to the regimens for all patients with evidence of bone involvement. *(Answer: D—Pamidronate)*

For more information, see Cheson BD: 12 Oncology: XV Chronic Lymphoid Leukemias and Plasma Cell Disorders. ACP Medicine Online (www.acpmedicine.com). Dale DC, Federman DD, Eds. WebMD Inc., New York, February 2003

Acute Leukemia

67. A 74-year-old white woman presents to you in clinic for routine follow-up. She has been your patient for several years. Her medical problems consist of hypertension and mild degenerative joint disease, for which she is receiving hydrochlorothiazide and nonsteroidal anti-inflammatory drugs (NSAIDs) as needed. On her last visit, her only complaint was of increasing fatigue, which she had been experiencing for several months. Results of routine laboratory tests at that time were as follows: white blood cell count, 7,500 cells/µl; hematocrit, 26%; mean cell volume, 96 fl; and platelet count, 485,000/µl. Follow-up laboratory studies revealed no vitamin B_{12} or folate deficiencies. Results of iron studies were also normal. Repeat laboratory values today reveal a persistent macrocytic anemia and an elevated platelet count. You schedule a bone marrow biopsy to further evaluate the patient's anemia; it reveals the presence of monolobulated and bilobulated micromegakaryocytes.

The presence of monolobulated and bilobulated micromegakaryocytes characterizes which of the following chromosomal abnormalities?

- ❑ **A. A deletion of the long arm of chromosome 5**

- ❑ **B. A translocation of chromosomes 15 and 17**
- ❑ **C. A translocation of chromosomes 9 and 22**
- ❑ **D. A deletion of the long arm of chromosome 9**

Key Concept/Objective: To know the clinical presentation of myelodysplastic syndrome (MDS)

Considerable data suggest that MDS results from combined defects of both stroma and hematopoietic stem cells. Several clinical syndromes that may have a more predictable natural history can now be defined. For example, a deletion of the long arm of chromosome 5 can be detected in some older patients, especially women, with a macrocytic, refractory anemia (RA). The platelet count is typically normal or elevated. The bone marrow picture in the RA with 5q⁻ syndrome is characterized by the presence of monolobulated and bilobulated micromegakaryocytes. Two thirds of these patients have RA or RA with ringed sideroblasts (RARS), and the remainder have RAEB (RA with excess of blasts). In those patients who have a del(5q) as their sole cytogenetic abnormality, MDS tends to follow a more benign course, although progression to acute myeloid leukemia (AML) may occur. *(Answer: A—A deletion of the long arm of chromosome 5)*

68. A 62-year-old woman well known to you comes to see you in clinic. Since the last time you saw her, she was admitted to the hospital and diagnosed with acute leukemia. She has been followed by a local hematologist and has undergone remission-induction chemotherapy. She is scheduled to begin postinduction consolidation therapy. She explains that she and the specialist are working toward a "complete remission" (CR) and wants to know if that means she will be cured.

Which of the following definitions of CR is most accurate?

- ❑ **A. Full recovery of normal peripheral blood counts; blast cells are undetectable in the bone marrow**
- ❑ **B. Full recovery of normal peripheral blood counts; bone marrow cellularity with less than 5% residual blast cells**
- ❑ **C. Full recovery of normal peripheral blood counts; bone marrow cellularity with less than 10% residual blast cells**
- ❑ **D. Full recovery of normal peripheral blood counts; bone marrow cellularity with less than 10% residual blast cells for a minimum of 1 year**

Key Concept/Objective: To understand the concept of CR in leukemia patients

The goal of remission-induction chemotherapy is the rapid restoration of normal bone marrow function. The term complete remission is reserved for patients who have full recovery of normal peripheral blood counts and bone marrow cellularity with less than 5% residual blast cells. Induction therapy aims to reduce the total-body leukemia cell population from approximately 10^{12} cells to below the cytologically detectable level of about 10^9 cells. The leukemia cells in some patients have high levels of primary drug resistance and will be refractory to courses of remission-induction chemotherapy. It is assumed, however, that even in CR a substantial burden of leukemia cells persists undetected, leading to relapse within a few weeks or months if no further therapy is administered. Postinduction or remission consolidation therapy, usually comprising several additional courses of chemotherapy, is designed to eradicate residual leukemia, allowing the possibility of cure. *(Answer: B—Full recovery of normal peripheral blood counts; bone marrow cellularity with less than 5% residual blast cells)*

69. A 52-year-old man presents to you in clinic as a new patient. It has been several years since he has seen a physician. He comes to you today because he has not been feeling well and he thinks something is wrong. He reports that for the past several weeks, he has been experiencing malaise, subjective weight loss, and fevers. He also reports some swollen lumps on his neck. Physical examination is notable for lymphadenopathy and splenomegaly. Laboratory data reveal a moderately decreased hemoglobin level, thrombocytopenia, and a moderate leukocytosis. You suspect acute lymphoblastic leukemia (ALL). Further studies confirm your suspicion. A *bcr-abl* fusion gene is identified.

Which of the following statements is the most accurate regarding cure of ALL?

- ❑ **A. A combination of vincristine, prednisone, and daunorubicin cures about one third of patients with Philadelphia positive (Ph$^+$) ALL**
- ❑ **B. A combination of L-asparaginase and cyclophosphamide cures about one third of patients with Ph$^+$ ALL**
- ❑ **C. Allogeneic stem cell transplantation cures about one third of patients with Ph$^+$ ALL**
- ❑ **D. There are currently no regimens that are known to cure this disease**

Key Concept/Objective: To know the regimen that is associated with cure of Ph$^+$ ALL

Ph$^+$ ALL is identified by the t(9;22)(q34;q22) or the *bcr-abl* fusion gene. It is currently the major challenge in curing ALL because it makes up 25% to 30% of adult cases and perhaps one half of B-lineage ALL. Approximately 70% of patients achieve CR, but the remission durations are markedly shorter (median, 7 months) for Ph$^+$ cases than for those without a Ph chromosome (remission of almost 3 years). As yet, no chemotherapy regimen alone appears to have the potential to cure this group of patients. In contrast, allogeneic stem cell transplantation cures about one third of patients with Ph$^+$ ALL. The probability of relapse after transplantation is approximately 30% to 50%, further attesting to the therapy-resistant nature of this disease. The treatment for Ph$^+$ ALL should include an intensive remission-induction chemotherapy program, followed by allogeneic stem cell transplantation in the first CR if a donor is available. Considerable interest exists in investigating new agents, especially the tyrosine kinase inhibitor imatinib mesylate, in this high-risk group of patients. *(Answer: C—Allogeneic stem cell transplantation cures about one third of patients with Ph$^+$ ALL)*

70. A 50-year-old man is referred to your clinic by the blood bank for a positive HTLV-I serology. He is healthy with no symptoms. He has donated blood for a workplace blood drive.

What advice would you give this patient at this time?

- ❑ **A. He has a 20% lifetime risk of developing leukemia**
- ❑ **B. He has a 40% lifetime risk of developing leukemia**
- ❑ **C. He is at increased risk for Burkitt lymphoma**
- ❑ **D. He is unlikely to have any medical problems associated with this virus**
- ❑ **E. He is at risk for developing an AIDS-like illness**

Key Concept/Objective: To be able to recognize that most patients exposed to the HTLV-I virus will not develop leukemia

Blood banks commonly screen donated blood for HTLV-1. This virus had been linked to acute T cell leukemia and cutaneous T cell lymphoma in adults. However, most people with antibodies to HTLV-I remain free of these associated diseases, which suggests a multifactorial process in the development of leukemia. Burkitt lymphoma is associated with Epstein-Barr virus. *(Answer: D—He is unlikely to have any medical problems associated with this virus)*

71. ***Which of the following groups has an increased incidence of acute leukemia?***

- ❑ **A. Men**
- ❑ **B. Persons of higher socioeconomic status**
- ❑ **C. Adults older than 50 years**
- ❑ **D. Whites**
- ❑ **E. All of the above**

Key Concept/Objective: To know the risk factors for acute leukemia

All of the groups listed have a higher risk of developing acute leukemia than does the general population. Other risk factors include Jewish ethnicity, prior exposure to ionizing radi-

ation (either through environmental exposure or as part of a treatment regimen), exposure to some industrial chemicals, several chemotherapy agents, a genetic predisposition, and the presence of specific diseases such as Down syndrome. *(Answer: E—All of the above)*

72. ***Which of the following statements is more commonly associated with acute myeloid leukemia (AML) than with ALL?***

- ❑ **A. It accounts for the majority of cases of acute leukemia in adults**
- ❑ **B. The CNS is a relatively common site of relapse**
- ❑ **C. Patients are more likely to have hepatosplenomegaly and lymphadenopathy at presentation**
- ❑ **D. Maintenance chemotherapy generally lasts 1 to 3 years**
- ❑ **E. The Philadelphia chromosome–positive (Ph^+) variant is more resistant to standard treatment**

Key Concept/Objective: To know the differences between AML and ALL in adults

AML accounts for about 80% of acute leukemias in adults and is most likely to present with hemorrhage or infection. Standard induction therapy with cytarabine and daunorubicin (7 + 3 regimen) is followed by consolidation chemotherapy but generally no long-term maintenance regimen. ALL typically presents with constitutional symptoms (fatigue, weight loss, night sweats), and organomegaly and lymphadenopathy are more likely to be present on exam. Because CNS involvement occurs in 5% of patients with ALL, CNS prophylaxis is a standard part of treatment, as is maintenance chemotherapy. Ph^+ ALL is less responsive to standard chemotherapy regimens. *(Answer: A—It accounts for the majority of cases of acute leukemia in adults)*

73. A 47-year-old man presents with gum bleeding, rectal bleeding, and fatigue. He is found to have disseminated intravascular coagulation (DIC). His white blood cell count is 27,000.

Which of the following conditions would best fit with this clinical presentation?

- ❑ **A. Burkitt cell ALL**
- ❑ **B. Acute promyelocytic leukemia (M3)**
- ❑ **C. Myelodysplastic syndrome**
- ❑ **D. AML in patients older than 65 years**
- ❑ **E. Ph^+ ALL**

Key Concept/Objective: To recognize acute promyelocytic leukemia as a distinct disease with a significant associated complication

DIC is frequently found at presentation or soon after induction of chemotherapy in patients with acute promyelocytic leukemia (FAB M3). Hemorrhage secondary to DIC is responsible for a high pretreatment or early-treatment mortality. DIC in this setting has been treated with heparin. Acute promyelocytic leukemia is unique in its response to all-*trans*-retinoic acid, which is used alone or in combination with more standard regimens for induction. *(Answer: B—Acute promyelocytic leukemia [M3])*

For more information, see Larson RA: 12 Oncology: XVI Acute Leukemia. ACP Medicine Online (www.acpmedicine.com). Dale DC, Federman DD, Eds. WebMD Inc., New York, July 2003

Chronic Myelogenous Leukemia and Other Myeloproliferative Disorders

74. A 55-year-old man presents to your clinic with complaints of generalized fatigue, weight loss, and abdominal discomfort with early satiety. On physical examination, the patient is afebrile and appears thin. His abdominal examination is notable for massive splenomegaly. No adenopathy is identified, and the liver is of normal size. A complete blood count (CBC) reveals a neutrophilic leukocytosis, and you suspect chronic myelogenous leukemia (CML).

Which of the following statements regarding CML is false?

- ❑ **A. CML is a myeloproliferative disorder (MPD) and represents a clonal disorder of the pluripotential hematopoietic stem cell**
- ❑ **B. The CBC often reveals thrombocytosis, neutrophilic leukocytosis, and basophilia**
- ❑ **C. The presence of the Philadelphia chromosome (Ph) is characteristic of CML and is a poor prognostic sign**
- ❑ **D. The three main phases of CML are the chronic phase, the accelerated phase, and the blast phase**

Key Concept/Objective: To understand the pathogenesis and clinical course of CML

MPDs represent clonal disorders of the pluripotential hematopoietic stem cell and include CML, polycythemia vera, essential thrombocythemia, myeloid metaplasia, and idiopathic myelofibrosis. CML accounts for 15% of all cases of leukemia in adults. Males are affected more often than females, and the median age at presentation is 45 to 55 years. CML is caused by the transforming capability of the protein products resulting from the Ph translocation t(9;22). Up to 95% of patients with CML express Ph, which results from a reciprocal translocation between the long arms of chromosomes 9 and 22. Patients with CML who do not have Ph translocation have a significantly worse prognosis than do patients who test positive for the *bcr-abl* gene. CML is characterized by expansion of myeloid progenitor cells at various stages of their maturation, by the premature release of these cells into the circulation, and by their tendency to home to extramedullary sites. Symptoms at presentation reflect the increase in mass and turnover of the leukemic cells. Patients may complain of lethargy and weakness, night sweats, and weight loss. Occasionally, the spleen enlarges, causing an increase in abdominal girth and abdominal discomfort. The prognosis for patients with CML has changed significantly in the past 2 decades. Patients who are diagnosed with chronic-phase CML can expect a median survival of 5 to 7 years. *(Answer: C—The presence of the Philadelphia chromosome [Ph] is characteristic of CML and is a poor prognostic sign)*

75. A 63-year-old woman presents to your clinic with a complaint of increasing abdominal girth; hepatosplenomegaly is detected on examination. CBC reveals a hematocrit of 52% and a platelet count of 900,000 cells/mm³. You suspect that she has polycythemia vera (PV).

Which of the following statements about PV is true?

- ❑ **A. The increase in red blood cell (RBC) mass is mainly the result of an increase in the level of erythropoietin**
- ❑ **B. Thrombotic complications are rare in PV**
- ❑ **C. To diagnose PV, independent determination of RBC mass and plasma volume by isotope dilution is mandatory**
- ❑ **D. The standard of care for treatment of PV is an aggressive chemotherapy regimen**

Key Concept/Objective: To understand the clinical presentation, diagnosis, and treatment of PV

PV is a clonal disorder of hematopoietic stem cells. Unlike in CML, however, no clear causative cytogenetic-molecular lesion has been identified. Expansion of RBC mass is caused by increased production by hypercellular bone marrow and is not dependent on serum levels of erythropoietin. Indeed, erythropoietin levels are typically low in patients with PV; this distinguishes PV from the secondary polycythemia associated with certain tumors (e.g., renal cell carcinoma and hepatocellular carcinoma) and with pulmonary, cardiac, and renal disorders. The clinical manifestations of PV are a consequence of the excessive proliferation of hematopoietic cell lines and are mainly characterized by microvascu-

lar and macrovascular thrombotic events. On physical examination, the most common findings in patients with PV are ruddy cyanosis, hepatosplenomegaly, conjunctival plethora, and hypertension. Unlike essential thrombocytopenia, venous and arterial thromboses occur with equal frequency in PV. Microvascular symptoms such as acroparesthesias, erythromelalgia, peripheral gangrene, and ischemic neurologic and visual disturbances are frequent. Particularly serious thrombotic events involve cerebral and coronary vessels; hepatic veins; the inferior vena cava (Budd-Chiari syndrome); and mesenteric vessels. The diagnosis of PV requires exclusion of secondary causes of increased red blood cell mass and blood volume. Independent determination of RBC mass and plasma volume by isotope dilution is mandatory. Phlebotomy, low-dose aspirin, and possibly hydroxyurea represent the best approach to treatment. *(Answer: C—To diagnose PV, independent determination of RBC mass and plasma volume by isotope dilution is mandatory)*

76. A 45-year-old man presents to your clinic with painful, unilateral swelling of the right lower extremity; he has been experiencing these symptoms for 48 hours. The patient has no known predisposing factors for deep vein thrombosis (DVT) and no family history of DVT. Ultrasonography reveals a femoral vein DVT. A CBC is obtained; the patient's platelet count is 1,200,000 cells/mm^3.

Which of the following statements regarding essential thrombocytosis (ET) is false?

- ❑ A. **In patients with ET, an elevation in the platelet count is caused by increased production by megakaryocytes in conjunction with normal platelet survival**
- ❑ B. **To diagnose ET, you must exclude iron deficiency, malignancies, inflammatory conditions, and infections**
- ❑ C. **The platelets in patients with ET are functional, and hemorrhage rarely occurs**
- ❑ D. **Unlike PV, ET rarely progresses; leukemia develops in only 3% to 4% of patients**

Key Concept/Objective: To understand the clinical presentation, diagnosis, and treatment of ET

The elevated platelet count in patients with ET is caused by increased production by megakaryocytes in conjunction with normal platelet survival. ET is diagnosed after secondary causes of elevated platelet counts (e.g., iron deficiency, malignancies, inflammatory conditions, and infections) have been excluded. Major thrombotic complications occur in 20% to 30% of patients. Thrombotic complications frequently manifest as DVT and pulmonary embolism. Thrombosis of hepatic veins leads to Budd-Chiari syndrome; thrombosis of renal veins can cause nephrotic syndrome. Erythromelalgia and digital ischemia constitute microvascular forms of arterial thrombosis in ET. Hemorrhagic events occur in up to 40% of patients, with the gastrointestinal tract, urinary tract, skin, eyes, and brain being possible bleeding sites. Individual patients can suffer from both thrombotic and hemorrhagic episodes. Unlike PV, ET rarely progresses, and leukemia develops in only 3% to 4% of patients. The correlation between the degree of thrombocytosis and the risk of thrombosis is poor. Untreated asymptomatic patients and those who are at low risk for thrombohemorrhagic complications (i.e., those with no history of thrombohemorrhagic episodes, those younger than 60 years, and those whose thrombocytosis is of shorter duration) may have the same life expectancy as an age-matched and sex-matched control group without ET. The indications for therapeutic intervention have to be considered carefully with regard to the risk of vascular complications. In general, treatment should be considered only in patients at high risk for thrombohemorrhagic events. *(Answer: C—The platelets in patients with ET are functional, and hemorrhage rarely occurs)*

77. A 52-year-old man is seen for annual examination. He reports increasing fatigue over the past 3 months, accompanied by a 10 lb weight loss and a sense of abdominal fullness. On examination, he is slightly pale, with dullness to percussion in the left upper quadrant of his abdomen. The remainder of his exam is normal, with no bruising or lymphadenopathy. A CBC reveals a WBC count of 117,000, predominantly neutrophils in all stages of maturation.

Which of the following other findings would you expect to see in this patient upon further evaluation?

- ❑ A. **Basophilia on peripheral smear**
- ❑ B. **A *BCR-ABL* translocation**
- ❑ C. **A Philadelphia chromosome**
- ❑ D. **A decreased leukocyte alkaline phosphatase (LAP) score**
- ❑ E. **All of the above**

Key Concept/Objective: To know the common laboratory findings in a patient with chronic myelogenous leukemia (CML)

CML is an acquired clonal stem cell disorder in which more than 90% of patients express the Philadelphia chromosome (a translocation between chromosomes 9 and 22) on cytogenetic analysis. Genetic material is exchanged between the *BCR* and *ABL* genes. Other common laboratory findings include a WBC count over 100,000, with a neutrophilic predominance, anemia, thrombocytosis, basophilia, and a decreased LAP score. *(Answer: E—All of the above)*

78. An active, otherwise healthy 32-year-old man with type 1 diabetes is found to have a hematocrit of 60%, a platelet count of 556,000, and a WBC count of 8,050 on routine blood work. These values were confirmed on three separate occasions. His examination is unremarkable except for a mildly elevated blood pressure, at 148/92 mm Hg. He has no hepatosplenomegaly or lymphadenopathy.

Which of the following would you expect to find in this patient on further evaluation?

- ❑ A. **An elevated erythropoietin level**
- ❑ B. **Splenomegaly on abdominal ultrasound**
- ❑ C. **An elevated transferrin saturation**
- ❑ D. **An oxygen saturation of < 92%**
- ❑ E. **Cytogenetic abnormalities**

Key Concept/Objective: To know the confirmatory tests and their expected results in a patient with polycythemia vera

Despite this patient's young age, polycythemia vera would best explain his laboratory values, lack of symptoms, and examination findings. The next step is to exclude other causes of an elevated RBC mass (pulmonary, renal, and hepatic disease), as well as to confirm the presence of polycythemia vera. This young man with diabetes should be screened for hemochromatosis, but hemochromatosis would not explain his constellation of hematologic findings. A normal oxygen saturation (expected in this healthy, asymptomatic man) and splenomegaly are two of the major diagnostic criteria for polycythemia vera. A normal clinical examination does not preclude the presence of splenomegaly, and an ultrasound should be ordered. Erythropoietin levels are low in polycythemia vera, differentiating it from many of the secondary causes of elevated RBC mass, and cytogenetic abnormalities are found in only 20% of polycythemia vera patients. Cytogenetic analysis is generally pursued because the presence of an abnormality confirms the diagnosis and can have prognostic and treatment implications. *(Answer: B—Splenomegaly on abdominal ultrasound)*

79. The patient in Question 78 is started on twice-weekly phlebotomy, and his hematocrit stabilizes at 39%.

Which of the following statements regarding this patient's prognosis is true?

- ❑ A. **His life expectancy will be unchanged as long as he maintains a normal hematocrit**
- ❑ B. **Addition of hydroxyurea to his treatment regimen could cure this disease**

❑ C. **Phlebotomy will reduce his risk for thrombotic complication**

❑ D. **His median expected survival time is 15 to 20 years**

❑ E. **He has a 50% chance of developing leukemia by the age of 40 years**

Key Concept/Objective: To know the common complications and prognostic factors in patients with polycythemia vera

The major complications of polycythemia vera are venous and arterial thrombosis, myelofibrosis ("spent phase"), and acute leukemia. Half of patients develop leukemia within 20 years of diagnosis. Although treatment can help reduce the risk of leukemic transformation and lower the rate of thrombosis, life expectancy will be significantly reduced in this young man. Low-dose aspirin and reduction of significantly elevated platelet counts with agents such as hydroxyurea are effective in controlling vascular complications. Phlebotomy does little to reduce the thrombotic risk. *(Answer: D—His median expected survival time is 15 to 20 years)*

For more information, see Faderi S, Kantarjian HM: 12 Oncology: XVII Chronic Myelogenous Leukemia and Other Myeloproliferative Disorders. ACP Medicine Online (www.acpmedicine.com). Dale DC, Federman DD, Eds. WebMD Inc., New York, April 2004

Head and Neck Cancer

80. A 37-year-old native Alaskan man presents with left-side otalgia of 2 months' duration. He has difficulty breathing through the left side of his nose. A nasopharyngeal mass is discovered; the mass is identified histologically as a lymphoepithelioma. He does not use cigarettes or alcohol.

Which of the following is true for this patient?

❑ A. **He should be given a course of trimethoprim-sulfamethoxazole**

❑ B. **He should have a chest CT scan**

❑ C. **Considering his age and smoking history, it is unlikely that this is a malignancy**

❑ D. **This may be a malignancy linked to a viral infection**

❑ E. **This is probably a malignant lymphoid cell tumor**

Key Concept/Objective: To know the distinction between endemic and sporadic nasopharyngeal carcinoma

Nasopharyngeal carcinoma occurs in two distinct forms. The most common is sporadic squamous cell carcinoma, usually seen in older patients who have a long history of smoking. A second endemic form is seen in Native Americans living in Alaska, Mediterraneans, and Southeast Asians. It is linked to Epstein-Barr virus, and it is likely that other risk factors are required as well. The lymphoid cells are normal T cells that infiltrate the epidermoid tumor. Antibiotics are not indicated in this case, nor is a chest CT scan, because this is neither a lymphoma nor a vasculitic or granulomatous process and therefore distant metastases are unlikely. *(Answer: D—This may be a malignancy linked to a viral infection)*

81. A 71-year-old man with a long history of tobacco and excessive alcohol use is found to have a 3 cm firm right anterior cervical lymph node. Fine-needle aspiration of the node reveals squamous cell carcinoma. He has no symptoms or obvious lesion to suggest the primary site.

What should be the next step in caring for this patient?

❑ A. **Watchful waiting**

❑ B. **Bone scan**

❑ C. **Initiation of treatment with node excision followed by radiation therapy**

❑ D. Induction chemotherapy with cisplatin and fluorouracil

❑ E. Panendoscopy under anesthesia with biopsy of sites at which primary head and neck cancers frequently occur

Key Concept/Objective: To understand the diagnosis of head and neck cancer with unknown primary site

The most common sites of cancers in this circumstance are the base of the tongue, the nasopharynx, and the piriform sinus. If no primary site can be identified, biopsies should be performed at these sites as part of the diagnostic and staging evaluation. If no primary site is discovered after these biopsies, treatment is based on the nodal stage. The goals of treatment for locoregional disease are cure and preservation of function. Chemotherapy may indeed be part of the initial treatment modality, but it should occur only after attempts are made to identify the primary site by biopsies performed under anesthesia. *(Answer: E—Panendoscopy under anesthesia with biopsy of sites at which primary head and neck cancers frequently occur)*

82. ***Which of the following statements about the treatment of head and neck cancer is true?***

❑ A. Cure is unlikely, even with early-stage disease

❑ B. Development of a second primary tumor after successful curative treatment of early-stage disease is rare

❑ C. Concomitant chemoradiotherapy has resulted in increased disease-free intervals and in some studies has increased survival

❑ D. Radical surgery is reserved for patients with recurrent disease

❑ E. Induction chemotherapy for locoregional disease has resulted in tumor shrinkage and preservation of the larynx as well as increased overall survival

Key Concept/Objective: To understand the treatment of head and neck cancer

Concomitant chemoradiotherapy involves sensitizing tumor cells to radiation by administering chemotherapy, usually cisplatin and fluorouracil, during radiation therapy. Use of concomitant chemoradiotherapy has led to improvements in the control of locoregional disease, with some studies suggesting an increase in the 3-year survival rate from 30% to 50%. Other studies have shown increased overall survival with concomitant chemoradiotherapy. This therapy may also lead to improvements in the preservation of organ function in patients who require less surgery. Concomitant chemoradiotherapy is now considered standard care for a majority of patients with locoregional disease. Early-stage disease is treated initially with either surgery or radiation therapy, depending on tumor location; this therapy results in a 60% to 90% cure rate. However, the risk of developing a second head and neck cancer is 3% to 5% per year. In recurrent or metastatic disease, chemotherapy is the standard approach for preserving quality of life while providing palliation. Induction chemotherapy leads to tumor shrinkage, laryngeal preservation, and decreased disease in areas other than the head and neck, presumably by eradicating micrometastases. However, survival is not improved with this modality because the locoregional control achieved is not better than that achieved with surgery and radiation therapy. *(Answer: C—Concomitant chemoradiotherapy has resulted in increased disease-free intervals and in some studies has increased survival)*

For more information, see Vokes EE: 12 Oncology: XVIII Head and Neck Cancer. ACP Medicine Online (www.acpmedicine.com). Dale DC, Federman DD, Eds. WebMD Inc., New York, November 2000

SECTION 13

PSYCHIATRY

Depression and Bipolar Disorder

1. A 56-year-old man is admitted to the coronary care unit and is diagnosed as having a non–Q wave myocardial infarction. The patient is aggressively managed and is clinically stable. During his admission, he describes to his treating physician that he has struggled with depression in the past but has been reluctant to share this with his local doctor. His recent symptoms include insomnia, unintentional weight loss, and depressed mood. He also has not been performing well at work and blames his poor performance on "being tired" and being incapable of concentrating. He has stopped playing golf with his friends on Saturday morning because it is not fun anymore.

Which of the following statements regarding depression is true?

- ❑ **A. The patient is not at increased risk for committing suicide**
- ❑ **B. Genetics plays no role in depression**
- ❑ **C. The incidence of depression decreases with age**
- ❑ **D. The mortality 6 months after a myocardial infarction is five times higher for depressed patients than for nondepressed patients**

Key Concept/Objective: To be able to recognize and treat depression in patients with medical problems

A broad array of antidepressants are available for the treatment of depression. Mood disorders are present in 50% to 70% of all cases of suicide, and patients with recurrent, serious depression (i.e., depression requiring hospitalization) have an 8% to 15% suicide rate. The strongest known risk factors for the development of depression are family history and previous episodes of depression. The risk of depressive disorders in first-degree relatives of patients with depression is two to three times that of the general population. If one parent has a mood disorder, a child's risk of a mood disorder is 10% to 25%; if both parents are affected, the risk roughly doubles. Depression is widespread in the elderly. Depression in late life is a serious public health concern; comorbidity of depression with other illnesses, both medical and psychiatric, is particularly problematic in older persons. The prevalence of depressive symptoms in those 65 years of age and older has been estimated to be 16.9%. Depression is a major risk factor for both the development of cardiovascular disease and death after an index myocardial infarction. The mortality 6 months after a myocardial infarction has been reported to be more than five times higher in depressed patients than in those without depression. *(Answer: D—The mortality 6 months after a myocardial infarction is five times higher for depressed patients than for nondepressed patients)*

2. A 73-year-old man who was recently diagnosed with depression returns for a follow-up visit. The patient was diagnosed 3 weeks ago and was started on fluoxetine. The patient reports no improvement in his depressive symptoms. He has a fixed income and does not want to pay for medication that is not effective. He is hopeful that something will work, and he says that his sister took sertraline and it "cured" her depression.

Which of the following statements concerning this patient is false?

- ❑ A. **Fluoxetine and other selective serotonin reuptake inhibitors (SSRIs) are safe in overdose**
- ❑ B. **Treatment is recommended for at least 4 to 6 weeks before efficacy is determined**
- ❑ C. **Sexual side effects are uncommon causes of poor compliance in patients being treated with SSRIs**
- ❑ D. **Therapy should be discontinued as soon as the patient reports improvement of depressive symptoms**

Key Concept/Objective: To know to inquire about sexual side effects in patients taking SSRIs

SSRIs offer several important advantages over the older medications. Perhaps most importantly, these medications are safe in overdose. The patient's medical history and personal or family history of response often help predict response and side effects. Treatment of depression is recommended for at least 4 to 6 weeks before a decision regarding efficacy can be made. Sexual side effects have been widely recognized as a major cause of poor compliance with SSRI regimens, particularly after improvement of depressed mood. Improvement of the illness should not be interpreted by the patient or the physician as indicating that antidepressants are no longer necessary. The continuation phase of treatment consists of 16 to 20 weeks of continued treatment (using the same antidepressant that was used in the acute phase) after remission, with the goal of preventing the relapses that typically occur in untreated patients. *(Answer: D—Therapy should be discontinued as soon as the patient reports improvement of depressive symptoms)*

3. A 36-year-old man with a history of bipolar disorder presents to a local emergency department in police custody. A family member called the police after the patient stole her credit card and charged almost $10,000 worth of clothes. The patient had locked himself in his home and is now accusing his family of being "out to get him." The police report that there were no drug paraphernalia in the home. The emergency department physician consults psychiatry for evaluation of mania with psychotic features and inpatient management. Results of laboratory testing on admission are all within normal limits.

Which of the following statements concerning pharmacologic therapy for this patient's mania is true?

- ❑ A. **Valproic acid appears most effective for classic bipolar disorder**
- ❑ B. **Carbamazepine is an approved treatment of acute mania**
- ❑ C. **Olanzapine has been shown to be an effective treatment of acute mania**
- ❑ D. **Evidence from clinical trials documents the efficacy of topiramate in acute mania**

Key Concept/Objective: To be familiar with different drugs available for the treatment of bipolar disorder and mania

Lithium is most effective in classic bipolar disorder, which consists of discrete episodes of mania and depression with symptom-free periods between episodes. Serum levels of lithium must be monitored. Valproic acid/divalproex sodium appears to be more effective for manias that are dysphoric or mixed and for patients who experience four or more episodes a year. Carbamazepine is not approved in the United States for the treatment of mania and may be associated with a number of pharmacokinetic drug-drug interactions because of its induction of microsomal P-450 enzymes. Olanzapine, an atypical antipsychotic agent, has been shown to be effective for the treatment of acute mania. Other atypical antipsychotics, including risperidone, quetiapine, ziprasidone, and aripiprazole, may be efficacious as well. Early evidence suggested that topiramate may be an effective mood stabilizer, but three randomized controlled clinical trials in

acute mania failed to demonstrate any efficacy. *(Answer: C—Olanzapine has been shown to be an effective treatment of acute mania)*

4. A 67-year-old man, 3 months after a myocardial infarction (MI), reports problems with severe insomnia. He cannot fall asleep easily and wakes up at about 4:30 A.M. each morning. He has had increased fatigue since his MI, is more forgetful, and has problems with concentration. His other medical problems include reflux esophagitis, benign prostatic hyperplasia (BPH), and a history of stroke with a related seizure disorder. Medications include aspirin, simvastatin, atenolol, and enalapril.

   Which of the following drugs would you recommend for treatment of this patient's symptoms?

   ❑ **A. Zolpidem**

   ❑ **B. Amitryptiline**

   ❑ **C. Nortryptiline**

   ❑ **D. Paroxetine**

   ❑ **E. Bupropion**

   Key Concept/Objective: To know how to select antidepressant medications for patients with multiple comorbid medical illnesses

   This patient has a major depression shortly after an MI. This is not uncommon; up to 20% to 30% of patients may develop depression after MI. This patient also has BPH and a history of a seizure disorder. Tricyclic antidepressants should be avoided because of the risk of cardiac arrhythmia, as well as the increased risk of urinary retention in this patient because of his BPH. Bupropion should be avoided because of his known seizure disorder. An SSRI (paroxetine in this case) is a safe choice, given his comorbid medical illnesses. *(Answer: D—Paroxetine)*

5. A 38-year-old man with a diagnosis of depression presents for follow-up. He has had a good response to treatment with sertraline but would like to stop treatment because of sexual side effects (delayed ejaculation). He has been on antidepressant therapy for 6 weeks.

   Which of the following would you recommend for this patient?

   ❑ **A. Stop sertraline**

   ❑ **B. Stop sertraline, begin paroxetine**

   ❑ **C. Stop sertraline, begin fluoxetine**

   ❑ **D. Stop sertraline, begin bupropion**

   ❑ **E. Stop sertraline, begin amitriptyline**

   Key Concept/Objective: To know the sexual side-effect profiles of antidepressant medications

   This patient is concerned about the sexual side effects he is experiencing from sertraline. He has been treated for only 6 weeks, which is too short a course for treatment of a major depression. Patients who discontinue treatment within the first 16 weeks of therapy are at much higher risk for relapse. Sexual side effects are a class effect of SSRIs and unlikely to be much reduced with fluoxetine or paroxetine. The antidepressant medications with the least likelihood of sexual side effects are bupropion, nefazodone, and mirtazapine. *(Answer: D—Stop sertraline, begin bupropion)*

6. A 49-year-old woman presents for follow-up of depression. She has been treated with fluoxetine for the past 12 weeks. She started on 20 mg a day and had only a minimal response. At 6 weeks her dose was raised to 40 mg. She reports that her fatigue has improved, and she is no longer suicidal. She still has marked anhedonia and problems with concentration. She reports that she has not been missing doses of her medication.

   Which of the following would you recommend for this patient?

- ❑ A. Stop fluoxetine; begin paroxetine
- ❑ B. Stop fluoxetine; begin psychotherapy
- ❑ C. Stop fluoxetine; refer for ECT
- ❑ D. Add lithium to current regimen
- ❑ E. Add buspirone to current regimen

Key Concept/Objective: To be able to recognize partial response to antidepressant therapy and to understand how to augment the response

This patient has had a partial response to treatment of her depression with fluoxetine. She has had an appropriate increase in dose from 20 mg to 40 mg and an appropriate interval (6 weeks) for observation of response at the higher drug dose. This patient is a good candidate for augmenting the response by the addition of another drug. The most common drugs used for this purpose are lithium and bupropion. *(Answer: D—Add lithium to current regimen)*

For more information, see Compton MT, Nemeroff CB, Rudorfer MV: 13 Psychiatry: II Depression and Bipolar Disorder. ACP Medicine Online (www.acpmedicine.com). Dale DC, Federman DD, Eds. WebMD Inc., New York, December 2003

Alcohol Abuse and Dependency

7. A 47-year-old man presents with cold symptoms. In giving his social history, the patient reports drinking six beers nightly to relieve stress. He admits to having been arrested once for driving while under the influence of alcohol, but he denies that there is any evidence of alcohol withdrawal or tolerance. He also denies having any thoughts of controlling his drinking or that he spends a great deal of time obtaining alcohol, using alcohol, or recovering from his drinking. He further denies having any psychological or physical problems related to his drinking.

Which of the following statements regarding this patient is false?

- ❑ A. This patient meets the criteria for alcohol abuse
- ❑ B. This patient does not meet the criteria for alcohol dependence
- ❑ C. This patient displays moderate drinking
- ❑ D. This patient displays at-risk drinking

Key Concept/Objective: To know the definitions of and criteria for alcohol-related conditions

The National Institute on Alcohol Abuse and Alcoholism has defined moderate drinking in terms of the average number of drinks consumed a day that places an adult at relatively low risk for developing alcohol-related health problems. For men younger than 65 years, moderate drinking is drinking an average of no more than two drinks a day. This 47-year-old male patient drinks six beers a day, and therefore C is the correct answer. For men older than 65 years and for all women, moderate drinking is defined as drinking less than two drinks a day. At-risk drinking occurs when those moderate drinking levels are exceeded or when the number of drinks consumed during a single occasion exceeds a specified amount (four drinks per occasion for men and three drinks per occasion for women). Alcohol abuse is defined as a maladaptive pattern of alcohol use leading to clinically significant impairment or distress, manifested in a 12-month period by one or more of the following problems: (1) failure to fulfill role obligations at work, school, or home; (2) recurrent use of alcohol in hazardous situations; (3) legal problems related to alcohol; and (4) continued use despite alcohol-related social problems. Alcohol dependence is manifested by a maladaptive pattern of use over a 12-month period that includes three or more of the following problems: (1) physiologic tolerance, characterized either by an increase in the amount of alcohol consumed or by a decrease in the effects of the amount of alcohol customarily consumed; (2) symptoms of withdrawal; (3) use of greater amounts of alcohol over a longer period than intend-

ed; (4) a persistent desire or unsuccessful attempts to control use; (5) a great deal of time spent obtaining alcohol, using alcohol, or recovering from use; (6) reducing important social, occupational, and recreational activities; and (7) continued use despite knowledge of physical or psychological problems. *(Answer: C—This patient displays moderate drinking)*

8. A 32-year-old woman is diagnosed with gastritis. She reports that she drinks four to five glasses of mixed drinks daily and has been arrested twice for driving while under the influence of alcohol. She reports that she becomes annoyed when her husband tells her to cut down on her drinking. She reports having periods of blackouts.

Which of the following statements regarding this patient is true?

❑ A. **A comorbid psychiatric condition of affective disorder is common for this type of patient**

❑ B. **This patient has an increased risk of accidents**

❑ C. **This patent has an increased risk of HIV infection**

❑ D. **All of the above**

Key Concept/Objective: To understand alcohol-related problems

Epidemiologic surveys have demonstrated high rates of psychiatric illness in persons diagnosed with alcohol abuse or dependence. The most common disorders are anxiety and affective and antisocial personality disorders. Patients with alcohol problems require careful evaluation for comorbid psychiatric symptoms and problems. Similarly, patients with psychiatric disorders are at high risk for having comorbid substance use disorders. Alcohol use is the leading cause of accidents (most notably, automobile accidents), injuries, and trauma (e.g., drownings, head injuries, burns, and spinal cord injuries). Alcohol use is associated with more severe injury in trauma patients. Alcohol use is associated with injuries and trauma related to acts of violence; such acts include assault and homicide, as well as the domestic abuse of children and spouses. HIV seroprevalence may be higher in patients with more severe impairment from alcohol, and women may be at especially increased risk. *(Answer: D—All of the above)*

9. A 44-year-old man comes in for a preventive health visit. He denies having any medical problems, and he is not on any medications. He denies smoking, but he drinks "socially." He denies having any alcohol-related problems.

For this patient, which of the following is the next step in screening for alcohol-related problems?

❑ A. **Inquire about the type, frequency, and quantity of alcohol use**

❑ B. **Administer a standardized questionnaire to detect alcohol problems**

❑ C. **Administer laboratory tests to detect alcohol-related medical problems**

❑ D. **Inquire about criteria that meet definitions of alcohol abuse, dependence, and alcoholism**

Key Concept/Objective: To understand the screening and diagnosis of alcohol-related problems

Easy-to-use techniques for screening patients for alcohol-use disorders are currently available. One such screening technique involves a four-step process for identifying and diagnosing alcohol-related problems. Step 1 is to inquire about current and past alcohol use in all patients. Steps 2 through 4 apply to all patients who report a history of alcohol use. In step 2, a more detailed history regarding quantity and frequency of alcohol use is obtained. In step 3, a standardized questionnaire is used to detect possible alcohol problems. Step 4 involves asking further questions with regard to potential alcohol problems. It is applied to those patients who were identified in steps 1 through 3 as having potential alcohol-related problems. Although not useful as screening tests for alcohol-use disorders, laboratory tests, such as liver enzyme assay, may be useful in

identifying undiagnosed alcohol-related medical problems. *(Answer: A—Inquire about the type, frequency, and quantity of alcohol use)*

10. A 54-year-old man presents with symptoms of alcohol withdrawal. He has hypertension, fever, diaphoresis, and agitation. He reports a recent episode of binge drinking, with his last drink having been consumed 8 hours ago. He is unsure of the quantity of alcohol that he consumed during this episode of binge drinking.

Which of the following pharmacologic therapies is the most appropriate to administer first?

- ❑ **A. Disulfiram**
- ❑ **B. Benzodiazepine**
- ❑ **C. Barbiturates**
- ❑ **D. Carbamazepine**

Key Concept/Objective: To understand the diagnosis and treatment of alcohol withdrawal symptoms

The benzodiazepines (e.g., chlordiazepoxide, diazepam, lorazepam, and oxazepam) are the safest and most effective medications for treatment of alcohol withdrawal. In addition to preventing or alleviating withdrawal symptoms, benzodiazepines may also decrease the incidence of seizures and possibly delirium tremens. Research has suggested that newer approaches using clonidine, beta blockers, and carbamazepine are effective in decreasing the severity of certain withdrawal symptoms but are not as effective as the benzodiazepines and presumably do not protect against seizures, as do benzodiazepines. Thus, these alternative treatments are generally considered to be adjuvants to benzodiazepines. Signs and symptoms of alcohol withdrawal, which can occur in alcohol-dependent persons who stop taking alcohol or who reduce their alcohol intake, include abnormalities in vital signs (e.g., tachycardia, hypertension, and fever), other symptoms of autonomic hyperactivity (e.g., tremor, diaphoresis, and insomnia), GI symptoms (e.g., nausea, vomiting, and diarrhea), and central nervous system effects (e.g., anxiety, agitation, hallucinations, seizures, and delirium). *(Answer: B—Benzodiazepine)*

For more information, see O'Connor PG: 13 Psychiatry: III Alcohol Abuse and Dependency. ACP Medicine Online (www.acpmedicine.com). Dale DC, Federman DD, Eds. WebMD Inc., New York, October 2001

Drug Abuse and Dependence

11. A 49-year-old man presents to your primary care clinic with his wife. His wife is concerned that her husband is "addicted" to alcohol. She wants him to be evaluated and treated because his father was an alcoholic. Over the past few months, he has been drinking alcohol more often, has received a traffic citation for driving under the influence of alcohol, and has missed days of work.

Which of the following statements regarding the Diagnostic and Statistical Manual of Mental Disorders—Text Revision (DSM-IVTR) definition of dependence is false?

- ❑ **A. Tolerance and withdrawal are criteria for dependence**
- ❑ **B. Dependence disorders encompass psychiatric states that resemble primary psychiatric syndromes but that occur only during periods of intoxication or withdrawal from a substance**
- ❑ **C. The inability to cut back when needed is a criterion**
- ❑ **D. Continued use of a substance despite problems is a criterion**

Key Concept/Objective: To understand the definition of dependence

The DSM-IV defines dependence as a condition of repetitive and intense use of a substance that results in repeated problems in at least three of seven areas of concern. Those problems must all occur within the same 12-month period. The categories of problems include tolerance and withdrawal (with the presence of either one justifying a diagnosis of dependence with a physiologic component), difficulty controlling use, an inability to cut back when needed, spending a lot of time taking the substance, failing to take part in important events to use the substance, and continuing use despite problems. In effect, the last of these indicates that the substance means more to the person than the problems it is causing. Substance-induced disorders encompass psychiatric states that resemble primary psychiatric syndromes (e.g., anxiety disorders, major depression, or schizophrenia) but that occur only during periods of intoxication or withdrawal from a substance. Substance-induced disorders improve rapidly and resolve completely within a few days or a month of stopping the use of the substance and can usually be treated with education, reassurance, and a cognitive-behavioral approach. *(Answer: B—Dependence disorders encompass psychiatric states that resemble primary psychiatric syndromes but that occur only during periods of intoxication or withdrawal from a substance)*

12. A 36-year-old woman enters the emergency department stating, "I just took too many pills." She says she wanted to commit suicide through overdose but has since changed her mind. She does not know what she took because she got the pills from her boyfriend's car. You have the nurse establish I.V. access, and you begin to assess the patient's vital signs.

Which of the following statements regarding the overdose of drugs of abuse and the management of overdose is false?

❑ A. A mild overdose with no significant change in vital signs is called intoxication and can be managed conservatively by putting the patient in a quiet room with a friend or relative

❑ B. An overdose of a stimulant can cause tachycardia, cardiac arrhythmias, hypertension, hyperthermia, and seizures

❑ C. Benzodiazepine overdose commonly causes pulmonary edema

❑ D. Opioid overdose can cause life-threatening decreases in respiratory rate, heart rate, and blood pressure

❑ E. Therapy for stimulant overdose can include intravenous benzodiazepines, cooling blankets, and intravenous nitroprusside

Key Concept/Objective: To understand common overdose states and their treatments

Intoxication involves changes in vital signs and alterations in mood and cognitive function caused by a drug. Provided that the vital signs are relatively normal, treatment of intoxication consists of controlling behavior by placing the person in a quiet room; having a friend or relative stay with the person, if possible; offering reassurance; and employing the judicious use of low doses of appropriate medications (e.g., benzodiazepines or antipsychotics). Overdoses are intoxications of such severity as to produce life-threatening changes in vital signs. As such, overdoses must be managed in an emergency department or an inpatient setting. Treatment begins with provision of general medical and psychological support, with an emphasis on normalizing vital signs and allowing the body to metabolize the drug. Depending on the drug category and the clinical manifestations, specific pharmacologic treatment may be indicated. Overdoses with stimulants typically produce tachycardia, cardiac arrhythmias, and potentially life-threatening elevations in blood pressure and body temperature; seizures may also occur. Treatment includes administration of intravenous fluids; administration of intravenous benzodiazepines for seizures; use of cooling blankets to control hyperthermia; and administration of intravenous phentolamine or nitroprusside for blood pressure control. High doses of opioids produce life-threatening decreases in respiratory rate, heart rate, and blood pressure; pulmonary edema or coma are possible. Patients who

have overdosed on benzodiazepines are treated with general supportive measures and an intravenous infusion of the antagonist flumazenil. *(Answer: C—Benzodiazepine overdose commonly causes pulmonary edema)*

13. A 49-year-old man who has a documented history of multiple substance abuse is brought to the emergency department after being "found down." I.V. access is obtained, and the patient undergoes volume resuscitation in the emergency department. After speaking with his family, it becomes evident that he is in a drug withdrawal state.

Which of the following statements regarding withdrawal states from drugs of abuse is false?

- ❑ **A. Stimulant withdrawal only requires general support; the patient will experience somnolence, hunger, an inability to concentrate, and mood swings**
- ❑ **B. Depressant withdrawal resembles alcohol withdrawal and comprises insomnia, anxiety, and an increase in most vital signs**
- ❑ **C. Opioid withdrawal is characterized by enhanced pain throughout the body, diarrhea, runny nose, cough, and a generalized flulike feeling**
- ❑ **D. The only viable option to manage opioid withdrawal is to administer another opioid such as methadone**

Key Concept/Objective: To understand the withdrawal states associated with common drugs of abuse

With some drugs, abrupt cessation after prolonged use is likely to result in rebound signs and symptoms that are the opposite of the drug's acute effects. The time course of the withdrawal syndrome depends mostly on the half-life of the drug involved. Patients undergoing withdrawal from stimulants require only general support. The most prominent acute difficulties include sleepiness; hunger; difficulty focusing attention; and mood swings, with prominent feelings of sadness and frustration. A withdrawal syndrome may occur after the prolonged consumption of high doses of illicit opioids, such as heroin, or of any prescription narcotic analgesic. Opioid withdrawal is characterized by enhanced pain throughout the body, diarrhea, runny nose, cough, and a generalized flulike feeling. In addition to the usual supportive social-model approach, opioid withdrawal states can be treated by readministering an opioid such as methadone. An alternative approach focuses on providing symptomatic relief with decongestants and antidiarrheal medications such as loperamide. Relief of some autonomic symptoms can be provided with an alpha blocker such as clonidine. The withdrawal syndrome associated with depressant drugs, such as benzodiazepines or barbiturates, resembles alcohol withdrawal and comprises insomnia, anxiety, and an increase in most vital signs. About 1% to 3% of patients experience a grand mal convulsion or delirium; this complication most often occurs in patients who concomitantly use more than one drug of abuse or who use high doses of depressants or in patients with medical disorders. The treatment for withdrawal from a depressant drug (other than alcohol) usually involves readministering the specific drug involved in the dependence and tapering it over about 5 days or 3 weeks, depending on the half-life of the drug. *(Answer: D—The only viable option to manage opioid withdrawal is to administer another opioid such as methadone)*

14. A 19-year-old man presents to the emergency department complaining of chest pain and palpitations of 2 hours' duration. He reports that he has no other medical history but has experienced these symptoms previously. On examination, he appears anxious. He has a pulse of 120 beats/min, and his blood pressure is 152/97 mm Hg. His ECG shows sinus tachycardia. A serum drug screen is positive for cocaine.

Which of the following is true for this patient?

- ❑ **A. Drug use anytime within the past 2 weeks can lead to a positive serum drug screen**
- ❑ **B. These symptoms may be a result of cocaine withdrawal**

❑ **C. These symptoms may be a result of cocaine dependence**

❑ **D. This patient has a risk factor for cocaine addiction**

Key Concept/Objective: To understand the characteristics of cocaine addiction

Addiction can be understood as a chronic medical illness. Addiction has identifiable risk factors, including genetic factors. The most well-established risk factors for addiction are family history and male sex. Serum and urine tests are useful when they are positive, but they are of limited utility when they are negative because of the short duration of detectability of cocaine (6 to 8 hours) and cocaine metabolites (2 to 4 days). Cocaine does not produce compensatory adaptations in brain regions that control somatic functions and therefore does not produce dependence. Dependence and, therefore, withdrawal are not produced by highly addictive compounds such as cocaine. *(Answer: D—This patient has a risk factor for cocaine addiction)*

15. A 45-year-old woman presents with complaints of back pain. She requests "something strong" for pain and states that various NSAIDs and nonnarcotic pain medications do not help her when she has pain. A review of her medical record shows a pattern of various musculoskeletal complaints, for which she has been given opiate-derivative pain medications on several occasions. She requests morphine for her back pain.

For this patient, which of the following statements is false?

❑ **A. Opiates can cause addiction**

❑ **B. Opiates can cause dependence**

❑ **C. Opiates function by blocking norepinephrine reuptake**

❑ **D. Pharmacologic therapy is available for treatment of opiate addiction**

Key Concept/Objective: To understand opiate abuse

All addictive drugs share the property of activating a subcortical brain circuit that normally functions to motivate the pursuit of goals with positive survival value, such as obtaining food and sexual partners. This circuit extends from the ventral tegmental area (VTA) of the midbrain to the nucleus accumbens (NAc), which is the ventral portion of the striatum and uses dopamine as its neurotransmitter. The opiates mimic endogenous opioid neurotransmitters (e.g., enkephalins), which disinhibit the VTA, leading to dopamine release, but can also act directly on the NAc, thus bypassing dopamine release. Opioids can produce physical dependence and withdrawal; detoxification from opioids is usually effected by substitution of a cross-reactive agent such as methadone or other long-acting opioids for heroin. For opiate detoxification, addition of alpha$_2$-adrenergic agonist compounds, such as clonidine, blocks emergent withdrawal symptoms and permits more rapid detoxification. *(Answer: C—Opiates function by blocking norepinephrine reuptake)*

16. A 47-year-old man with hypertension, diabetes, and a 20-pack-year history of cigarette smoking requests assistance in smoking cessation. He has tried to quit several times in the past but has always resumed smoking within a week.

Which of the following has the best results for smoking cessation?

❑ **A. Nicotine replacement therapy**

❑ **B. Behavioral therapy and counseling**

❑ **C. Bupropion therapy**

❑ **D. A combination of all of the above**

Key Concept/Objective: To understand the principles of smoking cessation

Cessation of cigarette smoking is aided by currently available pharmacotherapies. Effective therapies, including nicotine replacement therapy in the form of nasal spray, inhaler, gum, or patch, as well as the atypical antidepressant bupropion (300 mg/day for 7 to 12 weeks), have shown a success rate of smoking cessation twice that of placebo. Although bupropion is an antidepressant, the presence or absence of depression does not influence its effectiveness for smoking cessation. The combination of a nicotine replacement therapy with bupropion may be more effective than either modality alone. The addition of behavior therapy and social support counseling to pharmacotherapy further increases the cessation rate. *(Answer: D—A combination of all of the above)*

For more information, see Shuckit MA: 13 Psychiatry: VI Drug Abuse and Dependence. ACP Medicine Online (www.acpmedicine.com). Dale DC, Federman DD, Eds. WebMD Inc., New York, May 2004

Schizophrenia

17. A 29-year-old male patient is referred to you by his psychiatrist for treatment of hypertension and diabetes. The patient denies having headaches, chest pain, shortness of breath, edema, blurry vision, or change in sensation of his extremities. His medical record describes his initial presentation of schizophrenia.

For this patient, which of the following statements is consistent with the clinical manifestations of schizophrenia?

- ❑ **A. The patient was known to have depression and mania with associated delusions**
- ❑ **B. The patient did not exhibit prodromal symptoms before his initial episode of acute psychosis**
- ❑ **C. Between psychotic episodes, no residual symptoms are present**
- ❑ **D. The patient had restricted affect, low drive, and a poverty of speech**

Key Concept/Objective: To understand the clinical manifestations of schizophrenia

The diagnosis of schizophrenia should be considered in a patient who presents with hallucinations and delusions. The presence of disorganized thought and behavior increases the likelihood of schizophrenia. In the absence of other known causes of such symptoms (e.g., substance abuse, temporal lobe epilepsy), the principal diagnostic task is to discriminate between severe mental illnesses. If the patient does not have a mood disorder and the psychotic symptoms are accompanied by restricted affect, low drive, and poverty of speech, the probability of schizophrenia is high. The diagnosis can be made with greatest confidence, however, on the basis of the longitudinal pattern of the disorder, which includes the occurrence of prodromal symptoms before the initial episode, residual symptoms between psychotic episodes, and psychotic episodes that cannot be attributed to mood disturbance (e.g., manic or depressive psychosis) or other known causes of psychotic behavior. *(Answer: D—The patient had restricted affect, low drive, and a poverty of speech)*

18. A 31-year-old woman presents to your office with a chief complaint of hearing voices. She says that she can hear people telling her, "You're a failure," and being very critical of her actions. She also relates that she believes she is being watched carefully by the FBI and that your conversation with her is probably being monitored. It is clear that she has psychotic features that are consistent with schizophrenia, but you also consider other disorders that can cause psychotic symptoms.

Which of the following statements regarding disorders that can cause psychotic symptoms is true?

❑ A. Depression and mania are not associated with psychotic features

❑ B. Schizotypal personality disorder is similar to schizophrenia in that people with this personality disorder have persistent psychotic symptoms

❑ C. Drug abuse is an uncommon cause of psychotic symptoms

❑ D. Rarely, a brain tumor or temporal lobe epilepsy may be misdiagnosed as schizophrenia; in such cases, MRI or electroencephalography can help make the diagnosis

Key Concept/Objective: To know the common disorders that can mimic schizophrenia and to know how to differentiate between them

Because schizophrenia is defined as a psychotic illness with functional impairments, distinguishing schizophrenia from normalcy is usually not difficult. However, differentiating schizophrenia from other disorders with psychotic features can be a challenge. Schizotypal personality disorder shares some of the clinical characteristics of schizophrenia, such as social and physical anhedonia, suspiciousness, magical thinking, blunting of affect and emotional experience, and poor functioning. However, schizotypal patients do not experience overt and persistent psychotic symptoms, although rare and brief psychotic symptoms may occur. In a patient with persistent psychosis, the differential diagnosis consists mainly of affective disorders with psychosis, substance abuse, and delusional disorders. Psychosis that coincides with depression is typically associated with such affective features as delusions of poverty or accusatory voices. Similarly, delusions of grandeur are common during manic episodes. Psychotic symptoms in affective disorders typically follow the emergence of depression or mania and fade once the affective symptoms recede. The history and toxicology screen can rule out psychosis caused by drug abuse, such as use of PCP or long-term abuse of steroids. Delusional disorder is diagnosed on the basis of nonbizarre, persistent, and circumscribed delusions in the absence of the other characteristics of schizophrenia. Rarely, neurologic conditions such as brain tumor or temporal lobe epilepsy may be misdiagnosed as schizophrenia. When such conditions are suspected, MRI and EEG can help with the diagnosis. *(Answer: D—Rarely, a brain tumor or temporal lobe epilepsy may be misdiagnosed as schizophrenia; in such cases, MRI or electroencephalography can help make the diagnosis)*

For more information, see Carpenter WT, Thaller GK: 13 Psychiatry: VII Schizophrenia. ACP Medicine Online (www.acpmedicine.com). Dale DC, Federman DD, Eds. WebMD Inc., New York, June 2004

Anxiety Disorders

19. A 37-year-old woman presents to the emergency department with chest pain. The pain started 20 minutes ago. It is severe and is located in her right chest; it does not radiate. Onset was not associated with physical activity. The patient also complains of shortness of breath, shakiness, palpitations, diaphoresis, and nausea. The patient has visited the hospital three times over the past 4 months with similar symptoms. She used to run 3 miles a day 3 days a week, but she has stopped running because of concerns of dying of a heart attack. Lately, she has been spending more time at home because she is concerned she would be helpless if she suffered a heart attack outside her house. One month ago, she underwent a stress test, the results of which were normal. The patient does not smoke; she drinks one glass of wine a night. Her father died of a heart attack when he was 60 years of age. On physical examination, the patient's heart rate is 130 beats/min; her respiratory rate is 28 breaths/min; diaphoresis and distal tremors are noted. The rest of the examination is unremarkable. An electrocardiogram shows sinus tachycardia.

Which of the following is the most likely diagnosis, and which therapeutic intervention constitutes first-line therapy for this disorder?

- ❑ **A. Panic disorder with agoraphobia; start a benzodiazepine**
- ❑ **B. Panic disorder without agoraphobia; start a selective serotonin reuptake inhibitor (SSRI)**
- ❑ **C. Panic disorder with agoraphobia; start cognitive-behavioral psychotherapy**
- ❑ **D. Panic disorder without agoraphobia; refer to psychiatry**

Key Concept/Objective: To understand the diagnosis and treatment of panic disorder

This patient has panic disorder with agoraphobia. The pathognomonic feature of panic disorder is unexpected panic attacks, which are characterized by sudden onset and rapid escalation of somatic symptoms referable to the autonomic nervous system (e.g., chest pain, shortness of breath, heart palpitations, and dizziness), along with fear and apprehension. The diagnosis of panic disorder requires recurrent panic accompanied by significant worry about panic, its consequences, or a change in usual behavior. Panic disorder has four common clinical presentations: physical symptoms, anxiety and tension, hypochondriachal concerns, and medical conditions such as asthma. Agoraphobia is a fear of situations in which the person would feel trapped or alone should a panic episode occur. Drug therapy can be markedly effective for panic disorder. SSRIs are first-line therapy for panic disorder. Targeted cognitive-behavioral psychotherapy is as effective as medication in treating panic disorder. *(Answer: C—Panic disorder with agoraphobia; start cognitive-behavioral psychotherapy)*

20. A 68-year-old man comes to your clinic for a follow-up visit. He was discharged from a local hospital 3 months ago after a long stay in the intensive care unit for multiple medical problems, including pneumonia that required mechanical ventilation for 3 weeks, acute renal failure, sepsis, and amputation of his right foot as a result of a vascular event. He requires home oxygen therapy, but he says his breathing is slowly improving. He has no active complaints. His wife says he has had insomnia since he was discharged from the hospital. She also says the patient has been waking up in the middle of the night sweating and very anxious. The patient has been having recurrent dreams in which he is hospitalized in the ICU.

Which of the following is the most likely diagnosis, and what therapy should be started for this patient?

- ❑ **A. Panic disorder; start an SSRI**
- ❑ **B. Posttraumatic stress disorder (PTSD); start an SSRI**
- ❑ **C. Generalized anxiety; start cognitive behavioral psychotherapy**
- ❑ **D. Hospital phobia; start a benzodiazepine**

Key Concept/Objective: To understand PTSD and its treatment

Diagnostic criteria for PTSD include exposure to an event that posed a risk of death or serious physical injury, along with subsequent symptoms of reexperiencing the event, avoidance, and arousal. Dissociative symptoms may also be present. In addition to violence, events that can trigger PTSD include frightening or painful medical illness or procedures. SSRIs are efficacious in the treatment of PTSD. An intensive form of cognitive-behavioral psychotherapy can also be effective. Panic disorder is characterized by recurrent panic attacks. Generalized anxiety is characterized by persistent excessive and uncontrollable worry about everyday life situations. Specific phobias are irrational fears, usually accompanied by avoidance of the feared stimulus. *(Answer: B—Posttraumatic stress disorder [PTSD]; start an SSRI)*

21. A 34-year-old man comes to your clinic complaining of a recurrent headache. The headache is located posteriorly and is constant, dull, and nonthrobbing. The patient says that it lasts for several hours and that the use of acetaminophen provides some relief. He has been experiencing these symptoms for the past 8 months. On review of systems, the patient reports that he has been having difficulty falling asleep at night and that he has been experiencing fatigue. He says he is concerned about the headaches. He describes himself as a stressed person but denies feeling depressed. The patient smokes cigarettes and drinks alcohol socially. His physical examination is unremarkable. Basic laboratory studies, including a complete blood count, a metabolic profile, and thyroid function tests, are normal.

What therapeutic intervention would you recommend for this patient?

- ❑ **A. Start a beta blocker for headache prophylaxis**
- ❑ **B. Start venlafaxine**
- ❑ **C. Start a benzodiazepine**
- ❑ **D. Reassurance**

Key Concept/Objective: To know the different presentations of generalized anxiety disorder (GAD), as well as its treatment

The defining characteristic of GAD is persistent excessive and uncontrollable worry about everyday situations. GAD can be highly debilitating and may predispose to the development of other anxiety or mood disorders. GAD is the most common anxiety disorder seen in primary care settings; patients often present with sleep disturbance or somatic symptoms such as muscle aches and tension headaches. GAD is similar to other anxiety disorders in that it often goes undiagnosed and untreated. Venlafaxine is considered by most experts to be the first-line treatment. SSRIs have been found efficacious, and benzodiazepines have also been used to treat GAD. However, these drugs are generally not used as first-line treatments. Although cognitive-behavioral psychotherapy for GAD has been less studied than for other anxiety disorders, this approach appears promising. *(Answer: B—Start venlafaxine)*

22. A 29-year-old medical resident is often late for daily rounds. When asked for an explanation, he blames the traffic and his need for taking care of different issues at home before coming to the hospital. It has been noticed that he disappears during rounds, and he has been found several times washing his hands for several minutes before coming back to rounds.

What is the most likely diagnosis for this resident, and what would be the best therapeutic intervention to try first?

- ❑ **A. Obsessive-compulsive disorder (OCD); start clomipramine**
- ❑ **B. Substance abuse; refer for psychotherapy**
- ❑ **C. Schizophrenia; start an atypical antipsychotic**
- ❑ **D. Social phobia; start an SSRI**

Key Concept/Objective: To understand OCD and its treatment

OCD is characterized by repeated intrusive thoughts, ideas, or images (obsessions) and by repeated ritualistic behaviors (compulsions). Affected individuals recognize the irrationality of their thoughts but are powerless to control them. OCD is diagnosed when obsessions and compulsions are present for at least an hour a day or at a level that interferes with functioning. It is important to note that this disorder is often associated with considerable shame, and patients who have it may be reluctant to reveal their habits. Serotonin-active antidepressants, including clomipramine, are the first-line agents for OCD. Fluoxetine, sertraline, fluvoxamine, paroxetine, and citalopram also have demonstrated efficacy in the treatment of OCD. Cognitive-behavioral therapy is also highly effective. Social phobia and substance abuse are in the differential diagnosis of this patient. However, the presence of ritualistic behaviors (washing of hands) makes OCD more likely. In this patient, no diagnostic criteria for schizophrenia are present. *(Answer: A—Obsessive-compulsive disorder [OCD]; start clomipramine)*

For more information, see Shear MK: 13 Psychiatry: VIII Anxiety Disorders. ACP Medicine Online (www.acpmedicine.com). Dale DC, Federman DD, Eds. WebMD Inc., New York, August 2003

SECTION 14

RESPIRATORY MEDICINE

Asthma

1. A 42-year-old man with a history of wheezing and shortness of breath is referred to your pulmonary clinic for management of asthma. The diagnosis of asthma was apparently based on symptoms and evidence of obstruction on pulmonary function testing.

During an episode of airflow obstruction, which of the following findings would be specific for a diagnosis of asthma in this patient?

❑ A. Depressed diffusing capacity of the lung for carbon monoxide (DL_{CO}) on pulmonary function testing

❑ B. A normal alveolar-arterial difference in oxygen ($A\text{-}aDO_2$) gradient

❑ C. Improvement after administration of an inhaled bronchodilator

❑ D. Improvement after administration of corticosteroids

❑ E. The episode is associated with ingestion of a nonsteroidal anti-inflammatory drug (NSAID)

Key Concept/Objective: To understand the differential diagnosis of asthma

DL_{CO} may be elevated in some patients with asthma, possibly because of greater recruitment of capillaries from higher pulmonary arterial pressure. Depression of DL_{CO} in the setting of pulmonary obstruction is characteristic of chronic obstructive pulmonary disease, not asthma. Because of ventilation-perfusion mismatching, an elevation in $A\text{-}aDO_2$ is common, but severe hypoxemia is rare. A normal $A\text{-}aDO_2$ gradient in the setting of obstruction and a finding of wheezes that are heard loudest over the neck and that are transmitted with less intensity to the lung periphery are suggestive of partial upper airway obstruction. Other factors that suggest upper airway obstruction are the patient's perception that the problem is in the throat, hoarseness, a cough that sounds unusual, and a history of trauma, surgery, or prolonged intubation of the upper airway. Cardiac asthma may improve after administration of an inhaled bronchodilator. Therefore, one should exercise caution in making a diagnosis of bronchospasm on the basis of bronchodilator responsiveness, especially in the acute setting. Similarly, corticosteroids can occasionally relieve symptoms of upper airway obstruction by decreasing edema. However, bronchospasm that is associated with ingestion of aspirin or NSAIDs is highly suggestive of asthma. Perhaps 10% to 20% of patients with asthma exhibit an idiosyncratic reaction to aspirin and other NSAIDs. Within 15 minutes to 4 hours, patients may experience significant worsening of airflow obstruction and nasal or ocular symptoms. *(Answer: E—The episode is associated with ingestion of a nonsteroidal anti-inflammatory drug [NSAID])*

2. You are caring for a young woman with asthma who has symptoms almost on a daily basis. Although her symptoms occur at various times during the day, they occur more frequently at night. Currently, her medical regimen consists only of a short-acting inhaled beta-adrenergic agonist for rescue. The patient is trying to become pregnant.

Of the following, which is the best therapeutic step to take next for this patient?

❑ A. A long-acting selective $beta_2$-adrenergic agonist should be added to her regimen

❑ B. A low-dose oral steroid should be added to her regimen

❑ C. An inhaled corticosteroid should be added to her regimen

❑ D. Theophylline should be added to her regimen

❑ E. Ipratropium bromide should be added to her regimen

Key Concept/Objective: To understand the fundamental principles of the management of asthma

This patient has moderate asthma, and her current medical regimen is insufficient. An inhaled corticosteroid should be added to her regimen. Patients with daily symptoms of airflow obstruction should use inhaled steroids regularly. Long-acting selective beta$_2$-adrenergic agonists should not be used in place of low-dose inhaled steroids, but they can often be used to reduce (though not eliminate) steroid use. If taken before bedtime, they may be particularly helpful in patients with prominent nocturnal symptoms because of their long duration of action. However, their safety during pregnancy has not been thoroughly evaluated. Patients who remain symptomatic despite use of inhaled corticosteroids and a combination of inhaled beta-adrenergic agonist, theophylline, and possibly ipratropium bromide may require alternate-day oral steroid therapy at the minimal dosage necessary to maintain the patient's symptoms at an acceptable level. Theophylline is less effective than the combination of a long-acting inhaled beta$_2$-adrenergic agonist and inhaled corticosteroids. Anticholinergic agents such as ipratropium bromide have modest bronchodilatory effect in patients with asthma and could be added in refractory cases. The primary indication for anticholinergic agents is chronic obstructive pulmonary disease. Incidentally, this patient should probably be advised to wait until her asthma is better controlled before becoming pregnant. During pregnancy, approximately one third of patients experience improvement in their symptoms of asthma, and one third remain stable, but in one third, symptoms worsen. Those with more severe asthma are at greater risk of their symptoms worsening. *(Answer: C—An inhaled corticosteroid should be added to her regimen)*

3. A 42-year-old bakery worker presents with a complaint of cough and wheezing; he has been experiencing these symptoms for the past 2 months. He has been working at the bakery for the past 2 years. You consider occupational asthma in your differential diagnosis.

Which of the following statements accurately characterizes the evaluation and treatment of this patient?

❑ A. Occupational asthma is unlikely because the patient was exposed to the work environment for almost 2 years before developing symptoms

❑ B. Asthma that persists after the patient stops going to the workplace excludes occupational asthma as the diagnosis

❑ C. Skin testing with a soluble extract of the suspected offending agent confirms a diagnosis of occupational asthma

❑ D. If a diagnosis of occupational asthma is made, the patient should be advised to take an inhaled short-acting beta$_2$-adrenergic agonist before and during work, as needed

❑ E. Onset of symptoms hours after leaving the workplace supports a diagnosis of occupational asthma

Key Concept/Objective: To understand the diagnosis and treatment of occupational asthma

The typical history of a patient with occupational asthma is that after the patient has spent a few months (but sometimes up to several years) at a job, he or she experiences coughing, wheezing, and chest tightness shortly after arriving at the workplace. In most cases, occupational asthma is cured by removal of the offending agent or transfer of the patient from the site of the offending agent. Transfer of the patient to a job that merely reduces rather than eliminates exposure does not effectively relieve symptoms. Trying to treat occupational asthma with beta agonists without having the patient avoid exposure to the offending agent is not recommended. In a few cases, symptoms

of occupational asthma continue for years after the patient has left the workplace. Skin testing with the appropriate soluble extracts assesses only for sensitization to the agent. Many workers exhibit positive results on skin testing but have no evidence of asthma. Some persons with occupational asthma report a delayed onset of asthmatic symptoms: symptoms begin hours after the patient leaves the workplace. This can make recognition of an association with an offending agent difficult. *(Answer: E—Onset of symptoms hours after leaving the workplace supports a diagnosis of occupational asthma)*

4. A 38-year-old woman with known long-standing asthma presents with cough, wheezing, and fever; chest x-ray reveals a right upper lobe infiltrate. The patient is admitted to the hospital. After several days of treatment with antibiotics, her symptoms do not improve, nor is improvement seen in the infiltrate. Her blood work reveals a normal white blood cell (WBC) count, but there is significant eosinophilia. You suspect the diagnosis of allergic bronchopulmonary aspergillosis (ABPA).

Which of the following statements regarding the diagnosis of this patient is false?

❑ **A. Chest x-ray characteristically shows central bronchiectasis**

❑ **B. The disease rarely occurs in patients with asthma**

❑ **C. Diagnostic criteria include eosinophilia, an elevation in total serum IgE level, a positive immediate skin-test reaction to *Aspergillus* antigen, and elevated levels of IgE and IgG antibodies specific to *Aspergillus***

❑ **D. The chronic form of the disease can mimic tuberculosis**

Key Concept/Objective: To be able to recognize ABPA

ABPA is caused by a hypersensitivity reaction to the colonization of the airways by *Aspergillus* species. The acute form of the disease is characterized by fever, flulike symptoms, and myalgias; it is often confused with acute bacterial pneumonia. The presence of sputum and blood eosinophilia is highly characteristic; sputum cultures are negative for pathogenic bacteria. The chest x-ray is characterized by pulmonary infiltrates with corresponding atelectasis of the affected segment or lobe. These findings are related to the presence of tenacious secretions with obstruction of the bronchial airways. Migratory pulmonary infiltrates are not uncommon. The chronic form of the disease is characterized radiologically by central bronchiectasis and upper lobe infiltrates with corresponding volume loss that mimics tuberculosis. The diagnostic criteria for ABPA include (1) repeated growth of *Aspergillus* species in culture; (2) positive skin-test reaction to *Aspergillus* antigen; (3) elevated total serum IgE level (> 1,000 ng/ml in patients not receiving steroids); and (4) elevated levels of IgG and IgE antibodies specific against *Aspergillus*. Systemic steroids are used in treatment. New data suggest that the use of itraconazole in combination with inhaled steroids may be useful. This disease is seen almost exclusively in patients with long-standing asthma; occasionally, ABPA is diagnosed in patients with cystic fibrosis. *(Answer: B—The disease rarely occurs in patients with asthma)*

5. A 45-year-old man comes to your office to establish primary care. He has had asthma since childhood, and he has been experiencing occasional wheezing, shortness of breath, and cough productive of yellow sputum. He cannot identify specific irritants that trigger his asthma. He does not engage in regular exercise. He lives with his wife and their two children in an apartment building and works in an auto-body shop. He has no nasal polyps, and his physical examination is unremarkable.

Which of the following statements about this patient's condition is most likely to be true?

❑ **A. Because he has no specific allergic precipitants (i.e., he has intrinsic asthma), he is more likely to respond to an inhaled steroid**

❑ **B. His occasional cough associated with yellow sputum is likely to be infectious in origin**

❑ C. The fact that his physical examination is normal should raise suspicion that his symptoms are caused by something other than asthma alone

❑ D. Occupational asthma is a strong possibility

❑ E. You should caution him against starting a regular exercise program, because this may worsen his asthma symptoms

Key Concept/Objective: To understand that occupational asthma is common and that patients with long-standing asthma may not be aware that an occupational irritant is contributing to their asthma

Occupational exposure plays a role in 10% of patients with asthma. Patients with asthma often experience delayed hypersensitivity reactions more than 12 hours after exposure; because of this, a patient who had asthma before starting a job may not be aware of a noxious irritant in the workplace. Workers in auto-body shops are at risk for occupational asthma caused by paint spray. The distinction between intrinsic and extrinsic asthma has no bearing on asthma management. Eosinophils and their debris often cause yellow discoloration of sputum even in the absence of infection. Patients often have a normal physical examination between exacerbations. Although exercise can trigger asthma, with appropriate therapy almost all patients with asthma can perform regular exercise without difficulty. *(Answer: D—Occupational asthma is a strong possibility)*

6. At your urging, the patient in Question 5 attempts to start exercising, but he finds that he develops shortness of breath soon after he finishes jogging.

   Which of the following statements about this patient is most correct?

   ❑ A. His shortness of breath may very well result from being out of shape

   ❑ B. He would benefit from use of ipratropium bromide before exercise

   ❑ C. He would benefit from use of a beta agonist before exercise

   ❑ D. He would benefit from use of theophylline before exercise

   ❑ E. He would benefit from use of an inhaled steroid before exercise

   Key Concept/Objective: To understand the appropriate therapy for exercise-induced asthma

   The most effective therapy for exercise-induced asthma is an inhaled beta agonist. Cromolyn is also effective, and newer leukotriene modifiers may also have a role. Theophylline, corticosteroids, and anticholinergics have no role in the treatment of exercise-induced asthma. This patient's symptoms are clearly not caused by deconditioning, because they occur only after he stops exercising. *(Answer: C—He would benefit from use of a beta agonist before exercise)*

7. The patient in Question 5 returns to clinic for follow-up 12 weeks later. He mentions that 7 days ago he had a headache, for which he took two aspirin. Later, as the headache began to subside, he also developed itchy eyes and an itchy throat.

   Which of the following statements about this patient is most correct?

   ❑ A. Because he does not have nasal polyps, it is unlikely that he has aspirin hypersensitivity

   ❑ B. He is likely to have similar reactions to all NSAIDs

   ❑ C. This reaction was the result of salicylate sensitivity, so ibuprofen should be safe for him to use

   ❑ D. This reaction suggests that he would not benefit from a leukotriene modifier

   ❑ E. A COX-2 inhibitor, such as celecoxib, is likely to be safe for him to use

Key Concept/Objective: To understand the relationship between asthma and aspirin hypersensitivity

Aspirin hypersensitivity can initially present with bronchoconstriction or other allergic symptoms. Cross-reactivity with other NSAIDs is almost universal, because the causal mechanism is likely mediated by COX. Therefore, all NSAIDs, including COX-2 inhibitors, are likely to cause a reaction. Despite the classic triad, asthma and aspirin hypersensitivity often coexist in the absence of nasal polyps. Leukotriene modifiers are likely to be more effective in patients with aspirin hypersensitivity because of their effect on the COX pathway. *(Answer: B—He is likely to have similar reactions to all NSAIDs)*

8. A 28-year-old woman seeks a second opinion for asthma that has been recently worsening. She has had asthma for the past 14 years, but over the past 6 months her symptoms have been more severe. In addition to wheezing, shortness of breath, and chest tightness, she has had intermittent fevers and flulike symptoms. She has been treated with multiple courses of antibiotics as well as increasing doses of inhaled steroids with no significant improvement. A chest x-ray shows patchy bilobar infiltrates, which are in different locations from those seen on a chest x-ray that she had 3 months ago. Serum *Aspergillus* serologies are very high.

Which of the following statements about this patient is false?

- ❑ **A. Her serum eosinophil count is probably elevated**
- ❑ **B. A sputum culture for *Aspergillus* is likely to be positive**
- ❑ **C. Any bronchial involvement is likely to be on the surface only, without tissue invasion**
- ❑ **D. She may need to be treated with systemic corticosteroids**
- ❑ **E. A trial of antifungal therapy will not be helpful**

Key Concept/Objective: To understand the pathophysiology, diagnosis, and treatment of allergic bronchopulmonary aspergillosis

Allergic bronchopulmonary aspergillosis is a hypersensitivity reaction to colonization of the airways by *Aspergillus*. Recent studies have shown that the combination of the antifungal itraconazole and inhaled steroids may be effective treatment. If they fail, systemic corticosteroids may be necessary. Allergic bronchopulmonary aspergillosis typically causes an elevated serum eosinophil count, and sputum cultures will test positive. It is very unlikely that there will be fungal tissue invasion. *(Answer: E—A trial of antifungal therapy will not be helpful)*

For more information, see Staton GW, Ingram RH Jr: 14 Respiratory Medicine: II Asthma. ACP Medicine Online (www.acpmedicine.com). Dale DC, Federman DD, Eds. WebMD Inc., New York, August 2002

Chronic Obstructive Diseases of the Lung

9. A 57-year-old patient who smokes cigarettes presents with chronic productive cough and persistent progressive exercise limitation that is a result of breathlessness.

For this patient, which of the following statements is true?

- ❑ **A. Significant airway obstruction occurs in only 10% to 15% of people who smoke**
- ❑ **B. The best tool for assessing the severity of obstruction is the ratio of forced expiratory volume in 1 second to forced vital capacity (FEV_1/FVC)**
- ❑ **C. Chronic bronchitis is a clinical diagnosis defined as the presence of cough and sputum production on most days for at least 3 consecutive months in a year**

❑ **D. Measurement of lung volumes in patients with chronic airway obstruction (CAO) uniformly reveals an increased residual volume and a decreased functional residual capacity (FRC)**

Key Concept/Objective: To understand the pathogenesis and pathophysiology of chronic obstructive pulmonary disease (COPD)

Chronic bronchitis and emphysema are by far the most common causes of chronic airflow obstruction. Chronic bronchitis is defined as the presence of cough and sputum on most days for at least 3 months of the year for a minimum of 2 years in succession. Emphysema is a destructive process involving the lung parenchyma and is defined in pathologic terms. Only 10% to 15% of smokers experience clinically significant airway obstruction. Although a low FEV_1/FVC and a decrease in expiratory flow rates prove obstruction, the best measurement for assessing the severity of the obstruction is FEV_1. Measurement of lung volumes uniformly reveals an increased residual volume (RV) and a normal to increased FRC. RV may be two to four times higher than normal because of slowing of expiratory flow and trapping of gas behind prematurely closed airways. FRC increases by two mechanisms: dynamic hyperinflation and activation of inspiratory muscles during exhalation. As a result, tidal breathing may take place at lung volumes as high as 1 to 2 L above normal levels. *(Answer: A—Significant airway obstruction occurs in only 10% to 15% of people who smoke)*

10. A 53-year-old man presents to establish primary care. He has a history of COPD and a 60 pack-year history of cigarette smoking. Currently, he smokes one pack of cigarettes a week. His COPD is currently managed with PRN albuterol administered with a metered-dose inhaler (MDI); a long-acting $beta_2$ agonist; and an inhaled corticosteroid. The patient experiences dyspnea with moderate exertion; otherwise, he is functional. The results of a complete blood count (CBC) and serum chemistry are unremarkable. Pulse oximetry is significant for an O_2 saturation of 96% on room air with no change after climbing and descending two flights of stairs. The patient says he would like to change his medications to nebulized bronchodilators. He also wonders which intervention is most likely to alter the natural history of his COPD.

For this patient, which of the following statements is true?

❑ **A. Long-term administration of oxygen will favorably alter the natural history of this patient's disease**

❑ **B. Probably the single most important intervention is to help this patient quit smoking**

❑ **C. Physical training programs have been shown to significantly increase the exercise capacity of patients with even far-advanced chronic bronchitis and emphysema; such programs lead to objective improvements in lung function, as measured by FEV_1**

❑ **D. Nebulized bronchodilators are generally of greater benefit than MDIs**

Key Concept/Objective: To understand the importance and the benefits of smoking cessation in patients with COPD

Of the therapeutic measures available for patients with chronic bronchitis and emphysema, only smoking cessation and long-term administration of supplemental oxygen to the chronically hypoxemic patient have been definitively shown to alter the natural history of the disease favorably; in this patient with normal O_2 saturation, administration of oxygen would be of no clinical benefit. Helping a patient to quit smoking is probably the single most important intervention; effective methods include counseling by physicians and nurses, use of nicotine replacement therapy, behavioral intervention (e.g., individual or group therapy), and several pharmacologic interventions (e.g., bupropion and nortriptyline). A variety of other therapies offer potential relief of symptoms in patients with COPD. These include the use of bronchodilators; anti-inflammatory therapy; administration of antibiotics during acute purulent exacerbations; pulmonary rehabilitation programs, including physical exercise and respiratory muscle

training; and, for patients with cor pulmonale, the use of diuretics. There is no evidence that nebulized bronchodilators are of greater benefit than properly administered dry-powder inhalers or MDIs used with a spacer. Physical-training programs, such as treadmill walking, significantly increase the exercise capacity of patients with even far-advanced chronic bronchitis and emphysema. These results have been achieved despite the fact that lung function, as reflected in such measurements as vital capacity and FEV_1, is not affected and that maximal heart rate is generally not reached during the training sessions. *(Answer: B—Probably the single most important intervention is to help this patient quit smoking)*

11. A 62-year-old man with a history of COPD (FEV_1, 38%) presents with worsening dyspnea, which now occurs at rest; purulent sputum; and wheezing of 6 days' duration. He has increased the use of his inhalers without experiencing an improvement of symptoms. He denies having fever, chills, or pleuritic chest pain. A chest x-ray does not demonstrate an acute process. The patient is admitted for treatment of an acute exacerbation of COPD.

Which of the following statements regarding the management of acute exacerbations of COPD is true?

- ❑ **A. The duration of symptoms and the risk of serious deterioration in lung function can be reduced by at least a 14- to 21-day course of broad-spectrum antibiotics**
- ❑ **B. The bronchodilator of choice in exacerbations of COPD is an anticholinergic such as ipratropium**
- ❑ **C. Oxygen supplementation should be adjusted to maintain oxygen saturation at 95% or greater**
- ❑ **D. In patients already receiving theophylline, measurement of the theophylline level is indicated because acute illness and some of the medications used to treat exacerbations can precipitate theophylline toxicity; however, there are no data that show that the addition of theophylline is beneficial for exacerbations of COPD**

Key Concept/Objective: To understand the treatment of an acute exacerbation of COPD

Acute exacerbations are often precipitated by respiratory infection. Such infections may be caused by viral or bacterial pathogens. In patients with symptoms of infection, the duration of symptoms and the risk of serious deterioration in lung function can be reduced by a 7- to 10-day course of broad-spectrum antibiotics. The bronchodilator of choice in exacerbations of COPD is a short-acting $beta_2$ agonist such as albuterol, mainly because of its rapid onset of action. Once short-acting $beta_2$-agonist therapy is started, inhaled anticholinergic therapy (e.g., ipratropium) should be initiated or increased. The dosage is usually 3 to 4 puffs but can be increased to 5 to 8 puffs every 3 to 4 hours. Oxygen supplementation should be adjusted to keep oxygen saturation around 90% to 92% to maintain tissue oxygenation while minimizing the risk of worsening hypercapnia. There are no data indicating that the addition of theophylline is beneficial for exacerbations of COPD. For patients already on theophylline, the theophylline level should be measured, because some of the medications used to treat COPD exacerbations can precipitate theophylline toxicity. *(Answer: D—In patients already receiving theophylline, measurement of the theophylline level is indicated because acute illness and some of the medications used to treat exacerbations can precipitate theophylline toxicity; however, there are no data that show that the addition of theophylline is beneficial for exacerbations of COPD)*

12. A 40-year-old man presents for evaluation of worsening dyspnea on exertion. He denies having a cough. He has a remote history of tobacco use and a significant family history of emphysema. The results of a CBC and serum chemistry panel are unremarkable. A chest x-ray demonstrates attenuation of the pulmonary vasculature, predominantly in the lower lobes. Pulmonary function tests are consistent with severe airway obstruction.

Which of the following statements regarding α_1-antitrypsin deficiency is true?

❑ **A. Serious liver disease, usually in the form of cirrhosis, occurs in up to one third of adults with α_1-antitrypsin deficiency**

❑ **B. The mean age at onset of dyspnea is 55 to 60 years in nonsmokers and approximately 10 years earlier in those who smoke**

❑ **C. In the United States, the prevalence of α_1-antitrypsin deficiency caused by a homozygous Pi^Z genotype is one in 3,000 persons**

❑ **D. The typical pathologic picture is a centriacinar emphysema with a basilar predominance**

Key Concept/Objective: To understand the pathophysiology, epidemiology, and clinical presentation of α_1-antitrypsin deficiency

In the United States, α_1-antitrypsin deficiency caused by a homozygous Pi^Z genotype occurs in one in 3,000 persons; the prevalence is lower in African Americans. Emphysema develops in at least 80% of patients with homozygous Pi^Z α_1-antitrypsin deficiency. The mean age at onset of dyspnea is 45 to 50 years in nonsmokers and approximately 10 years earlier in those who smoke. The typical pathologic picture is panacinar emphysema, but as many as 25% to 30% of nonsmoking patients and 60% of cigarette smokers report symptoms of chronic bronchitis as well. Many of the patients have evidence of enhanced airway reactivity. A significant incidence of bronchiectasis is detected by high-resolution CT scanning. Involvement of the lower lobes often predominates, perhaps because of increased neutrophil traffic and release of neutrophil elastase in the lower lung fields. The radiographic manifestation of this phenomenon is most commonly attenuation of the pulmonary vasculature to the lower lobes; in more advanced cases, basilar bullae may be seen. Serious liver disease, usually in the form of cirrhosis, occurs in 5% to 10% of adults with α_1-antitrypsin deficiency and may provide a clue to the underlying enzyme deficiency in some patients. *(Answer: C—In the United States, the prevalence of α_1-antitrypsin deficiency caused by a homozygous Pi^Z genotype is one in 3,000 persons)*

13. A 67-year-old man presents to your clinic for evaluation of dyspnea. He reports that his breathing has been worsening for years. He has a 100-pack-year history of cigarette smoking. His physical examination is notable for obesity, prolonged expiratory phase with faint wheezing, jugular veinous distention to the mandible, hepatosplenomegaly; and 2+ bilateral lower extremity edema.

Which of the following would NOT be characteristic of this patient with type B COPD?

❑ **A. Mild to moderate hypoxia with normal to slightly decreased arterial carbon dioxide tension (P_aCO_2)**

❑ **B. Cough with sputum production**

❑ **C. Progression to cor pulmonale; abnormal depression of arousal responses to hypoxia and hypercapnia during sleep**

❑ **D. Increased resistance to airflow in both phases of the respiratory cycle**

Key Concept/Objective: To know the clinical factors for differentiating and identifying COPD type A patients (pink puffers) from type B patients (blue bloaters)

Type A patients exhibit dyspnea with only mild to moderate hypoxemia (arterial oxygen tension [P_aO_2] levels are usually > 65 mm Hg) and maintain normal or even slightly reduced P_aCO_2 levels. These patients are sometimes referred to as pink puffers; they tend to be thin, to experience hyperinflation at total lung capacity, and to be free of signs of right heart failure. The pink puffer usually has severe emphysema. Type B patients have marked hypoxemia and peripheral edema resulting from right heart failure. These patients, who are sometimes called blue bloaters, typically exhibit cough and sputum production. They have frequent respiratory tract infections, experience chronic carbon dioxide retention (P_aCO_2 > 45 mm Hg), and have recurrent episodes of cor pulmonale. The blue bloater may also have pathologic evidence of severe emphysema; in addition, the blue bloater suffers from inflammation of large and small airways and

possible defects in ventilatory control. *(Answer: A—Mild to moderate hypoxia with normal to slightly decreased arterial carbon dioxide tension [P_aCO_2])*

14. A 67-year-old man with a history of emphysema presents with a complaint of worsening dyspnea and cough that is productive of yellow-colored sputum. On pulmonary function testing, his FEV_1 is 45%. Arterial blood gas measurements were performed several months ago. The baseline value for P_aO_2 was 53 mm Hg, and the carbon dioxide tension (PCO_2) on room air was normal.

There is evidence showing improved survival for which of the following interventions (in addition to smoking cessation)?

- ❑ A. **Use of broad-spectrum antibiotics**
- ❑ B. **Use of corticosteroids**
- ❑ C. **Home oxygen therapy**
- ❑ D. **Lung volume reduction surgery**
- ❑ E. **Bronchodilator therapy**

Key Concept/Objective: To understand that only smoking cessation and long-term administration of supplemental oxygen have been definitively shown to change the natural history of emphysema

Reviews and guidelines on the treatment of CAO have been published, but they disagree on recommendations. Suboptimal prescription of and adherence to appropriate therapies further complicate the management of CAO. Of the therapeutic measures available for patients with chronic bronchitis and emphysema, only smoking cessation and long-term administration of supplemental oxygen to the chronically hypoxemic patient have been definitively shown to favorably alter the natural history of the disease. A variety of other therapies offer potential relief of symptoms in patients with CAO. These include the use of bronchodilators; anti-inflammatory therapy; the administration of antibiotics during acute purulent exacerbations; pulmonary rehabilitation programs, including physical exercise and respiratory muscle training; and, for patients with cor pulmonale, the use of diuretics. A randomized, multicenter clinical trial comparing lung volume reduction surgery with continued medical treatment in 1,218 patients with severe emphysema found that the surgery increased the chance of improved exercise capacity but did not confer a survival advantage, except in patients who had both predominantly upper lobe emphysema and low exercise capacity after rehabilitation. Broad-spectrum antibiotics, corticosteroids, and bronchodilators help improve symptoms, not long-term survival. *(Answer: C—Home oxygen therapy)*

15. A 40-year-old man presents to your clinic for evaluation of dyspnea. The patient is a nonsmoker and reports a slow progression of breathlessness. He also reveals that several of his family members were diagnosed with emphysema early in life, but he is confused because they were nonsmokers.

Which of the following statements concerning α_1-antitrypsin deficiency is true?

- ❑ A. **Emphysematous changes do not occur in the lower lobes of the lung**
- ❑ B. **α_1-Antitrypsin deficiency is not associated with cirrhotic liver disease**
- ❑ C. **α_1-Antitrypsin deficiency is not associated with a family history of emphysema in nonsmokers**
- ❑ D. **Purified α_1-antitrypsin is commercially available for treatment**
- ❑ E. **α_1-Antitrypsin levels higher than 40% of normal do not afford protection against the development of emphysema**

Key Concept/Objective: To know the clinical characteristics of α_1-antitrypsin deficiency and potential therapy to prevent disease progression

Emphysema develops in at least 80% of patients with homozygous Pi^Z α_1-antitrypsin deficiency. The mean age at onset of dyspnea is 45 to 50 years in nonsmokers and

approximately 10 years earlier in those who smoke. The typical pathologic picture is panacinar emphysema, but as many as 25% to 30% of nonsmoking patients and 60% of cigarette smokers report symptoms of chronic bronchitis as well. Many of the patients have evidence of enhanced airway reactivity. High-resolution CT scanning has detected a significant incidence of bronchiectasis in these patients. Involvement of the lower lobes often predominates, perhaps because of increased neutrophil traffic and the release of neutrophil elastase in the lower lung fields. The most common radiographic manifestation of this phenomenon is attenuation of the pulmonary vasculature to the lower lobes; in more advanced cases, basilar bullae may be seen. Features that would suggest α_1-antitrypsin deficiency as the cause of a particular patient's emphysema would thus include a family history of emphysema (especially among nonsmokers), the onset of symptoms at 30 to 50 years of age, the development of significant emphysema in a nonsmoker, and basilar predominance of the radiographic abnormalities. Serious liver disease, usually in the form of cirrhosis, occurs in 5% to 10% of adults with α_1-antitrypsin deficiency and may provide a clue to the underlying enzyme deficiency in some patients. It is thought that α_1-antitrypsin levels higher than 40% of normal afford protection against the development of emphysema. For patients with homozygous Pi^Z deficiency, consideration should be given to administration of purified α_1-antitrypsin, which is commercially available for replacement therapy. *(Answer: D—Purified α_1-antitrypsin is commercially available for treatment)*

16. A 37-year-old woman is referred to you for evaluation of dyspnea, purulent cough, and recurrent pneumonia. The patient has a childhood history of recurrent pneumonia. She has no known contacts with persons with tuberculosis, and a test for the presence of purified protein derivative (PPD) is negative. She has smoked a pack of cigarettes each day for 15 years. Pulmonary function tests were interpreted as indicating mild airflow obstruction.

Which of the following features does NOT favor a diagnosis of bronchiectasis over a diagnosis of emphysematous lung disease in this patient?

- ❑ **A. Chronic cough and dyspnea without purulent sputum production**
- ❑ **B. Tramlines noted on plain chest radiographs**
- ❑ **C. Clinical improvement from broad-spectrum antibiotics and drainage**
- ❑ **D. Massive hemoptysis**
- ❑ **E. Clubbing of the digits**

Key Concept/Objective: To understand that clubbing is a feature of bronchiectasis, not chronic airflow obstruction

Factors in the patient's history, such as chronic cough and sputum purulence originating from a serious respiratory tract infection, often in childhood, strongly suggest the diagnosis of bronchiectasis. Bronchiectasis may be seen on the plain chest radiograph in a number of different patterns. Occasionally, the thickened walls of a dilated bronchus can be visualized as the bronchus courses with its longitudinal axis perpendicular to the x-ray beam. These parallel lines are approximately 1 mm thick and are referred to as tramlines. Airflow obstruction is generally the main abnormality seen on pulmonary function tests. The mainstays of therapy for bronchiectasis (including cystic fibrosis [CF] and primary ciliary dyskinesia), as for any chronic suppurative disease, are administration of antibiotics and drainage. Massive hemoptysis (200 ml of blood over a 24-hour period) can occur as a complication of bronchiectasis. Clubbing of the digits occurs in the majority of patients with significant bronchiectasis and is a valuable diagnostic clue, especially since clubbing of the digits is not a manifestation of CAO. *(Answer: A—Chronic cough and dyspnea without purulent sputum production)*

17. A 21-year-old woman with a history of CF who previously received health care services at a local children's hospital now presents to your office to establish care as an adult.

Which of the following statements about CF is false?

❑ A. The median survival for women with CF is 28.3 years

❑ B. The majority of patients with CF possess the ΔF508 mutation, leading to an abnormal CF transmembrane regulator (CFTR)

❑ C. Impaired clearance of secretions leads to recurrent pulmonary infections and bronchiectasis

❑ D. Exocrine pancreatic function is maintained

❑ E. Diagnosis can be made by the sweat chloride test or by genetic testing

Key Concept/Objective: To understand the diagnosis and clinical manifestations of CF

Although CF is an inherited disease that usually manifests itself in early childhood, a discussion of the condition in the context of general adult medicine is worthwhile for two reasons. First, increasing numbers of children with CF are now surviving into young adulthood: the median survival in the United States is 31.1 years in men and 28.3 years in women. Second, some patients have a variant form of the disease in which symptoms first appear during adolescence or adulthood. The genetic defects responsible for CF have been identified. The CF locus is on the long arm of chromosome 7, and it codes for a 1,480 amino acid polypeptide that has been named the CF transmembrane regulator (CFTR). In 70% of patients with CF, the 508th amino acid of this sequence is missing (ΔF508). It is likely that impaired tracheobronchial clearance of the abnormal secretions leads to widespread mucous plugging of airways, resulting in secondary bacterial infection, persistent inflammation, and consequent generalized bronchiectasis. Extrapulmonary manifestations may also suggest the diagnosis of CF. Prominent among these findings are pancreatic insufficiency with consequent steatorrhea, recurrent partial intestinal obstruction caused by abnormal fecal accumulation (the so-called meconium ileus equivalent), heat prostration, hepatic cirrhosis, and aspermia in men. The diagnosis can be established by abnormal results on a sweat test performed in a qualified laboratory using pilocarpine iontophoresis. In persons younger than 20 years, a sweat chloride level exceeding 60 mEq/L confirms the diagnosis; a value exceeding 80 mEq/L is required for diagnosis in persons 20 years of age or older. With the identification of the gene for CF, genetic screening has become available. *(Answer: D—Exocrine pancreatic function is maintained)*

18. A 53-year-old man with a 60-pack-year history of cigarette smoking presents with complaints of productive cough and dypsnea. He reports that for the past 3 months, he has been treated for bronchitis with antibiotics, but his symptoms have not resolved. Over the past several weeks, he has experienced progressive dypsnea on exertion. He denies having any chest discomfort or any other significant medical history. Currently, he is not taking any medications. His lung examination shows wheezing that resolves with expectoration of phlegm. Chest x-ray shows hyperinflation. Initial pulmonary function tests show the patient's FEV_1 to be 55% of the predicted value. Arterial blood gas measurements are as follows: P_aO_2, 75 mm Hg; alveolar carbon dioxide tension (P_ACO_2), 55 mm Hg.

Which of the following is NOT true for this patient?

❑ A. If this patient continues to smoke, his FEV_1 value will continue to decrease two to three times faster than normal

❑ B. If this patient stops smoking, the rate of decline in expiratory flow reverts to that of nonsmokers, and there may be a slight improvement in FEV_1 during the first year

❑ C. This patient would be expected to have evidence of extensive panacinar emphysema

❑ D. This patient would be expected to have increased RV, increased FRC, and normal or increased total lung capacity (TLC)

❑ E. This patient is at risk for right-sided heart failure

Key Concept/Objective: To understand the progression of chronic bronchitis and emphysema

Panacinar emphysema is common in patients with α_1-antitrypsin deficiency. Centriacinar emphysema is commonly found in cigarette smokers and is rare in nonsmokers. Centriacinar emphysema is usually more extensive and severe in the upper lobes. In most cigarette smokers, a mixture of centriacinar and panacinar emphysema develops. In healthy nonsmokers, FEV_1 begins declining at about 20 years of age and continues at an average rate of about 0.02 to 0.04 L/yr. In smokers with obstructive lung disease, FEV_1 decreases, on average, two to three times faster than normal. When persons with mild to moderate airflow obstruction stop smoking, the rate of decline in expiratory flow reverts to that observed in nonsmokers, and there may be a slight improvement in FEV_1 during the first year. Measurement of lung volumes uniformly reveals an increased RV and a normal to increased FRC. RV may be two to four times higher than normal because of slowing of expiratory flow and gas trapping behind prematurely closed airways. TLC is normal or increased. One group of patients (type A) exhibit dyspnea with only mild to moderate hypoxemia (P_aO_2 levels are usually > 65 mm Hg) and maintain normal or even slightly reduced P_ACO_2 levels. They are sometimes referred to as pink puffers. The other clinical group of patients (type B) are sometimes called blue bloaters; they typically exhibit cough and sputum production, frequent respiratory tract infections, chronic carbon dioxide retention (P_ACO_2 > 45 mm Hg), and recurrent episodes of cor pulmonale. In the type B patient, both alveolar hypoxia and acidosis (secondary to chronic hypercapnia) stimulate pulmonary arterial vasoconstriction, and hypoxemia stimulates erythrocytosis. Increased pulmonary vascular resistance, increased pulmonary blood volume, and, possibly, increased blood viscosity (resulting from secondary erythrocytosis) all contribute to pulmonary arterial hypertension. In response to long-term pulmonary hypertension, cor pulmonale generally develops: the right ventricle becomes hypertrophic, and cardiac output is increased by means of abnormally high right ventricular filling pressures. *(Answer: C—This patient would be expected to have evidence of extensive panacinar emphysema)*

19. A 43-year-old female patient with chronic bronchitis associated with a 40-pack-year history of cigarette smoking presents for a routine appointment. Although she has a productive cough on a daily basis, she denies having any dypsnea and is currently not taking any medication.

Which of the following measures will most alter the natural progression of this patient's disease?

- ❑ **A. Daily bronchodilator use alone**
- ❑ **B. Daily corticosteroid use alone**
- ❑ **C. Daily prophylactic antibiotic**
- ❑ **D. Daily pulmonary rehabilitation**
- ❑ **E. Smoking cessation**

Key Concept/Objective: To know key treatment measures for chronic bronchitis and emphysema

Of the therapeutic measures available for patients with chronic bronchitis and emphysema, only smoking cessation and long-term administration of supplemental oxygen to the chronically hypoxemic patient have been shown to alter the natural history of the disease favorably. Helping a patient to quit smoking is probably the single most important intervention. Most patients with chronic bronchitis and emphysema who are given a sufficiently strong bronchodilating medication will exhibit at least a 10% increase in maximal expiratory airflow. Dyspneic patients should be given a trial of bronchodilators even if pulmonary function testing shows that they do not manifest significant bronchodilation, because bronchodilator responsiveness may vary over time. Given the underlying pathophysiology of emphysema, corticosteroids would be expected to provide little benefit, because tissue destruction is the basic disease mechanism. Only some patients derive significant benefit from corticosteroids. Clinical trials of daily antibiotic use in patients with mild chronic airflow obstruction demonstrated that neither the degree of disability nor the rate of progression of disease was significantly altered by this intervention. Intermittent antibiotic administration is indicated for acute episodes of clinical worsening marked by increased dyspnea, excessive sputum production, and sputum purulence. Physical-training programs, such as treadmill walk-

ing, significantly increase the exercise capacity of patients with even far-advanced chronic bronchitis and emphysema. *(Answer: E—Smoking cessation)*

20. A 23-year-old male college student with no history of cigarette smoking presents with a complaint of productive cough that has not improved with three courses of antibiotics. He reports some intermittent wheezing and dyspnea, which have worsened over the past 2 days, but he has no fever. He states that he has had various recurrent respiratory infections ever since childhood. On examination, his chest x-ray shows diffuse increased markings with cystic spaces predominantly in the upper lobes and hyperinflation. Further testing reveals an abnormal sweat chloride test.

Which of the following is the most likely diagnosis for this patient?

❑ **A. Cystic fibrosis**

❑ **B. Bronchiolitis obliterans**

❑ **C. Asthma**

❑ **D. α_1-Antitrypsin deficiency**

Key Concept/Objective: To understand the presentation of cystic fibrosis in adults

Although cystic fibrosis is an inherited disease that usually manifests itself in early childhood, increasing numbers of children with cystic fibrosis are now surviving into young adulthood, and some patients have a variant form of the disease in which symptoms first appear during adolescence or adulthood. The chest radiograph may strongly suggest the diagnosis of cystic fibrosis. The generalized bronchiectasis manifests itself as a diffuse increase in interstitial markings, and discrete bronchiectatic cysts are often visible; typically, involvement of the upper lobes predominates. The diagnosis can be established by abnormal results on a sweat test. Bronchiolitis is considered a disease of childhood. Bronchiolitis obliterans is a rare cause of chronic airflow obstruction in adults but can occur after inhalation of toxic gases (e.g., chlorine and nitrogen dioxide) and as an idiopathic phenomenon. Emphysema develops in at least 80% of patients with homozygous Pi^Z α_1-antitrypsin deficiency. The mean age at onset of dyspnea is 45 to 50 years in nonsmokers and approximately 10 years earlier in those who smoke. *(Answer: A—Cystic fibrosis)*

21. A 56-year-old male industrial worker presents with concern of possible exposures that can cause lung disease. He has never smoked and is currently asymptomatic.

Which of the following diseases does NOT have an occupational exposure etiology?

❑ **A. Chronic bronchitis**

❑ **B. Bronchiolitis obliterans**

❑ **C. Bronchiectasis**

❑ **D. Silo-filler's disease**

Key Concept/Objective: To know the risk factors and pathophysiology of bronchiectasis

Bronchiectasis is a chronic suppurative disease of the airways that if sufficiently widespread may cause chronic airflow obstruction. Bronchiectasis is a localized, irreversible bronchial dilatation caused by a destructive inflammatory process involving the bronchial walls. Necrotizing bacterial or mycobacterial infection is thought to be responsible for most cases of bronchiectasis. Adult-onset bronchiectasis may result from an untreated or inadequately treated bronchopneumonia that is caused by virulent organisms such as staphylococci or gram-negative bacilli. Prolonged exposure to respirable dusts in the work environment has long been recognized as a cause of so-called industrial or occupational bronchitis in nonsmoking workers engaged in occupations such as coal or gold mining, textile manufacturing, and cement and steel making. Bronchiolitis obliterans can occur with inhalation of toxic gases (e.g., chlorine and nitrogen dioxide). Silo-filler's disease is an example of bronchiolitis obliterans resulting from toxic gas inhalation of nitrous oxides. *(Answer: C—Bronchiectasis)*

For more information, see Staton GW: 14 Respiratory Medicine: III Chronic Obstructive Diseases of the Lung. ACP Medicine Online (www.acpmedicine.com). Dale DC, Federman DD, Eds. WebMD Inc., New York, November 2004

Focal and Multifocal Lung Disease

22. A 31-year-old healthy man who has no significant medical history or current complaints presents to your office with concern about an abnormal chest x-ray that was taken at a local health fair. He has neither constitutional nor pulmonary symptoms. He reports no toxic exposures or family history of lung diseases. The physical examination is unremarkable. On review of the chest x-ray, a 1 cm focal lesion with central calcification is seen in right middle lobe. There are no previous films available for comparison.

    Which of the following describes the most appropriate treatment plan for this patient?

    - ❑ **A. Although asymptomatic, this patient requires thoracic surgery consultation and open lung biopsy**
    - ❑ **B. Given his young age and the appearance of the nodule, no further workup is necessary at this time; follow-up chest x-ray in 6 to 12 months is recommended**
    - ❑ **C. Bronchoscopy with airway inspection and likely transbronchial biopsy will probably yield a diagnosis; if bronchoscopy is unrevealing, the patient should be referred to thoracic surgery**
    - ❑ **D. Placement of purified protein derivative, examination of sputum for malignant cells (sputum cytology), and a high-resolution chest computed tomographic scan should be performed promptly, and the patient should be referred to thoracic surgery consultation for open lung biopsy**

    Key Concept/Objective: To understand the management of a single pulmonary nodule on chest x-ray

    The management of a patient with a solitary lung nodule on chest x-ray can be challenging. In almost all cases, it should be assumed that the nodule is malignant. A benign etiology can be assumed if a chest radiograph taken 2 or more years earlier shows the lesion to have been the same size as or larger than it is currently. Such a situation could arise if the lesion went unrecognized on the initial film. Patients 35 years old or younger who are asymptomatic can also be managed in a conservative manner; otherwise, a thorough evaluation would be indicated. There are also classic benign patterns of calcification that obviate further assessment of single small nodules. For granulomas, such patterns include dense, perfectly central targets of calcium, ring calcification, and solid, dense calcification of the whole nodule. Given this patient's young age and central calcification, follow-up chest x-ray is the most prudent approach to management. *(Answer: B—Given his young age and the appearance of the nodule, no further workup is necessary at this time; follow-up chest x-ray in 6 to 12 months is recommended)*

23. A 42-year-old white man whose medical history is unknown presents to the clinic with shortness of breath of new onset. He reports decreased appetite, malaise, and cough with minimal sputum. He also states that he feels warm at night. He has been almost completely bed-bound for the past week. Physical examination is unremarkable except that the patient appears older than his stated age and has decreased breath sounds in the left apex. A chest radiograph shows infiltrates on both the right and left apices; no cavitations are noted. There is also ipsilateral hilar adenopathy.

    Which of the following statements is true regarding this patient's chest radiograph?

    - ❑ **A. Pneumococcal and other bacterial pneumonias can be ruled out, given the multifocal pattern of infiltrates**
    - ❑ **B. In light of the clinical presentation, reactivation of pulmonary tuberculosis seems likely; however, the lack of cavitations rules out this diagnosis**

❑ C. Given the vague complaints of this patient and the findings on chest radiography, the differential diagnosis should include bacterial pneumonia, reactivation tuberculosis, pulmonary thromboembolic disease, and sarcoidosis

❑ D. Radiographic changes such as these, if caused by malignancy, are certainly metastatic and do not originate in the lung parenchyma

Key Concept/Objective: To understand the radiologic changes seen with tuberculosis and multifocal infiltrates

Most disorders that cause single infiltrates can also cause multiple infiltrates. For example, *S. pneumoniae* pneumonia and other bacterial pneumonias are occasionally multifocal; most viral pneumonias and pneumonias caused by *Legionella* species and *Mycoplasma* are commonly multifocal or diffuse. Pulmonary thromboembolism and sarcoidosis can also produce multifocal infiltrates. Reactivation tuberculosis is often multifocal. Bilateral infiltrates in the upper lung zones are most characteristic of reactivation tuberculosis. The upper lung zones are favored sites because a higher ratio of ventilation to perfusion results in higher local oxygen tension, which enhances growth of *Mycobacterium tuberculosis*. The apical and posterior segments of the upper lobes are most commonly involved, followed by the apical-posterior segments of the lower lobes. Cavitation is frequent, but even in the absence of cavitation, the diagnosis of tuberculosis should be considered when multifocal infiltrates are present. Alveolar cell carcinoma and Hodgkin disease usually present as focal infiltrates; however, they can also exhibit a pattern of multifocal infiltrates. Metastatic lesions to the lung are usually seen as ill-defined opacities without a lobar or segmental distribution. *(Answer: C—Given the vague complaints of this patient and the findings on chest radiography, the differential diagnosis should include bacterial pneumonia, reactivation tuberculosis, pulmonary thromboembolic disease, and sarcoidosis)*

24. A 43-year-old African-American woman who has had asthma for 16 years presents to your walk-in clinic with progressive dyspnea, chills, and productive cough. Physical examination reveals a thin woman in moderate distress. She is afebrile but has mild tachypnea and tachycardia. Lung examination reveals moderate air movement, diffuse wheezes, and egophony in the left upper lung zone without change in tactile fremitus. Chest radiography shows a segmental infiltrate of the left upper lobe with fingerlike shadows and dilated central bronchi.

Which of the following diagnoses best explains the constellation of clinical findings and radiologic changes?

❑ A. Allergic bronchopulmonary aspergillosis

❑ B. Alvelolar cell carcinoma with endobronchial invasion

❑ C. Bronchiolitis obliterans organizing pneumonia (BOOP)

❑ D. Caplan syndrome

Key Concept/Objective: To understand the differential diagnosis of a segmental infiltrate and the classic presentation of allergic bronchopulmonary aspergillosis

Allergic bronchopulmonary aspergillosis, which is also associated with asthma, is a hypersensitivity disease that primarily affects the central airways. Immediate and delayed hypersensitivity to *Aspergillus* are involved in the pathogenesis of this disorder. Onset of disease occurs most often in the fourth and fifth decades, and virtually all patients have long-standing atopic asthma. Even those few patients who do not have a history of documented asthma exhibit airflow obstruction when they present with this disorder. The typical patient has a long history of intermittent wheezing, after which the illness evolves into a more chronic and more highly symptomatic disorder with fever, chills, pulmonary infiltrates, and productive cough. The chest x-ray may show a segmental infiltrate or segmental atelectasis, most commonly in the upper lobes. Caplan syndrome is characterized by pulmonary nodules; it is seen exclusively in patients with rheumatoid arthritis. The constellation of long-standing asthma, wheezing on physical examination, and the presence of central dilated bronchi are not asso-

ciated with either alveolar cell carcinoma or BOOP. In the patient with typical symptoms, the branching, fingerlike shadows from mucoid impaction of dilated central bronchi are pathognomonic of allergic bronchopulmonary aspergillosis. *(Answer: A—Allergic bronchopulmonary aspergillosis)*

For more information, see Ingram RH Jr: 14 Respiratory Medicine: IV Focal and Multifocal Lung Disease. ACP Medicine Online (www.acpmedicine.com). Dale DC, Federman DD, Eds. WebMD Inc., New York, December 2002

Chronic Diffuse Infiltrative Lung Disease

25. A 42-year-old African-American woman who works as a physician's assistant presents to your office with progressive dyspnea and a nonproductive cough. After a careful history is obtained, no occupational or toxic exposures are readily identified. The patient is concerned that her symptoms are secondary to idiopathic pulmonary fibrosis (IPF). The physical examination is unremarkable. Chest radiography shows prominent hilar adenopathy with a diffuse interstitial process. The working diagnosis is sarcoidosis. You obtain the patient's consent for a bronchoscopy and transbronchial biopsy, but she tells you she thinks an open lung biopsy is necessary for a diagnosis of sarcoidosis.

What is the correct response to this patient with regard to the appropriate workup of sarcoidosis?

- ❑ A. **"You are right, I will consult a thoracic surgeon."**
- ❑ B. **"You are right, but in regard to any interstitial lung process, one should always have a transbronchial biopsy before open lung biopsy."**
- ❑ C. **"No, open lung biopsy is a last resort in the workup of interstitial lung diseases."**
- ❑ D. **"No; given your chest x-ray and other factors, sarcoidosis is the likely diagnosis; yield from transbronchial biopsy should be around 90%."**

Key Concept/Objective: To understand the diagnostic approach to sarcoidosis

Given the demographics of this patient—a middle-aged African-American woman—sarcoidosis is a very likely diagnosis. This patient's chest x-ray indicates that she has stage II sarcoidosis; patients with stage II sarcoidosis have a 90% chance of having their diagnosis confirmed by transbronchial biopsy. The biopsy will show noncaseating granulomas. In general, transbronchial biopsy is most useful in the diagnosis of sarcoidosis or diffuse infiltrative lung diseases of infectious cause. If the working diagnosis is neither infection nor sarcoidosis, then lung biopsy would likely be indicated. Open lung biopsy is a very invasive procedure and should be reserved for other types of diffuse infiltrative lung disease. *(Answer: D—"No; given your chest x-ray and other factors, sarcoidosis is the likely diagnosis; yield from transbronchial biopsy should be around 90%.")*

26. A 38-year-old white man is referred to you for treatment of sarcoidosis. The patient reports that he has decreased exercise tolerance as well as a chronic cough. The patient has an 11-year history of injecting drug abuse. He brings records from his previous physician, which include a report of negative results on an HIV test, a chest x-ray report that reads, "diffuse interstitial process without hilar adenopathy," and a pathology report of noncaseating granulomas that gave sarcoidosis as the final diagnosis.

Of the following, which is the most appropriate approach to the treatment of this patient?

- ❑ A. **Start prednisone, 60 mg q.d., and taper over 6 weeks**
- ❑ B. **Inform the patient that given his chest x-ray findings, he has a 65% chance of spontaneous remission**
- ❑ C. **Assess arterial blood gases; if the patient is not hypoxic, schedule a follow-up appointment in 3 to 6 months**
- ❑ D. **Obtain a biopsy specimen for further testing**

Key Concept/Objective: To understand the differential diagnosis of illicit drug abuse and sarcoidosis

This patient's demographics do not support the diagnosis of sarcoidosis; however, that diagnosis should not be ruled out. The pathologic changes in the lung seen with injecting drug abuse are secondary to talc, which is used as "filler," most commonly with heroin. Given this patient's history, the biopsy specimen should be examined under polarizing light; talc particles are characteristically seen with this technique. No treatment should be initiated until the proper diagnosis has been made. Patients with stage III sarcoidosis have a 33% chance of spontaneous resolution in 2 years. Although measurement of arterial blood gases is not contraindicated, this is clearly not the most appropriate step to take next in this patient's workup. It is important to note that heroin per se is not associated with diffuse lung injury. *(Answer: D—Obtain a biopsy specimen for further testing)*

27. A 64-year-old white man presents to your office with a 1-year history of worsening dyspnea on exertion and mild cough, described as nonproductive. The patient has no other complaints. He reports he may have been exposed to asbestos when he was in his 20s, while working in a shipyard. The patient has never smoked. He has been treated with several inhaled beta agonists, without any improvement. The physical examination is significant for dry inspiratory crackles and clubbing of his digits. A chest x-ray shows a diffuse infiltrative process, without adenopathy or effusions. Ultimately, the patient undergoes an open lung biopsy, which shows minimal inflammatory round cell infiltrate, widening of alveolar septa, and fibrosis with fibroblastic foci.

What is the most likely diagnosis for this patient?

- ❑ **A. Bronchiolitis obliterans organizing pneumonia (BOOP)**
- ❑ **B. Desquamative interstitial pneumonitis (DIP)**
- ❑ **C. Idiopathic pulmonary fibrosis (IPF)**
- ❑ **D. Acute interstitial fibrosis (Hamman-Rich syndrome)**

Key Concept/Objective: To understand the diagnosis and prognosis of IPF

This patient's history and presentation is classic of IPF—an insidious loss of pulmonary function and the absence of signs or symptoms of a systemic process. His biopsy specimen report describes usual interstitial pneumonitis (UIP), which is characteristic of IPF. Besides a chest x-ray, high-resolution CT of the chest and pulmonary function testing are useful noninvasive ways to evaluate patients; however, an open lung biopsy is ultimately needed for diagnosis in the majority of patients. Older patients may be spared the morbidity of open lung biopsy if they have a classic presentation and features suggestive of IPF on transbronchial biopsy. Survival is usually 2 to 3 years after diagnosis has been made. Although multiple medicinal therapies have been tried, none to date have improved survival in this patient population. Lung transplantation is a good option, and patients should be referred once the diffusing capacity of the lung for carbon monoxide (DL_{CO}) has dropped below 40%. Patients with DIP are usually younger; biopsy in these patients reveals a homogeneous pattern of involvement and characteristic pigmented alveolar macrophages. In patients with Hamman-Rich syndrome, cough and dyspnea rapidly progress to significant respiratory compromise. The onset of BOOP is more acute, and systemic symptoms such as fever and malaise are not uncommon; microscopic findings are distinct in BOOP. *(Answer: C—Idiopathic pulmonary fibrosis [IPF])*

28. A 34-year-old white man presents to the emergency department with a cough of abrupt onset, fever, and chest pain. He has no significant medical history. He is admitted to the intensive care unit, where his respiratory distress worsens to the point that he requires intubation. The patient's chest radiograph shows diffuse, patchy ground-glass opacities and intralobular septal thickening. Bronchoscopy with bronchoalveolar lavage (BAL) shows copious amounts of grossly turbid exudates in the airways with material that tests positive with periodic acid–Schiff (PAS) reagent on pathologic examination.

What is the most likely diagnosis for this patient?

❑ A. Alveolar proteinosis

❑ B. Löffler syndrome

❑ C. Diffuse alveolar hemorrhage

❑ D. Lymphangioleiomyomatosis

Key Concept/Objective: To understand the diagnosis of alveolar proteinosis

Clinical presentations of patients with alveolar proteinosis can vary greatly. The condition may progress, remain stable, or resolve spontaneously. Some patients are asymptomatic; others have severe respiratory insufficiency. Most patients present with gradually progressive exertional dyspnea and cough that is usually unproductive. Diagnosis is made with BAL, which shows grossly turbid exudates in the airways and PAS-positive material on pathologic examination. Löffler syndrome is characterized by transient and migratory infiltrates on chest x-ray and a predominance of eosinophils on BAL. Diffuse alveolar hemorrhage is associated with a history of hemoptysis or is evidenced by bleeding at the time of BAL. Lymphangioleiomyomatosis affects women only. *(Answer: A—Alveolar proteinosis)*

29. A 76-year-old Iranian woman with hypertension and chronic back pain presents with a nonproductive cough of 5 months' duration and progressive dyspnea on exertion, which she has been experiencing for 2 months. She denies other symptoms, including weight loss, fever, and night sweats. Her medications include gabapentin, triamterene-hydrochlorothiazide, atenolol, and premarin. Her examination is normal. An x-ray done in clinic reveals diffuse interstitial infiltrates without adenopathy or effusion.

Which of the following is the most likely diagnosis for this patient?

❑ A. Drug-induced infiltrative lung disease

❑ B. Tuberculosis

❑ C. Sarcoidosis

❑ D. Idiopathic pulmonary fibrosis

❑ E. Pulmonary lymphangitic carcinomatosis

Key Concept/Objective: To be able to differentiate the natural history, associated symptoms, and x-ray findings of common causes of infiltrative lung diseases

Given the absence of a causative medication, systemic symptoms, hilar adenopathy, or pleural effusion, the gradually progressive cough and dyspnea in this older patient is most likely being caused by idiopathic pulmonary fibrosis. Lymphagitic carcinomatosis and tuberculosis are typically subacute; these disorders are associated with systemic symptoms and can present as pleural effusions. Because idiopathic pulmonary fibrosis is a diagnosis of exclusion, screening for breast and colon cancer and administering a PPD test are appropriate steps in this patient's evaluation. Although sarcoidosis does not typically present in the elderly, it can do so. Stage III sarcoidosis (diffuse infiltrative lung disease without adenopathy) is a less common form of sarcoidosis than the other stages and is often associated with extrapulmonary manifestations. *(Answer: D—Idiopathic pulmonary fibrosis)*

30. A 28-year-old Asian man presents with a nonproductive cough of 3 weeks' duration and progressive dyspnea on exertion. His dyspnea became acutely worse today. He denies having other symptoms, including fever and weight loss. He used intravenous cocaine on three occasions. He works on the docks unloading cargo ships. He is on no medications but smokes one pack of cigarettes a day. Chest x-ray shows bilateral interstitial infiltrates and a small left pneumothorax.

Which of the following would be initial therapy for this patient?

❑ A. Erythromycin

❑ B. Prednisone

❑ C. Dapsone

❑ D. **Trimethoprim-sulfamethoxazole**

❑ E. **Smoking cessation**

Key Concept/Objective: To know that Pneumocystis carinii *pneumonia (PCP) is a common cause of subacute diffuse interstitial lung disease, especially in the setting of pneumothorax*

This patient most likely has PCP, given the subacute clinical course, the pneumothorax, and this patient's risk factors for HIV. Even had the patient not been forthcoming with his risk factors, PCP would still be the presumptive diagnosis until another cause was identified. A pneumothorax in the setting of diffuse infiltrative lung disease is a clue to eosinophilic granuloma, PCP, and lymphangiomatosis. Eosinophilic granuloma (pulmonary histiocytosis X) occurs in patients between the ages of 20 and 40 years and is associated with smoking. *(Answer: D—Trimethoprim-sulfamethoxazole)*

31. A 23-year-old black woman fell while snowboarding and hurt her ribs. She denies having had any symptoms before her fall. Her examination reveals chest wall tenderness but no adenopathy, skin lesions, or organomegaly. An x-ray done to look for a rib fracture reveals bilateral hilar adenopathy.

Which of the following would be appropriate as initial therapy for this patient?

❑ A. **Isoniazid**

❑ B. **Itraconazole**

❑ C. **Prednisone**

❑ D. **Chloroquine**

❑ E. **Observation**

Key Concept/Objective: To know the presentation and differential diagnosis of stage I sarcoidosis

This asymptomatic young woman most likely has sarcoidosis. The differential diagnosis includes lymphoma, tuberculosis, histoplasmosis, and other granulomatous infections. In the absence of systemic symptoms or examination findings, these other diseases are unlikely. Skin tests for both tuberculosis and histoplasmosis should be performed; if the results are negative, no further workup would be needed at this point. In the absence of symptoms or hypercalcemia, this patient can be observed clinically without initial intervention. She has a 75% chance of clinical remission over the next 2 years. *(Answer: E—Observation)*

32. A 45-year-old dairy farmer reports that he experiences coughing and wheezing immediately upon entering the barn each morning. These symptoms resolve after returning home each evening.

Which of the following is the most likely diagnosis for this patient?

❑ A. **Acute hypersensitivity pneumonitis**

❑ B. **Acute interstitial pneumonia**

❑ C. **Allergen-induced bronchospasm**

❑ D. **Lymphocytic interstitial pneumonia**

❑ E. **Eosinophilic granuloma**

Key Concept/Objective: To understand the course of hypersensitivity pneumonitis

The differential diagnosis for symptoms that come and go in conjunction with exposure to an unidentified causative agent includes hypersensitivity pneumonitis and irritant- or allergen-induced lung irritation. Hypersensitivity pneumonitis is mediated by the complement pathway and takes 4 to 8 hours to develop after antigenic exposure. Antigen-induced bronchospasm is mediated by histamines and occurs soon after exposure. *(Answer: C—Allergen-induced bronchospasm)*

For more information, see Staton GW, Ingram RH Jr: 14 Respiratory Medicine: V Chronic Diffuse Infiltrative Lung Disease. ACP Medicine Online (www.acpmedicine.com). Dale DC, Federman DD, Eds. WebMD Inc., New York, November 2004

Ventilatory Control during Wakefulness and Sleep

33. A 64-year-old man with known severe chronic obstructive pulmonary disease is admitted to the hospital with worsening shortness of breath and green sputum production. He is known to require home oxygen therapy. He is given nebulized bronchodilators, antibiotics, intravenous methylprednisolone, and high-flow oxygen therapy. Although his bronchospasm is resolving and his respiration is less labored, you notice a decreased sensorium. Arterial blood gas measurements confirm the presence of hypercapnia and hypoxia.

Which of the following statements regarding the physiology of ventilatory control is false?

- ❑ **A. The central neural network is composed of medullary neurons, pontine neurons, and the nucleus tractus solitarius (NTS)**
- ❑ **B. Carotid and aortic bodies are peripheral chemoreceptors that are stimulated primarily by hypocapnia**
- ❑ **C. Cerebrospinal fluid can decrease its pH in response to increased levels of arterial carbon dioxide tension (P_aCO_2) to stimulate cells on the ventral medullary surface**
- ❑ **D. Mechanoreceptors in the upper airway, chest wall, and lung detect mechanical deformation and temperature changes that result from inhalation and exhalation**

Key Concept/Objective: To understand the key concepts of the physiology of ventilatory control

Ventilation is a critical function for eliminating carbon dioxide and acquiring oxygen. The control system for ventilation not only optimizes gas exchange but also serves a role in acid-base homeostasis, speech, deglutition, defecation, and postural adjustments. Inhalation and exhalation begin with the discharge properties of putative pacemaker neuronal groups located in the medulla. This neural network is embedded in a system of adjacent medullary neurons, pontine neurons, and regions such as the NTS that receive neural impulses through lung inflation, lung deflation, blood pressure, and other afferent systems. The intensity of the activity of medullary neurons is affected by chemoreceptors. The peripheral chemoreceptors—the carotid and aortic bodies—are highly vascular collections of specialized sensory cells. The carotid bodies are located bilaterally at the bifurcations of the common carotid arteries; the aortic bodies are situated anterior and posterior to the arch of the aorta and left main pulmonary artery. The peripheral chemoreceptors are stimulated primarily by a low arterial oxygen tension (P_aO_2), although hypercapnia, acidemia, and, possibly, hyperthermia may influence the gain of the response to hypoxemia. Impulses travel from the carotid and aortic bodies to the NTS via sensory ganglia and the afferent nerves that follow along the ninth and 10th cranial nerves, respectively. Increases in P_aCO_2 stimulate cells on the ventral medullary surface, primarily by lowering the pH of the medullary extracellular fluid. Specialized sensory cells (mechanoreceptors) located in the upper airway, chest wall, and lung detect mechanical deformation and temperature changes resulting from inhalation and exhalation. *(Answer: B—Carotid and aortic bodies are peripheral chemoreceptors that are stimulated primarily by hypocapnia)*

34. A 43-year-old man comes to your office for evaluation of a dry cough and worsening shortness of breath of 3 months' duration. He denies having orthopnea, paroxysmal nocturnal dyspnea, or lower extremity edema. He has no history of smoking or cardiac disease. On examination, the patient is tachypneic, but all other vital signs are normal. There is no clubbing, and the cardiac examination is normal, but you notice Velcro-like crackles at both lung bases. Arterial blood gas measurements reveal hypoxemia, hypocarbia, and a respiratory alkalosis. High-resolution CT scanning of the chest reveals diffuse interstitial infiltrates.

Which of the following statements regarding ventilatory drive is false?

- ❑ A. Interstitial lung diseases can be accompanied by hyperventilation that results from a rapid, shallow breathing pattern
- ❑ B. Adaptation to chronic hypoventilation in sleep apnea, chronic obstructive pulmonary disease (COPD), neuromuscular disease, and chest wall disease my depress responsiveness to CO_2
- ❑ C. Metabolic causes of hypoventilation may include metabolic alkalosis, deficiency of thyroid hormone, and excess sedative or narcotic agents
- ❑ D. Hyperventilation caused by progesterone stimulation is the result of an increase in both tidal volume and respiratory rate

Key Concept/Objective: To understand ventilatory drive

Interstitial lung diseases (e.g., pulmonary fibrosis) increase resting ventilation and lower P_aCO_2 as a result of increased activity of lung receptors (probably C fibers). The hyperventilation that accompanies pulmonary edema, pneumonia, interstitial disease, and the acute respiratory distress syndrome is a rapid, shallow breathing pattern that results from activation of these lung receptors. Hyperventilation is regularly produced by exposure to high altitude or other hypoxic environments; metabolic acidosis; pregnancy and conditions associated with elevated progestational hormones; anxiety states; and mildly toxic doses of salicylates, amphetamines, or other drugs that stimulate the central nervous system. Unlike the hyperventilation associated with parenchymal lung disease, the hyperventilation that occurs during progesterone stimulation (such as occurs during pregnancy) and metabolic acidosis is associated with an increase in tidal volume and little increase in respiratory rate. Hypoventilation occurs when alveolar ventilation is insufficient to eliminate metabolically produced CO_2. Metabolic causes of hypoventilation may include metabolic alkalosis, deficiency of thyroid hormone, and excess doses of sedative and narcotic agents. As hypoventilation becomes chronic, adaptation of receptors, of central inspiratory neurons, of metabolic alkalosis, or of all three may occur. Adaptation to chronic hypoventilation in sleep apnea, COPD, neuromuscular disease, and chest wall disease may eventually reduce responsiveness to CO_2 and depress ventilation during rest. *(Answer: D—Hyperventilation caused by progesterone stimulation is the result of an increase in both tidal volume and respiratory rate)*

35. A 55-year-old man presents to your clinic for evaluation of chronic headache and daytime sleepiness. His wife reports a long history of snoring, and the patient is concerned that he might have sleep apnea because he is overweight and his brother was recently diagnosed with sleep apnea.

Which of the following statements regarding sleep apnea is false?

- ❑ A. There are three categories of sleep apnea: central, obstructive, and mixed
- ❑ B. Patients with sleep apnea are not at increased risk for developing hypertension
- ❑ C. Sleep apnea has a genetic component
- ❑ D. Patients who have a short mandible and a round head are predisposed to apnea

Key Concept/Objective: To understand risk factors for and potential complications of sleep apnea

Three patterns of apnea, or cessation of breathing, can be observed during sleep. These apneas are defined as episodes of a reduction in airflow of more than 80% that occur for more than 10 seconds. Apneas may be classified as central (or nonobstructive), obstructive, or mixed. Certain measures are used to quantify respiratory disturbances during sleep. The apnea-hypopnea index (AHI) is the total number of apneas and hypopneas that occur during sleep, divided by the hours of sleep time. In communities

in the United States, 9% to 12% of women and 27% to 35% of men may have an AHI higher than 5—a number often quoted as a threshold value for normality; however, many people with an AHI higher than 5 have no symptoms or apparent illness. If the definition of illness is the presence of daytime sleepiness or cardiovascular complications such as hypertension, the estimates are that approximately 2% of women and 4% of men have symptomatic sleep-disordered breathing (SDB). Snoring is generally considered a predisposing feature for the development of SDB and sleep apnea. Sleep apnea has a genetic component. Symptoms relating to apnea occur two to four times more often in family members of affected patients than in a control population. Individuals with craniofacial features of a short mandible and round head are predisposed to snoring, apneas, or both. There are familial traits in hypercapnic and hypoxic sensitivity; these could relate to the tendency to breathe periodically during sleep. Sleep apnea is more common in stroke patients. *(Answer: B—Patients with sleep apnea are not at increased risk for developing hypertension)*

For more information, see Strohl KP: 14 Respiratory Medicine: VI Ventilatory Control during Wakefulness and Sleep. ACP Medicine Online (www.acpmedicine.com). Dale DC, Federman DD, Eds. WebMD Inc., New York, December 2003

Disorders of the Chest Wall

36. A 43-year-old white man with a history of diabetes and hypertension presents to your office for a routine follow-up visit. He complains of increasing dyspnea on exertion but denies having cough or edema. The patient has a long history of morbid obesity. His body mass index is 35 kg/m^2. You initiate a workup for his dyspnea on exertion that includes pulmonary function tests, arterial blood gas measurements, an echocardiogram, and assessment of his hematocrit and serum chemistries.

Which of the following statements regarding obesity and its impact on respiratory function is true?

- ❑ **A. In the absence of other primary lung illness, the major impact of obesity on respiration is as an obstructive respiratory defect**
- ❑ **B. Obesity typically causes an increase in functional residual capacity (FRC)**
- ❑ **C. The key therapy for patients with respiratory problems related to obesity is to decrease their physical activity to a level that is comfortable for the patient**
- ❑ **D. Obese patients may experience significant dyspnea during exercise because of the increased work required to move the heavy chest and abdomen and because of overall poor conditioning**

Key Concept/Objective: To know the implications of obesity on respiratory function

Obesity has several marked effects on respiratory function and can be a cause of severe respiratory disease. Obesity imposes a restrictive load on the thoracic cage, both directly, because weight has been added to the rib cage, and indirectly, because the large abdominal panniculus impedes the motion of the diaphragm when the person is supine. In the absence of other primary lung illnesses, obstructive respiratory disease is not a prominent feature of obesity-related respiratory disease. Obesity characteristically causes a decrease in FRC because of the increased load applied to the chest wall. Weight loss is the most important therapy for patients with respiratory problems related to obesity. Conservative measures for weight loss, such as improving diet and moderate exercise, should be the initial approach. Decreasing physical activity would likely induce further weight gain and worsening of aerobic conditioning. Obese patients may experience significant dyspnea during exercise, because of the increased work required to move the heavy chest and abdomen and because of overall poor conditioning. *(Answer: D—Obese patients may experience significant dyspnea during exercise because of the increased work required to move the heavy chest and abdomen and because of overall poor conditioning)*

37. A 21-year-old white woman with kyphoscoliosis visits your office to establish primary care. She recently moved to the area and states that she has been relatively healthy and was provided appropriate vaccinations and screenings by her previous physician. She developed scoliosis during her early teenage years. She denies having knowledge of any previous complications from her condition. She asks you to explain her condition and its possible complications.

Which of the following statements regarding kyphoscoliosis is true?

- ❑ **A. The two distinct forms of costovertebral skeletal abnormalities—scoliosis and kyphosis—do not typically occur together in a given patient**
- ❑ **B. Approximately 80% of cases of kyphoscoliosis are idiopathic**
- ❑ **C. Idiopathic kyphoscoliosis is most commonly a congenital abnormality or an abnormality that develops in the aged population**
- ❑ **D. The incidence of kyphoscoliosis is distributed equally between the sexes**

Key Concept/Objective: To know the features of idiopathic kyphoscoliosis

Kyphoscoliosis is an illness that can be associated with mild to severe respiratory compromise. The two basic types of costovertebral skeletal deformity—scoliosis, a lateral curvature with rotation of the vertebral column, and kyphosis, an anterior flexion of the spine—are usually found in combination. Approximately 80% of cases of kyphoscoliosis are idiopathic. Idiopathic kyphoscoliosis commonly begins in late childhood or early adolescence and may progress in severity during these years of rapid skeletal growth. Idiopathic kyphoscoliosis is not to be confused with kyphoscoliosis caused by a known underlying condition, such as osteoporosis or compression fractures in elderly patients. The incidence of kyphoscoliosis in females is four times higher than that in males. *(Answer: B—Approximately 80% of cases of kyphoscoliosis are idiopathic)*

38. A 37-year-old man arrives at your emergency center by ambulance shortly after being involved in a motor vehicle accident. The emergency medical technician (EMT) reports that the patient is hemodynamically stable with minimal external blood loss and no loss of consciousness. The EMT reports that the patient appears to be in moderate to severe respiratory distress; the patient has a respiratory rate of 40 breaths/min and an O_2 saturation of 78% while receiving supplemental oxygen at a rate of 3 L/min by nasal cannula. On physical examination, you note a remarkable 15 cm right anterolateral chest contusion. The contused segment appears to move paradoxically with respect to respiration. The patient has clear bilateral breath sounds in the upper and lower regions of both lungs.

Which of the following statements regarding flail chest injury is most accurate for this patient?

- ❑ **A. In young, otherwise healthy patients, a large flail chest segment is not a life-threatening injury**
- ❑ **B. The most appropriate step to take next in treatment of this patient is to provide supplemental oxygen by 100% nonrebreathing mask to attain O_2 saturations greater than 90%**
- ❑ **C. The most appropriate step to take next in the treatment of this patient is to provide positive pressure ventilation**
- ❑ **D. The most appropriate step to take next in the treatment of this patient is to order and evaluate a stat portable chest x-ray to rule out a tension pneumothorax**

Key Concept/Objective: To understand emergent therapy of flail chest segment with respiratory failure

Flail chest is an acute process that may lead to life-threatening abnormalities of gas exchange and mechanical function. This patient is in acute respiratory failure as a result of the massive chest-wall trauma and resultant flail segment. Stability of the thoracic cage is necessary for the muscles of inspiration to inflate the lung. In flail chest, a locally compliant portion of the chest wall moves inward as the remainder of the thoracic

cage expands during inhalation; the same portion then moves outward during exhalation. Consequently, tidal volume is diminished because the region of lung associated with the chest wall abnormality paradoxically increases its volume during exhalation and deflates during inhalation. The result is progressive hypoxemia and hypercapnia. Multiple rib fractures, particularly when they occur in a parallel vertical orientation, can produce a flail chest. The degree of dysfunction is directly proportional to the volume of lung involved in paradoxical motion. Patient management may be complicated by other manifestations of trauma to the chest, such as splinting of ventilation because of pain, contusion of the underlying lung, or hemothorax or pneumothorax. Positive-pressure inflation of the lung or negative pressure applied to the chest wall corrects the abnormality until more definitive stabilization procedures can be undertaken. Supplemental O_2 by face mask will not alleviate the patient's paradoxical chest movement and loss of tidal volume. For this patient, the most appropriate step to take next is to provide positive-pressure ventilation, preferably with endotracheal intubation. A chest x-ray is needed in this patient, but ventilatory resuscitation should take precedence. The fact that the patient has good bilateral breath sounds and is hemodynamically stable would make a significant tension pneumothorax unlikely. *(Answer: C—The most appropriate step to take next in the treatment of this patient is to provide positive pressure ventilation)*

39. A 51-year-old man presents to your office for evaluation of a nonproductive cough and a "scratchy" throat. He has no significant medical history but does have a 50-pack-year history of cigarette smoking. He states that his cough and mild sore throat started 3 weeks ago when he developed a "head cold" and that he has had a persistently runny nose since. After further questioning, you come to the conclusion that it is likely that this patient's cough is secondary to postnasal drip following his upper respiratory infection. Because of his significant smoking history, you order a routine chest x-ray, which is interpreted as being normal except for an elevated right hemidiaphragm. You suspect a diaphragmatic paralysis, which is verified by a sniff test.

Which of the following statements regarding diaphragmatic paralysis is true?

- ❑ **A. With bilateral diaphragmatic paralysis, degrees of dyspnea tend to be unrelated to body position**
- ❑ **B. In otherwise healthy patients, unilateral diaphragmatic paralysis will typically present as acute onset of orthopnea and dyspnea on exertion**
- ❑ **C. The underlying cause of bilateral diaphragmatic paralysis is almost exclusively trauma related**
- ❑ **D. Most cases of unilateral diaphragmatic paralysis are the result of neoplastic invasion of the phrenic nerve**

Key Concept/Objective: To know the characteristics of unilateral and bilateral diaphragmatic paralyses

Diaphragmatic paralysis is a relatively common finding. Most cases of unilateral diaphragmatic paralysis are the result of neoplastic invasion of the phrenic nerve. Compression or destruction of the phrenic nerve by surgery, trauma, or enlargement of lymph nodes or aneurysmal vessels may also cause the condition. Bilateral diaphragmatic paralysis can result from a number of causes, including cervical and thoracic surgery, cold cardioplegia for cardiac surgery, trauma, multiple sclerosis, and neuralgic amyotrophy. Orthopnea may be a prominent symptom in the setting of bilateral diaphragm dysfunction. With the patient supine, the hydrostatic force of the abdominal contents pushes the patient's diaphragm into the thorax. Negative intrapleural pressure generated by the accessory muscles causes the diaphragm to be sucked further into the thorax during inspiration, producing a paradoxical inward motion of the upper abdomen as the thorax expands. As a result, mechanical and gas exchange abnormalities similar to those seen in flail chest develop. Unilateral diaphragmatic paralysis is most often detected as an asymptomatic radiographic finding. In the absence of associated pleuropulmonary disease, most adult patients with unilateral diaphragmatic paralysis but without a coexisting pulmonary disease remain asymptomatic. *(Answer:*

D—Most cases of unilateral diaphragmatic paralysis are the result of neoplastic invasion of the phrenic nerve)

40. An 82-year-old woman who resides in a nursing home presents to your office for routine evaluation. She has severe kyphoscoliosis secondary to osteoporosis, and she has been hospitalized twice for pneumonia.

Which of the following is NOT important in the prevention of respiratory compromise in this patient?

- ❑ **A. Immunization with influenza vaccine**
- ❑ **B. Early treatment of respiratory tract infections**
- ❑ **C. Avoidance of central nervous system depressants**
- ❑ **D. Nocturnal oxygen therapy**
- ❑ **E. Yearly pulmonary function testing to monitor progress**

Key Concept/Objective: To understand outpatient management of kyphoscoliosis-induced respiratory disorders

Kyphoscoliosis is the most common disorder of the chest wall that produces ventilatory failure. Approximately 80% of cases are idiopathic, first manifesting in late childhood and early adolescence; the other 20% are caused by neuromuscular disorders. Females are four times more likely to develop this deformity than males. The deformities worsen with age. Immunization with influenza and pneumococcal vaccines, early treatment of respiratory infections, avoidance of CNS depressants, and use of nocturnal oxygen therapy can prolong life and enhance quality of life in these patients. There is no evidence that yearly pulmonary function testing will affect the disease process or provide any added information for intervention. *(Answer: E—Yearly pulmonary function testing to monitor progress)*

41. A 36-year-old black man presents to the emergency department after a motor vehicle accident. Except for some minor scrapes, he is asymptomatic; however, his chest x-ray reveals an elevated left hemidiaphragm.

Which of the following tests can confirm the diagnosis?

- ❑ **A. Determination of DL_{CO} on pulmonary function testing**
- ❑ **B. Arterial blood gas measurements**
- ❑ **C. Sniff test**
- ❑ **D. Pulse oximetry**
- ❑ **E. CT scan of the chest**

Key Concept/Objective: To understand the evaluation and diagnosis of a patient with unilateral diaphragmatic paralysis

Unilateral diaphragmatic paralysis is most often detected as a radiographic finding in an asymptomatic patient. Although most cases are the result of neoplastic invasion of the phrenic nerve, it is also commonly seen in postoperative patients, in patients with trauma, or in idiopathic cases. The sniff test involves asking the patient to perform a sudden, forceful inspiration. The diaphragmatic movements can be viewed under fluoroscopy; with unilateral diaphragmatic paralysis, the affected side of the diaphragm ascends into the thorax. This movement is in the opposite direction of the normal side. Such a finding confirms the diagnosis of diaphragmatic paralysis. *(Answer: C—Sniff test)*

42. A 26-year-old woman presents to the emergency department with shortness of breath, which has been progressively increasing for several days. She has also been experiencing increasing weakness and double vision. She notes a worsening of her symptoms at the end of the day, and she has noticed weakness while brushing her hair. Her physical examination is unrevealing.

Which of the following neuromuscular disorders is most likely the cause of this patient's symptoms?

- ❑ A. Guillain-Barré syndrome
- ❑ B. Bilateral diaphragmatic paralysis
- ❑ C. Myasthenia gravis
- ❑ D. Duchenne muscular dystrophy
- ❑ E. Amyotrophic lateral sclerosis (ALS)

Key Concept/Objective: To be able to differentiate between the multiple neuromuscular disorders that affect respiratory function

Guillain-Barré syndrome usually presents as an ascending paralysis. Although bilateral diaphragmatic paralysis would explain this patient's shortness of breath, the proximal muscle weakness and ocular symptoms would remain unexplained. Duchenne muscular dystrophy is an X-linked disorder that exclusively affects males. Its symptoms are present by 3 to 5 years of age, and patients are usually wheelchair bound by 12 years of age. The majority of patients with ALS present clinically with progressive asymmetrical weakness, fasciculations, and prominent muscle atrophy. The distal musculature is primarily involved. Myasthenia gravis is an autoimmune disorder that affects the neuromuscular junction: specifically, the postsynaptic acetylcholine receptor. Patients usually present with intermittent symptoms that are usually worse at the end of the day. Respiratory failure may occur; in myasthenia crisis, the patient requires a ventilator. *(Answer: C—Myasthenia gravis)*

For more information, see Staton GW, Ingram RH Jr: 14 Respiratory Medicine: VII Disorders of the Chest Wall. ACP Medicine Online (www.acpmedicine.com). Dale DC, Federman DD, Eds. WebMD Inc., New York, December 2003

Respiratory Failure

43. A 41-year-old woman presents to the emergency department for evaluation of shortness of breath. She is currently undergoing therapy for newly diagnosed breast cancer. She states that she was in her usual state of health until she began to experience acute shortness of breath 2 hours ago. For the past 2 hours, she has also been experiencing sharp right chest pain on inspiration. She denies having fever, chills, or cough. Results of physical examination are as follows: heart rate, 130 beats/min; respiratory rate, 30 breaths/min; a loud second heart sound; and there is mild pretibial pitting edema of the left lower extremity. Results of blood gas measurements are as follows: normal pH; arterial carbon dioxide tension (P_aCO_2), 17 mm Hg; arterial oxygen tension (P_aO_2), 70 mm Hg; and hemoglobin O_2 saturation, 95%. The patient is started on anticoagulation therapy with heparin, and a helical CT scan of the chest is ordered.

Which of the following statements regarding acute hypoxemic respiratory failure is true?

- ❑ A. This patient has no significant $\dot{V}/\dot{Q}$ mismatching because her hemoglobin saturation is normal
- ❑ B. In patients with ARDS, shunting is the major physiologic derangement resulting in hypoxemia
- ❑ C. Pure alveolar hypoventilation is the most common pathophysiologic cause of acute hypoxemia
- ❑ D. Shunting and $\dot{V}/\dot{Q}$mismatching respond similarly to inhalation of 100% O_2

Key Concept/Objective: To know the clinical characteristics of common causes of hypoxemia

Patients with ARDS can have diffusion impairments that contribute to hypoxemia, but shunting is the more important physiologic derangement in this disorder. The alveolar-arterial oxygen gradient or difference (A-aDO_2) is used to identify $\dot{V}/\dot{Q}$ mismatching when the measured P_aO_2 is normalized by hyperventilation. $\dot{V}/\dot{Q}$ mismatching is the most common pathophysiologic cause of acute hypoxemia. It develops when there is a decrease in ventilation to normally perfused regions of the lung, a decrease in perfusion to normally ventilated regions of the lung, or some combination of a decrease in both

ventilation and perfusion. Shunting can be differentiated from $\dot{V}/\dot{Q}$ mismatching on the basis of the differences in the response to inhalation of 100% oxygen. *(Answer: B—In patients with ARDS, shunting is the major physiologic derangement resulting in hypoxemia)*

44. A 74-year-old male patient of yours who has severe COPD presents to your office for the evaluation of worsening shortness of breath. The patient has smoked two packs of cigarettes daily for the past 50 years. Through home oxygen therapy, he receives oxygen at a rate of 2 L/min. He states that he was in his usual state of health until 2 days ago, when he developed worsening shortness of breath, particularly with exertion. He also complains of mild substernal "burning" pain with exertion. He denies having orthopnea, edema, or palpitations. His hemoglobin O_2 saturations are 92% on 2 L of oxygen provided by nasal cannula. Results of blood gas measurements are as follows: pH, 7.38; P_aCO_2, 80 mm Hg; and P_aO_2, 70 mm Hg. ECG shows lateral T wave inversions; otherwise, ECG results are unremarkable.

For this patient, which of the following statements regarding hypercapnic respiratory failure is true?

- ❑ **A. This patient should be admitted to the hospital because he has acute hypercapnic respiratory failure and will likely require mechanical ventilatory support**
- ❑ **B. As with acute hypoxemia, the effects of hypercapnia on the central nervous system are typically irreversible**
- ❑ **C. Acute hypercapnic respiratory failure is defined as a P_aCO_2 greater than 45 to 50 mm Hg along with respiratory acidosis**
- ❑ **D. Acute elevation in P_aCO_2 to 80 or 90 mm Hg is generally well tolerated, but levels in excess of 100 mm Hg often produce neurologic signs and symptoms**

Key Concept/Objective: To understand the clinical effects and the management of acute and chronic hypercapnia

Acute hypercapnic respiratory failure is defined as a P_aCO_2 greater than 45 to 50 mm Hg along with respiratory acidosis. Signs and symptoms of hypercapnia depend not only on the absolute level of P_aCO_2 but also on the rate at which the level increases. A P_aCO_2 above 100 mm Hg may be well tolerated if the hypercapnia develops slowly and acidemia is minimized by renal compensatory changes, as is the case with this patient. Acute elevation in P_aCO_2 to 80 to 90 mm Hg may produce many neurologic signs and symptoms, including confusion, headaches, seizures, and coma. A careful neurologic examination of a patient with acute hypercapnia may reveal agitation, coarse tremor, slurred speech, asterixis, and, occasionally, papilledema. These effects of hypercapnia on the central nervous system are fully reversible, unlike the potentially permanent neurologic sequelae that are associated with acute hypoxemia. *(Answer: C—Acute hypercapnic respiratory failure is defined as a P_aCO_2 greater than 45 to 50 mm Hg along with respiratory acidosis)*

45. A 52-year-old man with severe emphysema presents to the emergency department with shortness of breath and altered mental status. A history is taken from the patient's wife. She states that the patient was in his usual state of health until 24 hours ago, when he awoke with fever and shortness of breath. Since that time, he has experienced worsening fever, cough, and sputum production. She states that the patient has been acting "very funny" for the past several hours. She does not believe the patient has come into contact with anyone who was sick, and she states that he receives oxygen at home at a rate of 3 L/min via nasal cannula. On physical examination, the patient's temperature is found to be 101.1° F (38.4° C). The oropharynx and mucous membranes are dry, and rales with egophony are heard at the left pulmonary base. Laboratory studies reveal leukocytosis with left shift. Results of arterial blood gas measurements are as follows: pH, 7.02; P_aCO_2, 80 mm Hg; and P_aO_2, 60 mm Hg.

Which of the following statements regarding the management of respiratory failure in patients with COPD is true?

- ❑ **A. The most common cause of acute respiratory deterioration in patients with COPD is cigarette smoking**

❑ B. **The first priority in the management of respiratory failure in these patients is to decrease P_aCO_2 to a normal value**

❑ C. **The level of P_aCO_2 at which ventilatory assistance becomes necessary is approximately 70 mm Hg for males and 60 mm Hg for females**

❑ D. **When invasive ventilation is required, P_aCO_2 levels should not be lowered to the normal range in patients with chronic hypercapnia**

Key Concept: To understand the management of respiratory failure in patients with COPD

The first priority is to achieve a P_aO_2 level of 50 to 60 mm Hg but no higher. Intubation should be performed if hemodynamic instability or somnolence occurs or if secretions cannot be cleared. It is important to remember that P_aCO_2 levels in patients with chronic hypercapnia should not be lowered to the normal range, because this could result in alkalemia, which increases the risk of cardiac dysrhythmias and seizures. In addition, overventilation for more than 2 to 3 days may result in renal restoration of the pH to normal. As a consequence, during subsequent trials of spontaneous ventilation, as the P_aCO_2 rises to the baseline hypercapnic level, the patient becomes acidemic or the patient's respiratory muscles become fatigued because of the greater minute ventilation required for the reset baseline pH and P_aCO_2. *(Answer: D—When invasive ventilation is required, P_aCO_2 levels should not be lowered to the normal range in patients with chronic hypercapnia)*

46. A 29-year-old man with AIDS is admitted to the hospital for worsening shortness of breath. He was in his usual state of health until 1 week ago, when he developed dyspnea on exertion, with cough productive of thick sputum. His dyspnea has worsened over the past week, and he has developed a fever as well. He denies having been in contact with sick persons. He states that he received treatment for "PCP" 1 year ago. He also states that his last $CD4^+$ T cell count was "less than 10." He is not currently taking any medications, because he cannot afford them. On his second day of hospitalization, he develops acute respiratory failure and is moved to the critical care unit, where he is intubated and undergoes mechanical ventilation.

Which of the following statements regarding complications of mechanical ventilation is true?

❑ A. **Ventilated patients with acute, worsening respiratory distress or oxygen desaturation should be disconnected from the ventilator; manual ventilation should be administered with an anesthesia bag and 100% oxygen**

❑ B. **Growth of cultures obtained by suctioning through an endotracheal tube leads to a reliable diagnosis of pneumonia in ventilated patients**

❑ C. **Subcutaneous emphysema is the most common life-threatening manifestation of barotrauma**

❑ D. **In a patient with whole-lung atelectasis, a chest radiograph will reveal increased opacity in the affected hemithorax, together with a contralateral tracheal shift**

Key Concept/Objective: To know the complications of mechanical ventilation

Worsening respiratory distress or arterial oxygen desaturation may develop suddenly as a result of changes in the patient's cardiopulmonary status or secondary to a mechanical malfunction. The first priority is to ensure patency and correct positioning of the patient's airway so that adequate oxygenation and ventilation can be administered during the ensuing evaluation. The patient should be disconnected from the ventilator, and manual ventilation should be administered with an anesthesia bag, using 100% oxygen. Tension pneumothorax is the most common life-threatening manifestation of barotrauma. Tension pneumothorax leads to worsening hypoxemia and decreased venous return with hypotension. With atelectasis of an entire lung, breath sounds are diminished or absent on the affected side, and the trachea is shifted toward that side. *(Answer: A—Ventilated patients with acute, worsening respiratory distress or oxygen desaturation should be dis-*

connected from the ventilator; manual ventilation should be administered with an anesthesia bag and 100% oxygen)

For more information, see Kollef MH: 14 Respiratory Medicine: VIII Respiratory Failure. ACP Medicine Online (www.acpmedicine.com). Dale DC, Federman DD, Eds. WebMD Inc., New York, September 2004

Disorders of the Pleura, Hila, and Mediastinum

47. A 43-year-old male nurse presents to your office for evaluation. For the past 2 months, he has experienced intermittent fever, night sweats, and a 20-lb weight loss. He denies having any cough or sputum production. The patient states that about 3 months ago, he tested positive on purified protein derivative (PPD) screening. He denies any drug abuse, nor does he report any HIV risk factors. The patient states that he was prescribed isoniazid, but he chose not to follow this regimen. His chest x-ray is remarkable only for a moderate left pleural effusion.

Which of the following statements regarding tuberculous pleuritis is true?

- ❑ **A. Pleural effusion is more often a manifestation of reactivation tuberculosis than of primary tuberculosis**
- ❑ **B. Without therapy, this patient's pleural effusion will likely persist for many years**
- ❑ **C. In most cases of this illness, pleural fluid cell differential will reveal greater than 85% neutrophils**
- ❑ **D. Acid-fast bacilli are rarely seen in pleural liquid, and cultures are positive in only 20% to 40% of patients**

Key Concept/Objectives: To understand the clinical features of tuberculous pleuritis and pleural effusion

Pleural effusion is more often a manifestation of primary tuberculosis than of reactivation tuberculosis. In patients with primary tuberculosis, untreated pleural effusions resolve spontaneously in approximately 2 to 4 months. However, active tuberculosis develops in two thirds of such patients during the ensuing 5 years. The pleural liquid is usually serous or serosanguineous. In most cases, the differential white cell count reveals lymphocytosis. Acid-fast bacilli are rarely seen in pleural liquid, and cultures are positive in only 20% to 40% of patients. However, closed-needle biopsy of the pleura reveals caseating or noncaseating granulomas in approximately 70% of cases and provides material that is culture positive in approximately 75% of cases. Thus, the total diagnostic yield, as determined on the basis of histopathology and culture, is 90% to 95%. *(Answer: D—Acid-fast bacilli are rarely seen in pleural liquid, and cultures are positive in only 20% to 40% of patients)*

48. A 21-year-old white man is admitted to the hospital. The patient reports that while jogging earlier that day, he developed acute right anterior chest pain that was significantly worsened by deep inspiration. His pain radiated to his left scapula. He also developed moderate shortness of breath. He denies having any fever or chills; he has not experienced any recent immobility, and he has no personal or family history of clotting disorders. The patient has smoked one pack of cigarettes a day for the past 3 years. A chest x-ray is normal except for a large left pneumothorax.

Which of the following statements regarding idiopathic spontaneous pneumothorax is true?

- ❑ **A. The peak incidence occurs in persons between 30 and 50 years of age; there is a strong female preponderance**
- ❑ **B. Patients are often tall and thin in stature and are often cigarette smokers**
- ❑ **C. Most patients with idiopathic spontaneous pneumothorax have subpleural basilar blebs**

❑ D. **Strenuous physical activity and airplane travel are frequent triggers for the development of idiopathic spontaneous pneumothorax**

Key Concept/Objectives: To understand the clinical features of idiopathic spontaneous pneumothorax

The peak incidence of idiopathic spontaneous pneumothorax is in persons between 20 and 30 years of age; the male-to-female ratio is approximately 5:1. Patients often have a tall, thin stature and very frequently are cigarette smokers. Although patients with idiopathic spontaneous pneumothorax are otherwise healthy, most have subpleural apical blebs, frequently associated with more diffuse centrilobular emphysema that is detectable by CT scan. Common misconceptions are that strenuous physical activity is frequently a trigger for the development of pneumothorax and that patients are at increased risk during airplane travel. In fact, most studies have found that the onset of symptoms of pneumothorax usually occurs at rest or during light activity. *(Answer: B—Patients are often tall and thin in stature and are often cigarette smokers)*

49. A 55-year-old man visits your office with a complaint of fatigue and increasing dyspnea on exertion. He has been experiencing these symptoms for 2 weeks. He denies having fever, chills, cough, or weight loss, and he has no significant cardiac history. He denies having been in contact with anyone who was ill. He recently quit smoking, after having smoked cigarettes for 35 years. He does have a history of alcoholism and chronic pancreatitis; the pancreatitis has been well controlled with analgesics and pancreatic enzyme replacement therapy. His serum chemistries and complete blood count are unremarkable. A chest x-ray reveals a large left pleural effusion. A diagnostic thoracentesis is performed.

Which of the following statements regarding laboratory studies of pleural fluid is true?

❑ A. **An elevated pleural fluid amylase level is uncommon in patients with a malignant pleural effusion**

❑ B. **Pleural fluid eosinophilia is diagnostic of a pulmonary parasitic infection**

❑ C. **A pleural liquid hematocrit that exceeds half the simultaneous peripheral blood hematocrit indicates frank bleeding into the pleural space and is diagnostic of a hemothorax**

❑ D. **A pleural effusion with a pH of 5.8 is suggestive of empyema**

Key Concept/Objective: To understand the clinical correlations of pleural fluid laboratory abnormalities

Determination of the pleural liquid amylase level is warranted in patients with unexplained left-sided pleural effusions, particularly in the presence of coexistent abdomi- [illegible] levels are also commonly [illegible] nancy. Pleural liquid eosinophilia is rarely the result of a fungal or parasitic infection. Much more commonly, the eosinophilia is a nonspecific finding; in some cases, it is thought to result from the previous introduction of air or blood into the pleural space. A pleural liquid hematocrit that exceeds half the simultaneous peripheral blood hematocrit indicates frank bleeding into the pleural space and is diagnostic of a hemothorax. In patients who have a pleural effusion associated with bacterial pneumonia (parapneumonic effusion), a pleural liquid pH of less than 7.0 is suggestive of an infected pleural space (empyema). A pH of 6.0 or less suggests esophageal rupture. *(Answer: C—A pleural liquid hematocrit that exceeds half the simultaneous peripheral blood hematocrit indicates frank bleeding into the pleural space and is diagnostic of a hemothorax)*

50. An 86-year-old man is admitted to the hospital for volume depletion and inability to care for himself. He has experienced a 30-lb weight loss over the past several months, and his appetite has been poor. His family reports that his mental status has been normal. He has a long history of tobacco and alcohol abuse. Routine blood work reveals the following: iron deficiency anemia, a blood urea nitrogen/creatinine ratio of 25, and a mildly elevated alkaline phosphatase level. Other findings are normal. Chest x-ray reveals a moderate left pleural effusion. Diagnostic thoracentesis yields 60 ml of milky white fluid.

Which of the following statements regarding chylothorax is true?

- ❑ A. **Mediastinal tumors are the most common cause of chylothorax**
- ❑ B. **There is no clinical correlation between lymphangiomyomatosis and chylothorax**
- ❑ C. **In most cases of chylothorax, the triglyceride concentration exceeds 400 mg/dl**
- ❑ D. **Chylous effusions will typically reaccumulate at the rate of 100 to 200 ml/day**

Key ConceptObjective: To know the clinical features of chylothorax

Various conditions can cause chylothorax. Mediastinal tumors are the most common cause, with lymphomas exceeding metastatic carcinomas in frequency. Chylothorax frequently occurs as a complication of the rare disease lymphangiomyomatosis. In most cases of chylothorax, the triglyceride concentration exceeds 110 mg/dl; exceptions usually are limited to patients in whom feedings have been withheld, such as postoperative patients. The major consequence of chylous effusions is the rapid and recurrent accumulation of liquid in the pleural space. Normally, the thoracic duct transports chyle at a rate of 1.5 to 2.5 L/day. In patients with chylothorax, much or all of this liquid may enter the pleural space. *(Answer: A—Mediastinal tumors are the most common cause of chylothorax)*

51. A 65-year-old female smoker presents to your office for evaluation of weight loss and general malaise. Physical examination is remarkable for cachexia, dullness to percussion with associated decreased breath sounds, and decreased tactile fremitus over the left lung base. You order a chest radiograph, which reveals a left-sided pleural effusion. Subsequent lateral decubitus films reveal that the effusion is free-flowing. You perform a thoracentesis and send the fluid to the laboratory for analysis.

Which of the following findings would NOT be consistent with an exudative pleural effusion or one resulting from lymphatic obstruction?

- ❑ A. **A ratio of pleural protein to serum protein greater than 0.5**
- ❑ B. **A ratio of pleural lactate dehydrogenase (LDH) to serum LDH greater than 0.6**
- ❑ C. **A pleural LDH concentration greater than two thirds of the upper limit of normal for serum LDH**
- ❑ D. **A pleural protein concentration of 1 g/dl**
- ❑ E. **A pleural cholesterol level greater than 60 mg/dl**

Key Concept/Objective: To know the criteria used to distinguish exudative pleural effusions from effusions resulting from lymphatic obstruction

If the pleural effusion does not appear macroscopically to be blood, pus, or chyle, then the diagnosis requires differentiating between an exudative process and a transudative process. Pleural effusions resulting from exudation or obstruction of lymphatic drainage typically have a protein concentration of 3 g/dl or greater. However, the following four criteria are more likely to correctly identify an exudative effusion: (1) a ratio of pleural protein to serum protein greater than 0.5; (2) a ratio of pleural LDH to serum LDH greater than 0.6; (3) a pleural LDH concentration greater than two thirds of the upper limit of normal for serum LDH; (4) a pleural cholesterol level greater than 60 mg/dl. The presence of any of these findings makes the diagnosis of an exudative effusion more likely. The absence of all four findings points toward a transudative effusion. *(Answer: D—A pleural protein concentration of 1 g/dl)*

52. A 60-year-old man suffers from chronic obstructive pulmonary disease (COPD). He is brought to see you urgently for chest pain and shortness of breath. He is obviously having difficulty breathing but is able to give some history. He states that he experienced the sudden onset of sharp right-sided chest pain just a few minutes before calling for an ambulance. The pain is associated with shortness of breath, but he denies having any wheezing, fever, chills, or cough. After examining the patient, you obtain a chest radiograph, which reveals a right-sided pneumothorax.

Which of the following physical examination findings is NOT consistent with the diagnosis of pneumothorax?

- ❑ **A. Hyperresonance to percussion on the affected side**
- ❑ **B. Distant or absent breath sounds on the affected side**
- ❑ **C. Expansion of the hemithorax on the affected side**
- ❑ **D. Increased tactile fremitus on the affected side**
- ❑ **E Diminished transmission of voice sounds on the affected side**

Key Concept/Objective: To know the physical examination findings associated with pneumothorax

The patient with pneumothorax should have decreased tactile fremitus on the affected side. All of the other findings discussed in the case are consistent with the diagnosis of pneumothorax. This case illustrates the most common symptoms of pneumothorax: chest pain and dyspnea. In addition, this patient is a good example of someone in whom pneumothorax should be suspected, given his sudden onset of chest pain and dyspnea in conjunction with his history of chronic airflow obstruction. The diagnosis is confirmed with a chest radiograph. *(Answer: D—Increased tactile fremitus on the affected side)*

53. A 32-year-old man develops a nonproductive cough and experiences some decrease in his exertional tolerance, secondary to dyspnea, and general malaise. He works as a lawyer for a large corporation. During your evaluation, you order a chest radiograph, which reveals bilateral hilar adenopathy.

What is the most likely diagnosis for this patient?

- ❑ **A. Lymphoma**
- ❑ **B. Metastatic cancer**
- ❑ **C. Tuberculosis**
- ❑ **D. Sarcoidosis**
- ❑ **E. Berylliosis**

Key Concept/Objective: To know the most common cause of bilateral hilar adenopathy and to know the differential diagnosis

The most common cause of bilateral hilar adenopathy is sarcoidosis, especially in those persons between 20 and 40 years of age. Lymphoma, tuberculosis, malignancy, and berylliosis should all be included as diagnostic possibilities. Lymphoma is often accompanied by lymphadenopathy at other sites, systemic symptoms, and anemia. When hilar adenopathy is a manifestation of metastatic disease, the primary malignancy is usually known or easily identifiable. Chronic granulomatous diseases such as tuberculosis and histoplasmosis usually present with unilateral rather than bilateral hilar adenopathy. It can be difficult to differentiate berylliosis from sarcoidosis; in the former, there is usually a history of occupational exposure to beryllium in the manufacture of alloys, ceramics, or high-technology electronics. *(Answer: D—Sarcoidosis)*

For more information, see Staton GW, Ingram RH Jr: 14 Respiratory Medicine: IX Disorders of the Pleura, Hila, and Mediastinum. ACP Medicine Online (www.acpmedicine.com). Dale DC, Federman DD, Eds. WebMD Inc., New York, February 2004

Pulmonary Edema

54. A 65-year-old man is admitted to the intensive care unit for mechanical ventilation. There are no family members available to discuss the patient's history or current care. On arrival at the emergency department, the paramedics told the staff that the patient was "found down" in the park and smelled of alcohol. His initial hemoglobin oxygen saturation was 60%, and respirations were labored; thus, the patient was urgently intubated. Results of physical examination are as follows: temperature, 95.4° F (35.2° C); heart rate, 120 beats/min; respiratory rate, 20 breaths/min on mechanical ventilatation; and diffuse rales heard bilaterally in the lung fields. The patient is generally disheveled, with poor hygiene. Chest x-ray reveals bilateral interstitial and alveolar infiltrates. ECG reveals Q waves throughout the precordial leads.

Which of the following statements regarding the differentiation between cardiogenic and noncardiogenic pulmonary edema is true?

❑ **A. A bat's-wing or butterfly pattern on chest x-ray is more typical of noncardiogenic than cardiogenic pulmonary edema**

❑ **B. Distinct air bronchograms are more common with cardiogenic pulmonary edema**

❑ **C. A widened vascular pedicle and an increase in the cardiothoracic ratio suggest cardiogenic pulmonary edema**

❑ **D. Pulmonary arterial catheterization will yield useful information in these patients and will decrease their overall mortality**

Key Concept/Objective: To know how to differentiate cardiogenic pulmonary edema from noncardiogenic pulmonary edema

Ancillary features that can be routinely visualized on an anteroposterior chest radiograph made with a portable x-ray machine may help differentiate cardiogenic from noncardiogenic pulmonary edema. A widened vascular pedicle and an increase in the cardiothoracic ratio suggest increased pulmonary capillary pressure; distinct air bronchograms are more common with noncardiogenic pulmonary edema. A predominantly perihilar distribution of pulmonary edema is common, and occasionally, there is a very sharp demarcation between the central area of pulmonary edema and the lung periphery, leading to a so-called bat's-wing or butterfly pattern. This pattern is more typical of cardiogenic than noncardiogenic pulmonary edema. Despite the logical appeal of the use of pulmonary arterial catheters, no beneficial effect on outcome has been attributed to their use. A study of a large number of patients in intensive care units has suggested that patients who had pulmonary arterial catheters had a higher mortality at a higher financial cost than patients who did not undergo catheterization. *(Answer: C—A widened vascular pedicle and an increase in the cardiothoracic ratio suggest cardiogenic pulmonary edema)*

55. A 61-year-old woman presents to the emergency department. She was in her usual state of health until 2 days ago, when she developed fever; a cough productive of rusty sputum; chills; and exertional dyspnea. She denies having any contact with sick persons, and she has otherwise been very healthy. Results of physical examination are as follows: temperature, 102.3° F (39.4° C); heart rate, 105 beats/min; respiratory rate, 30 breaths/min; blood pressure, 80/42 mm Hg; hemoglobin oxygen saturation on room air, 84%; hyperdynamic precordium noted; jugular veins, flat; rales, heard diffusely in bilateral lung fields; and egophony noted, with increased fremitus in the right midlung zone. Laboratory data reveal leukocytosis with a left shift; thrombocytopenia; anemia with schistocytes; elevated coagulation parameters; mild renal insufficiency; and a moderate metabolic acidosis with an elevated anion gap. Chest x-ray reveals a diffuse alveolar filling process with focal consolidation of the right middle lobe. In the emergency department, the patient's respiratory failure worsens, and she is urgently intubated.

Which of the following statements regarding the diagnosis and management of acute respiratory distress syndrome (ARDS) is true?

❑ **A. There are high levels of neutrophils and their secretory products in the bronchoalveolar lavage liquid of patients with ARDS**

❑ **B. The alveolar filling process of ARDS affects all lung units equally**

❑ **C. Gas exchange in ARDS is characterized initially by hypoxemia that is refractory to increasing concentrations of inspired oxygen, implying the presence of $\dot{V}/\dot{Q}$ mismatching**

❑ **D. Respiratory failure is the most common cause of death in patients with ARDS**

Key Concept/Objective: To understand the diagnosis and management of ARDS

In ARDS patients, the underlying inflammatory response causes high levels of neutrophils and their secretory products in bronchoalveolar lavage liquid; this characteristic distinguishes noncardiogenic from cardiogenic edema. Typically, portable anteroposterior chest radiography reveals a diffuse and homogeneous alveolar filling process. When examined by CT, however, the air-space filling pattern frequently appears less homogeneous. Radiographs with the patient in the supine position typically show a greater degree of consolidation in posterior lung zones than in anterior lung zones. Gas exchange in ARDS is characterized initially by hypoxemia that is refractory to increasing concentrations of inspired oxygen, implying the presence of increased intrapulmonary shunting. Sepsis is the most common cause of death during the course of illness. As a result of state-of-the-art ventilatory-support techniques, respiratory failure is the cause of death in fewer than 20% of cases—a fact that highlights the importance of dysfunction of other organ systems in causing morbidity and mortality. *(Answer: A—There are high levels of neutrophils and their secretory products in the bronchoalveolar lavage liquid of patients with ARDS)*

56. A 65-year-old man presents to the emergency department complaining of progressive shortness of breath and lower leg swelling. Evaluation reveals increased jugular venous pressure, bilateral crackles, an S_3 gallop, and moderate lower extremity edema. Arterial blood gas assessment reveals hypoxemia. A chest radiograph shows cardiomegaly and bilateral pulmonary edema.

What is the most common cause of cardiogenic pulmonary edema?

- ❑ **A. Renal failure**
- ❑ **B. Left ventricular dysfunction**
- ❑ **C. Mitral valve disease**
- ❑ **D. Pulmonary venous obstruction**

Key Concept/Objective: To understand the most common cause of cardiogenic pulmonary edema

Cardiogenic pulmonary edema is caused by increased capillary pressure (hydrostatic forces); fluid accumulates first in the airways, then in the alveolar interstitium, and finally in the alveolar space. The most common cause of cardiogenic pulmonary edema is left ventricular dysfunction. In congestive cardiomyopathy, the systolic performance of the left ventricle is impaired, the ventricle is dilated, and left ventricular end-diastolic pressure (LVEDP) is increased. The rise in LVEDP leads to an increase in pulmonary capillary pressure. *(Answer: B—Left ventricular dysfunction)*

57. The family of a 72-year-old female patient meets with you to discuss her condition. The patient was admitted to the intensive care unit with ARDS 2 days ago and has required mechanical ventilation and vasopressors. They ask you about her prognosis.

Which of the following is NOT a factor associated with a worse prognosis?

- ❑ **A. Age less than 65 years**
- ❑ **B. Higher number of organ systems in failure**
- ❑ **C. Higher number of days of organ-system failure**
- ❑ **D. Longer duration of positive pressure ventilation**

Key Concept/Objective: To know the factors associated with a worse prognosis for patients with ARDS

ARDS is frequently part of a systemic inflammatory response syndrome. This highlights the importance of multiple organ systems in the course of the disease. Factors associated with higher mortality in patients suffering from ARDS include a higher number of organ systems in failure, a higher number of days of organ-system failure, and age

greater than 65 years. A longer duration of positive pressure ventilation is associated with a worse pulmonary functional outcome. The most common cause of death in patients with ARDS is sepsis. *(Answer: A—Age less than 65 years)*

For more information, see Staton GW, Ingram RH Jr: 14 Respiratory Medicine: X Pulmonary Edema. ACP Medicine Online (www.acpmedicine.com). Dale DC, Federman DD, Eds. WebMD Inc., New York, September 2004

Pulmonary Hypertension, Cor Pulmonale, and Primary Pulmonary Vascular Diseases

58. A 34-year-old woman with a diagnosis of primary pulmonary hypertension returns for evaluation. She has had a progressive increase in her dyspnea over the past 6 months. She has had marked fatigue for the past 4 months. Last month, she developed hoarseness. Evaluation by an otolaryngologist led to a diagnosis of Ortner syndrome. One week ago, she had onset of chest pain and an episode of syncope.

Of the symptoms this patient has had, which one suggests the worst prognosis?

- ❑ **A. Chest pain**
- ❑ **B. Dyspnea**
- ❑ **C. Fatigue**
- ❑ **D. Syncope**
- ❑ **E. Hoarseness**

Key Concept/Objective: To know the symptoms of pulmonary hypertension and their prognostic significance

All of the symptoms listed are associated with pulmonary hypertension. Chest pain can mimic angina pectoris, and hoarseness can occur because of compression of the recurrent laryngeal nerve by enlarged pulmonary vessels (Ortner syndrome). Syncope and right heart failure generally occur later in the course of illness and are associated with a poorer prognosis. *(Answer: D—Syncope)*

59. A 32-year-old man comes to your office for a job-related injury. His family history is remarkable for two relatives who had "internal bleeding" in their 40s. On examination, you notice multiple small telangiectasias on his lips, skin, and oral mucosa. His fingernails appear slightly clubbed. Chest x-ray reveals several small, perfectly round nodules in both lungs.

Which of the following is the most accurate statement about this patient's condition?

- ❑ **A. He is likely to develop pulmonary hypertension and right heart failure**
- ❑ **B. Orthopnea is common in this disorder**
- ❑ **C. He has an increased risk of stroke and brain abscess**
- ❑ **D. His pulmonary function tests will show significant restrictive disease**
- ❑ **E. There is no need to consider treatment if he remains asymptomatic**

Key Concept/Objective: To be able to recognize hereditary hemorrhagic telangiectasia and to know its consequences

In this disorder, there are often numerous arteriovenous malformations (AVMs) in the lungs and elsewhere in the body. Such patients have an artificially low pulmonary resistance because a substantial fraction of blood may be shunting through the AVMs. Although the presence of AVMs generally does not lead directly to pulmonary hypertension, occasionally pulmonary hypertension is seen in association with AVM therapy; that is, if AVMs are resected, one can develop pulmonary hypertension because of vascular remodeling and an abrupt increase in resistance once the AVMs are no longer able to shunt blood. Orthopnea is actually unusual in this disorder; classically, patients have

increased dyspnea when standing up, a symptom called platypnea. Pulmonary function tests are generally normal except for a slightly diminished diffusing capacity of lung for carbon monoxide (DL_{CO}). The long-term risk associated with the disease is largely the possibility that a clot or organism could embolize through one of these malformations directly to the brain. This makes treatment of asymptomatic patients controversial, but some favor it to prevent negative neurologic outcomes. *(Answer: C—He has an increased risk of stroke and brain abscess)*

60. ***Which of the following statements is true regarding primary pulmonary hypertension?***

- ❑ A. Right heart failure is a contraindication to lung transplantation
- ❑ B. Calcium channel blockers are not effective therapy
- ❑ C. Subcutaneous epoprostenol is a safe and effective treatment
- ❑ D. Five-year survival is roughly similar with medical therapy and lung transplantation
- ❑ E. Prognosis is excellent with early treatment

Key Concept/Objective: To understand the management of primary pulmonary hypertension

Primary pulmonary hypertension is a challenging and rare disease with a poor prognosis; 5-year survival is around 50% for both medical therapy and transplantation. Right heart failure often improves with a single-lung transplant and is not considered a contraindication to transplantation. Both calcium channel blockers and epoprostenol have been shown to be effective, and both can cause significant rebound pulmonary hypertension if stopped abruptly. Because of epoprostenol's short half-life (3 to 6 minutes), it is delivered by continuous I.V. infusion, and complications from the pump or vascular access devices cause significant problems. *(Answer: D—Five-year survival is roughly similar with medical therapy and lung transplantation)*

For more information, see Staton GW, Ingram RH Jr: 14 Respiratory Medicine: XI Pulmonary Hypertension, Cor Pulmonale, and Primary Pulmonary Vascular Diseases. ACP Medicine Online (www.acpmedicine.com). Dale DC, Federman DD, Eds. WebMD Inc., New York, March 2003

SECTION 15

RHEUMATOLOGY

Introduction to the Rheumatic Diseases

1. A 56-year-old man presents for evaluation in a primary care clinic. He has a 2-day history of right ankle swelling and pain. He reports experiencing discomfort with ambulation and when driving an automobile. On further questioning, he denies experiencing a recent trauma, although he does recall spraining his ankle approximately 10 years ago. On examination, the patient's temperature is 99.9° F (37.7° C). His right ankle is warm to palpation and reveals an effusion. With passive range of motion of the right ankle, significant pain is elicited.

   Which of the following is the most appropriate step to take next in the treatment of this patient?

   - ❑ A. **Check the serum uric acid level; if elevated, initiate therapy with indomethacin and colchicine**
   - ❑ B. **Obtain a plain radiograph of the right ankle to assess for structural damage or chondrocalcinosis**
   - ❑ C. **Perform arthrocentesis of the right ankle, with analysis of the synovial fluid**
   - ❑ D. **Treat with ibuprofen and have the patient return to clinic in 1 week if his symptoms do not improve**

   Key Concept/Objective: To understand the importance of synovial fluid analysis in the evaluation of a patient with acute monoarthritis

   In this patient, the acute onset of symptoms, low-grade fever, and lack of trauma warrant a prompt evaluation; empirical therapy will not provide a definitive diagnosis and could potentially result in a serious illness, such as septic arthritis, being missed. Joint aspiration should be performed with aseptic technique as a part of the evaluation of every case of acute monoarthritis. Analysis of the synovial fluid includes a WBC count and differential, appropriate cultures and stains for microorganisms, and polarized-light microscopy. The WBC count in the synovial fluid is useful in distinguishing inflammatory from noninflammatory arthritis: levels greater than 2,000/mm^3 are consistent with inflammation. Patients with crystal-induced arthritis usually have counts in excess of 30,000/mm^3. The finding of monosodium urate or calcium pyrophosphate dihydrate crystals on polarized-light microscopy is pathognomonic for gout and pseudogout, respectively; the absence of crystals does not exclude these diagnoses. The serum level of uric acid is of little use in diagnosing gouty arthritis. Twenty percent of patients with gout have normal uric acid levels, and most persons with elevated levels never develop gouty arthritis. Plain radiography is most useful in patients with significant trauma that suggests the possibility of fracture, in those who experience a sudden loss of function, and in those with symptoms that do not improve despite appropriate treatment. This patient did not have any recent trauma and was still able to bear weight (although it did cause pain). Chondrocalcinosis would suggest the diagnosis of pseudogout, but the most appropriate initial evaluation of a patient with a monoarticular arthritis is arthrocentesis. *(Answer: C—Perform arthrocentesis of the right ankle, with analysis of the synovial fluid)*

2. ***Which of the following statements regarding immunologic tests is true?***

❑ A. As a class, immunologic tests are highly sensitive and specific

❑ B. The use of arthritis panels, in which many serologic tests are bundled together, can increase the likelihood of diagnosing a rheumatic disease

❑ C. Low titers of antinuclear antibody (ANA) are uncommon in young women

❑ D. Rheumatoid factor positivity in healthy persons increases with age

Key Concept/Objective: To understand that immunologic tests are not useful as screening tests

As a class, immunologic tests have low specificity and only moderate sensitivity. They are more expensive than other clinical laboratory tests, and the results are less reproducible. Immunologic tests should never be used as screening tests; their greatest utility occurs when the pretest probability of disease is high. The misuse of immunologic tests frequently confounds the diagnosis and leads to unnecessary rheumatology referrals. The use of so-called arthritis panels, in which many serologic tests are bundled together, increases the likelihood of an abnormal test result occurring in a patient without rheumatic disease; such panels should be avoided. It is common for young women to test positive for ANA; approximately 32% of young women will test positive for ANA at low titers. A positive ANA in and of itself is by no means diagnostic of systemic lupus erythematosus. The probability of testing positive for rheumatoid factor increases with age even in healthy persons. Additionally, conditions other than rheumatoid arthritis can be associated with elevations in rheumatoid factor; because of this, a positive test result for rheumatoid factor is not diagnostic of rheumatoid arthritis. A careful and detailed history is the most important part of the evaluation of a patient with arthritis. Laboratory findings should be evaluated in the context of the information obtained by a detailed history and physical examination. Diagnoses of rheumatic diseases should not be based solely on the findings of immunologic tests. *(Answer: D—Rheumatoid factor positivity in healthy persons increases with age)*

3. A 56-year-old woman with a history of rheumatoid arthritis presents to clinic with symmetrical pain and swelling of her wrists and metacarpophalangeal joints. She reports morning stiffness, and she notes that it now takes her 4 hours to "loosen up" in the morning. Recently, this has caused her much distress, because she has had increasing difficulty with bathing and dressing herself. The patient has been treated with ibuprofen in the past and expresses concern that her condition will continue to decline.

Of the following, which is the most appropriate statement to make to this patient at this time?

❑ A. "Your disease will likely progress and further limit your function regardless of what we do at this point."

❑ B. "I recognize your concern; we have very effective treatments available that may prevent progression of your disease and help you regain function."

❑ C. "I'll have you talk with our social worker about getting a home health nurse to assist you at home."

❑ D. "We now have effective medications that can cure rheumatoid arthritis; don't worry."

Key Concept/Objective: To recognize the importance of patient education regarding the effectiveness of treatment as a critical component in the care of the patient with a rheumatic disease

Patients who present with complaints of joint pain often express the opinion that nothing can be done for their arthritis. One of the most important things the physician can do is to correct this misconception. It is important that the patient understands that treatment greatly improves the condition of most patients with arthritis. Educating the patient about the effectiveness of treatment is the first step toward a successful outcome. It is important to provide realistic goals regarding the effectiveness of treatment options. Very effective therapies for rheumatoid arthritis have been available for 20 years, such that long-term outcome has distinctly improved. New treatments with biologic agents that block the inflammatory cytokines tumor necrosis factor–α and interleukin-1 are very effective, have a rapid onset of action, and prevent radiographic progression of disease. To date, there is

no therapy available that is curative of rheumatoid arthritis. This case illustrates the importance of obtaining a functional assessment as a part of the history. After pain, loss of function is of the greatest concern to the patient. Patients with significant functional impairment should be asked more detailed questions about routine activities of daily living. *(Answer: B—"I recognize your concern; we have very effective treatments available that may prevent progression of your disease and help you regain function.")*

4. A 48-year-old man with a history of rheumatoid arthritis presents to clinic complaining of left wrist pain and swelling. He has been maintained on prednisone and methotrexate. The patient expresses frustration with this flare, because he had been doing very well the past few months. Vital signs are significant for a temperature of 100.6° F (38.1° C).

Which of the following statements regarding the evaluation of this patient is most accurate?

❑ A. **The affected joint should be examined; the examination should include appropriate maneuvers in an attempt to reproduce the patient complaint**

❑ B. **Frank redness of the skin overlying the left wrist is always present if the pain is secondary to inflammation**

❑ C. **Increased temperature of the skin overlying the left wrist is common in inflammatory arthritis and is best detected by palpation with the palms**

❑ D. **Arthrocentesis of the left wrist is not indicated, because the patient is known to have rheumatoid arthritis**

Key Concept/Objective: To understand the components and findings of the joint examination in a patient with inflammatory arthritis

By looking at and palpating the joints, the physician can identify the exact anatomic structures that are the source of the patient's pain and decide whether the pain is caused by inflammation. A goal of the examination is to reproduce the patient's pain, either by motion of the joint or by palpation. Frank redness of the skin overlying a joint is unusual; however, increased temperature, best detected by palpation with the backs of the fingers (not the palms), is common and, when present, indicates inflammation. Palpation for tenderness may reveal whether the problem lies within the joint or is discretely localized to an overlying bursa or tendon sheath. Arthrocentesis of the left wrist should be performed as part of the evaluation of this patient. When patients with established rheumatoid arthritis have fever and an apparent flare, joint infection should be excluded by joint aspiration because septic arthritis occurs more frequently in such patients. *(Answer: A—The affected joint should be examined; the examination should include appropriate maneuvers in an attempt to reproduce the patient complaint)*

For more information, see Ruddy S: 15 Rheumatology: I Introduction to the Rheumatic Diseases. ACP Medicine Online (www.acpmedicine.com). Dale DC, Federman DD, Eds. WebMD Inc., New York, March 2005

Rheumatoid Arthritis

5. A 41-year-old woman comes in for a checkup. You diagnosed her with rheumatoid arthritis (RA) several years ago when she presented with bilateral metacarpophalangeal joint swelling with stiffness and fatigue. The course of this patient's disease has been mild, and the patient has been maintained on nonsteroidal anti-inflammatory drugs (NSAIDs) and methotrexate therapy. Today she is doing well; she has minimal pain and functional impairment. She asks you about the cause of RA. This stimulates you to read about current evidence regarding the pathogenesis of this illness.

Which of the following statements regarding the pathogenesis of RA is false?

❑ A. **Damage to bone and cartilage by synovial tissue and pannus is mediated by several families of enzymes, including serine proteases and cathepsins**

❑ B. IgG rheumatoid factor is most commonly detected in patients with RA

❑ C. Interaction of rheumatoid factors with normal IgG activates complement and thereby starts a chain of events that includes production of anaphylatoxins and chemotactic factors

❑ D. Although many cytokines are involved in the pathogenesis of RA, tumor necrosis factor–α (TNF-α) and interleukin-1 (IL-1) are major pathogenic factors

Key Concept/Objective: To understand the pathogenesis of RA

Damage to bone and cartilage by synovial tissue and pannus is mediated by several families of enzymes, including serine proteases and cathepsins. The most damaging enzymes are the metalloproteinases (e.g., collagenase, stromelysin, and gelatinase) and cathepsins (especially cathepsin K), which can degrade the major structural proteins in the joint. IgM rheumatoid factor is most commonly detected; IgG and, less frequently, IgA rheumatoid factors are also sometimes found. The presence of IgG rheumatoid factor is associated with a higher rate of systemic complications (e.g., necrotizing vasculitis). Interaction of rheumatoid factors with normal IgG activates complement and thereby starts a chain of events that includes production of anaphylatoxins and chemotactic factors. Macrophage- and fibroblast-derived cytokines (e.g., IL-1, IL-6, TNF-α, and granulocyte-macrophage colony-stimulating factor) are abundantly expressed in the rheumatoid joint. Although many of these cytokines are involved in the pathogenesis of RA, TNF-α and IL-1 are major pathogenic factors; both can induce synoviocyte proliferation, collagenase production, and prostaglandin release. *(Answer: B—IgG rheumatoid factor is most commonly detected in patients with RA)*

6. A 29-year-old woman visits your office for the evaluation of painful hand swelling. She was in her usual state of health until 2 months ago, when she began to notice moderate morning hand pain. The pain seems to be worsening. She states that her hands are stiff and painful each morning, but they tend to improve over the course of the day. Her pain is localized to the knuckles of both hands. She denies having any rash, difficulty breathing, fevers, or other joint pains. The only notable finding on her physical examination is boggy edema and tenderness to palpation of her metacarpophalangeal joints and proximal interphalangeal joints. She has no wrist pain or deformity. Laboratory test results are normal except for a mild normocytic anemia and an elevated CRP. The patient tests negative for serum rheumatoid factor.

Which of the following statements regarding the diagnosis of RA is true?

❑ A. The typical initial presentation of RA is isolated arthritis of large joints such as the knee or ankle

❑ B. The diagnosis of RA is confirmed by joint stiffness, which is a specific finding for the illness

❑ C. RA tends to cause marked erythema of the involved joints

❑ D. Classically, RA is a symmetrical arthritis

Key Concept/Objective: To know the typical features of RA

Small joints of the hands and feet are usually involved at the outset, although large joints (e.g., knees and ankles) are sometimes affected first. In about 10% of cases, monoarthritis of a large joint can presage progression to polyarticular RA. Most patients experience some degree of joint stiffness, especially in the morning after awakening, which may accompany or precede joint swelling or pain. These symptoms are hallmarks of disease activity and help distinguish RA from noninflammatory diseases such as osteoarthritis. However, joint stiffness and swelling are not specific for RA and can occur with other types of inflammatory arthritis. Unlike acute inflammatory arthritides (e.g., gout or septic arthritis), RA tends not to cause marked erythema, and swelling usually does not extend far beyond the articulation. Classically, RA is symmetrical. When RA is progressive and unremitting, nearly every peripheral joint may eventually be affected, although the thoracic, lumbar, and sacral spine are usually spared. *(Answer: D—Classically, RA is a symmetrical arthritis)*

7. A 48-year-old female patient of yours with moderately severe RA presents for a scheduled visit. She is very satisfied with her current therapy and feels that joint pains, swelling, and stiffness have all improved over the past 3 months. Her energy level has also improved, and she has recently planted a large flower garden. Her only complaint today is that she can't "catch her breath" when she works in her garden. Her shortness of breath is worsened by exertion, and she now states that she experiences shortness of breath while ambulating in her house. Over the past week, she has developed pain in her right chest; the pain worsens with exertion or with deep inspiration. Physical examination is noteworthy for decreased breath sounds, decreased fremitus, dullness to percussion, and a pleural rub of the right basilar lung field. Chest radiography confirms the diagnosis of rheumatoid lung disease.

Which of the following statements regarding rheumatoid lung disease is true?

- ❑ A. **The most common form of lung involvement is pleurisy with effusions**
- ❑ B. **Rheumatoid effusions typically have a glucose concentration of greater than 50 mg/dl**
- ❑ C. **RA is not a reported cause of cavitary lung disease**
- ❑ D. **Rheumatoid lung disease with fibrosis typically causes an obstructive ventilatory defect with a decreased carbon dioxide diffusion rate**

Key Concept/Objective: To know the key features of rheumatoid lung disease

The most common form of lung involvement in RA is pleurisy with effusions. Evidence of pleuritis is often found at postmortem examination, but symptomatic pleurisy occurs in fewer than 10% of patients. Clinical features include gradual onset and variable degrees of pain and dyspnea. The effusions generally have protein concentrations greater than 3 to 4 g/dl, as well as glucose concentrations lower than 30 mg/dl; the latter finding has been ascribed to a primary defect in glucose transport. Rheumatoid nodules occur in the pulmonary parenchyma and on the pleural surface. They range in size from just detectable to several centimeters in diameter. They may be single or multiple. At times, the nodules cavitate. Such nodules can be difficult to distinguish radiologically from tuberculous or malignant lesions and often require further evaluation, including biopsy. Progressive, symptomatic interstitial pulmonary fibrosis that produces coughing and dyspnea in conjunction with radiographic changes of a diffuse reticular pattern (i.e., honeycomb lung) is usually associated with high titers of rheumatoid factor. The lesion is histologically indistinguishable from idiopathic pulmonary fibrosis. Chest radiographs show pleural thickening, nodules, diffuse or patchy infiltrates, and a restrictive ventilatory defect that is characterized by a decreased carbon dioxide diffusion rate. *(Answer: A—The most common form of lung involvement is pleurisy with effusions)*

8. A 35-year-old woman returns for a follow-up visit. The patient has been receiving a cyclooxygenase-2 (COX-2) selective NSAID for RA, with only minimal improvement in her symptoms. She continues to have significant pain and morning stiffness in her hands and wrist. Her fatigue is stable and without improvement. She has been reading about the many available therapies for RA and feels that she now needs additional therapy. You explain that the NSAID was only the starting point for her medical therapy and that you agree that it is time to change her therapy.

Which of the following statements regarding accepted medical therapy of RA is false?

- ❑ A. **An acceptable escalation in this patient's therapy would be to begin methotrexate at the recommended starting dose**
- ❑ B. **The antimalarial drug hydroxychloroquine is useful as early second-line therapy for RA**
- ❑ C. **An acceptable escalation in this patient's therapy would be to replace her current therapy with infliximab monotherapy**
- ❑ D. **The conventional wisdom is that glucocorticoids neither alter the course of the disease nor affect the ultimate degree of damage to joints or other structures**

Key Concept/Objective: To understand medical therapy for RA

Advancement from NSAIDs to second-line agents is recommended if (1) symptoms have not improved sufficiently after a short trial of NSAIDs, (2) the patient has aggressive seropositive disease, or (3) there is radiographic evidence of erosions or joint destruction. The trend today is for more aggressive treatment, and the majority of patients require additional pharmacotherapy. Most patients require rapid advancement from NSAIDs to a second-line agent, most often methotrexate. In the United States, most rheumatologists prefer to increase the methotrexate dosage rapidly to 20 to 25 mg/wk and then add another agent within 2 to 3 months if necessary. The antimalarial drug hydroxychloroquine is useful as early second-line therapy for RA. Its response rate is lower than that of methotrexate, and less improvement is seen; however, its relative safety makes it an ideal choice for patients with mild early disease or as an additive agent in combination therapy. Infliximab is used in combination with methotrexate; this appears to permit long-term use of infliximab with less formation of neutralizing antibodies. Infliximab is administered by intravenous infusion; the recommended dose is 3 to 10 mg/kg every 8 weeks. As with etanercept and all TNF inhibitors, the drug must be used with care in the presence of infections. The conventional wisdom is that glucocorticoids neither alter the course of the disease nor affect the ultimate degree of damage to joints or other structures. *(Answer: C—An acceptable escalation in this patient's therapy would be to replace her current therapy with infliximab monotherapy)*

9. A 60-year-old man is diagnosed with RA after several months of joint pain, swelling, and stiffness. His disease has been progressing and involves numerous joints. The patient tests positive for rheumatoid factors and rheumatoid nodules. He is concerned about his prognosis.

Which of the following is associated with a favorable course for a patient with RA?

- ❑ A. **Age greater than 40 years**
- ❑ B. **Acute onset in a few large joints**
- ❑ C. **Insidious onset of disease**
- ❑ D. **Positive rheumatoid factor**

Key Concept/Objective: To know the major prognostic factors in RA

In approximately 75% of patients with RA, the disease waxes and wanes in severity over a number of years. Other patients have complete remission. A favorable course and long remissions are associated with age less than 40 years, acute onset restricted to a few large joints, disease duration less than 1 year, and negative test results for rheumatoid factors. An unfavorable prognosis is associated with insidious onset, constitutional symptoms, the rapid appearance of rheumatoid nodules, the appearance of bone erosions early in the course of disease, and high titers of rheumatoid factors. Patients with the most aggressive form of the disease experience a significant loss in quality of life and a shortened life expectancy. Early aggressive management with disease-modifying agents is clearly indicated for patients with an unfavorable prognosis. *(Answer: B—Acute onset in a few large joints)*

10. A 35-year-old woman has been seeing you for treatment for RA for several years. Her disease is currently well controlled, but she is anxious about her future. She has read extensively about RA and recently learned that patients with the disease die at a younger age than other persons. She asks you about this and about which diseases most commonly cause death in patients with RA.

What is the most common cause of death in patients with RA?

- ❑ A. **Cardiovascular disease**
- ❑ B. **Leukemia**
- ❑ C. **Infection**
- ❑ D. **Non-Hodgkin lymphoma**

Key Concept/Objective: To understand that mortality is higher in patients with RA and to be able to identify the leading causes of death in patients with RA

Patients with RA die at earlier ages than those without the disease. The leading cause of death in patients with RA is cardiovascular disease (40% to 45% of deaths); this increase in

cardiovascular mortality may be related to the chronic inflammation caused by the disease and to the potential for vascular disease associated with treatments such as glucocorticoids. Malignancy accounts for 15% of deaths in these patients; infections account for 10%. There is an increased incidence of lymphoproliferative diseases such as non-Hodgkin lymphoma and Hodgkin disease in patients with RA. *(Answer: A—Cardiovascular disease)*

11. A 34-year-old woman with a 5-year history of rheumatoid arthritis presents for routine follow-up. She has been taking sulfasalazine, 1 g b.i.d., and naproxen, 500 mg b.i.d. She complains of 1 to 2 hours of morning stiffness and mild swelling of multiple PIP and MCP joints. Physical examination (in early afternoon) reveals mild synovitis of the MCPs and PIPs of both hands and difficulty making a full fist. She also has synovitis of multiple MTP joints. X-rays demonstrate small erosions in the joints of the hands and feet that seem to have progressed since last year.

What therapy would you recommend for this patient's arthritis?

❑ **A. Continue the current therapy**

❑ **B. Increase sulfasalazine to 3 g/day**

❑ **C. Add prednisone, 5 mg/day**

❑ **D. Add hydroxychloroquine, 400 mg/day**

❑ **E. Add oral methotrexate, 7.5 mg/wk**

Key Concept/Objective: To understand the treatment of progressive rheumatoid arthritis

To prevent the development of erosive joint changes, the standard of treatment for rheumatoid arthritis has become much more aggressive. This patient on sulfasalazine has developed further x-ray changes, and the next step for most rheumatologists would be to add methotrexate to the regimen to gain more control of the synovitis that is damaging her joints. The dose could be increased to as much as 25 mg/wk, if needed, to control her disease. More than 2 g/day of sulfasalazine is rarely more effective but is potentially more toxic. Low-dose prednisone may help her symptoms but would not affect the disease process. Finally, hydroxychloroquine, although safe, has less disease-modifying power than methotrexate. Recently, the combination of methotrexate, sulfasalazine, and hydroxychloroquine has been shown to be an effective combination in resistant disease and could be used if the addition of methotrexate is insufficient. *(Answer: E—Add oral methotrexate, 7.5 mg/wk)*

12. A 62-year-old woman comes to clinic complaining of right eye pain and redness. It has been present for several weeks and is getting worse. She has a history of rheumatoid arthritis and has been on hydroxychloroquine, 400 mg/day, and prednisone, 5 mg/day, for several years. On examination, the eye is very red, with a violaceous hue to the sclera. Gentle finger pressure over the eyelid onto the globe is painful.

Which of the following should be the next step in the care of this patient?

❑ **A. Add an ocular lubricant to her regimen**

❑ **B. Prescribe corticosteroid ocular drops**

❑ **C. Stop the hydroxychloroquine immediately**

❑ **D. Increase the prednisone to 20 mg/day**

❑ **E. Call for an ophthalmology appointment**

Key Concept/Objective: To be able to recognize serious eye disease in rheumatoid arthritis

Patients with rheumatoid arthritis may have a variety of eye problems, including dry eye, episcleritis, and scleritis. Dry eye is rarely serious and is treated with eyedrops and lubricants. Episcleritis is inflammation of superficial vessels and is generally not a threat to vision; scleritis is caused by inflammation of the deeper vessels and can lead to loss of vision. Differentiation of the two is based on the more violaceous hue of the sclera in scleritis—caused by inflammation around the sclera vessels—and pain on pressure over the closed lid onto the globe, which is not seen in episcleritis. Confirmation can be done by

slit-lamp examination. Scleritis comes in different forms, and treatment decisions are best made in conjunction with an ophthalmologist. The most serious form of scleritis can lead to scleromalacia perforans, which usually leads to blindness in the affected eye. Hydroxychloroquine can cause eye disease, notably retinopathy, but there are no superficial manifestations. *(Answer: E—Call for an ophthalmology appointment)*

13. A 55-year-old man comes to your clinic with a persistent cough. He had a viral syndrome 3 weeks ago that has cleared, but he continues to have a nonproductive cough. Past medical history is significant for seropositive rheumatoid arthritis and a 25-pack-year history of smoking. Current medications include leflunomide, 10 mg/day, and prednisone, 5 mg/day. Physical examination is significant for mild ulnar deviation of the fingers and fibular deviation of the toes, but little active synovitis. Rheumatoid nodules are present over the extensor surface of both forearms near the elbows. Chest x-ray reveals a 2 cm × 2 cm pulmonary nodule in the right upper lobe but is otherwise normal. Old films are not available.

Which of the following should be the next step in the care of this patient?

- ❑ **A. Reassure and treat symptomatically**
- ❑ **B. Increase the leflunomide to 20 mg/day**
- ❑ **C. Repeat the chest x-ray in 3 months**
- ❑ **D. Perform a CT scan to evaluate the lesion further**
- ❑ **E. Schedule a transbronchial biopsy**

Key Concept/Objective: To understand the evaluation of pulmonary nodules in patients with rheumatoid arthritis

Patients with rheumatoid arthritis, particularly men with subcutaneous nodules who are smokers, are prone to developing rheumatoid nodules in the lung. These lesions are generally well circumscribed. They can be of various sizes, may be single or multiple, and tend to be peripheral in location. Unfortunately, those patients who are at risk for rheumatoid lung nodules are also at risk for lung cancer, and pulmonary nodules in patients with rheumatoid arthritis should be considered potentially malignant. A CT scan of the chest is the most reasonable first step to evaluate location and the presence of adenopathy. In most cases, a biopsy will be necessary for histologic evaluation. *(Answer: D—Perform a CT scan to evaluate the lesion further)*

14. A 35-year-old woman comes to clinic for follow-up of rheumatoid arthritis and to evaluate a new rash on the lower extremities. She was diagnosed with rheumatoid arthritis 5 years ago on the basis of joint pain and a positive rheumatoid factor, but the rheumatoid factor has been intermittently positive since then. Current medications include methotrexate, 7.5 mg/wk, and ibuprofen, 400 mg t.i.d. Physical examination is significant for the lack of synovitis in the small joints of the hands and feet and the presence of palpable purpura on both lower extremities. Biopsy of the purpura reveals leukocytoclastic vasculitis.

Which of the following would be the most useful serologic test to clarify this patient's illness?

- ❑ **A. Antineutrophil cytoplasmic antibodies**
- ❑ **B. Antinuclear antibody reflexive panel**
- ❑ **C. Hepatitis C antibody with PCR if positive**
- ❑ **D. Hepatitis B antibodies, including anticore**
- ❑ **E. Repeat the testing for rheumatoid factor**

Key Concept/Objective: To be able to recognize the mimicking of rheumatoid arthritis by hepatitis C infection

Patients with hepatitis C infection may have polyarthralgias or polyarthritis that can resemble rheumatoid arthritis. To make matters even more problematic, rheumatoid factor is present in many patients with hepatitis C, especially in the setting of mixed cryoglobulinemia. The rheumatoid factor, as part of the cryoglobulin, may not be present in the serum if it is collected and allowed to clot at room temperature. Cryoglobulins will

aggregate and clot if subjected to temperatures generally lower than 100.4° F (38° C). If rheumatoid arthritis is suspected, the specimen should be allowed to clot in a 38° C water bath and then checked for rheumatoid factor. Patients with hepatitis C should in general avoid potentially hepatotoxic drugs such as methotrexate. *(Answer: C—Hepatitis C antibody with PCR if positive)*

15. A 45-year-old woman with a 10-year history of rheumatoid arthritis comes to clinic with a 3-day history of right knee pain and swelling. She cannot bend the knee without severe discomfort. She has also noted a mild increase in pain and swelling of the small joints of her hands and feet. Current medications include methotrexate, 15 mg/week, prednisone, 5 mg/day, and ibuprofen, 600 mg t.i.d. Physical examination reveals ulnar deviation of the fingers, with 1+ synovitis of the MCPs and PIPs, hammer toe deformities, and fibular deviation of the toes, also with 1+ synovitis. The right knee has a significant effusion, is erythematous, and is warm to the touch. She resists attempts to flex and extend the knee. X-rays of the knee show mild, diffuse joint-space narrowing, unchanged from films taken last year.

Which of the following should be the next step in the care of this patient?

- ❑ A. **Increase prednisone to 30 mg/day for 1 week, then taper**
- ❑ B. **Increase the dose of methotrexate to 17.5 mg/week**
- ❑ C. **Order an MRI to evaluate the knee for internal derangement**
- ❑ D. **Perform arthrocentesis and give colchicine, 0.6 mg t.i.d.**
- ❑ E. **Perform arthrocentesis and then admit for I.V. antibiotics**

Key Concept/Objective: To be able to recognize septic arthritis in a patient with underlying rheumatoid arthritis

Patients with rheumatoid arthritis are at increased risk for septic arthritis. The most common joint affected by septic arthritis is the knee. Clues to an underlying septic arthritis in this patient include severe joint pain (rare in rheumatoid joints), erythema (also rare), and a joint that is much more symptomatic than the rest. Patients with rheumatoid arthritis may not have the usual systemic symptoms of fever and chills because of the anti-inflammatory medications that are used to treat the chronic arthritis. In general, it is important to have a high degree of suspicion; when in doubt, rule out septic arthritis. The mortality is as high as 20% for septic monoarthritis in patients with underlying rheumatoid arthritis and up to 50% if more than one joint is infected. *(Answer: E—Perform arthrocentesis and then admit for I.V. antibiotics)*

For more information, see Firestein GS: 15 Rheumatology: II Rheumatoid Arthritis. ACP Medicine Online (www.acpmedicine.com). Dale DC, Federman DD, Eds. WebMD Inc., New York, July 2004

Seronegative Spondyloarthropathies

16. A 27-year-old man comes to your office asking that you evaluate him for the possibility of having ankylosing spondylitis. His older brother has recently been diagnosed with ankylosing spondylitis, and he has learned on the Internet that ankylosing spondylitis runs in families. He is completely asymptomatic, and his physical examination, including a careful examination of his back, sacroiliac joints, and heart, is unremarkable. You consider ordering a test to assess for the presence of the HLA-B27 allele.

In which patients is testing for HLA-B27 indicated?

- ❑ A. **Any male patient under the age of 35 years who presents with chronic back pain (i.e., pain persisting over 6 months) should be assessed for HLA-B27 as part of the routine workup**
- ❑ B. **HLA-B27 testing is never indicated**
- ❑ C. **All first-degree relatives of patients with a confirmed diagnosis of ankylosing spondylitis should be screened for possible disease with HLA-B27 testing**

❑ **D. Only those patients whose clinical presentation and examination are consistent with ankylosing spondylitis but whose radiographic testing is negative should undergo HLA-B27 testing**

Key Concept/Objective: To understand the role of HLA-B27 in the diagnosis of ankylosing spondylitis

The diagnosis of ankylosing spondylitis is based on the following modified New York criteria: (1) low back pain of at least 3 months' duration that is alleviated with exercise and is not relieved by rest; (2) restricted lumbar spinal motion; and (3) decreased chest expansion relative to normal values for age and sex. In addition, the patient must have definitive radiographic evidence of sacroiliitis. HLA-B27 is not required for the diagnosis. The lack of specificity of HLA-B27 in asymptomatic patients precludes its use in this patient. Infrequently, a patient can present with clinical stigmata of disease without radiographic evidence of disease. After other primary disease processes have been ruled out, such as reactive arthritis, psoriasis, or inflammatory bowel disease, it is reasonable to test for HLA-B27. In this subgroup of patients, follow-up sacroiliac radiographic abnormalities will eventually evolve; this may take as long as 10 years. *(Answer: D—Only those patients whose clinical presentation and examination are consistent with ankylosing spondylitis but whose radiographic testing is negative should undergo HLA-B27 testing)*

17. A 28-year-old white man presents as a walk-in patient to your clinic. He reports a 5-day history of right-sided knee pain and bilateral ankle pain. He also thinks his back has been "a little stiff." He reports no trauma or previous joint ailments, nor does he have a family history of hematologic diseases or joint disorders. He reports mild fever subjectively, no visual changes or eye pain, and very mild and intermittent dysuria. On physical examination, the patient is found to have mild effusion in his right knee, without overt inflammation, and bilateral tenderness of his Achilles tendons. Genital examination is significant for shallow ulcerations on the glans of the penis upon foreskin retraction.

Which of the following statements regarding this patient is true?

❑ **A. The diagnosis of reactive arthritis is highly unlikely given the absence of evidence of uveitis or urethritis in either the history or the physical examination**

❑ **B. Normal gut flora have a prominent role in the pathogenesis of this disease process**

❑ **C. A careful sexual history should be obtained, and testing for *Chlamydia trachomatis* (i.e., culture or molecular probe assay) should be completed**

❑ **D. Oral ciprofloxacin should be prescribed for this patient**

Key Concept/Objective: To understand the pathogenesis and the classic presentation of reactive arthritis

The presence of an asymmetrical arthritis and balanitis circinata in this patient is highly suggestive of reactive arthritis, one of the seronegative spondyloarthropathies. Reactive arthritis was originally defined as the triad of nongonococcal urethritis, conjunctivitis, and arthritis. It is now recognized that most patients present with arthritis alone and have no clinical evidence of urethritis or conjunctivitis. Reactive arthritis provides the strongest evidence of bacterial pathogenesis in the spondyloarthropathies. Enteric infections by pathogens such as *Shigella flexneri, Salmonella* (many species), *Yersinia enterocolitica, Y. pseudotuberculosis,* and *Campylobacter jejuni* have all been implicated as triggers of the disease (epidemic or postenteric form), especially in HLA-B27–positive persons. Similarly, sexually acquired infections with *Chlamydia trachomatis* and perhaps *Ureaplasma urealyticum* may cause reactive arthritis (endemic or postvenereal form). HLA-B27 is found in 63% to 75% of patients with both forms of reactive arthritis and confers a relative risk of approximately 37. Because the symptoms associated with *Chlamydia* genital infections can be subtle, a careful sexual history should be obtained; testing for *Chlamydia* should be pursued if a history of venereal exposure or genitourinary symptoms is obtained. Early treatment of genitourinary infections with appropriate antibiotics (tetracycline or erythromycin) has been shown to reduce the likelihood of subsequent reactive arthritis; however, even early

antibiotic use in patients with gastroenteritis does not appear to prevent reactive arthritis. A blinded, placebo-controlled trial of the use of tetracycline for the treatment of reactive arthritis demonstrated that the duration of disease was shortened only in patients who had *Chlamydia*-induced disease. *(Answer: C—A careful sexual history should be obtained, and testing for* Chlamydia trachomatis *[i.e., culture or molecular probe assay] should be completed)*

18. A 49-year-old white male patient of yours comes to you with hand pain of new onset. His medical history is significant only for hypertension, which is well controlled. He has experienced hand pain and swelling intermittently for the past 6 months, but this has hardly interfered with his daily activities. He indicates that the second and third distal interphalangeal joints on his right hand and the fourth distal interphalangeal joint on his left hand give him the most trouble. He reports no trauma or repetitive activities. Physical examination reveals fingers that are markedly swollen and inflamed but are remarkably nontender on palpation. Range of motion is preserved. Skin examination reveals no rash; however, the scalp has several small areas of silver scaling.

Regarding this patient, which of the following statements is true?

- ❑ **A. This patient likely has rheumatoid arthritis, given the joints that are involved**
- ❑ **B. Psoriatic arthritis is highly unlikely, given the fact that there is no history of psoriasis and the lack of extensive skin changes consistent with psoriasis**
- ❑ **C. Radiographic changes characteristic of this patient's condition include a pencil-in-cup appearance and periostitis**
- ❑ **D. Gold, penicillamine, and hydoxychloroquine are considered first-line agents in the treatment of this patient**

Key Concept/Objective: To know the classic presentation of psoriatic arthritis and to understand the radiographic changes and treatment options

An inflammatory arthropathy attributable to psoriasis appears in 5% to 7% of patients with the skin disease, especially in those whose nails are affected. In general, there is little relation between joint disease and the severity of skin involvement. In fact, psoriatic skin lesions may be found only after careful scrutiny of scalp, umbilicus, or gluteal regions, and nail pitting or other changes may be the only clues supporting a diagnosis of psoriatic arthritis. Asymmetrical oligoarthritis of both small and large joints is the most common form of psoriatic arthritis. Involvement of the distal interphalangeal joints and sausage-shaped toes or fingers are highly suggestive signs. A disparity is often noted between clinical appearance and subjective symptoms; overtly involved joints may be largely asymptomatic, unlike the concordance usually found in rheumatoid arthritis. A characteristic change is the whittling of the distal ends of phalanges, giving the joints a so-called pencil-in-cup appearance, which is radiographically distinctive for psoriatic arthritis. Periostitis, bony erosions, and joint effusions are also common and so are diagnostically useful. *(Answer: C—Radiographic changes characteristic of this patient's condition include a pencil-in-cup appearance and periostitis)*

19. A 21-year-old man who has experienced low back pain for the past 5 months comes to the clinic for evaluation. The pain wakes him at night, but by getting up and moving around he is able to go back to sleep. He has stiffness in the arm that lasts for 1 hour or so and is lessened by a hot shower. He also complains of right groin pain, which has the same character as the back discomfort. His only previous musculoskeletal problem was a prolonged bout of Achilles tendonitis 3 months ago. His father has had back problems for years. Ibuprofen, 1,200 mg/day, gives him little relief. Recent x-rays of the lumbar spine and pelvis were interpreted as being normal.

Of the following, which is the best step to take next in the management of this patient?

- ❑ **A. Determine erythrocyte sedimentation**
- ❑ **B. Evaluate for the presence of *HLA-B27* gene**
- ❑ **C. Perform bone scan of the spine and pelvis**

- ❑ **D. Perform CT scan of the sacroiliac joints**
- ❑ **E. Start a regimen of indomethacin, 50 mg t.i.d.**

Key Concept/Objective: To understand the diagnosis of ankylosing spondylitis

This patient has classic inflammatory low back pain. In addition, he appears to have involvement of the hip and enthesitis (inflammation where connective tissue inserts into bone) of the heel. Analgesic doses of ibuprofen are minimally effective because anti-inflammatory dosages of NSAIDs (i.e., dosages in the upper level of the dosing range) are usually necessary to achieve any symptomatic improvement in ankylosing spondylitis. Indomethacin at a dosage of 50 mg t.i.d. would be anti-inflammatory, but a response is not diagnostic. Determination of the erythrocyte sedimentation rate may confirm the inflammatory nature of the symptoms; the presence of *HLA-B27* is not diagnostic but might suggest the presence of a spondyloarthropathy. A bone scan is not specific, and the sacroiliac joints normally take up the radiotracer used in a bone scan. A CT scan of the sacroiliac joints can demonstrate early bony and cartilage changes not visible on regular x-rays—in this case, CT would be the best method of diagnosis. *(Answer: D—Perform CT scan of the sacroiliac joints)*

20. A 44-year-old woman complains of pain and swelling of the right ankle and foot. The symptoms have been present for 4 weeks and are generally worse in the morning. She had an episode of right knee swelling and pain 2 years ago that seemed to have responded to a course of NSAIDs. Her medical history is significant for hypertension, treated by hydrochlorothiazide, 25 mg/day, and mild scalp psoriasis, treated by tar shampoo. On physical examination, the blood pressure is 130/84 mm Hg, there are several small patches of hyperkeratosis in the scalp, the right ankle has a moderate effusion, and there is dactylitis of the second and fourth toes on the right foot.

Which of the following should be the next step in treating this patient?

- ❑ **A. Perform arthrocentesis of the right ankle and send fluid for culture**
- ❑ **B. Perform arthrocentesis of the right ankle and send fluid for crystal analysis**
- ❑ **C. Order x-rays of the foot and ankle to look for evidence of joint erosions**
- ❑ **D. Test for rheumatoid factor to evaluate for possible early rheumatoid arthritis**
- ❑ **E. Start the patient on piroxicam, 20 mg/day, and have her return in 1 month**

Key Concept/Objective: To be able to recognize psoriatic arthritis

This patient has classic psoriatic arthritis. The diagnosis is based on clinical presentation, because there are no definitive diagnostic tests. The oligoarticular nature of this patient's arthritis, along with the presence of dactylitis (sausage digits) and scalp psoriasis, makes the differential diagnosis short indeed. Piroxicam is a potent anti-inflammatory, and use of this agent is a reasonable first step in addressing the arthritis. *(Answer: E—Start the patient on piroxicam, 20 mg/day, and have her return in 1 month)*

21. A 30-year-old man who recently experienced an attack of uveitis is referred by an ophthalmologist for evaluation for possible underlying systemic disease. The patient's episode of uveitis involved the left eye and lasted 3 weeks; the uveitis responded to topical corticosteroids. The patient denies having any pulmonary symptoms, diarrhea, urethritis, peripheral joint pain or swelling, or recent low back pain. When he was in his early 20s, he was involved in a car accident and for several years after experienced low back pain. He is an avid soccer player but has had to avoid playing recently because of plantar fasciitis of the right foot. On examination, the eyes are without inflammation, the lungs are clear, there is no peripheral joint swelling and no tenderness over the sacroiliac joints, the Schober test demonstrates 3 cm of distraction, and there is tenderness in the right heel at the insertion of the plantar fascia.

Which of the following would be the most useful step to take next in the evaluation of this patient?

- ❑ A. **Posteroanterior and lateral chest x-rays**
- ❑ B. ***HLA-B27* determination**
- ❑ C. **Pelvic outlet view of the sacroiliac joints**
- ❑ D. **Lateral x-ray of the heel**
- ❑ E. **GI consult for sigmoidoscopy**

Key Concept/Objective: To be able to recognize systemic disease underlying uveitis

The differential diagnosis of unilateral uveitis includes ankylosing spondylitis, Reiter syndrome, and inflammatory bowel disease. Many cases, however, are idiopathic. Sarcoidosis typically causes bilateral uveitis. This patient has symptoms that suggest an underlying spondyloarthropathy. The most useful test would be a pelvic outlet view of the sacroiliac joints, particularly given this patient's history of low back pain. Determination of the presence of *HLA-B27* would be useful only to further the suspicion of an underlying spondyloarthropathy. The foot film might demonstrate the presence of enthesitis, but it would not be as diagnostic of spondyloarthropathy as it would be of sacroiliitis. *(Answer: C—Pelvic outlet view of the sacroiliac joints)*

22. A 48-year-old man with longstanding ankylosing spondylitis is brought to the emergency department after a minor rear-end motor vehicle accident. He is complaining of neck pain. Plain films of the neck demonstrate advanced ankylosing spondylitis with a bamboolike cervical spine. No fracture is seen, and the neurologic examination is normal.

Which of the following would be the most useful step to take next for this patient?

- ❑ A. **Reassure and follow up in 1 week**
- ❑ B. **Prescribe a mild muscle relaxant**
- ❑ C. **Place in a rigid collar and refer**
- ❑ D. **Order an MRI of the cervical spine**
- ❑ E. **Place in immediate cervical traction**

Key Concept/Objective: To be able to recognize post-trauma cervical fracture in ankylosing spondylitis

Patients with longstanding ankylosing spondylitis and bamboo-type spine are at risk for fracture through the fused disk space. Such a fracture may lead to an unstable spine and myelopathy. This condition is difficult to recognize with plain x-rays, and the best course of action would be to evaluate the cervical spine for the presence of a disk-space fracture through a more sensitive diagnostic approach, such as MRI. If a fracture is demonstrated, immediate neurosurgical or orthopedic spinal surgery consultation is required. *(Answer: D—Order an MRI of the cervical spine)*

For more information, see Arnett FC: 15 Rheumatology: III Seronegative Spondyloarthropathies. ACP Medicine Online (www.acpmedicine.com). Dale DC, Federman DD, Eds. WebMD Inc., New York, November 2002

Systemic Lupus Erythematosus

23. A 24-year-old woman presents to your clinic as a new patient. She complains of fatigue, and she has experienced a 10 lb weight loss over the past several months. On review of systems, she admits to moderate myalgias and arthralgias. She denies having any rash involving her face, but she has occasionally noted a rash on her hands. She also experiences pain and skin changes in cold weather. She reports some mild dyspnea and pain on inspiration. Blood work reveals a WBC of 2,500 with a relative lymphopenia. The serum antinuclear antibody (ANA) titer is 1:80; the anti–double-stranded DNA antibody assay is negative, as is anti-Smith (anti-Sm) antibody assay; the anti-ribonucleoprotein (anti-RNP) assay is positive with a high titer. Urinalysis is normal.

This clinical picture with the given serologies is most consistent with which of the following rheumatologic disorders?

- ❑ **A. Systemic lupus erythematosus (SLE)**
- ❑ **B. Dermatomyositis**
- ❑ **C. Mixed connective tissue disease (MCTD)**
- ❑ **D. Undifferentiated connective tissue disease (UCTD)**

Key Concept/Objective: To understand that lupuslike symptoms may present as part of an overlap syndrome

Some patients have symptoms suggestive of lupus (most commonly, arthritis, pleuritic chest pain, and cytopenia) but lack the specific diagnostic criteria for lupus (e.g., butterfly rash, glomerulonephritis, high-titer anti-dsDNA, or anti-Sm antibody). Other patients have lupuslike symptoms together with findings suggestive of rheumatoid arthritis, dermatomyositis, or scleroderma. Those with no definable serology and a nondescript clinical picture are defined as having UCTD. Other patients have inflammatory myositis, Raynaud phenomenon, and sclerodactyly together with very high titer antibodies to the ribonucleoprotein antigen (U1 RNP) and no anti-DNA or anti-Sm antibody. This set of findings is defined as MCTD. The differentiation of SLE from UCTD, MCTD, and Sjögren syndrome depends on the extent and pattern of different organ involvement (glomerulonephritis is rare in all these disorders except lupus) and on the accompanying serologic abnormalities. This patient presents with several complaints consistent with a connective tissue disease, including serositis, arthralgias, myalgias, and a nonspecific skin rash affecting predominantly the hands. The combination of a low-titer ANA and negative anti-dsDNA and anti-Sm makes the diagnosis of SLE questionable. More importantly, the presence of high-titer anti-RNP is consistent with the diagnosis of MCTD. *(Answer: C—Mixed connective tissue disease [MCTD])*

24. A 31-year-old woman comes to your clinic for follow-up. For the past several years, her lupus has been well controlled without systemic medications. She is employed full-time, and she and her husband have been contemplating pregnancy. Last month, however, she presented to your office complaining of fever, severe arthralgias, myalgias, and a diffuse erythematous rash. The pregnancy test was negative. Results of urinalysis and renal function testing were normal. After a failed trial of NSAIDs, you started her on prednisone, 60 mg/day. At follow-up, she reports that all of her symptoms have improved significantly.

Of the following, what is the most appropriate step to take next in the treatment of this patient?

- ❑ **A. Discontinue her steroids and try another trial of NSAIDs**
- ❑ **B. Taper her steroids and add high-dose oral calcium and vitamin D**
- ❑ **C. Taper her steroids and add high-dose calcium, vitamin D, and a bisphosphonate**
- ❑ **D. Discontinue her steroids and switch to oral cyclophosphamide**

Key Concept/Objective: To understand the importance of bone-protective therapies and the contraindications to those therapies for patients on long-term steroid regimens

This patient has experienced a flare of her SLE. She had a good response to high-dose corticosteroids and is likely to require steroid therapy for the next several months. High-dose corticosteroid therapy is used for patients with severe systemic symptoms, renal disease, or other visceral disease that is potentially life-threatening. Treatment should be initiated in split doses during the day, maintained for 4 to 6 weeks, and then tapered; too-early reduction in the dosage usually results in recurrence of disease activity. Osteoporosis follows long-term corticosteroid therapy with sufficient frequency that all patients receiving such therapy should receive prophylaxis for this complication. High-dose oral calcium, vitamin D, and a bisphosphonate are the primary preventive measures; estrogen replacement may be considered in postmenopausal women who do not have antiphospholipid antibody. Because this woman desires to become pregnant, she should not be given an oral bisphosphonate. The decision to start an agent such as cyclophosphamide should be considered

when the patient is not responding to steroids or has severe renal disease. Furthermore, cyclophosphamide can cause infertility and be teratogenic if used inadvertently during pregnancy. *(Answer: B—Taper her steroids and add high-dose oral calcium and vitamin D)*

For more information, see Lockshin MD: 15 Rheumatology: IV Systemic Lupus Erythematosus. ACP Medicine Online (www.acpmedicine.com). Dale DC, Federman DD, Eds. WebMD Inc., New York, December 2002

Scleroderma and Related Diseases

25. A 32-year-old white man with known scleroderma presents for evaluation. On physical examination, you see that his blood pressure is elevated (165/105 mm Hg). The other findings of the physical examination are unchanged from before. The patient's creatinine level is 1.5 mg/dl (baseline, 0.8 mg/dl); urinalysis shows trace protein and 5 to 10 red cells. You are concerned about the possibility of scleroderma renal crisis.

Which of the following statements regarding this patient is false?

- ❑ **A. The patient should be treated with a thiazide diuretic**
- ❑ **B. The patient's symptoms are associated with microangiopathic hemolytic anemia**
- ❑ **C. It is likely that this patient has received high-dose steroids in the past**
- ❑ **D. This patient is at risk for oliguric renal failure**
- ❑ **E. Unless this patient receives aggressive treatment, his prognosis is poor**

Key Concept/Objective: To be able to recognize scleroderma renal crisis and understand its management

Scleroderma renal crisis is a dreaded complication of diffuse scleroderma. It can occur rapidly and is more likely to be seen in patients with rapidly progressive skin disease. Hypertension of new onset, in conjunction with proteinuria and microscopic hematuria, is highly characteristic. In more severe cases, patients present with malignant hypertension and microangiopathic hemolytic anemia. Scleroderma renal crisis was the most common cause of death among patients with diffuse scleroderma until the advent of angiotensin-converting enzyme (ACE) inhibitors. Use of short-acting agents such as captopril is indicated. Because the response to therapy seems to be better when the creatinine level is less than 3 mg/dl, the diagnosis needs to be made promptly, and therapy should be instituted quickly. Recovery of normal renal function has been documented in patients requiring dialysis who received ACE inhibitors. *(Answer: C—It is likely that this patient has received high-dose steroids in the past)*

26. A 35-year-old woman known to have long-standing scleroderma comes to you complaining of worsening constipation. She has been experiencing constipation for the past several months; recently, her constipation has become associated with abdominal pain and very hard stools. On occasion she has vomited.

Which of the following is NOT a gastroenterologic complication of scleroderma?

- ❑ **A. Pneumatosis intestinalis**
- ❑ **B. Esophageal dysmotility, gastroparesis, and intestinal pseudo-obstruction**
- ❑ **C. Colonic diverticulosis**
- ❑ **D. Sjögren syndrome**
- ❑ **E. Achalasia**

Key Concept/Objective: To be aware of the different manifestations of scleroderma in the GI tract

Although not completely understood, scleroderma-associated lesions of the GI tract appear to be the result of autonomic nerve dysfunction of the GI tract. In time, this autonomic nerve dysfunction leads to smooth muscle atrophy and eventually irreversible muscle

fibrosis of the gut. As a consequence, hypomotility of the esophagus, stomach, and small and large intestine are seen in patients with systemic sclerosis. Esophageal dysmotility is associated with reflux and, eventually, strictures and even changes associated with Barrett esophagus. Involvement of the stomach and small intestine is associated with gastroparesis and pseudo-obstruction, respectively. The presence of wide-mouth diverticula is pathognomonic of scleroderma. The lower two thirds of the esophagus show an absence of peristaltic waves and incompetence of the lower esophageal sphincter. Achalasia is characterized by an increase, not a decrease, in activity of the lower esophageal sphincter. *(Answer: E—Achalasia)*

For more information, see Moxley G: 15 Rheumatology: V Scleroderma and Related Diseases. ACP Medicine Online (www.acpmedicine.com). Dale DC, Federman DD, Eds. WebMD Inc., New York, March 2004

Idiopathic Inflammatory Myopathies

27. A 34-year-old woman presents to your clinic complaining of weakness of 1 month's duration and shortness of breath of 2 weeks' duration. She says her weakness is worse when she tries to comb her hair or when she tries to stand up from a sitting position. She does not have any significant medical history, and she is not taking any medications or over-the-counter drugs. Her family history is unremarkable. On physical examination, the patient has a hyperkeratotic rash on her hands. The strength of her legs and arms is 5/5 distally and 3/5 proximally. A chest x-ray shows the presence of interstitial infiltrates. You suspect her symptoms are caused by an inflammatory myopathy. You order muscle enzyme levels and a muscle biopsy; the findings are consistent with your presumed diagnosis. You also order testing of autoantibody levels to better categorize her disease.

This patient is likely to test positive for which of the following antibodies?

- ❑ **A. Antimitochondrial antibodies**
- ❑ **B. Antibodies against aminoacyl-transfer RNA (tRNA) synthetases**
- ❑ **C. Antibodies against signal recognition particle (SRP)**
- ❑ **D. Antibodies against Mi-2**

Key Concept/Objective: To know the antibodies that correlate with different clinical pictures in idiopathic inflammatory myopathies

Autoantibodies to nuclear and cytoplasmic antigens are found in as many as 90% of patients with an inflammatory myopathy. These antibodies are often useful in differentiating inflammatory myopathies from diseases that are not autoimmune disorders. Some of these antibodies are nonspecific and can be seen in several autoimmune disorders. About 25% of patients with inflammatory myositis test positive for antinuclear antibodies. Autoantibodies that are in large part directed against cytoplasmic ribonucleoproteins have been designated as myositis-specific autoantibodies (MSA) and are present in 30% of the patients. These antibodies tend to correlate with some specific clinical presentations, responses to therapy, and prognoses. Three groups of patients can be defined by the MSA specificities. The first group is defined by the presence of antibodies directed against aminoacyl-tRNA synthetases. These patients are generally characterized by an acute onset of muscle disease, with a high incidence of associated interstitial lung disease. They may also have arthritis and a hyperkeratotic rash on the hands, known as mechanic's hands. This description fits the patient presented in this case. The second group includes patients with anti-SRP antibodies; these patients tend to have an abrupt onset of weakness, and they may have cardiac disease. The third group is identified by the presence of antibodies against Mi-2; these patients have a dermatomyositis with the so-called shawl sign. *(Answer: B—Antibodies against aminoacyl-transfer RNA [tRNA] synthetases)*

28. A 58-year-old man is seen in your clinic for the first time. He says he has not seen a doctor in 5 years. He has no significant medical history. He says he has decided to see a doctor because over the past 2 years he has noticed some weakness of his arms and legs. He says these symptoms were not bothering him initially but that, over the past few months, he has noticed more weakness in his left arm. He is not taking any medications. On physical examination, there is no rash; his strength is 5/5 on the right side of his body, 5/5 in his left leg, and 3/5 in his left arm. His distal strength and proximal strength are quite similar. Neurologic examination results are otherwise normal. His creatine kinase (CK) level is moderately elevated.

Which of the following is the most likely diagnosis for this patient?

- ❑ **A. Dermatomyositis**
- ❑ **B. Polymyositis**
- ❑ **C. Sarcoidosis**
- ❑ **D. Inclusion body myositis (IBM)**

Key Concept/Objective: To understand the presentation of inclusion body myositis

This patient is a middle-aged man with slow-onset muscle weakness. Dermatomyositis is defined by the presence of an inflammatory myopathy and a characteristic rash. Polymyositis is characterized by weakness that is symmetrical and predominantly proximal, and the clinical course is more aggressive than the one described here. Sarcoidosis can cause a myopathy but usually is accompanied by other manifestations that are absent here. This patient's symptoms are more consistent with IBM. The pattern of severity of muscle weakness in IBM differs from that seen in other idiopathic inflammatory myopathies. In addition to the presence of proximal weakness, distal muscles may be involved, and in some cases, muscle abnormalities are asymmetrical. Unlike most of the other inflammatory muscle disorders, IBM affects more men than women. Response to treatment is generally poor. Electron microscopy may be required to demonstrate the inclusion bodies that define IBM. *(Answer: D—Inclusion body myositis [IBM])*

29. A 40-year-old woman with polymyositis comes to your office for an initial visit. She was diagnosed 3 months ago and was placed on prednisone, 1 mg/kg/day. She says her strength has recovered significantly since she started therapy. She comes to visit you because she recently moved to your town. She has no other significant medical history; she has no allergies, and she is taking no medications other than prednisone. She has a family history of diabetes. Her physical examination shows minimal proximal weakness.

Which of the following would be the best therapeutic intervention at this time?

- ❑ **A. Continue steroids at the same dose for 3 more months and then proceed with a slow taper**
- ❑ **B. Start tapering the steroids and start methotrexate or azathioprine**
- ❑ **C. Discontinue the steroids and start cyclophosphamide**
- ❑ **D. Order a muscle biopsy to see if the patient is in remission**

Key Concept/Objective: To understand the treatment of idiopathic inflammatory myopathies

Corticosteroids are the mainstay of initial therapy for the inflammatory myopathies. Most patients with documented muscle inflammation should be started on these drugs at relatively high doses (1 mg/kg/day). A standard approach has been to maintain this dosage for up to 3 months or until clinical improvement occurs. After this initial period of high-dose therapy, the dose can be consolidated into a single morning dose and then tapered so that the total daily dose is reduced by 20% to 25% each month; a maintenance dose of 5 to 10 mg daily should be reached in about 6 to 8 months. The addition of second-line drugs to the prednisone regimen is now recommended within the first 3 months of initiating treatment. The most commonly used second-line agents for the treatment of inflammatory myopathy are methotrexate and azathioprine. Azathioprine and methotrexate have similar efficacy in these disorders, and the choice of which to use may depend on tolerability or other comorbid conditions. Cyclophosphamide may be useful in the treatment of the antisynthetase syndrome with interstitial lung disease and in children with vasculitis-related complications of dermatomyositis. There is no indication in this case for the use of cyclophosphamide. After the diagnosis is made and the therapy is started, the response to therapy in patients with idiopathic inflammatory myopathies is followed clinically and

with assessment of muscle enzyme levels; a muscle biopsy is usually not necessary in this setting. *(Answer: B—Start tapering the steroids and start methotrexate or azathioprine)*

30. A 35-year-old woman comes to your office complaining of weakness and fatigue that has lasted for about 2 months. She has found it difficult to get up from a chair, and brushing her hair has become more problematic. In addition, she has developed blanching of the hands with exposure to cold, as well as stiffness of the hands, wrists, and feet lasting for 1 to 2 hours in the morning. She can no longer wear her wedding ring because of finger swelling. She also notes that she gets out of breath easily after climbing just one flight of stairs. On examination, she has evidence of proximal muscle weakness; synovitis of the MCPs, PIPs, wrists, and MTPs; and rales at the lung bases. There is no evidence of rash or lower extremity edema, and cardiac examination is normal. You suspect a connective tissue disease, and indeed, the screening ANA is positive at a titer of 1:640.

What additional antinuclear test will be most useful diagnostically for this patient?

❑ **A. Anti–Scl-70**

❑ **B. Anti-dsDNA**

❑ **C. Anti-SSA**

❑ **D. Anti–Jo-1**

❑ **E. Anti-Sm**

Key Concept/Objective: To know the extramuscular manifestations of polymyositis associated with Jo-1 antibodies

Patients with polymyositis frequently have extramuscular manifestations. One of the most common is pulmonary fibrosis. Almost 70% of patients with pulmonary fibrosis will have the autoantibody Jo-1 in their serum. Anti–Jo-1 is one of the antisynthetase antibodies currently found only in patients with myositis. Besides pulmonary fibrosis, the antisynthetase syndrome includes Raynaud phenomenon, polyarthritis, and, in some cases, so-called mechanic' s hands. The last condition causes cracked and fissured skin on the hands. Anti-dsDNA and anti-Sm are autoantibodies found only in systemic lupus erythematosus, anti-Scl-70 is seen in patients with scleroderma, and anti-SSA is found in patients with either systemic lupus erythematosus or Sjögren syndrome. *(Answer: D—Anti–Jo-1)*

31. A 50-year-old woman with a 6-month history of polymyositis complains of increasing weakness. After diagnosis, she was started on 60 mg of prednisone a day, which has been tapered to 30 mg/day. The initial CK was 3,000 mg/dl, but 3 weeks ago it was only slightly elevated to 400 mg/dl (normal, greater than or equal to 275 mg/dl). Examination demonstrates cushingoid facies, 4/5 proximal muscle strength, and no abnormal heart or lung findings. Current CK is 375 mg/dl.

Of the following, which is the best step to take next in the treatment of this patient?

❑ **A. Increase prednisone to 60 mg/day and reevaluate in 2 weeks**

❑ **B. Refer to surgery for biopsy of one of the quadriceps muscles**

❑ **C. Decrease prednisone to 20 mg/day and reevaluate in 2 weeks**

❑ **D. Add methotrexate, 7.5 mg/wk**

❑ **E. Refer to physical therapy to initiate strengthening exercises**

Key Concept/Objective: To be able to recognize steroid myopathy

This patient with polymyositis has evidence of steroid myopathy. There is an increasing sense of proximal weakness without any increase in the CK. The best way to determine whether steroid myopathy is contributing to the weakness is to try a steroid taper and see if the weakness improves. If so, a second-line agent such as methotrexate would be useful, although even methotrexate may take several weeks to months to be effective. Biopsy of the muscle may show type 2 fiber atrophy typical of steroid myopathy, but in the setting of polymyositis, the diagnosis may be difficult to interpret. *(Answer: C—Decrease prednisone to 20 mg/day and reevaluate in 2 weeks)*

32. A 34-year-old woman complains of weakness, fatigue, hair loss, and numbness of the fingers. Her symptoms began 4 months ago, soon after the delivery of her second child. While visiting her mother, she saw her mother' s physician for the above complaints and was found to have a CK of 600 mg/dl. She was told to see her local physician on returning home for evaluation of possible polymyositis. On examination, blood pressure is 90/60 mm Hg; pulse is 60 beats/min; hair appears thin; lungs and heart are normal; muscle strength is 5/5 in both the proximal and distal groups; and Phalen testing is positive at both wrists.

Of the following, which is the best test to perform next in the evaluation of this patient?

- ❑ **A. Electromyogram (EMG) study**
- ❑ **B. Sensitive TSH**
- ❑ **C. Aldolase**
- ❑ **D. ANA panel**
- ❑ **E. Repeat CK**

Key Concept/Objective: To know that the differential diagnosis of polymyositis includes hypothyroidism

Hypothyroidism can cause all of the symptoms experienced by this patient as well as an elevated CK. CK levels generally do not reach those seen in inflammatory myositis. Rheumatologic manifestations of hypothyroidism include arthralgias and even joint swelling, myalgias and muscle cramps, carpal tunnel syndrome (which this patient has), and nonspecific paresthesias. *(Answer: B—Sensitive TSH)*

33. A 54-year-old woman with a recent diagnosis of dermatomyositis is referred to you for further evaluation. She has read that dermatomyositis can be associated with malignancy. She has recently had a thorough physical examination, chest x-ray, stool screening for occult blood, mammogram, and pelvic examination, all of which were deemed unremarkable.

What would you recommend to this patient?

- ❑ **A. Reassure her with regards to malignancy**
- ❑ **B. Set up a routine-visit schedule for screening**
- ❑ **C. Suggest that a CEA be checked today**
- ❑ **D. Suggest that a CA-125 and transvaginal ultrasound be performed**
- ❑ **E. Suggest that a colonoscopy be done soon**

Key Concept/Objective: To understand the relationship between dermatomyositis and malignancy

It is generally accepted that patients with dermatomyositis are at increased risk of malignancy, the relative risk of which is approximately four to five times that of control groups. Cancers of the ovary, lung, lymphatic system, and hematopoietic system are overrepresented in patients with dermatomyositis. In women older than 40 years with dermatomyositis, the risk of ovarian cancer is 20 times that of the general population. Ovarian tumors are notoriously hard to find early. The most recent recommendations for detecting them in patients with dermatomyositis include a careful gynecologic examination, measurement of CA-125, and transvaginal ultrasound at 3- to 6-month intervals. *(Answer: D—Suggest that a CA-125 and transvaginal ultrasound be performed)*

34. A 45-year-old man is referred to you for a workup of muscle weakness. He presented 2 months ago with proximal weakness and an elevated CK of 4,000 mg/dl. A recent biopsy showed no abnormalities. On examination, the patient has 4/5 strength in the proximal muscles and 5/5 strength distally; otherwise, the examination is normal.

Of the following, which is the best step to take next in the management of this patient?

- ❑ **A. Order an MRI of the quadriceps muscles**
- ❑ **B. Order an EMG study of the proximal muscles**
- ❑ **C. Refer the patient to a muscular dystrophy clinic**

❑ D. **Repeat CK after patient has a period of rest**

❑ E. **Perform the ischemic forearm test**

Key Concept/Objective: To understand the use of MRI in improving the diagnostic accuracy of biopsy

Involvement of muscles in polymyositis is often patchy. In recent years, the use of MRI of the proximal muscles has demonstrated the patchy nature of the disease and aided in the localization of biopsy. This is the most likely reason for this patient's normal biopsy. An MRI scan will probably demonstrate the extent and location of muscle disease, and rebiopsy of involved sites will most likely demonstrate myositis. *(Answer: A—Order an MRI of quadriceps muscles)*

For more information, see Olsen NJ, Brogan BL: 15 Rheumatology: VI Idiopathic Inflammatory Myopathies. ACP Medicine Online (www.acpmedicine.com). Dale DC, Federman DD, Eds. WebMD Inc., New York, January 2003

Systemic Vasculitis Syndromes

35. A 47-year-old woman presents to your clinic complaining of crampy abdominal pain and diarrhea; she also has been experiencing progressive dyspnea on exertion and constant chest pain that is worse when she leans forward. She has had these symptoms for the past several days. She also reports arthralgias and has now developed a rash. On physical examination, the patient is mildly tachypneic, but her vital signs are otherwise stable. Pulmonary examination reveals dullness to percussion and decreased breath sounds over the right lower lung field, with no egophony. Cardiac and abdominal examinations are unremarkable. Lower extremities are notable for purpura and trace edema below the knees. Chest x-ray reveals a right pleural effusion. Evaluation of her diarrhea reveals an eosinophilic gastroenteritis. You suspect that her underlying problem is Churg-Strauss syndrome (CSS).

Which of the following components of this patient's medical history would be most supportive of the diagnosis of CSS?

❑ A. **A preceding streptococcal or viral infection**

❑ B. **Chronic sinusitis**

❑ C. **Bronchial asthma**

❑ D. **Polymyalgia rheumatica**

Key Concept/Objective: To understand the importance of history in the diagnosis of Churg-Strauss syndrome

CSS displays clinical similarities to Wegener granulomatosis (WG) in terms of organ involvement and pathology, especially in patients with upper or lower airway disease or glomerulonephritis. CSS can follow a rapidly progressive course. CSS differs most strikingly from WG in that the former occurs in patients with a history of atopy, asthma, or allergic rhinitis, which is often ongoing. In the prevasculitic atopy phase, as well as during the systemic phase of the illness, eosinophilia is characteristic and often of striking degree (≥ 1,000 eosinophils/mm^3). When eosinophilia is present in WG, it is usually more modest (~500 eosinophils/mm^3). Chronic sinusitis can be seen in both CSS and WG, although it is more characteristic in the latter than the former. Polymyalgia rheumatica is not associated with either CSS or WG; there is, however, a clear association between polymyalgia rheumatica and temporal arteritis. A preceding streptococcal or viral infection has been seen occasionally with both WG and CSS. *(Answer: C—Bronchial asthma)*

36. A 54-year-old man is brought to the emergency department by his family. They report that several days ago, the patient began complaining of arthralgias, myalgias, and subjective fevers. He thought that he had the flu and remained home from work. Yesterday he developed swelling and a rash on his legs. According to his family, yesterday evening the patient started acting funny, and today he has been somewhat confused. On physical examination, the patient's temperature is 99.5° F (37.5° C); his heart rate is 93 beats/min, and his blood pressure is 154/85 mm Hg. He is able to answer questions but is easily distracted during the examination. Pulmonary, cardiovascular, and abdominal examinations are normal. On musculoskeletal examination, petechiae and purpura are noted on the upper and lower extremities, with 1+ pitting edema in the lower extremities. Laboratory values reveal a white blood cell count of 24,000, a platelet count of 550,000, and a hematocrit of 35%. Blood urea nitrogen and creatinine levels are 120 mg/dl and 4.5 mg/dl, respectively. You admit the patient to the hospital for further workup. Renal biopsy reveals pauci-immune glomerulonephritis. A serum test for perinuclear antineutrophil cytoplasmic antibodies (p-ANCAs) with antimyeloperoxidase specificity is positive.

Which of the following vasculitides is most likely responsible for this man's illness?

- ❑ **A. Polyarteritis nodosa (PAN)**
- ❑ **B. Allergic granulomatous angiitis**
- ❑ **C. Microscopic polyangiitis (MPA)**
- ❑ **D. Wegener granulomatosis (WG)**

Key Concept/Objective: To know the clinical presentation and laboratory findings for MPA

Glomerulonephritis, particularly rapidly progressive glomerulonephritis, and alveolar hemorrhage are common in MPA and absent, by definition, in classic PAN. Constitutional symptoms such as fever, asthenia, and myalgias are common in both PAN and MPA. Elevated acute-phase reactants, thrombocytosis, leukocytosis, and the anemia of inflammatory disease are common, although they are not uniformly present. The diagnosis of MPA and PAN should ideally be based on histopathologic demonstration of arteritis and the clinical pattern of disease. A biopsy specimen of clinically involved, nonnecrotic tissue that demonstrates the presence of arteritis of muscular arteries is the ideal supportive finding for the diagnosis of arteritis of a medium-sized vessel, but such a finding is not always possible. The presence of serum p-ANCA with antimyeloperoxidase specificity (found in 60% of MPA patients) supports the clinical diagnosis of MPA, but p-ANCA is not specific for this disease. ANCAs are not characteristic of PAN. The renal biopsy tissue in MPA, as in WG and CSS, does not contain extensive immune complexes on immunofluorescent staining and electron microscopy (so-called pauci-immune glomerulonephritis). *(Answer: C—Microscopic polyangiitis [MPA])*

37. A 14-year-old girl is brought in to the emergency department by her parents. They report high spiking fevers that began several days ago. They also report that the patient has complained of headaches and aching joints and that today she developed a rash. On physical examination, the patient's temperature is 103.2° F (39.5° C), her heart rate is 110 beats/min, and her blood pressure is 125/70 mm Hg. You note nonexudative conjunctivitis and an erythematous, dry oropharynx. Pulmonary and cardiac examinations are unremarkable except for tachycardia. Her distal limbs are notable for mild swelling. Skin examination reveals a diffuse, polymorphous rash with some plaques. You seriously suspect Kawasaki disease (KD) and begin administration of I.V. immunoglobulin and aspirin.

The morbidity and mortality of KD is associated with which of the following complications?

- ❑ **A. Overwhelming sepsis caused by encapsulated organisms**
- ❑ **B. Central hypertension and stroke**
- ❑ **C. Glomerulonephritis and renal failure**
- ❑ **D. Coronary artery aneurysms and thrombosis**

Key Concept/Objective: To know the life-threatening complications of KD

The morbidity and mortality (< 3%) of KD is overwhelmingly associated with the development of inflammatory coronary artery aneurysms, most of which are asymptomatic at the time of formation. Aneurysms may be detected by echocardiography. Thrombosis can occur in the aneurysms, resulting in direct or embolic coronary artery occlusion. Coronary events may occur weeks or even many years after the febrile illness. A baseline echocardiogram should be obtained at the time of the acute illness and should be repeated 2 and 6 weeks later. Early recognition of the disease and treatment with intravenous immunoglobulin and aspirin have significantly decreased the frequency of aneurysm formation and thrombotic coronary events. Renal compromise is distinctly unusual in KD. *(Answer: D—Coronary artery aneurysms and thrombosis)*

38. An 18-year-old woman comes to your clinic complaining of a rash on her legs. She reports having crampy abdominal pain and aching joints for several days. She also reports that the rash began yesterday evening and was worse this morning, and she complains that her skin is itchy. Her medical history is significant only for an upper respiratory infection 2 or 3 weeks ago that resolved spontaneously. She is otherwise healthy. Physical examination is notable only for trace edema and purpura, noted on both lower extremities. You suspect small vessel vasculitis. You perform a skin biopsy, which stains positively for IgA-containing immune complexes.

This biopsy finding is most consistent with which of the following diseases?

❑ **A. Henoch-Schönlein purpura**

❑ **B. Urticarial vasculitis**

❑ **C. CSS**

❑ **D. WG**

Key Concept/Objective: To know the clinical presentation and pathologic findings of Henoch-Schönlein purpura

Cutaneous involvement can occur in many of the primary or secondary vasculitic syndromes. Large, medium-sized, or small vessel occlusion can cause livedo, Raynaud phenomenon, or necrosis. Purpura is the most common manifestation of small vessel vasculitis. Small vessel vasculitis, particularly when associated with infections, is frequently associated with immune complex deposition. Vasculitis primarily involving the postcapillary venules has been termed hypersensitivity vasculitis in older literature. Primary small vessel vasculitis may be limited to the skin or may be associated with visceral involvement, including alveolar hemorrhage; intestinal ischemia or hemorrhage; and glomerulonephritis. Purpura tends to occur in recurrent crops of lesions of similar age and is more pronounced in gravity-dependent areas. Biopsy is useful in excluding causes of nonvasculitic purpura such as amyloidosis, leukemia cutis, Kaposi sarcoma, T cell lymphomas, and cholesterol or myxomatous emboli. Tissue immunofluorescent staining is useful to support the diagnosis of Henoch-Schönlein purpura (specifically, IgA staining), systemic lupus erythematosus, or infection (the percentage of cases with positive results on immunofluorescent staining is not known). Patients with WG and CSS can present with purpura; however, they do not exhibit IgA deposits in the immunoflourescence stains. Urticarial vasculitis is a disease that affects the skin exclusively; very rarely, patients present with interstitial lung disease but not articular or abdominal complaints, as seen in this patient. *(Answer: A—Henoch-Schönlein purpura)*

For more information, see Mandell BF: 15 Rheumatology: VIII Systemic Vasculitis Syndromes. ACP Medicine Online (www.acpmedicine.com). Dale DC, Federman DD, Eds. WebMD Inc., New York, August 2003

Crystal-Induced Joint Disease

39. A 67-year-old man comes to your clinic to establish care. He has a history of hypertension, gout, obesity, and hyperlipidemia. He denies alcohol abuse. He tells you that he has not had a "gout flare" in several years and takes no medicines for this condition. His medications include a dihydropyridine calcium channel blocker and a statin. He does not take aspirin. You order routine laboratory studies, including assessment of the uric acid level. All laboratory results are normal.

For this patient, which of the following statements regarding gout is false?

❑ **A. Hyperuricemia must be present to make a diagnosis of gout**

❑ **B. This patient likely has secondary gout**

❑ **C. Gout is primarily a disease of middle-aged men**

❑ **D. Obesity, alcohol intake, high blood pressure, and an elevated serum creatinine level correlate with elevation of the serum uric acid level and the development of gout**

❑ E. **In 80% to 90% of patients with primary gout, hyperuricemia is caused by underexcretion of uric acid in the presence of normal renal function**

Key Concept/Objective: To understand that although hyperuricemia is associated with gout, it does not always lead to the development of gout

The development of gout tends to be associated with chronically increased levels of serum uric acid. However, a substantial minority of patients with acute gout will have normal uric acid levels, and hyperuricemia does not always lead to the development of gout. Gout is often classified as primary or secondary. Gout associated with an inborn problem in metabolism or decreased renal excretion without other renal disease is referred to as primary gout, whereas gout associated with an acquired disease or use of a drug is called secondary gout. In both primary and secondary gout, chronic hyperuricemia may be the result of overproduction of uric acid caused by increased purine intake, synthesis, or breakdown, or it may be the result of decreased renal excretion of urate. Gout is predominantly a disease of middle-aged men, but there is a gradually increasing prevalence in both men and women in older age groups. In most studies, the annual incidence of gout in men is one to three per 1,000; the incidence is much lower in women. Additional factors that correlate strongly with serum urate levels and the prevalence of gout in the general population include serum creatinine levels, body weight, height, blood pressure, and alcohol intake. Hyperuricemia can result from decreased renal excretion or increased production of uric acid. In 80% to 90% of patients with primary gout, hyperuricemia is caused by renal underexcretion of uric acid, even though renal function is otherwise normal. *(Answer: A—Hyperuricemia must be present to make a diagnosis of gout)*

40. A 74-year-old man presents to your clinic with a 2-day history of pain in his right great toe. You suspect gout and recommend treatment. You order laboratory studies, and the patient's serum uric acid level is found to be elevated. Before leaving your office, the patient asks you what he should expect in the future concerning this disease.

In counseling this patient about the clinical presentation and course of this condition, which of the following statements is false?

❑ A. **Initial attack of gout is monoarticular in 85% to 90% of cases, and half of these cases will involve the first metatarsophalangeal joint**

❑ B. **The presence of fever and the involvement of multiple joints effectively rules out the diagnosis of gout**

❑ C. **If the patient's hypouricemia is not treated, there is at least a 75% chance of further attacks within 2 years and a 90% chance within 10 years**

❑ D. **Without treatment for hyperuricemia, the patient will likely develop tophi within 12 years**

❑ E. **Chronic gout eventually progresses to articular destruction, including bony erosions that may have the radiographic appearance of punched-out lesions of periarticular bone, often with an overhanging edge that can be distinguished from rheumatoid arthritis**

Key Concept/Objective: To understand that gout may involve multiple joints and be associated with fever

Acute gouty arthritis is usually characterized by a sudden and dramatic onset of pain and swelling, usually in a single joint. This condition occurs most often in lower extremity joints and evolves within hours to marked swelling, warmth, and tenderness. The initial attack of gout is monoarticular in 85% to 90% of patients. At least half of initial attacks occur in the first metatarsophalangeal joints (a condition known as podagra), but other joints of the foot may be involved simultaneously or in subsequent attacks. Other lower extremity joints, including the ankles and knees, are often affected; in more advanced gout, attacks may occur in upper extremity joints, such as the elbow, wrist, and small joints of the fingers. Polyarticular gout occurs as the initial manifestation in about 10% to

15% of patients and may be associated with fever. After the initial attack of gout subsides, the clinical course may follow one of several patterns. A minority of patients never have another attack of gout, and some may not have another attack for several years. Most patients, however, have recurrent attacks over the ensuing years. In a study conducted before the use of hypouricemic agents, 78% of patients had a second attack within 2 years and 93% had a second attack within 10 years. Persistent hyperuricemia with increasingly frequent attacks of gout eventually leads to joint involvement of wider distribution, as well as chronic joint destruction as a result of deposition of massive amounts of urate in and around joints. Without therapy to lower serum uric acid levels, the average interval from the first gouty attack to the development of chronic arthritis or tophi is about 12 years. Erosive bony lesions may be seen on x-rays as well-defined, punched-out lesions in periarticular bone, often associated with overhanging edges of bone. These erosions are usually 5 mm or more in diameter and are larger than those seen in rheumatoid arthritis. Bone mineralization appears to be generally normal in chronic tophaceous gout, and periarticular osteopenia, which is seen in rheumatoid arthritis, is usually not present. The distribution of destructive joint disease in gout is often asymmetrical and patchy. *(Answer: B—The presence of fever and the involvement of multiple joints effectively rules out the diagnosis of gout)*

41. A 77-year-old male patient of yours presents to your clinic for evaluation of right knee pain. He has had recurrent gout in this knee, and his current symptoms are consistent with previous presentations. This patient has many medical problems, which include congestive heart failure, chronic kidney disease, and hypertension. Three months ago, the patient was admitted to the hospital for upper gastrointestinal bleeding; he was found to have peptic ulcer disease. His medications include a daily dose of colchicine, but he admits that he has not taken his medications today because of the pain and mild nausea. The patient is noticeably uncomfortable. His examination is notable only for marked swelling and erythema of the right knee and the presence of an effusion.

Which of the following treatment strategies should be prescribed for this patient's gouty attack?

- ❑ A. **Nonsteroidal anti-inflammatory drugs (NSAIDs), such as indomethacin**
- ❑ B. **Colchicine, 0.6 mg to 1.2 mg initially and then 0.6 mg every 2 hours until the flare resolves**
- ❑ C. **Allopurinol**
- ❑ D. **Cyclooxygenase-2 inhibitors**
- ❑ E. **Arthrocentesis followed by administration of an intra-articular steroid to provide immediate relief**

Key Concept/Objective: To understand the management of acute gouty attacks in patients with multiple comorbidities

Treatment of acute gout should be initiated as early in the attack as possible. Agents available for terminating the acute attack include colchicine, NSAIDs, adrenocorticotropic hormone (ACTH), and corticosteroids. Each agent has a toxicity profile, with advantages and disadvantages applicable to individual circumstances. This patient's overall health and coexistent medical problems, particularly renal and gastrointestinal disease, dictate the choice among these approaches. Corticosteroids and ACTH have been used more often in recent years in patients with multiple comorbid conditions, because of the relatively low toxicity profile of these agents. Colchicine has been used for centuries to treat acute attacks of gout. Given in oral dosages of 0.6 to 1.2 mg initially, followed by 0.6 mg every 2 hours, colchicine begins relieving most attacks of gout within 12 to 24 hours. However, most patients experience nausea, vomiting, abdominal cramps, and diarrhea with these dosages. Colchicine should be given more cautiously in elderly patients and should be avoided in patients with renal or hepatic insufficiency and in patients who are already receiving long-term colchicine therapy. NSAIDs are useful in most patients with acute gout and remain the agents of choice for young, healthy patients without comorbid diseases. The use of all NSAIDs is limited by the risks of gastric ulceration and gastritis, acute renal failure, fluid retention, interference with antihypertensive therapy, and, in older patients, problems with mentation. Cyclooxygenase-2–specific NSAIDs should be useful in treating acute gout and possibly for long-term prophylaxis in patients at risk for gastrointestinal toxicity from the currently available NSAIDs but are not without risk in patients with renal

insufficiency and congestive heart failure. The use of intra-articular steroids after arthrocentesis is extremely useful in providing relief, particularly in large effusions, in which the initial aspiration of fluid results in rapid relief of pain and tightness in the affected joint. The dosage of the steroid triamcinolone depends on the size of the joint; dosages range from 5 to 10 mg for small joints of the hands or feet to 40 to 60 mg for larger joints, such as the knee. Systemic corticosteroids may also be useful in patients for whom colchicine or NSAIDs are inadvisable and for patients with polyarticular attacks. *(Answer: E—Arthrocentesis followed by administration of an intra-articular steroid to provide immediate relief)*

42. A 55-year-old man presents with a painful swollen right great toe. He reports a previous similar attack 3 months ago. The pain is severe, even with minimal pressure from his sock or bed sheet. The medical history includes reflux esophagitis, GI bleeding, and COPD. Laboratory results include the following: uric acid, 8.8; Ca, 9.3; Na, 144; K, 5.0; BUN, 26; Cr, 2.9; and Glu, 96.

What is the best treatment option for this patient?

- ❑ **A. Indomethacin, 50 mg p.o., t.i.d**
- ❑ **B. Prednisone taper**
- ❑ **C. Rofecoxib, 25 mg p.o., q.d.**
- ❑ **D. Allopurinol, 300 mg p.o., q.d.**
- ❑ **E. Acetaminophen, 1 g p.o., q.i.d.**

Key Concept/Objective: To appreciate comorbid conditions when selecting treatment for acute gout

This patient's acutely painful great toe is suggestive of gout. His uric acid level is high, which is consistent with this diagnosis. Appropriate treatment would be either oral prednisone or steroids injected into the joint. He should not receive NSAIDs because he has renal insufficiency. Rofecoxib, a COX-2 inhibitor, can also be detrimental to renal function and should not be used in this setting. Allopurinol is not indicated for the acute treatment of gout. *(Answer: B—Prednisone taper)*

43. A 54-year-old man presents with an attack of gout. He had his first attack 6 months ago; gout was confirmed by joint aspiration that revealed uric acid crystals. Three months later, he had a second attack, which involved his knee and left great toe. The medical history includes hypertension, reflux esophagitis, and psoriasis. The patient reports drinking one glass of wine once a week. Medications include omeprazole, lisinopril, hydrochlorothiazide, and triamcinolone ointment.

What would you recommend for this patient to prevent future episodes of gout?

- ❑ **A. Stop all alcohol use**
- ❑ **B. Stop hydrochlorothiazide**
- ❑ **C. Begin allopurinol**
- ❑ **D. Begin probenecid**
- ❑ **E. Begin colchicine**

Key Concept/Objective: To understand that hydrochlorothiazide is a common trigger for elevated uric acid and gout

This patient has had several attacks of gout over a 6-month period. Hydrochlorothiazide can decrease uric acid excretion and raise uric acid levels, triggering attacks of gout. Before considering use of prophylactic medications in this patient, it would be appropriate to withhold the hydrochlorothiazide and see whether the gout attacks stop. Alcohol consumption can also precipitate attacks, but this patient's infrequent alcohol use is unlikely to be the cause of his gout attacks. *(Answer: B—Stop hydrochlorothiazide)*

44. A 51-year-old man presents for primary care. He has no major medical problems. He brings with him old records that include results of lab testing done a year ago. Those results were as follows: Na, 139; K, 4.2; Cl, 100; HCO_3, 26; BUN, 12; Cr, 1.0; uric acid, 10.2. Laboratory tests are repeated, and the results are normal, with the exception of a uric acid measurement of 10.4.

What would you recommend for this patient?

- ❑ A. **No therapy**
- ❑ B. **Allopurinol**
- ❑ C. **Probenecid**
- ❑ D. **Colchicine**
- ❑ E. **Aspirin**

Key Concept/Objective: To understand that asymptomatic hyperuricemia does not need therapy

This patient has asymptomatic hyperuricemia. There is no need to treat asymptomatic patients with hypouricemic agents. They should be followed closely for the development of gout or renal stones. If either condition develops, it would be appropriate to consider treatment. *(Answer: A—No therapy)*

45. A 61-year-old man presents with a swollen, warm, tender left knee. He has had three episodes of gout this year, which were treated successfully with indomethacin. He is started on a 1-week course of indomethacin.

What other therapy would be appropriate to start?

- ❑ A. **Prednisone, 40 mg q.d. for 3 days**
- ❑ B. **Probenecid, 1 g p.o., b.i.d.**
- ❑ C. **Colchicine, 0.6 mg p.o., b.i.d.**
- ❑ D. **Allopurinol, 300 mg p.o., q.d.**
- ❑ E. **Acetaminophen, 1 g p.o., b.i.d.**

Key Concept/Objective: To understand how and when to start prophylactic medications for gout

This patient presents with an acute attack of gout. He has had several episodes in the past year. It would be appropriate to treat him with indomethacin for the acute attack and to begin medication to decrease the risk of another attack in the near future. Colchicine, 0.6 mg once or twice a day, prevents recurrent attacks in 80% of patients with gout. It should be started in conjunction with acute treatment (NSAIDs or steroids) and continued for 1 to 2 months. Colchicine should also be used when urate-lowering drug therapy is initiated. This patient should not receive allopurinol or probenecid during the acute attack because both of these agents can worsen the acute attack. There is no need to add prednisone to the indomethacin being used for acute treatment. *(Answer: C—Colchicine, 0.6 mg p.o., b.i.d.)*

For more information, see Wise C: 15 Rheumatology: IX Crystal-Induced Joint Disease. ACP Medicine Online (www.acpmedicine.com). Dale DC, Federman DD, Eds. WebMD Inc., New York, March 2001

Osteoarthritis

46. A 51-year-old white woman presents to your primary care clinic for evaluation of knee pain. She states that the pain has been progressing gradually for at least a year. The patient denies having had any trauma. She also states that she has not experienced any erythema, point tenderness, fevers, or chills, nor has she lost the ability to ambulate. However, she occasionally notes some swelling of the joint. Physical examination is notable for the absence of joint instability, fever, redness, edema, or warmth. You suspect that the patient has osteoarthritis.

Which of the following statements regarding osteoarthritis is false?

- ❑ A. **In patients older than 50 years, men are more commonly affected than women**
- ❑ B. **In most patients with primary osteoarthritis, involvement is limited to one or a small number of joints or joint areas**
- ❑ C. **Intra-articular fractures and meniscal tears can lead to osteoarthritis years after the injury**

❑ D. **Most patients with radiographic changes consistent with osteoarthritis have few symptoms or functional limitations**

Key Concept/Objective: To understand the epidemiology and etiology of osteoarthritis

Osteoarthritis is a common form of arthritis characterized by degeneration of articular cartilage and reactive changes in surrounding bone and periarticular tissue. The disease process results in pain and dysfunction of affected joints and is a major cause of disability in the general population. Patients without a specific inflammatory or metabolic condition known to be associated with arthritis who have a history of specific injury or trauma are considered to have primary osteoarthritis. In most patients, involvement is limited to one or a small number of joints or joint areas. Secondary osteoarthritis has been associated with several conditions that cause damage to articular cartilage through a variety of mechanisms, including mechanical, inflammatory, and metabolic processes. Acute trauma, particularly intra-articular fractures and meniscal tears, can result in articular instability or incongruity and can lead to osteoarthritis years after an injury. Osteoarthritis is the most common type of arthritis, and it is one of the most common causes of disability and dependence in the United States. Fortunately, most patients with radiographic changes found in population-based surveys have few symptoms or functional limitations. Men and women tend be affected equally by osteoarthritis in middle age, but after the age of 50 years, women are more commonly affected than men. *(Answer: A—In patients older than 50 years, men are more commonly affected than women)*

47. A 32-year-old man presents to your clinic for management of hypertension. He states that his mother and father and many of their siblings have arthritis, and he wants to know if he will get arthritis, too. He has no current complaints of arthritis or arthralgias, and his joint examination is normal.

Which of the following statements regarding risk factors for osteoarthritis is false?

❑ A. **Age and presence of osteoarthritis are positively correlated**

❑ B. **Despite many well-designed studies, an association between obesity and osteoarthritis has not been established**

❑ C. **Bone mineral density and the presence of osteoarthritis are positively correlated**

❑ D. **A family history of osteoarthritis is common in patients with osteoarthritis**

Key Concept/Objective: To understand the risk factors for osteoarthritis

A number of risk factors are believed to contribute to the development of primary osteoarthritis, including age, obesity, joint malalignment, bone density, hormonal status, nutritional factors, joint dysplasia, trauma, occupational factors, and hereditary factors. Age is the factor most strongly associated with radiographic and clinically significant osteoarthritis, with an exponential increase seen in more severely involved joints. Obesity is clearly associated with osteoarthritis of the knee. The increased load carried by obese persons and the alterations in gait and posture that redistribute the load contribute to cartilage damage. A study in young men suggested that each increase in weight of 8 kg results in a 70% increase in the risk of symptomatic arthritis of the knee in later years. This association is particularly high in patients with varus malalignment of the knee, and obese patients with malalignment are at risk for more rapid progression of established osteoarthritis in the knee. Most of the association of obesity with osteoarthritis of the knee appears to be related to environmental, rather than genetic, factors. An association between increased bone density and osteoarthritis has been noted in several studies. Women with osteoporosis and hip fractures have a decreased risk of osteoarthritis, and those affected by osteoarthritis have significantly increased bone density. This negative association suggests that soft subchondral bone absorbs impact and protects articular cartilage better than dense bone. Many patients with osteoarthritis have a family history of the disorder, and multiple genetic factors may be responsible in various forms of osteoarthritis. In women, osteoarthritis with finger joint involvement is probably the best-recognized form of arthritis with familial associations, but hereditary factors are also

important in osteoarthritis of the hip. *(Answer: B—Despite many well-designed studies, an association between obesity and osteoarthritis has not been established)*

48. A 64-year-old white woman presents to the clinic with a 3- to 4-month history of worsening right hand pain. She denies undergoing any trauma or injury, and she states that her pain is worse at the base of the thumb. On physical examination, the patient has bony enlargement of her distal and proximal interphalangeal joints. The carpometacarpal joint of the right thumb is exquisitely painful to motion, but there is no overlying erythema or edema.

Which of the following statements regarding the clinical manifestations and diagnostic tests for osteoarthritis is true?

- ❑ **A. The most commonly involved joints are the wrists, the metacarpophalangeal joints, the elbows, the shoulders, and the ankles**
- ❑ **B. The ESR is usually elevated, and it is common to find an elevated leukocyte count (> 2,000 cells/mm^3) in the synovial fluid**
- ❑ **C. Synovial effusions may be present; erythema and warmth suggest the presence of coexistent crystal-induced inflammation or other conditions**
- ❑ **D. Morning stiffness can occur with osteoarthritis and typically will last longer than 1 hour**

Key Concept/Objective: To understand the clinical manifestations of osteoarthritis and the diagnostic tests used in the workup

Typical symptoms of osteoarthritis include pain, stiffness, swelling, deformity, and loss of function. Pain is usually chronic and localized to the involved joint or joints or referred to nearby areas. Pain may be mild or moderate early in the disease but tends to worsen gradually over many years. Most of the pain is made worse with activity and improves with rest. Morning stiffness is not as prolonged as it is in patients with inflammatory diseases; morning stiffness in patients with osteoarthritis usually lasts less than an hour. Physical findings in osteoarthritis include crepitus, pain on motion, bony enlargement, and periarticular tenderness. Synovial effusions may be present, particularly in the knee. Erythema and warmth are unusual and should suggest the presence of coexistent crystal-induced inflammation or other conditions. Osteoarthritis has a characteristic pattern of involvement in most patients. Frequently involved joints include the distal and proximal interphalangeal joints and the first carpometacarpal joints in the hands; the cervical and lumbar spine; the hips; the knees; and, less commonly, the small joints of the feet or the acromioclavicular joint. The wrists, metacarpophalangeal joints, elbows, shoulders, and ankles are usually not affected unless there is a history of injury to the specific joint, occupational overuse, or an underlying condition that might be a cause of secondary osteoarthritis. Characteristic radiographic features are usually considered essential for diagnosis but should be corroborated by the presence of compatible symptoms. Laboratory studies are useful in the evaluation of patients with osteoarthritis only in that they help to exclude other diagnoses. Thus, the ESR, rheumatoid factor, and routine hematologic and biochemical parameters should be normal in patients with osteoarthritis unless the osteoarthritis is attributable to comorbid conditions. Synovial fluid from involved joints is noninflammatory, with leukocyte counts of less than 2,000 cells/mm^3 in most patients. Typical radiographic findings in osteoarthritis include joint space narrowing, subchondral bone sclerosis, subchondral cysts, and osteophytes (bony spurs). *(Answer: C—Synovial effusions may be present; erythema and warmth suggest the presence of coexistent crystal-induced inflammation or other conditions)*

49. A 46-year-old woman presents with complaint of pain, stiffness, and swelling in her right hand; these symptoms have persisted for several months. She denies experiencing any past or recent trauma to her hand or having any other significant medical history. On examination, she has tenderness on several of her distal and proximal interphalangeal joints and a Heberden node on the index finger.

Which of the following is the most likely diagnosis?

❑ A. Primary osteoarthritis

❑ B. Secondary osteoarthritis

❑ C. Erosive osteoarthritis

❑ D. Rheumatoid arthritis

Key Concept/Objective: To understand the classification of various forms of arthritis

Erosive osteoarthritis is characterized by polyarticular involvement of the small joints of the hand and tends to occur more often in middle-aged and elderly women. Patients without a specific inflammatory or metabolic condition known to be associated with arthritis and without a history of specific injury or trauma are considered to have primary osteoarthritis. Secondary osteoarthritis has been associated with several conditions that cause damage to articular cartilage through a variety of mechanisms, including mechanical, inflammatory, and metabolic processes. Rheumatoid arthritis can usually be distinguished from osteoarthritis on the basis of a different pattern of joint disease, more prominent morning stiffness, and soft tissue swelling and warmth on physical examination. *(Answer: C—Erosive osteoarthritis)*

50. A 50-year-old man presents with complaints of right knee pain and swelling of 4 days' duration. He reports no new injury, but several years ago he underwent arthroscopic surgery in that knee for a meniscal tear. Since the time of his surgery, he has experienced intermittent pain in his knee when he "overdoes it," but he has not previously experienced swelling in his knee. On examination, there is moderate effusion in the patient's right knee, and range-of-motion assessment elicits crepitus and pain.

Which of the following may be found on radiographic examination of this patient's right knee?

❑ A. Joint space narrowing

❑ B. Subchondral bone sclerosis

❑ C. Osteophytes

❑ D. All of the above

Key Concept/Objective: To understand the common radiographic findings of osteoarthritis

Typical radiographic findings in osteoarthritis include joint space narrowing, subchondral bone sclerosis, subchondral cysts, and osteophytes (bony spurs). Joint space narrowing, resulting from loss of cartilage, is often asymmetrical and may be the only finding early in the disease process. In weight-bearing joints such as the knees, narrowing may be seen only in a standing view and may be missed in a film obtained in the recumbent position. In more chronic disease, the hypertrophic features of subchondral sclerosis and osteophyte formation become more prominent, and subluxations or fusion of the joint may become apparent in more severely affected joints. In the small interphalangeal joints of the fingers, central erosions may be seen within the joint space. *(Answer: D—All of the above)*

51. A 33-year-old morbidly obese man presents for a routine physical examination. He reports pain in his knees, which he has been experiencing for several months and for which he takes acetaminophen. He denies undergoing any trauma to either knee. He also denies having any other past or present medical problems. On examination, both knees have crepitus with range-of-motion assessment, and the right knee has a small effusion.

Which of the following statements regarding this patient is false?

❑ A. This patient has an increased risk of osteoarthritis of the knees

❑ B. This patient should be counseled regarding dietary vitamin C and D supplementation

❑ C. Analysis of the synovial fluid would show an absence of inflammation, with leukocyte counts below 2,000 cells/mm^3

❑ D. This patient would be expected to have an elevated erythrocyte sedimentation rate (ESR)

Key Concept/Objective: To understand the risk factors for and characteristics of nonpharmacologic measures for osteoarthritis

The ESR, rheumatoid factor level, and routine hematologic and biochemical parameters should be normal in patients with osteoarthritis unless the osteoarthritis is attributable to comorbid conditions. Laboratory studies are useful in the evaluation of patients with osteoarthritis only in that they help to exclude other diagnoses. Synovial fluid from involved joints is noninflammatory, with leukocyte counts being under 2,000 cells/mm^3 in most patients. A number of risk factors are believed to contribute to the development of primary osteoarthritis, including age, obesity, bone density, hormonal status, nutritional factors, joint dysplasia, trauma, occupational factors, and hereditary factors. Obesity is clearly associated with osteoarthritis of the knee. The increased load carried by obese patients and the alterations in gait and posture that redistribute the load contribute to cartilage damage. Nonpharmacologic measures that have the potential to improve outcomes in osteoarthritis include patient education, physical and occupational therapy assessment and interventions, exercise, weight loss, and dietary vitamin D and C supplementation. Epidemiologic studies have suggested a role for adequate dietary vitamin C and D intake in reducing the risk of progression of established osteoarthritis. *(Answer: D—This patient would be expected to have an elevated erythrocyte sedimentation rate [ESR])*

52. A 67-year-old woman presents with pain and stiffness in various joints of her hands; these symptoms have persisted for several months. She denies experiencing any trauma to her hands. She also denies having any other relevant medical history. She states that she takes aspirin when she has pain. On examination, she has swelling on several proximal interphalangeal joints in both hands and has Bouchard nodes in two joints.

Which of the following is the most appropriate first-line pharmacologic treatment for this patient?

❑ **A. Acetaminophen**

❑ **B. Opioids**

❑ **C. Steroids**

❑ **D. Cyclooxygenase-2 (COX-2) NSAIDs**

Key Concept/Objective: To understand the pharmacologic therapies for osteoarthritis

Acetaminophen in doses up to 3,000 to 4,000 mg daily should be prescribed initially in most patients with osteoarthritis. The primary goal of drug therapy in osteoarthritis is to relieve pain. In some patients, simple analgesics may be as effective as NSAIDs. Opioids are generally avoided in osteoarthritis but may be useful in selected patients. Opioids should be used with caution in elderly patients. Tramadol, a centrally acting analgesic with dual mechanisms, may give relief comparable to that achieved with acetaminophen and codeine. Topical capsaicin may be useful in some patients, particularly those with involvement of the knees and hands. NSAIDs are useful in osteoarthritis mostly for their analgesic effects, although anti-inflammatory effects may have some clinical significance. NSAIDs are associated with an increased risk of gastric ulcers and bleeding, particularly in patients with a history of GI disease. The recently available COX-2–specific NSAIDs celecoxib and rofecoxib have been shown to reduce endoscopic gastritis and ulcers as well as serious GI complications when compared to the previously available nonselective COX inhibitors. *(Answer: A—Acetaminophen)*

For more information, see Wise C: 15 Rheumatology: X Osteoarthritis. ACP Medicine Online (www.acpmedicine.com). Dale DC, Federman DD, Eds. WebMD Inc., New York, January 2005

Back Pain and Common Musculoskeletal Problems

53. A 67-year-old African-American man comes to your office with low back pain. He has been experiencing progressive back pain for the past 2 weeks. He believes these symptoms started after he lifted a 20-lb box. His medical history is unremarkable. Review of systems is significant for a weight loss of 10 lb over the past 6 months and urinary hesitancy. Physical examination reveals tenderness to percussion over L5 and a nodular, enlarged prostate. The neurologic examination is normal.

Of the following, which is the most appropriate step to take next in the treatment of this patient?

- ❑ **A. Start nonsteroidal anti-inflammatory drugs (NSAIDs) and have the patient come back to your clinic only if the pain persists**
- ❑ **B. Prescribe bed rest for 1 week**
- ❑ **C. Obtain imaging studies**
- ❑ **D. Start opiates and muscle relaxants**

Key Concept/Objective: To be able to identify patients with acute back pain who are at risk for serious underlying conditions

For patients with acute back pain, the initial history should be used to identify those who are at risk for serious underlying conditions, such as fracture, infection, tumor, or major neurologic deficit. The initial physical examination should include evaluation for areas of localized bony tenderness and assessment of flexion and straight leg raising. This patient has symptoms and signs that suggest the presence of a malignancy. He has experienced weight loss, and there is bony tenderness and a nodular prostate. In this clinical scenario, imaging is indicated to evaluate for the possibility of metastatic disease to the spine. For the treatment of acute back pain, NSAIDs and mild analgesics may be useful for symptom control. Muscle relaxants and opiates should be used sparingly. Spinal manipulation or specific exercise programs may also be effective in acute back pain. Over 90% of patients will improve within 1 month. Strict bed rest should be kept to a minimum, and continuation of normal activities should be enforced. *(Answer: C—Obtain imaging studies)*

54. A 42-year-old male postal worker presents to your clinic asking for a second opinion regarding the management of his chronic low back pain. The pain started 4 months ago. The pain is located in his lower back; it does not radiate. The patient denies having any weakness or sensory deficits. The pain is worse when he walks or when he lifts weights, and it is interfering with his work. The patient's medical history and review of systems are unremarkable. He has tried over-the-counter acetaminophen and ibuprofen, without relief. Recently, he saw another physician, who ordered a magnetic resonance imaging scan. The report describes a bulging disk on L4-5 with no signs of spinal cord compression. On the basis of that study, the patient was told he needed surgery. On physical examination, there is diffuse tenderness in his lower back, and a leg-raising test is negative. The neurologic examination, including sphincter tone, is normal.

How would you manage this patient?

- ❑ **A. Prescribe an NSAID at a higher dosage than previously used, educate the patient about low back pain, and recommend physical therapy**
- ❑ **B. Order a repeat MRI because the results do not fit with the physical examination**
- ❑ **C. Refer to a neurosurgeon for surgical repair of his herniated disk**
- ❑ **D. Recommend that the patient apply for disability because of his chronic pain**

Key Concept/Objective: To understand the management of chronic back pain

A herniated lumbar disk should be considered in patients with back pain who have symptoms of radiculopathy, as suggested by pain radiating down the leg with symptoms reproduced by straight leg raising. MRI may be necessary to confirm a herniated disk, but findings should be interpreted with caution, because many asymptomatic persons have disk abnormalities. This patient has no signs of radiculopathy. Also, the MRI reports a bulging disk with no signs of compression: a finding that is frequently seen in healthy persons. Surgery would be indicated if there were signs of radiculopathy and the MRI showed a herniated disk with evidence of spinal compression; however, this is not the situation in this case. A repeat MRI is not indicated, because it is unlikely that a herniated disk is the cause of this patient's symptoms, given the clinical evidence. The management of chronic back pain is complex. Patients should undergo physical therapy, an exercise program, and an education program that emphasizes proper ergonomics for lifting and other activities. Light normal activity and a regular walking program should be encouraged. Encouraging

the patient to apply for disability before trying different therapeutic interventions is not appropriate. Judicious use of NSAIDs and mild analgesics may improve patient function and outcome. *(Answer: A—Prescribe an NSAID at a higher dosage than previously used, educate the patient about low back pain, and recommend physical therapy)*

55. A 55-year-old woman with a history of rheumatoid arthritis presents to the emergency department complaining of right elbow pain. The pain started 4 days ago and has become progressively worse, to the point where it is now difficult for her to move her elbow. She has also felt febrile. On physical examination, the patient's temperature is 98.8° F (37.1° C), there are signs of chronic rheumatoid arthritis on her hands, and there is a 3 × 3 cm area of indurated swelling over the tip of her elbow. This area is tender to palpation and is warm and erythematous. The passive range of motion of the elbow is preserved.

What is the appropriate step to take next in the treatment of this patient?

❑ **A. Start NSAIDs and follow up within a week**

❑ **B. Aspirate the fluid to rule out infection or crystal-induced disease**

❑ **C. Order an MRI to evaluate the degree of joint damage**

❑ **D. Inject steroids to the area**

Key Concept/Objective: To be able to recognize different causes of olecranon bursitis

Olecranon bursitis presents as a discrete swelling with palpable fluid over the tip of the elbow. Olecranon bursitis may be secondary to trauma, rheumatoid arthritis, crystal-induced disease (e.g., gout or pseudogout), or infection. This patient's clinical presentation should raise concern about an infectious process. She may have had a fever previously. On examination, she has an indurated, tender, erythematous area over her elbow. The ability to perform passive range of motion of the elbow makes the possibility of synovial infection unlikely; however, aspiration of the bursae is indicated to rule out infection and crystal-induced disease. Infectious bursitis, usually caused by gram-positive skin organisms, is accompanied by heat, erythema, and induration. When infection is suspected, prompt aspiration and culture of the fluid are mandatory. Antibiotics should be started empirically, and the bursae should be reaspirated frequently until the fluid no longer reaccumulates and cultures are negative. NSAIDs and steroids should not be started until the fluid has been examined, because of the risk of underlying infection. MRI is not indicated at this point, because the clinical picture is consistent with bursitis. *(Answer: B—Aspirate the fluid to rule out infection or crystal-induced disease)*

56. A 31-year-old obese man presents to your clinic with a 2-week history of right foot pain. The pain is located on his posterior heel. There is no history of trauma. The pain is worse when standing in the morning and when walking after sitting down for a period. On physical examination, there is tenderness to palpation on the heel area. The rest of the physical examination is normal.

Which of the following is the most likely cause of this patient's symptoms?

❑ **A. Previous unrecognized traumatic event**

❑ **B. A deformity of the arch of his foot**

❑ **C. Peripheral neuropathy**

❑ **D. Plantar fasciitis**

Key Concept/Objective: To know the causes of hindfoot pain

Plantar fasciitis is one of the most common causes of hindfoot pain. Patients report pain over the plantar aspect of the heel and midfoot that worsens with walking. Localized tenderness along the plantar fascia or at the insertion of the calcaneus is helpful in diagnosis. Plantar fasciitis is associated with obesity, pes planus, and activities that stress the plantar fascia. It may also be seen in systemic arthropathies such as ankylosing spondylitis and Reiter syndrome. Although radiographic spurs in the affected area are common, they may also be seen in asymptomatic persons and are therefore not diagnostic. In this case, the constellation of symptoms, obesity, and physical examination findings are consistent with the diagnosis of plantar fasciitis. Careful examination usually helps distinguish between

Achilles tendinitis and plantar fasciitis. Therapy for plantar fasciitis is usually conservative and includes the use of orthotic devices (heel wedges), stretching exercises, and judicious use of NSAIDs. Heel spurs can be seen on plain radiography; however, their role in the pathogenesis of plantar fasciitis is unclear. *(Answer: D—Plantar fasciitis)*

For more information, see Wise C: 15 Rheumatology: XII Back Pain and Common Musculoskeletal Problems. ACP Medicine Online (www.acpmedicine.com). Dale DC, Federman DD, Eds. WebMD Inc., New York, December 2002

Fibromyalgia

57. A 34-year-old woman returns to your office for a routine follow-up visit. You diagnosed her as having fibromyalgia 3 years ago, when she presented with multiple tender points of muscle and tendons, marked sleep disturbance, recurrent headaches, fatigue, and chronic generalized pain. You have also treated her for generalized anxiety disorder and depression. Today, she states that her generalized pain is slightly improved. She is sleeping better, and her energy level has improved. She remembers that just before her pain syndrome started 3 years ago, she fell down her neighbor's doorsteps. She asks you if you agree that this fall is the likely cause of her current pain syndrome.

Which of the following statements regarding fibromyalgia is true?

- ❑ A. **Fibromyalgia most commonly occurs in middle-aged men**
- ❑ B. **Fibromyalgia is considered to be a purely somatic disease; social or psychological factors have little bearing on the disease**
- ❑ C. **The type of pain associated with fibromyalgia is typically nociceptive or neuropathic**
- ❑ D. **Fibromyalgia patients often have fixed beliefs that minor traumatic events or exposure to pathogens, chemicals, or other physical agents caused their illness**

Key Concept/Objective: To know the general features of fibromyalgia

Fibromyalgia is a chronic syndrome that occurs predominantly in women. It is marked by generalized pain, multiple defined tender points, fatigue, disturbed or nonrestorative sleep, and numerous other somatic complaints. Fibromyalgia becomes more common after 60 years of age but also occurs in children. The cause of fibromyalgia is unknown. Despite extensive research, no definitive organic pathology has been identified. Psychological factors associated with chronic distress appear to be very important. In fibromyalgia, negative psychological elements constituting stress and distress are major contributors to the development of increased pain sensitivity and myriad other symptoms. There are four principal categories of pain: nociceptive, neuropathic, psychogenic, and chronic pain of complex etiology. Chronic pain of complex etiology is the type of pain characteristic of fibromyalgia. Fibromyalgia patients often have fixed beliefs that minor traumatic events, pathogens, chemicals, or other physical agents caused their illness. *(Answer: D—Fibromyalgia patients often have fixed beliefs that minor traumatic events or exposure to pathogens, chemicals, or other physical agents caused their illness)*

58. A 27-year-old woman visits your clinic as a new patient. She was in very good health until 1 year ago, when she developed severe neck, shoulder, and hip pain. Her primary physician has completed an extensive workup for rheumatologic disorders; the patient has brought the data from that workup with her today. The patient is in constant pain and has difficulty sleeping; she also has a "nervous stomach" and chronic diarrhea, and she feels that her "memory is slipping." Her pains are so constant and severe that she has had to resign her job as a schoolteacher. Her social history reveals that she was divorced 1 year ago and is a single parent of three children.

Which of the following statements regarding the historical diagnosis of fibromyalgia is true?

- ❑ A. **Cognitive complaints, such as difficulty with concentration and memory, are notably absent in patients with fibromyalgia**
- ❑ B. **Fibromyalgia does not lead to functional impairment**

❑ C. **Regional pain syndromes, such as headache, temporomandibular joint syndrome, or irritable bowel syndrome, are uncommon in fibromyalgia**

❑ D. **Pain is the hallmark of fibromyalgia**

Key Concept/Objective: To understand important historical elements in patients with fibromyalgia

Cognitive complaints, such as difficulties with concentration and memory, may be prominent in fibromyalgia. Functional impairment is usually present, at least in patients with fibromyalgia who seek care. Patients report difficulty performing usual activities of daily living; in addition, they avoid exercise—indeed, patients with fibromyalgia are fearful of exercise. Regional pain syndromes, such as headache, temporomandibular joint syndrome, or irritable bowel syndrome, are extremely common in fibromyalgia. It is essential that the physician not automatically attribute all such symptoms to fibromyalgia, however, because fibromyalgia frequently coexists with other organically defined disorders. Pain is the hallmark of fibromyalgia. The pain radiates diffusely from the axial skeleton and is localized to muscles and muscle-tendon junctions of the neck, shoulders, hips, and extremities. *(Answer: D—Pain is the hallmark of fibromyalgia)*

59. A 35-year-old woman presents to your office with the complaints of severe joint pain, joint swelling, muscle aches, insomnia, and severe fatigue. All of her symptoms started 3 months ago when she lost her job as an executive assistant. She denies having fever or chills, unprotected sexual contact, morning stiffness, or gastrointestinal or urinary symptoms. On physical examination, diffuse swelling of the patient's metacarpophalangeal joints and wrists is noted. The patient has an erythematous rash on her face. She has significant pain at 12 of the 18 tender points, and there is a mild reduction in strength in all extremities. Her physical examination is otherwise normal.

Which of the following statements regarding the physical examination findings of fibromyalgia is false?

❑ A. **Evidence of synovitis, objective muscle weakness, or other definite physical or neurologic signs suggests the presence of either a comorbid disease or an alternative diagnosis**

❑ B. **When assessing tender points, palpation is performed with the thumb, using approximately 4 kg of pressure**

❑ C. **For an accurate diagnosis, the examiner must confirm pain at all 18 tender points**

❑ D. **Useful tests in fibromyalgia include antinuclear antibody (ANA), complete blood count (CBC), erythrocyte sedimentation rate (ESR), C-reactive protein (CRP), thyroid-stimulating hormone (TSH), creatine kinase (CK), aspartate aminotransferase (AST), and alanine aminotransferase (ALT)**

Key Concept/Objective: To know the important components of the physical examination of a patient with fibromyalgia

Evidence of synovitis (e.g., joint effusion, warmth over the joint, pain on joint motion), objective muscle weakness, or other definite physical or neurologic signs suggest the presence of either comorbid disease or an alternative diagnosis. Eighteen specific tender points have been identified in fibromyalgia. A patient with fibromyalgia will have pain, not just tenderness, on palpation at many of these tender points. Palpation is performed with the thumb, using approximately 4 kg of pressure—about the pressure necessary to blanch the examiner's thumbnail. Attempting to confirm pain at all 18 tender points is not necessary for diagnosis and is inconsiderate toward patients, many of whom find tender-point palpation quite distressing. Useful tests in fibromyalgia include the following: ANA, CBC, ESR, CRP, TSH, CK, AST, and ALT. Tests for Lyme disease, Epstein-Barr virus infection, and endocrinologic status are usually unnecessary. *(Answer: C—For an accurate diagnosis, the examiner must confirm pain at all 18 tender points)*

For more information, see Winfield JB: 15 Rheumatology: XIII Fibromyalgia. ACP Medicine Online (www.acpmedicine.com). Dale DC, Federman DD, Eds. WebMD Inc., New York, July 2004